Dendrimers: A Themed Issue in Honor of Professor Donald A. Tomalia on the Occasion of His 85th Birthday for His Outstanding Achievements in Advancing the Field of Dendrimers

Dendrimers: A Themed Issue in Honor of Professor Donald A. Tomalia on the Occasion of His 85th Birthday for His Outstanding Achievements in Advancing the Field of Dendrimers

Guest Editors

Zofia Urbanczyk-Lipkowska
Anne-Marie Caminade

MDPI

Basel • Beijing • Wuhan • Barcelona • Belgrade • Novi Sad • Cluj • Manchester

Guest Editors
Zofia Urbanczyk-Lipkowska
Institute of Organic Chemistry
Polish Academy of Sciences
Warsaw
Poland

Anne-Marie Caminade
Laboratoire de Chimie
de Coordination
Centre National de la
Recherche Scientifique
Toulouse
France

Editorial Office
MDPI AG
Grosspeteranlage 5
4052 Basel, Switzerland

This is a reprint of the Special Issue, published open access by the journal *Pharmaceutics* (ISSN 1999-4923), freely accessible at: https://www.mdpi.com/journal/pharmaceutics/special_issues/8R566V9SMG.

For citation purposes, cite each article independently as indicated on the article page online and as indicated below:

Lastname, A.A.; Lastname, B.B. Article Title. *Journal Name* **Year**, *Volume Number*, Page Range.

ISBN 978-3-7258-4849-2 (Hbk)
ISBN 978-3-7258-4850-8 (PDF)
https://doi.org/10.3390/books978-3-7258-4850-8

Cover image courtesy of Anne-Marie Caminade

Contents

About the Editors

Zofia Urbanczyk-Lipkowska

Zofia Urbanczyk-Lipkowska was PhD DSc, Group Leader, and Professor (Crystallochemistry and Chemistry of Dendrimers) at the Institute of Organic Chemistry of the Polish Academy of Sciences in Warsaw (Poland) until her death on 22 January 2024. She was a researcher at the University of Minnesota (USA) for two years, and she was also an Invited Professor at the Stevens Institute of Technology, Hoboken, New Jersey (USA). She co-authored about 200 publications, was awarded the Knight's Cross of the Order of Merit for Invention of the Kingdom of Belgium (2007) and the Professor Mirosław J. Mossakowski Medal (2009), and was a laureate of the Polish Prize for Intelligent Development (2019).

Anne-Marie Caminade

Anne-Marie Caminade is Director of Research Exceptional Class (Emeritus) at the Laboratoire de Chimie de Coordination of the CNRS in Toulouse, France, where she was previously Deputy Director (2021–2024). She is a phosphorus chemist, and the creator of the phosphorus dendrimers. She is the co-author of about 575 publications (hindex = 83), of 18 patents, and the editor of 4 books. She is a Member of the European Academy of Sciences and of the Academia Europaea. She has received many awards, including most recently the Knight of the Legion of Honor (France, 2021), awards from the four most important Chemistry Societies in the EU (SCF France, GDCh Germany, RSEQ Spain, and SCI Italy with the prestigious Luigi Sacconi medal), and from the French Academy of Sciences (2024).

Preface

This Reprint is dedicated to the 85th birthday of Prof. Dr. Donald A. Tomalia, who is the creator of the PAMAM (poly(amidoamine)) dendrimers, and of the name "dendrimers". He played a key role in establishing the place of dendrimers in polymer chemistry and in nanosciences, and he inspired several generations of researchers around the world.

I would also like to dedicate this reprint to the memory of Prof. Dr. Zofia Urbanczyk-Lipkowska, who proposed the idea for this Special Issue, but who sadly passed away on 22 January 2024. She truly was a very kind person, and her death came as a great shock to all her friends in the dendrimer community.

This Reprint displays the recent advances in the field of dendrimers and dendritic structures, with emphasis on diverse biological and pharmaceutical properties, written by many of the major contributors to the field. It contains four reviews and nine original research papers, of which six concern special dendritic structures such as Janus dendrimers and dendrons.

The four reviews concern first a reflection on the beginning, past, present, and future of dendrimers in pharmaceutic, medicine, and life science (D. A. Tomalia). Three other reviews concern ferrocene-based dendritic drugs, inducing the Fenton mechanism to kill cancer cells (D. Astruc et al.), dendrimers functionalized with boron clusters for boron neutron capture therapy (BNCT) against cancers (A.M. Caminade et al.), and dendrimers used in vivo as drug carriers (V. Ceña et al.).

The six research papers about special dendritic architectures first concern a large library of amphiphilic Janus dendrimers derived from renewable plant phenolic acids for the targeted delivery of mRNA and for the storage of vaccines (D. Weissman, V. Percec et al.). Five different biological uses of dendrons are then displayed. Polypropylene imine dendrons equipped with doxorubicin and antibody were tested against prostate cancer cells (M.C. Daniel et al.); polyglycerol dendrons and block copolymers were used to form micelles in water and to encapsulate doxorubicin against cancer cells (E. Mohammadifar, R. Haag et al.); carbosilane dendrons were used to encapsulate and deliver different drugs (ibuprofen, lidocaine, procaine, or diclofenac) (M. Valiente, R. Gomez et al.); carbosilane dendrons cross-linked with dithiol polymers formed hydrogels suitable for drug release (S. Garcia-Gallego et al.); and PAMAM dendrons were associated with human serum albumin and studied both experimentally and theoretically (E. Laurini, S. Pricl et al.).

The three research papers about dendrimers concern PAMAM dendrimers. Generation 6 hydroxyl-terminated PAMAM dendrimers were functionalized with some peptides for the treatment of wet age-related macular degeneration in the eyes (R.M. Kannan et al.); PAMAM dendrimers functionalized with phenylalanine were loaded with protoporphyrin IX and paclitaxel and tested against cancer cells (C. Kojima et al.); and PAMAM dendrimers functionalized with amoxicillin were used in the decoration of silica nanoparticles, to afford a tool in the diagnosis of allergy to betalactam antibiotics (M. I. Montañez, Y. Vida et al.).

In conclusion, I wish to thank all the authors who contributed their work, and in so doing made this Special Issue a success. I also wish to thank the staff of *Pharmaceutics* for their excellent support throughout the editorial process.

Zofia Urbanczyk-Lipkowska and Anne-Marie Caminade
Guest Editors

pharmaceutics

Editorial

Dendrimers: A Themed Issue in Honor of Professor Donald A. Tomalia on the Occasion of His 85th Birthday, Recognizing His Outstanding Achievements in Advancing the Field of Dendrimers

Anne-Marie Caminade [1,2]

[1] Laboratoire de Chimie de Coordination (LCC-CNRS) 205 Route de Narbonne, CEDEX 4, 31077 Toulouse, France; anne-marie.caminade@lcc-toulouse.fr

[2] LCC-CNRS, Université de Toulouse, CNRS, 31077 Toulouse, France

As the main pioneer in the field of dendrimers, a term that he coined in 1985 in reference to their tree-like structure, Prof. Donald A. Tomalia has inspired several generations of researchers worldwide. I am very happy to announce that our *Pharmaceutics* Special Issue callout dedicated to his 85th birthday was a great success, with 13 contributions, including several from the main players in the field and even a remarkable review by Prof. Donald A. Tomalia himself [1].

On the other hand, this launch also brings sadness, because the idea of this Special Issue was proposed by Prof. Zofia Urbanczyk-Lipkowska, who very unfortunately passed away on 22 January 2024. The announcement of her death was a great shock for me. I had known Zofia for a long time, as she had been involved in work on peptide dendrimers since 2003. We met several times at congresses about dendrimers, as well as in Poland, and we became friends. She really was a very kind person, as emphasized by the "In Memoriam" contribution of Donald A. Tomalia in the paper that he wrote for this Special Issue [1]. Rest in peace, Zofia—your friends will never forget you.

This Special Issue of *Pharmaceutics* contains 13 papers, 4 reviews and 9 research articles, that illustrate the diversity of dendrimers, dendrons, and dendritic structures. Their diverse potential uses, such as in pharmaceutical sciences, against cancers, in macular degeneration in the eyes, for vaccines, in drug delivery, and in diagnosis, are emphasized. This Special Issue provides an up-to-date overview and the latest results in relation to dendrimers as bio-tools.

The review written by D.A. Tomalia [1] is an important and thought-provoking contribution, reflecting on the beginning, past, present, and future of dendrimers in pharmaceutics, medicine, and the life sciences, told over 40 pages. It begins with an historical perspective on the beginnings of dendrimers, in which D.A. Tomalia played a major role, in particular with the elaboration of the PAMAM (polyamidoamine) dendrimers and the creation of the name dendrimers. The review continues with the concept of critical nanoscale design parameters (CNDPs), which he elaborated to classify and predict the characteristics of nanoparticles, including dendrimers. The last part explores anticipated new applications for dendrimers and predicts the roles that they could be playing in ten years' time (2034) as advanced nano-pharmaceuticals for drug delivery and imaging.

The review by D. Astruc et al. [2] concerns ferrocene-based drugs, with an emphasis on their delivery using nanosystems, micelles, metal–organic frameworks (MOFs), polymers, and dendrimers. One of the main advantages of ferrocenes in pharmacy is that they induce the production of reactive oxygen species (ROS). The main ROS generated by ferrocenes is the OH· radical, produced by Fenton catalysis, which is the reaction of Fe^{2+} with H_2O_2 and is particularly suitable for killing cancer cells.

The review by A.M. Caminade et al. [3] is about the biological properties of dendritic structures functionalized with boron clusters. These compounds are potentially useful in the treatment of cancers using boron neutron capture therapy (BNCT), the efficiency of which is directly correlated with the number of boron atoms. The BNCT method starts from ^{10}B, a nonradioactive natural element, which is irradiated with low-energy thermal neutrons to generate high-linear-energy transfer particles that are suitable for killing cancer cells. Boronated dendrimers increased the mean survival time in BNCT in vivo experiments.

The review by V. Ceña et al. [4] concerns the in vivo applications of dendrimers as drug carriers. It describes, firstly, experiments carried out on cancer cells, and then in vivo experiments, mainly in mice, in the treatment of diverse diseases, such as cancers, neurodegenerative diseases, infections, and ocular diseases, but also as diagnostic agents. The very few clinical trials carried out with dendrimer formulations up until now are also presented.

The quite large paper by D. Weissman, V. Percec et al. [5] present an extensive paper comprising 50 pages and 166 pages of Supporting Information. It concerns the synthesis of large libraries of amphiphilic Janus dendrimers, derived from renewable plant phenolic acids, and their use in the targeted delivery of mRNA. The screening of these libraries using the CNDP principles demonstrated that the precise location of the functional groups can induce the targeting of precise organs, including the liver, spleen, lymph nodes, and lungs. These Janus dendrimers can also facilitate the handling and storage of vaccines, such as COVID-19 mRNA vaccines.

The paper by M.C. Daniel et al. [6] concerns the use of PPI (polypropylene imine) dendrons equipped with a disulfide (thioctic acid) at the focal point for their attachment to gold nanoparticles. The dendrons are functionalized on their surface either with doxorubicin or with azides. Both dendrons are then linked to gold nanoparticles (NPs), and a few azides are reacted with an EphA2-targeting antibody fragment to target the prostate cancer cell PC3. These dendronized gold NPs were tested and were found to be very efficient (IC_{50} = 0.9 nM) against PC3 cancer cells.

The paper by R.M. Kannan et al. [7] describes the grafting of some integrin-binding ALG-1001 peptides to generation 6 hydroxyl-terminated PAMAM dendrimers to provide a potential alternative treatment against wet age-related macular degeneration in the eyes. This disease is characterized, in particular, by the abnormal growth of blood vessels. This dendrimer has been found to be suitable for protecting ALG-1001 against degradation by proteinases and induces significant reductions in CNV lesion areas (choroidal neovascularization or the creation of new blood vessels) in vivo in rat eyes.

The paper by E. Mohammadifar, R. Haag et al. [8] concerns both a polyglycerol dendron G2 functionalized with cholesterol at the core and dendritic structures consisting of a block copolymer of the type poly(G1-polyglycerol dendron methacrylate)-block-poly(cholesterol methacrylate). Both the dendron and the dendronized copolymer form micelles in water. Cell viability studies on A549 cells demonstrated that the dendron is toxic, but not the copolymer. The encapsulation of doxorubicin (DOX) by the copolymer induced the accumulation of DOX in the cell nucleus.

In the study by M. Valiente, R. Gomez et al. [9], cholesterol was also grafted to the core of carbosilane dendrons (G1 to G3) equipped with ammonium terminal groups. Another series of dendrons, with d-α-tocopherol (vitamin E) as the focal point, were also synthesized. The cell toxicity was in the range of 10–20 μM for both families. They formed micelles in water, which were used for the encapsulation of drugs (such as ibuprofen, lidocaine, procaine, or diclofenac), the release of which was studied.

The paper by S. Garcia-Gallego et al. [10] concerns small carbosilane dendrons and dendrimers bearing alkene functions and their use as cross-linkers by "thiol-ene" coupling with dithiol polymers to produce hydrogels. The nature of the hydrogel depends on the type of polymers, affording either non-swelling (propylene glycol and Pluronics L31 and L61) or high-swelling (polyethylene glycol and Pluronics L35) hydrogels with thermo-responsive behavior. These hydrogels are suitable for drug release, as illustrated with caffeic acid.

The paper by E. Laurini, S. Pricl et al. [11] describes a PAMAM dendron with two alkyl chains as a tail and primary amines as terminal functions, and its association with human serum albumin (HAS), which plays a crucial role in pharmacokinetics. This interaction is studied both experimentally (via fluorescence spectroscopy, circular dichroism, calorimetry, dynamic light scattering, and zeta potential) and theoretically (through computational simulations at the atomistic level using the AMBER22 main program CPPTRA).

The paper by C. Kojima et al. [12] concerns both PAMAM dendrimers and dendrigraft polylysine (DGL), functionalized with phenylalanine (Phe), and their association with Jurkat cells, a T-cell model. The strength of the association is higher with functionalized DGL than with PAMAM, but the functionalized DGL is insoluble in water, and thus unsuitable as a drug carrier. Model drugs (protoporphyrin IX and paclitaxel) loaded in PAMAM-Phe exhibit similar toxicities against Jurkat cells than free drugs.

The paper by M. I. Montañez, Y. Vida et al. [13] is also about PAMAM dendrimers, exploring their use in the decoration of silica NPs and when functionalized with amoxicillin. Free amoxicillin is used in routine diagnosis, as it is assumed to conjugate to a carrier present in blood, but it does not afford information on the size and composition of these conjugates. The nanocomposite can specifically activate basophils more efficiently than free amoxicillin, making it an accurate tool in the diagnosis of allergy to betalactam antibiotics.

To conclude, from myself and from all the contributors to this Special Issue of *Pharmaceutics*, Don, I wish you a happy birthday and a long and happy life.

Conflicts of Interest: The author is a shareholder in IMD-Pharma.

References

1. Tomalia, D. Dendrimers, Dendrons and the Dendritic State. Reflection on the Last Decade with Expected New Roles in Pharma, Medicine and the Life Sciences. *Pharmaceutics* **2024**, *16*, 1530. [CrossRef]
2. Ornelas, C.; Astruc, D. Ferrocene-Based Drugs, Delivery Nanomaterials and Fenton Mechanism: State of the Art, Recent Developments and Prospects. *Pharmaceutics* **2023**, *15*, 2044. [CrossRef]
3. Caminade, A.-M.; Milewski, M.; Hey-Hawkins, E. Dendritic Structures Functionalized with Boron Clusters, in Particular Carboranes, and Their Biological Properties. *Pharmaceutics* **2023**, *15*, 2117. [CrossRef]
4. Sztandera, K.; Rodriguez-Garcia, J.L.; Cena, V. In Vivo Applications of Dendrimers: A Step toward the Future of Nanoparticle-Mediated Therapeutics. *Pharmaceutics* **2024**, *16*, 439. [CrossRef]
5. Lu, J.; Atochina-Vasserman, E.N.; Maurya, D.S.; Shalihin, M.I.; Zhang, D.; Chenna, S.S.; Adamson, J.; Liu, M.; Shah, H.U.R.; Shah, H.; et al. Screening Libraries to Discover Molecular Design Principles for the Targeted Delivery of mRNA with One-Component Ionizable Amphiphilic Janus Dendrimers Derived from Plant Phenolic Acids. *Pharmaceutics* **2023**, *15*, 1572. [CrossRef] [PubMed]
6. Dockery, L.T.; Daniel, M.-C. Targeted Doxorubicin-Loaded Dendronized Gold Nanoparticles. *Pharmaceutics* **2023**, *15*, 2103. [CrossRef] [PubMed]
7. Wu, T.; Liu, C.; Kannan, R.M. Systemic Dendrimer-Peptide Therapies for Wet Age-Related Macular Degeneration. *Pharmaceutics* **2023**, *15*, 2428. [CrossRef] [PubMed]
8. Romero, J.F.; Herziger, S.; Cherri, M.; Dimde, M.; Achazi, K.; Mohammadifar, E.; Haag, R. Dendritic Glycerol-Cholesterol Amphiphiles as Drug Delivery Systems: A Comparison between Monomeric and Polymeric Structures. *Pharmaceutics* **2023**, *15*, 2452. [CrossRef] [PubMed]
9. Mencia, G.; Algar, S.; Lozano-Cruz, T.; Munoz-Fernandez, M.A.; Gillies, E.R.; Cano, J.; Valiente, M.; Gomez, R. Carbosilane Dendritic Amphiphiles from Cholesterol or Vitamin E for Micelle Formation. *Pharmaceutics* **2024**, *16*, 451. [CrossRef] [PubMed]
10. Munoz-Sanchez, S.; Barrios-Gumiel, A.; de la Mata, F.J.; Garcia-Gallego, S. Fine-Tuning the Amphiphilic Properties of Carbosilane Dendritic Networks towards High-Swelling Thermogels. *Pharmaceutics* **2024**, *16*, 495. [CrossRef] [PubMed]
11. Cavalieri, G.; Marson, D.; Giurgevich, N.; Valeri, R.; Felluga, F.; Laurini, E.; Pricl, S. Molecular Ballet: Investigating the Complex Interaction between Self-Assembling Dendrimers and Human Serum Albumin via Computational and Experimental Methods. *Pharmaceutics* **2024**, *16*, 533. [CrossRef] [PubMed]

12. Shiba, H.; Hirose, T.; Sakai, A.; Nakase, I.; Matsumoto, A.; Kojima, C. Structural Optimization of Carboxy-Terminal Phenylalanine-Modified Dendrimers for T-Cell Association and Model Drug Loading. *Pharmaceutics* **2024**, *16*, 715. [CrossRef] [PubMed]
13. Calvo-Serrano, S.; Matamoros, E.; Cespedes, J.A.; Fernandez-Santamaria, R.; Gil-Ocana, V.; Perez-Inestrosa, E.; Frecha, C.; Montanez, M.I.; Vida, Y.; Mayorga, C.; et al. New Approaches for Basophil Activation Tests Employing Dendrimeric Antigen-Silica Nanoparticle Composites. *Pharmaceutics* **2024**, *16*, 1039. [CrossRef] [PubMed]

pharmaceutics

MDPI

Review

Dendrimers, Dendrons, and the Dendritic State: Reflection on the Last Decade with Expected New Roles in Pharma, Medicine, and the Life Sciences

Donald A. Tomalia [1,2,3]

[1] The National Dendrimer & Nanotechnology Center, NanoSynthons LLC, Mt. Pleasant, MI 48858, USA; donald.tomalia@gmail.com; Tel.: +1-989-317-3737
[2] Department of Chemistry, University of Pennsylvania, Philadelphia, PA 19104, USA
[3] Department of Physics, Virginia Commonwealth University, Richmond, VA 23284, USA

Abstract: This perspective begins with an overview of the major impact that the dendron, dendrimer, and dendritic state (DDDS) discovery has made on traditional polymer science. The entire DDDS technology is underpinned by an unprecedented new polymerization strategy referred to as step-growth, amplification-controlled polymerization (SGACP). This new SGACP paradigm allows for routine polymerization of common monomers and organic materials into precise monodispersed, dendritic macromolecules (i.e., dendrons/dendrimers) with nanoscale sizes and structure-controlled features that match and rival discrete in vivo biopolymers such as proteins and nucleic acids (i.e., DNA, siRNA, mRNA, etc.). These dendritic architectures exhibit unprecedented new intrinsic properties widely recognized to define a new fourth major polymer architecture class, namely: Category (IV): dendrons, dendrimers, and random hyperbranched polymers after traditional categories: (I) linear, (II) cross-linked, and (III) simple-branched types. Historical confusion over the first examples of the structure confirmed and verified cascade, dendron, dendrimer, and arborol syntheses, while associated misuse of accepted dendritic terminology is also reviewed and clarified. The importance of classifying all dendrons and dendrimers based on branch cell symmetry and the significant role of critical nanoscale-design parameters (CNDPs) for optimizing dendritic products for pharma/nanomedicine applications with a focus on enhancing stealth, non-complement activation properties is presented. This is followed by an overview of the extraordinary growth observed for amphiphilic dendron/dendrimer syntheses and their self-assembly into dendritic supramolecular assemblies, as well as many unique applications demonstrated in pharma and nanomedicine, especially involving siRNA delivery and mRNA vaccine development. This perspective is concluded with optimistic expectations predicted for new dendron and dendrimer application roles in pharma, nanomedicine, and life sciences.

Keywords: dendrons; dendrimers; PAMAM; CNDP; dendrimersomes; Janus dendrimers; PEG alternatives; supramolecular dendrimers; amphiphilic dendrimers; mRNA delivery vectors

---

In Memoriam of Professor Zofia Urbanczyk-Lipkowska

There are no words to describe the personal emotions and sadness felt upon the loss of our dear friend, dendrimer colleague/scientist, and co-organizer of this 85th birthday-themed tribute, Professor Zofia Urbanczyk-Lipkowska (*deceased 22 January 2024). I knew Zofia for nearly 2 decades since being invited as a lecturer and guest of the Polish Academy of Sciences in 2008. At that time, Zofia and her husband Andrei hosted me and my wife Janet for a week in Warsaw. We soon became aware of their warm, generous, and kind-hearted manners, which quickly united us as friends and kindred spirits.

Both Janet and I have always been curious historians with a special interest in the culture and history of Poland. Andrei and Zofia shared the amazing history of Warsaw both pre- and post-WWII and the origin/evolution of the Polish Academy of Sciences, and they introduced us to several obscure but brilliant Polish artists whose paintings still adorn our home to this day. After Andrei's passing, it was obvious that his loss was immense to Zofia as she immersed herself more deeply into her poly(peptide) science. However, she had an inexplicable new curiosity about the dendritic state and certain possibilities. It was through this mutual and shared interest in the dendritic state that I enjoyed such a long and enduring friendship with Zofia. She had always impressed me as a very hard-working, articulate, and outstanding poly(peptide) scientist with a certain hidden curiosity in dendrimer chemistry. That curiosity was soon revealed as Zofia shared a unique and unexpected scientific concept/dream that I considered to be both stunning and quite ambitious at the time. She proposed the synthesis and evaluation of specific poly(peptide) dendrimers (i.e., asymmetrical branch-cell type), which she felt would function as excellent structural mimics of certain natural membranolytic peptides known to exhibit unique anti-microbial activity (AMPs). Needless to say, with her typical, highly disciplined, articulate, and focused approach, she completed the synthesis of her novel dendrimer AMP mimics and determined they exhibited highly effective anti-microbial properties in record time [1]. This remarkable "scientific breakthrough", based on the cleverly engineered key critical nanoscale-design parameters (CNDPs) of asymmetric branch-celled dendrimers, allowed Zofia to produce the first dendritic examples of low-toxicity, high-potency antimicrobial agents against clinical isolates of antibiotic-resistant *ESBL E. coli* strains. The discovery of these effective new dendritic agents against such multi-drug-resistant pathogens was widely recognized as a seminal breakthrough. This amazing work convinced me that Zofia was indeed an extraordinary, creative, and brilliant scientist who, without pause, earned my deepest respect and admiration.

It is with a "heavy and saddened heart" that I dedicate this modest but sincere "dendritic perspective" to Professor Zofia Urbanczyk-Lipkowska, a truly kind, generous, and sensitive human being, as well as a very creative and visionary scientist of the highest intellect. We are all very saddened by her loss, as well as knowing there are undoubtedly many more scientific visions and contributions that Zofia would have shared that now will remain incomplete. They could have enriched the dendrimer community and the sciences, as well as humanity in general. Zofia will truly be missed by all of us!

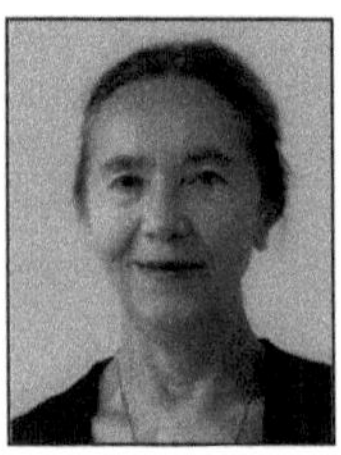

Prof. Dr. Zofia Urbancyzyk-Lipkowska.

1. Prologue

The ultimate hope for all major new discoveries, such as Dendrimers, Dendrons, and the Dendritic State (DDDS), is that such a "scientific breakthrough" will serve humanity in some significant manner, as well as advance and translate into an important technology platform for enhancing the human condition by fulfilling many unmet needs in society, such as a more sustainable world food supply, better human health, increased longevity, or a generally improved quality of life worldwide.

My optimism for this hope and dream has been substantially heightened and reassured after reading the 12 outstanding contributions to the 85th birthday Dendrimer-themed special issue of *Pharmaceutics*. I am truly grateful to my dear friends and DDDS colleagues Prof. Zofia Urbanczyk-Lipkowska (Polish Academy of Science, Warsaw, Poland) and Prof. Anne-Marie Caminade (CNRS, Toulouse), who so skillfully mentored and organized this special-themed issue on Dendrimers. It was especially pleasing and exciting to note the progress and many new advancements described in these excellent scientific contributions coauthored by many highly recognized pioneers and colleagues from the DDDS community, including: V. Percec/D. Weissman [2], D. Astruc/C. Ornelas [3], A.-M. Caminade [4], R. Haag [5], R. Kannan [6], M.-C. Daniel [7], V. Cena [8], C. Kojima [9], J. Rodrigues, F. de la Mata [10], M.A. Munoz-Fernandez/E.R. Gillies/R. Gomez [11], S. Pricl [12], S. Calvo-Serrano, E. Matamoros, E. Perez-Inestrosa, C. Mayorga, M.J. Torres [13], and others. I am truly humbled, deeply honored, and very pleased by this extraordinary 85th birthday-themed tribute and will remain eternally grateful to each of you for your sincere and magnificent effort. This is an exceedingly thoughtful and meaningful gift to receive for my 85th birthday, 5 September, 2023, which I coincidentally shared with John Dalton on the occasion of his 257th birthday (born 5 September 1766).

2. Reflections on the Dendron, Dendrimer, and Dendritic State (DDDS) Discovery

2.1. Several Major Consequences/Advancements Resulting from the DDDS Discovery

In my humble and subjective opinion, several unexpected consequences resulting from the DDDS discovery that have benefited the major sciences and other disciplines should include the following:

(a) The DDDS discovery initiated a major paradigm shift in the polymer science area based on an unprecedented, multi-step, iterative polymerization strategy referred to as step-growth, amplification-controlled polymerization (i.e., SGACP).

Historically, polymer science has evolved into three major architectural categories; namely: (I) linear, (II) cross-linked, and (III) simple branched-type polymers. These traditional macromolecular architectures are derived from the assembly of monomers via two major polymerization or molecular weight-amplification strategies, namely: (1) chain-like addition polymerizations (i.e., free-radical, anionic, cationic propagations, etc.) or (2) step-growth, condensation polymerizations. In either case, one has very little control over absolute molecular weight homogeneity (i.e., polydispersity) and virtually no control over resulting macromolecular structures. As such, current polydispersity values for most commercial polymers generally range from 2–10. In contrast, these discrete dendron/dendrimer-type macromolecules exhibit very enhanced homogeneity features with polydispersity values of M_w/M_n = 1.05–1.005 and allow substantial macromolecular structure control. These values are significantly better compared to the best known traditional living polymerization protocols. For example, as reported by Matyjaszewski, et al. [14], ATRP-type living free-radical polymerization results in M_w/M_n = 1.2–1.3 and allows very little control over resulting macromolecular structures.

(b) The DDDS discovery has revealed a very versatile polymerization strategy for the synthesis of precise, amplification, and structure-controlled dendritic macromolecules using common organic monomers and reagents.

The resulting dendritic macromolecules possess monodispersity and structure control rivaling that are observed for natural biological polymers (e.g., proteins, enzymes, RNA, DNA, etc.). All original poly(L-lysine) dendrons (i.e., Denkewalter type) and poly(amidoamine) (PAMAM) dendrons and dendrimers (i.e., Tomalia type) are examples of unprecedented, new dendritic architectures and structures (i.e., dendrimers, dendrons, etc.) created via "step-growth, amplification-controlled polymerization" (i.e., SGACP) protocols. Using common organic reagents such as α-amino acids, ethylene diamine, acrylates, or acrylonitrile monomers with SGACP-type protocols has produced these unprecedented new dendritic macromolecular structures. The Denkewalter poly(L-lysine) (PLL dendron)- and Tomalia, poly(amidoamine) (PAMAM) dendrimer)-type structures represent the first examples of well-characterized/confirmed structures required for the historical verification of the DDDS discovery.

(c) Precise, amplification and structure-controlled dendritic macromolecules made possible with SGACP protocols offer extraordinary nanoscale property benefits to pharma, nanomedicine, and life sciences.

Dendrons and dendrimers allow unlimited access to vast libraries of precise, dendritic nanoscale, and macromolecular nanoparticles (i.e., NPs) that either mimic or possess equivalent dimensions observed for important natural polymers (i.e., proteins, nucleic acids, etc.), as well as many in vivo cellular or physiological compartments (i.e., 1–500 nm). Furthermore, the ability to engineer and modify these dendritic NPs as a function of their critical nanoscale parameters (CNDPs) (i.e., size, shape, surface chemistry, flexibility/rigidity, elemental composition, and architecture) is an invaluable feature for optimizing structures to fit specific application needs, especially for personalized pharma or nanomedicine.

(d) These unique dendritic macromolecules exhibit unprecedented new properties that define a major new polymer architecture class, namely: Category (IV): dendrimers, dendrons, and hyperbranched dendritic polymers.

The iconic Berzelius hypothesis that states new molecular architecture creates new intrinsic properties has been fulfilled. A broad range of diverse, structure-controlled, dendritic macromolecules have been synthesized by these SGACP strategies and shown to exhibit a plethora of unexpected intrinsic properties, behavior, and associated phenomena. These new architecturally driven dendritic properties have been extensively characterized and demonstrated to fulfill many new applications, especially as active pharma ingredients (APIs), delivery vectors for targeted therapy, nucleic acid vaccine vectors, or in vivo bioimaging nano-devices in nanomedicine. These new architecturally driven dendritic properties have been extensively characterized and shown to exhibit unique utility in a wide variety of unprecedented applications. Collectively, these new dendritic structures/properties define the fourth-newest major polymer architecture category; namely: **Category (IV):** dendrimers, dendrons, hyperbranched and other dendritic polymers after traditional (I) linear, (II) cross-linked, and (III) simple-branched polymers as illustrated in Figure 1.

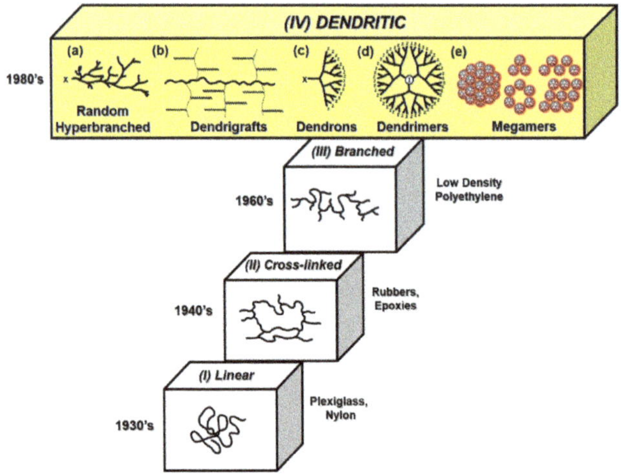

Figure 1. A chronology of the three major traditional polymer architectures with widely recognized applications, leading to the fourth new major Category (IV) of dendritic polymers: (**a**) random hyperbranched, (**b**) dendrigrafts, (**c**) dendrons, (**d**) dendrimers, and (**e**) megamers [15,16]. Reprinted and adapted with permission from Ref. [15]. Copyright 2002, John Wiley & Sons.

The importance of these major polymer architecture categories is readily apparent by noting historical Nobel laureate recognition associated in the past for pioneering work involving the first three traditional major architecture classes, namely: Categories (I), (II), and (III) as illustrated in Figure 2.

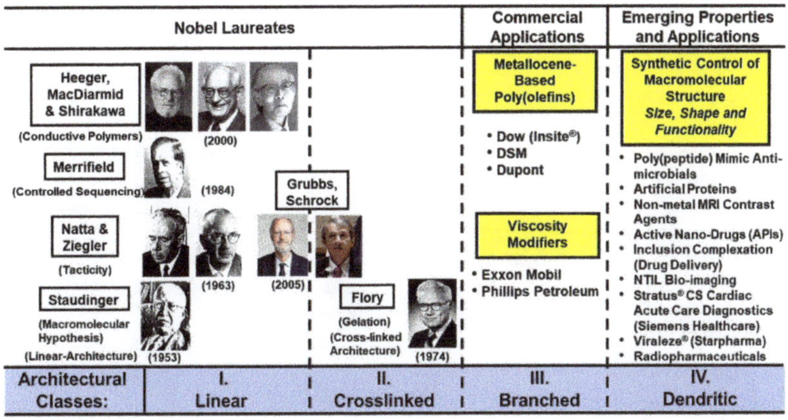

Figure 2. Nobel recognition, commercial applications, and new emerging properties for the four major polymer architectures. Reproduced with permission from Ref. [17]. Copyright 2013, Springer-Verlag Berlin Heidelberg.

2.2. Clarification of Historical Confusion Surrounding First Confirmed Examples of Authentic Non-Macromolecular and Macromolecular Dendrons and Dendrimers

A cursory survey of current literature and key archives (i.e., Wikipedia, etc.) reveals an alarming level of misinformation and confusion surrounding the general perception of the first historical examples of structure-confirmed and verified dendron/dendrimer syntheses. This confusion appears to result largely from a lack of accurate historical information and improper use of currently accepted IUPAC dendron/dendrimer terminology [18], as well as a plethora of incorrect or misused information. Such confusion has resulted in a distorted historical perspective concerning key contributions and specific examples that provided the first unequivocal confirmation of dendron and dendrimer structures considered to be absolutely critical and essential for the final acceptance of this seminal DDDS discovery.

A very small sampling of such examples is described below:

Example 1: "Vögtle and his team (1978) reported the formation of the first non-skid chain-like and cascade-like molecules with the topology of the molecular cavity, which is considered the earliest dendritic polymer form. The term "hyperbranched polymer" was first coined by Kim and Webster in 1988 in reference to the synthesis of soluble hyperbranched polyphenylene. This term was later used to describe the structure of dendrimers" [19].

Example 2: "Since the first dendrimer was reported in 1978 by Fritz Vögtle, dendrimer research has grown exponentially, from synthesis to application in the past four decades" [20].

Example 3: "The term "dendrimer" was coined by the polymer chemist Donald Tomalia from the Greek "dendra" for tree and "meros" for part of at Dow Chemical in Midland, Michigan. Afterwards, in 1978, at the University of Bonn, Fritz Vögtle's group synthesized dendrimers for the very first time when they tinkered with multi-functional branches ......" [21].

These excerpts and a brief account of this historical confusion merely document the "tip of the iceberg". My greatest concern is that the historical integrity of the DDDS discovery for future generations of young dendritic scientists will be irretrievably lost or diminished, if not properly monitored and corrected. It is from this important perspective, as well as our common mission to strive for uncompromised integrity in all of our scientific endeavors by pursuing the "truth" (i.e., verified structure confirmations) and seeking accurate historical information with steadfast objectivity, that I share earlier critical DDDS research information made available to me by the Dow Chemical Company, Midland, MI, USA.

Recent access to officially released, confidential Dow Chemical Company dendrimer patent documents reveals a much clearer perspective concerning the actual synthesis and confirmation of first cascade structure examples, as reported by Vögtle, et al. in 1978 [22] (i.e., often erroneously referred to as the first examples of dendrimer structures). This important new Dow information, generated from 1990–1992, was in response to a final dendrimer/dendron patent rejection, wherein the 1978 Vögtle cascade publication was cited as prior art. Unfortunately, this important Vögtle reference was not discovered by Dow until the late 1980s. Widely recognized as a supramolecular scientist, Vögtle may have inadvertently caused the obscurity of this reference by comingling and introducing this extraordinary cascade structure/synthesis topic into one of his typical supramolecular articles. As such, all early literature searches failed to detect this important cascade synthesis reference. In fact, the only dendron/dendrimer-associated literature reference known to exist was the 1981 Denkewalter patent [23], which had been readily eliminated earlier as non-equivalent prior art.

As such, Dow expected all 8–10 Dow patent applications under examination in 1988 by the Japan National Patent Office (JNPO) would be granted without any difficulty. That said, a JNPO literature search was the first to reveal the obscure and undetected Vögtle cascade synthesis/structure reference, which had been missed by essentially all interested parties in this area [22]. This single reference was cited as prior art and led to final rejections of all Dow dendrimer patent applications in Japan.

In a final effort to overcome this negative JNPO decision, the Dow Chemical Co. Patent Department was directed to organize and fund a 1-year investigation entitled: cascade synthesis/structure reproducibility study. The objective of this effort was to determine if all cascade synthesis results, as well as reported cascade structures, could be reproduced and verified as reported by Vögtle in 1978. This Dow-funded investigation involved a neutral third party of highly qualified scientific experts who were directed to re-examine and confirm the reproducibility of cascade poly(propyleneimine) (PPI) structures as reported by Vögtle in the journal *Synthesis* [22]. Dow selected two well-recognized, organic synthesis experts, namely: Dr. Christoph Rickert, Ph.D. (ETH, Switzerland) and Dr. Lars Piehler, Ph.D. (Stanford University) for this 1-year funded investigation to determine the synthetic reproducibility of Vögtle's cascade poly(propyleneimine) (PPI) structures. These Dow reproducibility study results are presented briefly below with more details available in the Supplementary Material Section.

As reported in this Dow-funded and officially certified cascade synthesis reproducibility study:

(1) There was "no evidence" that any multi-directional core (i.e., ethylenediamine core) derived true dendrimers could be synthesized or obtained by the Vögtle procedures published in 1978.

(2) The Dow study confirmed that only simple, low-molecular-weight di-directional benzylamine core-initiated dendritic-type structures could be synthesized and isolated according to Vögtle's 1978 procedures. More specifically, only three low-molecular-weight benzylamine core-initiated dendritic cascade structures could be synthesized and confirmed. As described in Scheme 1, only the di-nitrile structure **1**; G = 0, MW: 213.3 Da; the di-amine structure **2**; G = 0; MW: 221.3 Da and the tetra-nitrile structure **3**; and G = 1.0, MW: 433.6 Da could be synthesized and confirmed. The structure **4**-tetra-amine, G = 1.0, MW: 439.6 Da could not be synthesized or detected using Vögtle's 1978 procedures.

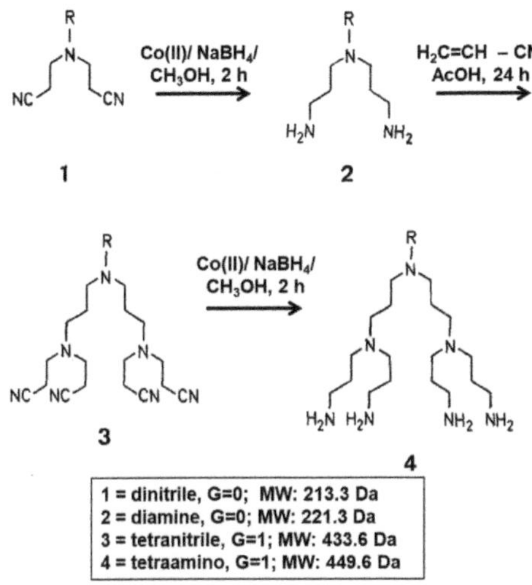

Scheme 1. The divergent iterative synthesis of a cascade dendrimer precursor structure **3**, where: R = benzyl. Reprinted and adapted with permission from Ref. [22]. Copyright 1978, Georg Thieme Verlag KG.

(3) All cascade structure product detection and confirmation were based on highly sensitive state-of-the-art mass spectrometry instrumentation (Electrospray Mass Spectrometer, Finnigan Model TSQ 700). It is very notable that no evidence could be obtained for the reproducibility of more complex multi-directional, dendrimer-based structures (i.e., structures 5b, 6b, 7b in the original Vögtle reference), resulting from a multifunctional initiator core such as ethylenediamine (EDA). (See as reported by Dr. C. Rickert and Dr. L Piehler in the certified documentation to the Dow Chemical Co. and disclosed in the Supplemental Section of this manuscript.)

(4) The essential absence of any meaningful product characterization data to support and confirm the cascade structures reported by Vögtle in 1978 was truly surprising. Absolutely no spectral data (i.e., FTIR, UV-vis, ^{1}H, ^{13}C-NMR) or chromatographic information (i.e., SEC, HPLC, etc.) were presented or reported to support these unprecedented cascade structures.

(5) The cascade product characterization and cascade structure confirmation were based solely on: (a) thin-layer chromatography (TLC) analyses, (b) standard C, H, N-elemental analyses, and (c) subjective interpretations of FAB mass spectrometry fragments. Vögtle reported that parent molecular ion masses for the cascade structures were either difficult or impossible to obtain, although these masses were detected routinely in the Dow study. Without any further activity in this cascade dendritic area from 1978–1993 (i.e.,~15 years), in 1993 [24], Vögtle mentioned that he had encountered substantial challenges with his 1978 cascade process that led to low cascade product yields, as well as characterization difficulties. These same Vögtle process difficulties were also noted by both Meijer, et al. [25] and Worner/Mülthaupt [26] later in 1993. Using their improved catalysts and revised processing conditions, Meijer and Worner/Mülhaupt independently reported obtaining very high cascade product yields via vastly improved protocols that proved suitable even for commercial production. For example, these new processing conditions allowed Worner/Mülhaupt to synthesize and isolate [(core: NH_3 initiated] tri-directional, poly(propyleneimine) (PPI) dendrimer precursors (i.e., G = 0–1; Mwt.= 176–530 Da), as well as macromolecular dendrimers (i.e., G = 2–4; Mwt.= 1167–5133 Da).

In view of the failure to reproduce Vögtle's results in the Dow-funded 1-year study, and the notable absence of critical product characterization/structure confirmation data in the 1978 Vögtle cascade synthesis article, the Japanese National Patent Office made an unprecedented decision to totally reverse their final patent-rejection decision. In fact, the JNPO accepted these Dow-funded reproducibility data as absolute evidence that no cascade, dendron, or dendrimer structures with MW > 433.6 Da had ever been synthesized or detected using the procedures as published by Vögtle in 1978. As a result, the Japanese National Patent Office officially granted all dendrimer and dendron patent claims to the Dow Chemical Company. This included all Tomalia PAMAM-type symmetrical branch-cell dendrimer and dendron structures possessing molecular weights higher than 433.6 Da (i.e., poly(propyleneimine) (PPI); tetra-nitrile; G = 1.0; MW = 433.6 Da).

In summary, the Dow Chemical Co.-funded "cascade reproducibility study" (1991–1992) provided important criteria for defining special terms such as true dendrimers and true dendrons. These terms were, accordingly, reserved for macromolecular, dendritic structures possessing MWts > 1000 Da. (i.e., generations > 2), whereas the term "cascade structures" was, accordingly, reserved for non-macromolecular, low-molecular-weight dendrimer precursor structures possessing MWts < 1000 Da.

A brief review of currently accepted terminology and corresponding dendritic structures is described in Figure 3 [27].

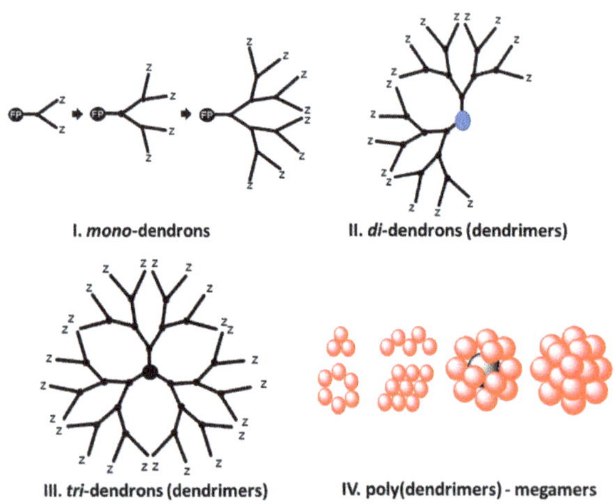

Figure 3. Structural designations for (**I**). monodendrons, (**II**). di-dendrons (dendrimers), (**III**). tri-dendrons (dendrimers), and (**IV**). poly(dendrimers)-megamers [28].

For historical clarification, very little product-characterization data or meaningful structure-verification work was reported by Vögtle in 1978. It was not until 1983–1985 that critical confirmation and structure verification of various unprecedented cascade, arborols, and, especially, true dendron/dendrimer structures were reported.

The initial verification/confirmation of these novel synthetic dendron or dendrimer macromolecular structures appeared to be a very daunting challenge. In fact, the extraordinary proposal that these dendritic structures were expected to exhibit mathematically predictable and controlled MWts as a function of specific growth stages (i.e., generations) was considered to be virtually impossible by many. For that reason, and many others, the critical urgency for providing unequivocal and compelling dendritic structure confirmations was of the highest importance. It was very quickly realized that both macromolecular and small molecule-analytical protocols had to be articulately combined and integrated into a holistic, self-consistent confirmation of these novel dendritic structures in order to support a compelling and unequivocal verification of these unprecedented dendritic structures, as well as their non-traditional properties and behavior [29].

A historical and annotated overview describing the first literature reports of analytical-characterization protocols that were required to verify these unprecedented dendritic structures and architectures is outlined below (see Figure 4) and discussed extensively elsewhere [30].

The first literature references and specific analytical protocols are described in Figure 4 below:

MW Amplification/Generation and Poly(dispersity) (Mw/Mn):

1. **Chromatography:** TLC [22], HPLC [31], SEC [31], electrophoresis (PAGE) [32]
2. **Nanoscale Sizes:** TEM [31,33], SEM [31], AFM [34,35], MS [31], SEC [31], electrophoresis (PAGE) [32], SAXS and SANS [36], Corey–Pauling–Koltun (CPK) models [31,37]
3. **Nanoscale Shapes:** AFM, TEM [31,33], SEM [31], fluorimetry [38], CPK models [31, 37]
4. **Interior Surface Chemistry:** FTIR [31], titrimetry [31], ^{1}H, ^{13}NMR [31], UV-vis [31], NIR [39]
5. **Mass Spectrometry:** MS-FAB [31], ESI [40,41], MALDI-TOF [42]
6. **Branching Ideality and Defects:** ^{1}H, NMR [31], ESI [40,41]
7. **Inclusion Complexation and Encapsulation:** Dialysis [43], NMR [31], UV-VIS [31], MS [31], EPR [38]
8. **Elemental Compositions:** C,H,N,O analyses [22], FTIR [31], NIR [39], UV-vis [31], titrimetry [31], electrochemical methods [31]
9. **Flexibility/Rigidity:** AFM [34,35], CPK models [31,37]

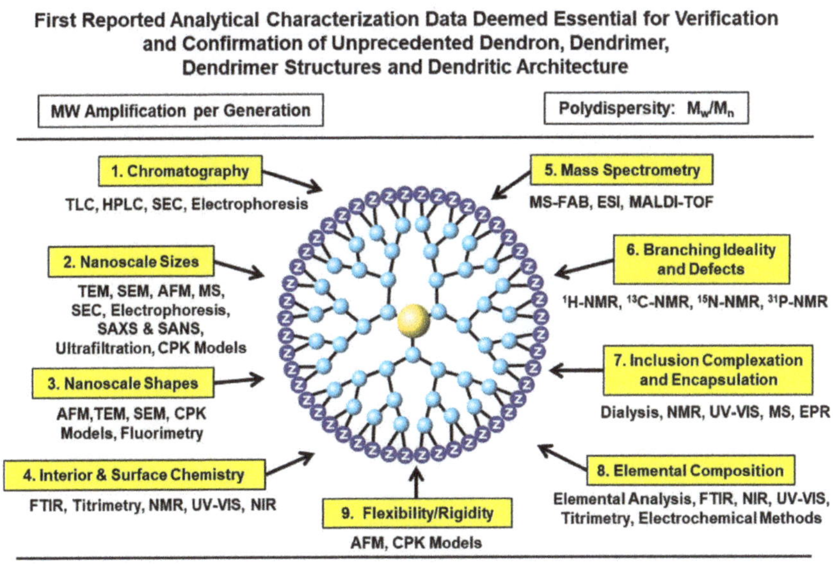

Figure 4. First reported analytical characterization data that led to confirmation of both symmetrical and unsymmetrical branch-cell dendrons, dendrimers, and megamers involved articulate documentation of critical nanoscale-design parameters (CNDPs) for these nanostructures.

A chronology of these first confirmed examples is described briefly below and as illustrated in Figure 5.

- **F. Vögtle, et al.** (1978) [22]: the first confirmed, low-molecular-weight, "symmetrical branch-cell", di-directional, (benzylamine core); oligo-(propyleneimine) cascade (OPI), "dendrimer precursor" structures (i.e., G = 0–1.0; MWt: 213.3–433.6 Da) using iterative, divergent synthesis with in situ branch-cell formation protocols. The 1978 Vögtle cascade synthesis was shown by the Dow-funded study to yield only a low MWt (i.e., 433.6 Da), symmetrical branch-cell, oligo-(propyleneimine) (OPI) dendrimer precursor (i.e., G = 1.0; nitrile terminated). There was no detectable evidence that the reported tetra-directional core (i.e., [EDA core], PPI dendrimers) had ever been synthesized in 1978 by Vögtle procedures. Note: This confirmation and verification are based on the Dow reproducibility study (1992) since essential cascade structure characterization documented in Synthesis (1978) was either not reported, considered non-critical to the cascade structure confirmation, or was not reproducible.

- **R. Denkewalter, et al.** (1981) [23]: the first confirmed macromolecular, uni-directional, (dibenzhydryl amine core); poly(L-lysine) (PLL), "asymmetrical branch-cell" dendron structures (i.e., G = 0–9; MW: 511 Da–233,600 Da) using iterative, divergent synthesis with (protect–deprotect) protocols.
- **D. Tomalia, et al.** (1983) [31,44]: the first confirmed macromolecular, uni-directional (diethanolamine (DEA) core); poly(amidoamine) (PAMAM), "symmetrical branch-cell", dendron structures (i.e., G = 0–7; MW: 445 Da~912 Da) using iterative, divergent synthesis, and (in situ branch-cell-formation) protocols.
- **D. Tomalia, et al.** (1983) [31]: the first confirmed macromolecular, tri-directional (NH_3 core) poly(amidoamine) (PAMAM), "symmetrical branch-cell" dendrimer structures (i.e., G = 0–7; MWts: 275 Da–43,451 Da) using iterative divergent synthesis and (in situ branch-cell-formation) protocols.
- **D. Tomalia, et al.** (1983) [31]: the first confirmed macromolecular, tetra-directional (EDA core) poly(amidoamine) (PAMAM),"symmetrical branch-cell" dendrimer structures (i.e., G = 0–7; MWts: 517 Da–116,493 Da) using iterative, divergent synthesis with (*in situ branch-cell-formation*) protocols.
- **D. Tomalia et al.** (1983) [31] (2000): the first confirmed examples of low-molecular-weight and high-molecular-weight, "symmetrical branch-cell" poly(dendrimers) referred to as "megamers". Both random-structure megamers [27] and controlled-structure megamers referred to as core-shell tecto(dendrimers) [45,46] have been synthesized, characterized, and confirmed.
- **G. Newkome, et al.** (1985) [47]: the first confirmed, low-molecular-weight, uni-directional (pentane focal point core): poly(amidoether) (PAmE),"symmetrical branch-cell" dendron/arborol-type structures (i.e., G = 0–2; MW: 303 Da–1130 Da) using a six-step divergent synthesis and a preformed branch-cell protocol.
- **Ranganathan, et al.** (1997) [48]: the first confirmed, di-directional (1,3-adamantane carbonyl core); poly(glutamic acid) (Glu peptidyl), "asymmetrical branch-cell" dendrimers and di-directional, (1,3-adamantane carbonyl core); poly(aspartic acid) (Asp), "asymmetrical branch-cell" dendrimers, respectively. These dendrimers were each synthesized by first constructing uni-directional poly(Glu) dendrons (G = 1–3) or uni-directional oly(Asp) dendrons (G = 1–3), respectively. After deprotection of the (-NH_2 end) focal point of the Glu or Asp dendrons, they were coupled to the 1,3-adamantane dicarbonyl chloride core in a convergent manner to obtain the respective Glu and Asp di-directional, asymmetrical branch-cell dendrimers.
- To our best knowledge, the first examples of asymmetrical branch-cell poly(dendrimer)-type megamers have not yet been synthesized or reported.

Earlier Dow–Tomalia evidence demonstrated the non-equivalency of Denkwalter's asymmetrical branch-cell dendrons/dendrimers compared to the Dow symmetrical branch-cell dendrimer and dendron structures. This non-equivalency is based on highly differentiated intrinsic properties that result due to branch-cell symmetry in each case. As such, it is critical to divide all known dendrons and dendrimers into two distinctly separate categories, namely: Category (I): symmetrical branch cell and Category (II): asymmetrical branch-cell structures. This important issue of classifying all known dendrons and dendrimers according to their branch cell symmetry is discussed extensively elsewhere [49] and described briefly in Section 2.3.

Historically, the first critical characterization examples that ultimately led to confirmation, verification, and acceptance of all recognized dendron, dendrimer, and megamer structures were reported by five early contributors in the DDDS area, as noted in Figure 5.

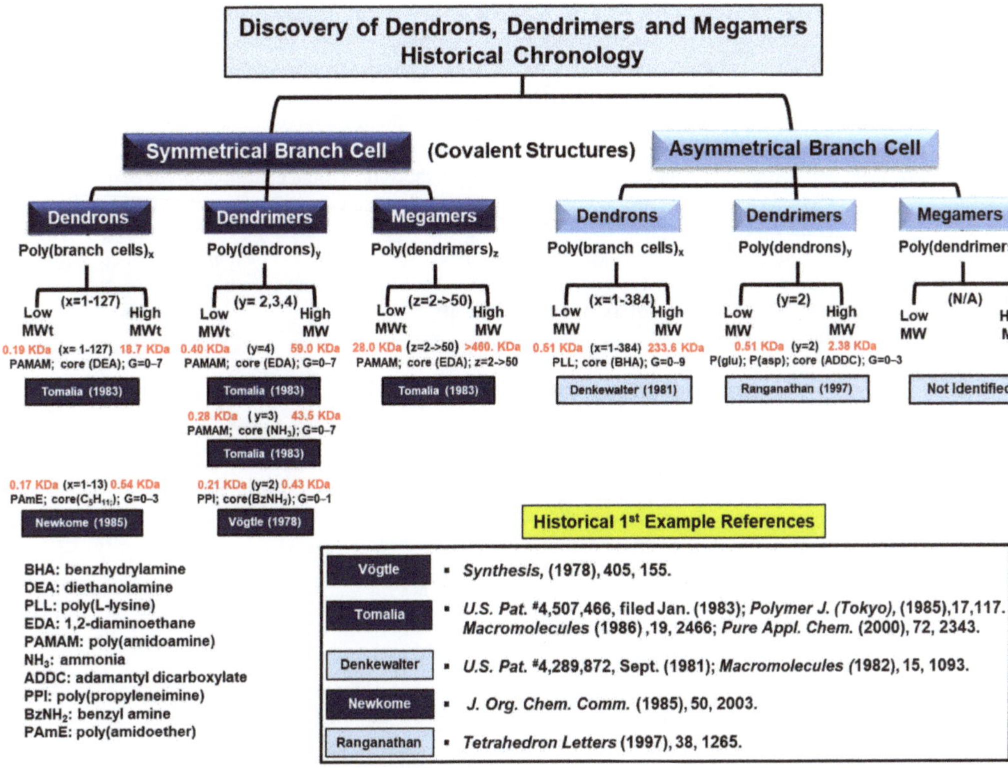

Figure 5. A chronology of historical first confirmed/verified examples of symmetrical and asymmetrical branch-cell dendrons, dendrimers, and megamers. First historical examples include: Vögtle [22], Tomalia [27,31,33,37,43], Denkewalter [23,50], Newkome [47], Ranganathan [48].

That said, one of the most compelling characterization protocols leading to ultimate dendritic structure confirmation and acceptance was unarguably the invention of electrospray ionization (ESI) for mass spectroscopy by John Fenn in 1989 [51]. The application of these ESI protocols to demonstrate mathematically predictable, precise molecular weights as a function of generation was compelling to even the most severe critics of the DDDS discovery. Other equally compelling contributions that verified the DDDS concept should also include the convergent synthesis of dendrimers first reported by Fréchet/Hawker [52–55] and independently by Neenan, et al. [56,57], as well as the integration of main-row hetero-elements such as phosphorous, silicon, boron, germanium, or bismuth into a wide range of important dendrimer compositions as reviewed by Majoral/Caminade [58,59].

2.3. *Why All Dendrons and Dendrimers Should Be Classified According to Branch Cell Symmetry*

A little-known fact related to the DDDS discovery is that all early Dow Chemical Co. patent applications (1981–1984) for Tomalia/Dewald dendrimer inventions were rejected by the U.S. Patent Office. Based on the obscurity of the 1978 Vögtle cascade structure reference, extensive literature searches did not reveal any conflicting prior art to the 1979 Tomalia/Dewald Dow discovery of poly(amidoamine) (PAMAM) compositions. A portfolio of 8–10 Dow patent applications filed to protect these unprecedented dendritic architecture/compositions was expected to be granted and allowed without any difficulty. Receiving these patent rejections was truly stunning and devastating to the Dow Chemical Company, Midland, MI, USA. This unexpected U.S. Patent Office action was based solely on a single R. Denkewalter U.S. Patent #4,289,872 (1981) [23] to the Allied Chemical Co., wherein, the U.S. Patent Office had deemed the Denkewalter dendritic structures to be equivalent to those in the Dow applications. This disappointing event immediately initiated an extensive study to determine if a true equivalency between Denkewalter and Tomalia-type dendritic structures really existed. The ensuing assessment and comparison clearly confirmed a total absence of equivalency between the conflicting Denkewalter and Tomalia structures. Non-equivalency was unequivocal based on dramatically differentiated intrinsic, physico-chemical properties observed in each case. Although a casual examination of each highly branched structure type suggested equivalent dendritic architecture, it was soon revealed that "branch-cell symmetry" controlled and defined essentially all observed intrinsic dendrimer properties in each case. This included fundamental properties such as densities, refractive indices, interior solvent-filled void space, an ability to form (guest–host) inclusion complexes, the presentation of terminal surface groups, etc. [60–63], with several fundamental differences as noted below in Figure 6.

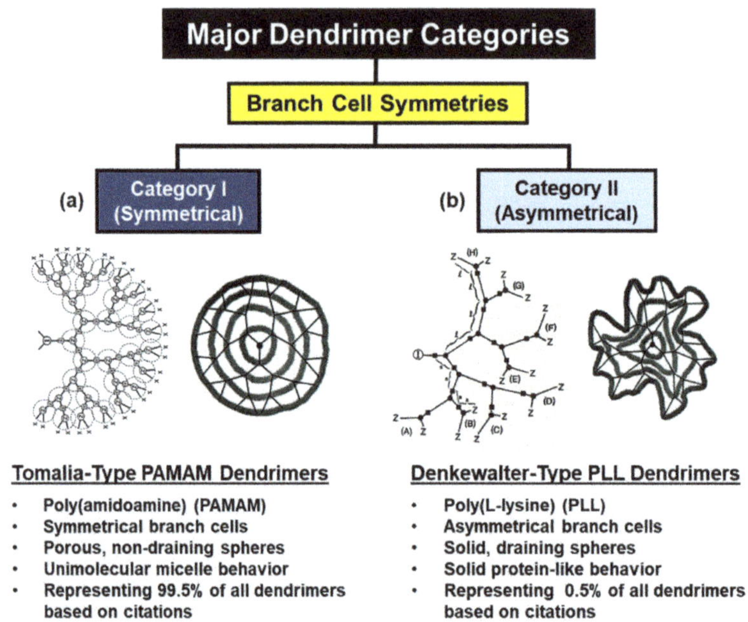

Figure 6. Classification of all dendrons and dendrimers according to branch-cell symmetry, namely: (**a**) Category (I): symmetrical branch cells represented by Tomalia-type PAMAM dendrimers, which are porous, non-draining spheroids that possess interior void space, exhibit guest–host inclusion complex-formation properties, and account for 99.5% of all literature citations. (**b**) Category (II): asymmetrical branch cells represented by Denkewalter-type PLL dendrimers, which are protein-like, solid draining spheres and account for 0.5% of all literature citations. Reprinted with permission from Ref. [49]. Copyright 2020, MDPI.

This critical demonstration of highly differentiated intrinsic properties observed for Category (I): symmetrical branch-cell dendrimers versus Category (II): asymmetrical branch-cell dendrimers clearly established the non-equivalency of Tomalia-type Category (I) and Denkewalter-type Category Type (II) dendrons/dendrimers, respectively. This differentiation led to the immediate allowance of all earlier Dow dendrimer patents, as well as literally dozens of subsequent patent applications in that area. These issues and details have been reviewed extensively elsewhere [49].

In retrospect, although this difference in dendron and dendrimer branch-cell symmetry (i.e., symmetrical vs. asymmetrical) appears to be minor, this subtle architecture difference truly confirms the power and importance of the Berzelius molecular architecture hypothesis, which states that any change in architecture at the molecular level, no matter how small or subtle, should be expected to produce entirely new intrinsic properties. Some of these intrinsic property differences are described in Figure 6.

This profound branch-cell symmetry effect has prompted an important and essential classification of all known dendrimer and dendron structures into two significant category types, namely: a major class of Category (I): symmetrical branch-cell structures and a minor group of Category (II): asymmetrical branch-cell structures. Denoting these major and minor branch-cell symmetry categories is based on the historical number of literature/patent citations documented for dendritic structures residing in Categories (I) and (II), respectively. A recent survey (i.e., patent and literature activity) of all known covalent dendrons and dendrimers has revealed a preponderance of activity (i.e., 99.5%) has focused on Category (I): symmetrical branch-cell dendrimers such as Tomalia and Newkome-type structures [64]. Meanwhile, Category (II): asymmetrical branch-cell dendrimers such as poly(peptide) and Denkewalter-type poly(L-lysine) dendrimers have received substantially less attention, but with recent indications that Category (II) activities may be increasing. In any case, we recommend the branch-cell symmetry classification of all covalent dendrons/dendrimers into Major Category (I) or Minor Category (II), respectively, as described in Figure 6.

That said, dramatically enhanced interest and activity have been observed in the asymmetrical branch-cell dendrimer area (i.e., poly(peptide) dendrimers). More specifically, this activity has been inspired and catalyzed based on recent new advancements in synthesis [64,65] and discovery of new intrinsic properties [66], as well as exciting new developments in a variety of medical applications, including dendritic mimics of multi-drug resistant anti-microbial peptides (AMPs) [1,67–69], anti-bacterial [70], anti-fungal, and anti-viral agents [64].

2.4. The Important Role of Critical Nanoscale-Design Parameters (CNDPs)

A brief survey of the 12 outstanding articles contributed to the current 85th birthday-themed issue on DDDS (2023-2024) has revealed the following interesting trends based on topics covered and discussed in Table 1.

Table 1. Recent trends and topics discussed in contributions to the Pharmaceutics 85th birthday-themed issue on DDDS (2023–2024).

Topics Covered and Discussed	Number of Articles/12
Dendron/dendrimer-CNDPs	12/12
Dendron/dendrimer targeted/drug delivery	8/12
Amphiphilic dendrons/dendrimers, supramolecular assemblies	7/12
Hetero-atom containing dendrimers/dendrons	3/12
Dendritic APIs; anti-(bacterial, viral, fungal, parasite, cancer, neurodegeneration)	3/12
Complement activation	1/12
Dendrimer-inorganic nanoparticle hybrids	1/12

Essentially every contributed article to this current special topics issue touches on some aspect of dendron and dendrimer-related critical nanoscale-design parameters (CNDPs) followed by targeted/drug delivery, amphiphilic/supramolecular assemblies, heteroatom-containing and dendritic APIs, etc.

Intrinsic nanoparticle property patterns based on the six CNDPs, such as size, shape, surface chemistry, flexibility/rigidity, architecture, and elemental compositions, have provided powerful and predictive guides for optimizing nanoparticle features. This concept was introduced as early as 2010 for dendrimers and all well-defined hard/soft nanoparticles (NPs) [63,71]. These special features are required for many nanomedicine applications, including their use as APIs, nanoscale vectors for MRI contrast agents, solubilization and encapsulation of drugs, or as site-specific, targeting agents for the delivery of small drugs/nucleic acids. Using these CNDP principles, the optimization of many pharmacokinetic and biodistribution, as well as excretion and nano-toxicology, properties have been demonstrated for a wide range of well-defined hard and soft nanoparticle platforms [71] as illustrated in Figure 7. The importance of exploiting CNDPs and their widespread use in nanomedicine has been discussed extensively elsewhere [72–74].

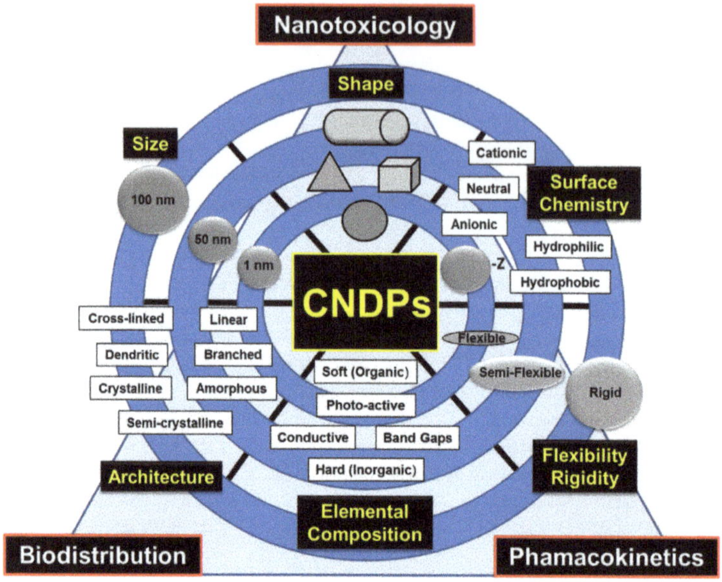

Figure 7. Six critical nanoscale-design parameters (CNDPs) and their important role in determining the nano-toxicity, pharmacokinetics, and biodistribution of well-defined, hard/soft nanoparticles (NPs) used in drug delivery and nanomedicine applications [28,63,72,73].

A specific and important application of these CNDP principles has recently been demonstrated by the simple modification of PAMAM dendrimer terminal surface moieties to render them (a) more bioavailable, (b) non-toxic, (c) NTIL fluorescent, and (d) stealth to innate immuno-responses.

Currently, one of the greatest challenges confronting nanomedicine is the in vivo delivery of therapeutic drug levels to disease sites with minimal collateral exposure to healthy tissue while avoiding innate immune system recognition [75]. Essentially all living organisms have evolved and survived by developing innate immune recognition strategies for eliminating deleterious pathogens or other foreign objects that may interfere with normal physiological processes. These innate immunological defenses involve both humoral and cellular recognition mechanisms and are generally referred to as the complement system. The complement system consists of specific soluble plasma proteins, as well as membrane-bound protein regulators/receptors that may be recruited to activate a cascade of reactions directed at the elimination of a pathogen/foreign object from the organism. The complement system utilizes a diverse repertoire of "pattern-recognition strategies" to identify dangerous pathogen signals. Activation signals associated with pathogens may include conserved microbial cell wall components, carbohydrate/protein, or other poly(hydroxyl)motifs. In general, any surface chemistry/moieties/features leading to serum protein adsorption (i.e., opsonization) will be expected to produce a strong immune response through complement activation. The complement system is an integral component of the innate immune system. It recognizes intruder danger signals primarily through pattern recognition, a process mediated by complement-sensing molecules such as IgG, IgM, and IgA class antibodies, C1q, mannose-binding lectin (MBL), ficolins, and properdin [75]. These recognition events are programmed to trigger various complementary cascade or activation sequences, which are generally recognized to follow any of three major courses, referred to as (1) the classical, (2) lectin, or (3) alternate-activation pathways. Inadvertent activation of the complement system will elicit acute reactions and pro-inflammatory responses, including anaphylaxis shock, which may be fatal. These complementary activation cascades are often observed following infusion or in vivo use of many nanomedicines, nanoparticles, or polymeric structures in animals and humans [75–77]. There is now growing evidence that these same nanoparticle-based CNDP principles may be applied to NP engineering strategies for avoiding in vivo innate immune recognition and complement activation (Figure 8).

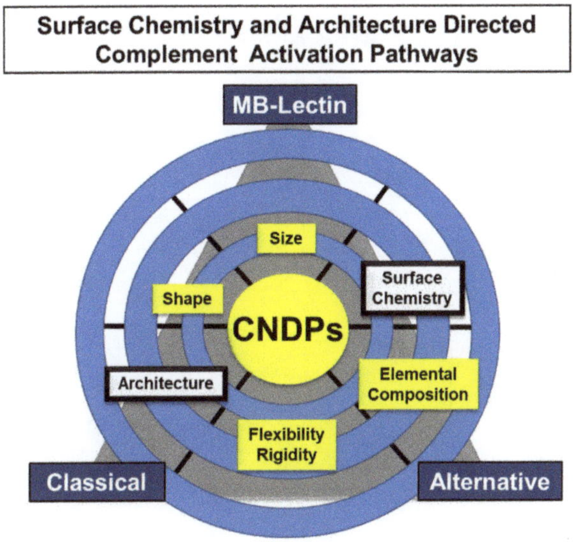

Figure 8. Six critical nanoscale-design parameters (CNDPs) and the important role that "surface chemistry" plays in determining stealth features and non-complementary activation properties for well-defined nanoparticles such as dendrimers.

A simple CNDP-surface chemistry modification of an important class of nanoparticle vectors such as PAMAM dendrimers has been shown to produce "stealth-like features" and exhibit non-complementary activation properties analogous to those observed for traditional PEGylated drugs and products. More specifically, the reaction of amine-terminated PAMAM dendrimers with dimethyl itaconate provides essentially quantitative conversions into 4-carbomethoxy pyrrolidone terminated dendrimers as illustrated in Scheme 2a. Considered to be analogous to PEGylation, this unique pyrrolidone modification of amine-terminated dendrimers is referred to as PYRROLIDONylation. Other demonstrated examples of PYRROLIDONylation by modification of dendrimer surface chemistry are illustrated in Scheme 2b. PYRROLIDONylation represents an alternative strategy to PEGylation and produces unprecedented examples of unique nanoscale materials that exhibit amazing non-complementary activation properties as predicted by Tomalia et al. [78], subsequently reported by Christensen/Klajnert–Maculewicz [79] and later demonstrated by Moghimi, et al. [80]. These "PYRROLIDONylation" products should be viewed as important and cost-effective alternatives to PEGylated products, which are currently under scrutiny due to recent confirmation that the "innate immune system" recognizes and produces detectable immuno-responses (i.e., antibodies) after repeated usage [81–83].

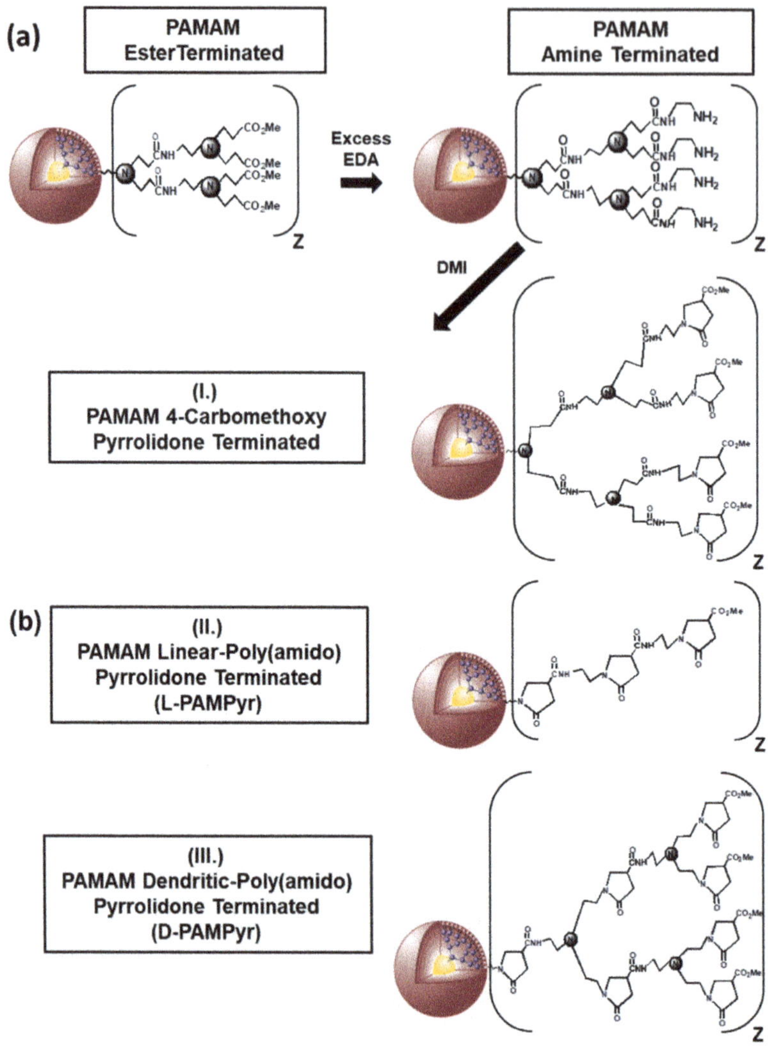

Scheme 2. (**a**) Unique modifications of amine-terminated PAMAM dendrimers with dimethyl itaconate (DMI) to produce stealth-like, non-complementary activating properties, (**b**) other examples of PYRROLIDONylation involving the modification of amine or pyrrolidone-terminated PAMAM dendrimers [78].

2.5. A Decade (2012–2022) of Expansion and Growth for Supramolecular Dendritic Structures (i.e., Dendrimersomes, Nano-Micelles, Dendri-Micelles, Supramolecular Dendrimers, etc.)

In addition to significant growth noted for traditional covalent-bonded dendritic structures over the past decade, explosive growth and expansion have occurred with supramolecular, non-bonded, dendritic structures and architecture. Many novel amphiphilic and Janus-type dendrons and dendrimers have been described by new terms/terminology (i.e., hybrid and supramolecular dendrimers). They have been self-assembled into a wide range of new dendritic supramolecular assemblies that exhibit unique and unprecedented properties [84–86].

The first peer-reviewed publication describing intrinsic supramolecular features of dendrimers appeared in 1988 [87,88]. Subsequent supramolecular perspectives of the "dendritic state" began to emerge as early as 1995. At that time, both Meijer, et al. [89] and Percec, et al. [90] recognized that amphiphilic dendrimeric entities did not self-assemble according to traditional Israelachvili-type amphiphilic surfactant rules [91] but produced new, unexpected dendritic, micelle-like assemblies. These unique, unprecedented dendritic self-assemblies appeared to result from the significantly larger hydrophilic, dendritic head component compared to the traditional dimensions of the hydrophobic linear tail components. Concurrently, Zimmerman, et al. [92] reported the first self-assembly of focal-point functionalized dendrons possessing suitable "hydrogen-bonding" features. These were the first examples of true supramolecular dendrimers. This seminal event was soon followed by the assembly of carboxylic acid functionalized focal-point dendrons around metal cations according to Fréchet, et al. [93], as well as the assembly of excess carboxylic acid-terminated shell reagents around a limited amount of amine-terminated PAMAM dendrimer to produce charge-neutralized carboxylic acid terminated core-shell tecto(dendrimer) precursors, which were then converted into their covalent form with carbodiimide reagents [45].

A variety of supramolecular issues related to dendrimers and dendrons included "all-or-nothing reactivity" with hydrophobes as a signature for de Gennes dense packing, for multivalent supramolecular dendrimer-drug interactions [94], aggregation of amphiphilic PAMAM dendrimers G = 0–3 [95], the mimicry of classical regular and inverse micelles, etc., while "guest–host" encapsulation properties were reviewed extensively elsewhere [95–97].

2.5.1. Amphiphilic Janus Dendrimers: Self Assembly into Dendrimersomes

Throughout the timeframe 2009–2014, a more intense interest began to emerge with a specific focus on dendritic amphiphilic entities, such as the first examples of Janus dendrimers, which appeared in a patent [98], amphiphilic Janus-type PAMAM dendrons, as well as other modified dendrimers (Figure 9). It involved a number of pioneering scientists, including Percec, Peng, Velder, et al. and others. It began with the pioneering work of Percec, et al. in 2009 [99–103]. This seminal work demonstrated that predictable nano-periodic, dendron-shape changes occurred as a function of the generation level. These predictable and quantized nano-patterns of hierarchical shape changes were manifested as unique dendron morphologies. These unique morphologies obtained as a function of the generation were readily defined as solid-angle dendron projections (α') when projected onto a plane (Figure 10). The α' angle is defined as the solid-angle projection of the dendron onto a plane and can be determined in all cases according to (α') = 360/μ, wherein μ is the number of dendrons in a specific column stratum or supramolecular sphere. Increasing the branching of a tapered-like dendron via a sequence change or an increase in generation number increases the α' and the fraction of the disk occupied in a columnar self-assembly. At a certain threshold, only disks are formed. Above this threshold, further branching results in congestion-induced deformation of the disk into a conical segment with diminished α'. Beyond this point, enhanced branching increases (α'), as well as the fraction of a sphere formed. These transformations are illustrated as a function of generation levels 1–7. Ultimately, an unimolecular spheroid should result at G = 8, as shown in Figure 10 [102].

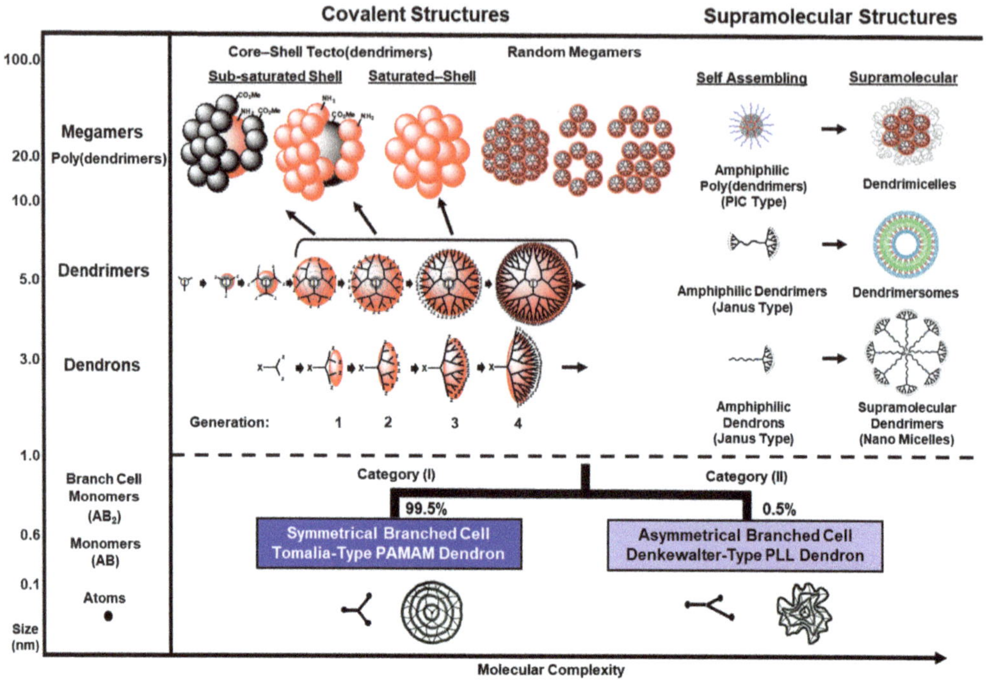

Figure 9. Various dendrons, dendrimers, and megamers as a function of known covalent and supramolecular structures. Proposed division of all known dendrons/dendrimers according to branch-cell symmetry, namely: the major Category (I) possessing symmetrical branch cells and the minor Category (II) possessing asymmetrical branch-cell structures.

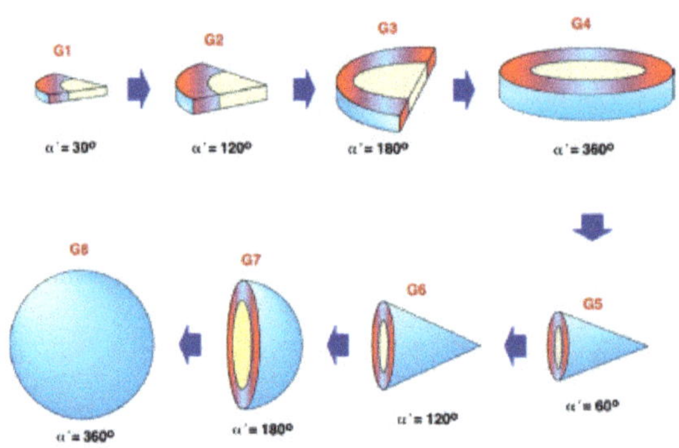

Figure 10. Hierarchical control of self-assembly via molecular solid angle. Reprinted with permission from Ref. [102]. Copyright 2000, American Chemical Society.

Within the context of this quantized and predictable behavior, Percec et al. [99] systematically investigated the effect of the generation number on the self-assembly of various amphiphilic dendrons. Using X-ray diffraction studies [102], it was revealed that G = 1 and G = 2 dendrons tended to form 2-D, flattened disc-like shapes that self-assembled into cylindrical columns. On the other hand, G = 3 dendrons underwent a congestion-induced shape change resembling a 3-D fragment of a sphere and tended to form spherical aggregations within a cubic lattice. In essence, it was confirmed by X-ray analysis that congestion-induced shape changes to produce a spheroid-like morphology should be expected to occur as a function of generation level. This was an amazingly concise alternative corroboration of a similar generation-dependent, congestion-induced shape change observed by Tomalia/Goddard et al. in 1989 [62]. Many of these first principles were subsequently applied by Percec et al. [99] to gain a deeper understanding of these nanoscale self-assemblies. They were then used in the development of extensive libraries describing the self-assembly modes and ultimate 3-D lattices formed by these amphiphilic dendrons. Extensive X-ray characterization and retro analyses of these 3-D lattice libraries have produced quantitative roadmaps for understanding critical dendron-structural parameters that direct these self-assembly patterns. This information now allows for an accurate a-priori prediction of final self-assembled structures one would expect based on certain critical nanoscale-design parameters. It has now been shown that these controlled CNDPs such as size, shape, surface chemistry, and flexibility [100] may be analyzed in the primary amphiphilic dendrimer structures and used for these predictions [100]. Historically, this was the first demonstrated example and proof that one could predict the final supramolecular-type assembly that would form with an accuracy of >85% [100]. These predictions were based on known dendrimer nano-periodic property patterns and the specific CNDP design of the Janus dendron. These results actually suggested and supported a concept for creating a Mendeleev-like nano-periodic table for well-defined dendron and dendrimer nanoparticles.

This seminal work was discussed in great detail with V. Percec on the occasion of a historical *IDS-6* dinner in Stockholm, Sweden (2009). This revelation clearly connected with my long-term interest in defining a unifying nano-periodic property concept for explaining the many pervasive nano-periodic property patterns that have been observed for discrete quantized nanoparticles that appear to mimic atoms, such as dendrimers, dendrons, etc. This Percec work appeared to be a "demonstration of concept" for a unified nano-periodic concept as proposed elsewhere in collaboration with physicists such as Prof. Shiv Khanna (VCU), et al. for other super atoms (i.e., nanoscale atom mimics) [104–106]. This seminal work by Percec clearly demonstrated the remarkable predictive power with >85% accuracy and potential implications for Percec's first predictive tables for the self-assembly of amphiphilic Janus dendrimers. Historically, these data may have fulfilled/validated our proposed nano-periodic concept for unifying well-defined quantized nanoparticles and represent the first example of a Mendeleev-like nano-periodic table. These issues have been discussed and described extensively elsewhere [17,104–106].

A preponderance of the earlier pioneering dendrimer work by Percec, et al. [99] in the 1990s had been focused on the self-assembly of amphiphilic dendrons. That effort subsequently evolved into the supramolecular assembly of amphiphilic dendrimers currently referred to as Janus dendrimers [19]. A Janus-type dendrimer is formed by linking two chemically differentiated features or components (i.e., a hydrophobic and hydrophilic domain) into a single dendrimer structure. Some of the earliest examples of surface-differentiated Janus dendrimers were reported by Hawker/Fréchet [54], as well as by Tomalia, et al. [107–109], as illustrated in Figure 11 below.

As early as 2010, Percec, et al. [109] reported the synthesis of a broad class of amphiphilic Janus dendrimers with typical structures, such as those illustrated in Figure 12. Over 11 distinct libraries consisting of more than 107 uncharged and cationically charged dendrimers were examined [109]. By simply injecting an ethanolic solution of Janus dendrimers into water, they obtained very uniform, robust populations of bilayer vesicle assemblies reminiscent of liposomes. These new unprecedented Janus dendrimer self-assemblies, which are in essence megameric assemblies (i.e., poly(dendrimers)) that have been coined—dendrimersomes and are as shown in Figure 12.

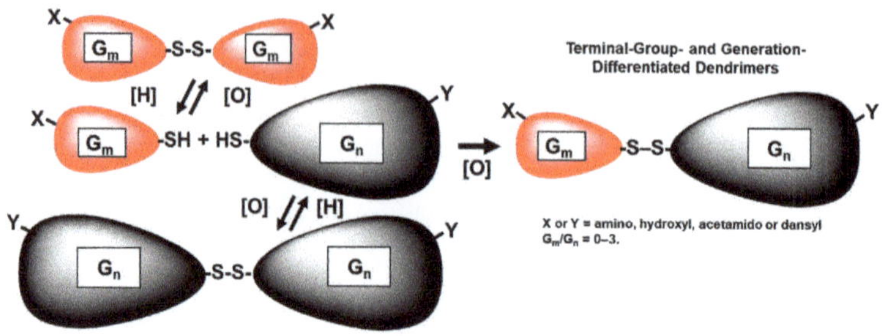

Figure 11. The first example of a Janus dendrimer was obtained by reduction and re-oxidation of two differentiated (i.e., surface and generation differentiated) cystamine core PAMAM dendrimers. Reprinted with permission from Ref. [16]. Copyright 2005, Elsevier [107].

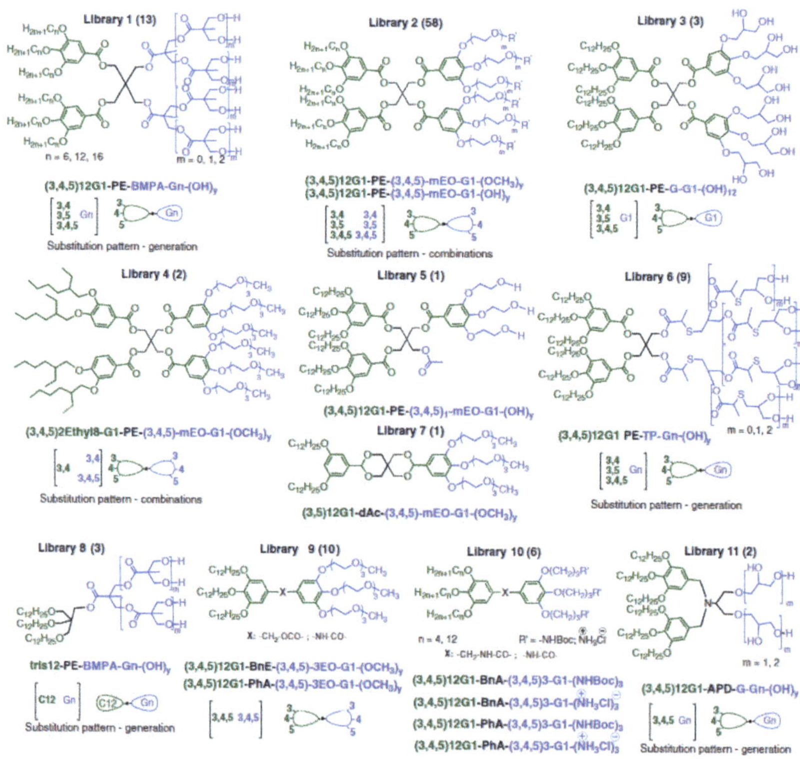

Figure 12. Various libraries of Percec-type Janus dendrimers suitable for self-assembly into dendrimersomes. Reprinted with permission of Ref. [109]. Copyright 2010, The American Association of the Advancement of Science.

It is readily apparent that these Janus dendrimers are powerful, structure-directing amphiphiles that exhibit greater versatility than simple lipids, surfactants, or block copolymers in their ability to produce uniform, robust, and highly predictable functional assemblies Figure 13. Based on specific dendrimersome CNDP features and associated principles, Percec was able to predict the type of supramolecular dendrimersome self-assembly structure that would result in an accuracy of >88%. This suggests the strong possibility for evolving a variety of unprecedented and predictive Mendeleev-like nano-periodic tables [101].

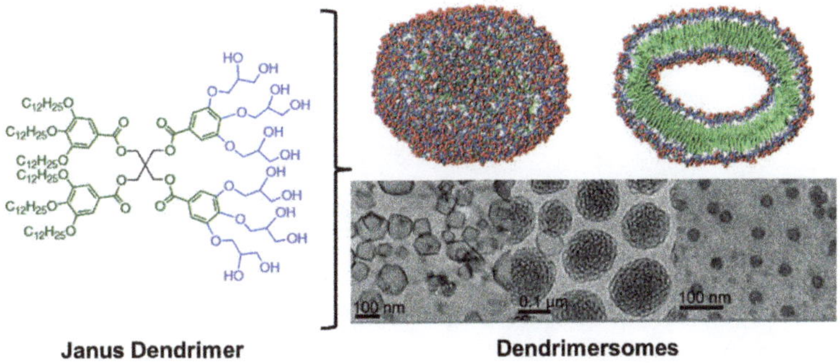

Figure 13. Self-assembly of a Percec-type Janus dendrimer into a dendrimersome. Reprinted and adapted with permission of Ref. [109]. Copyright 2010, The American Association of the Advancement of Science.

A wide range of diverse Janus-type dendrimer structures have been synthesized. A small sampling of these Janus-type dendrimer libraries reveals that unique structures such as "twin–twin", "single–single", and "twin–mixed" carbohydrate-presenting entities have been made, as illustrated in Figure 14. Depending on the structure of the Janus dendrimer precursor, at least four major dendrimersome topologies were obtained, as illustrated in Figure 15.

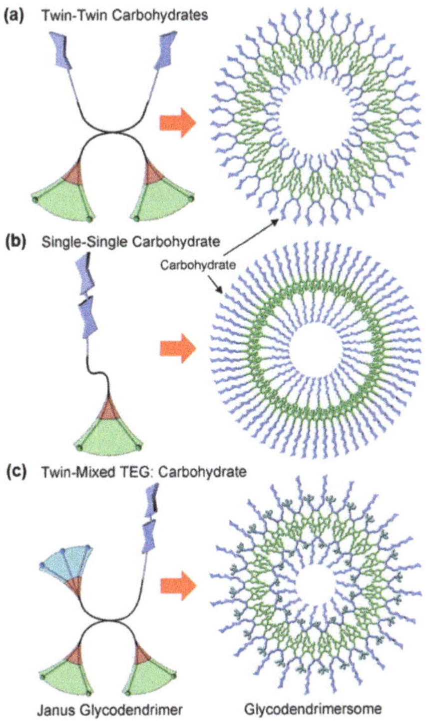

Figure 14. Various "twin–twin", single–single", and "twin–mixed" carbohydrate presenting structures and libraries. Color code: hydrophilic blue, hydrophobic green, aromatic red. Reprinted with permission from Ref. [110]. Copyright 2014, John Wiley & Sons.

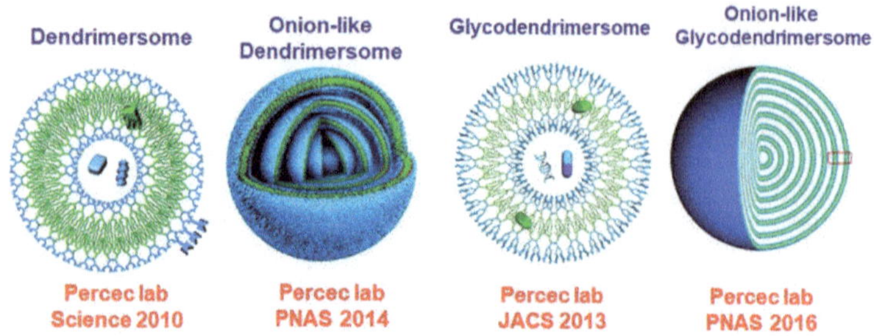

Figure 15. Four major categories of Percec-type dendrimersomes. Reprinted and adapted with permission from [111]. Copyright 2023, MDPI.

These unique dendrimersome assemblies have been recently demonstrated to play a critical role in new simplified, one-component protocols for the delivery of mRNA in future vaccines, as described later.

2.5.2. Amphiphilic, Janus Dendrons: Self-Assembly into Supramolecular Dendrimers (i.e., Dendrimeric Nano-Micelles)

As early as 2012, L. Peng, et al. [112] developed a groundbreaking and innovative clickable modular component approach for producing self-assembling amphiphilic PAMAM dendrons. This approach involved combining clickable azide and alkyne components. Using these modular components (Figure 16), a wide range of "click-synthesized" amphiphilic PAMAM dendrons may be rapidly synthesized as shown in Figure 17.

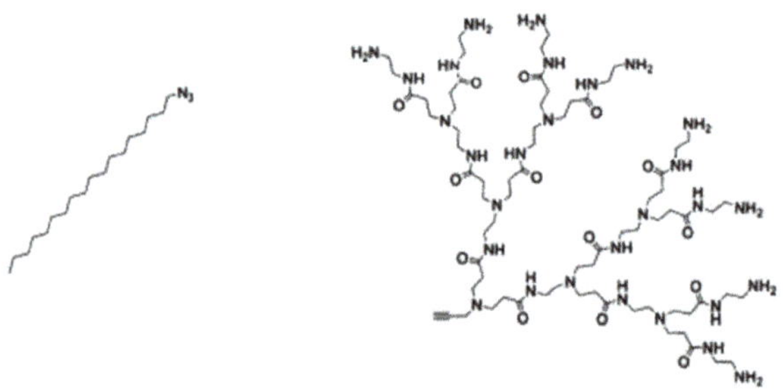

Figure 16. Hydrophobic azide and hydrophilic alkyne click chemistry precursors to Peng-type amphiphilic dendrons. Reprinted with permission from Ref. [112]. Copyright 2012, John Wiley & Sons.

These module-clicked amphiphilic Janus PAMAM dendrons could be readily designed and rapidly synthesized according to CNDP engineering principles described in Section 2.3. The desired amphiphilic PAMAM dendrons were readily synthesized in a modular fashion by performing Sharpless-type click coupling of various hydrophilic PAMAM dendrons (i.e., G = 0–3) possessing suitable alkyne focal-point modifications (i.e., hydrophilic-head components) with various azide-modified hydrophobic alkanes (i.e., hydrophobic-tail components) to create large libraries of hydrophilic head-hydrophobic tail and amphiphilic PAMAM dendrons. An abbreviated series of these clickable components with TEMs, as shown in Figure 17.

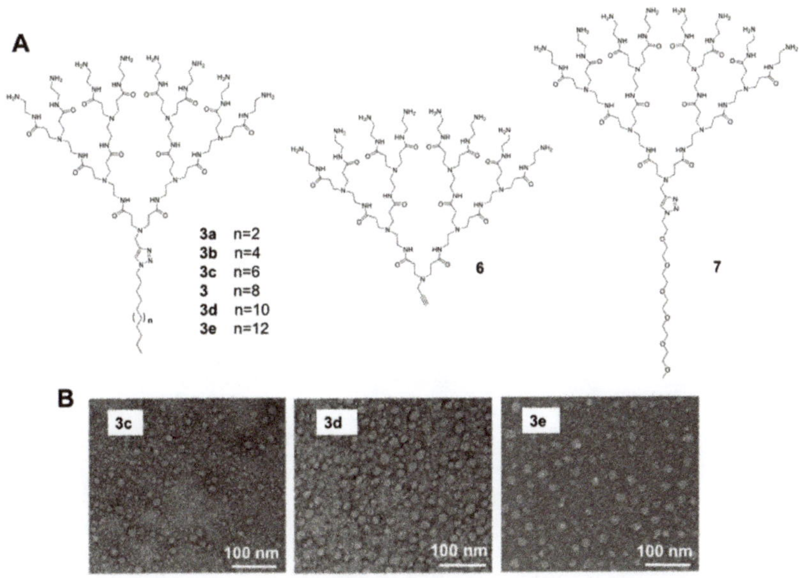

Figure 17. (**A**) Various Peng-type amphiphilic PAMAM dendrons, (**B**) TEMs observed after self-assembly into their respective supramolecular dendrimers, **3c**, **3d,** and **3e** (i.e., nano-micelles). Reprinted and adapted with permission from Ref. [113]. Copyright 2016, John Wiley & Sons.

Chen/Peng et al. have demonstrated that these amphiphilic Janus dendrons readily self-assemble into a wide variety of specific generational-level supramolecular dendrimers (i.e., some refer to them as dendrimeric nano-micelles). These supramolecular dendrimers appeared to mimic the generational-level features and properties of traditional covalently derived dendrimers, G = 4–6, which are generally more onerous and time-consuming to synthesize (Figure 18).

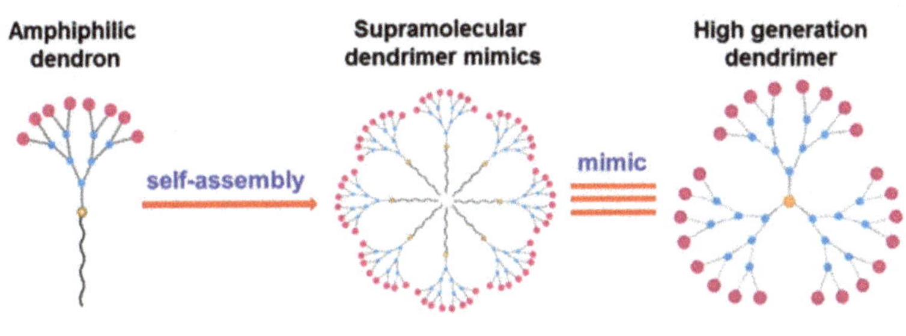

Figure 18. The self-assembly of amphiphilic dendrons into supramolecular dendrimers and proposed mimicry of covalent dendrimers. Reprinted with permission from Ref. [113]. Copyright 2016, John Wiley & Sons.

2.5.3. Amphiphilic Dendrimers: Self-Assembly into Dendrimicelles

In an effort to produce modified dendrimer assemblies containing encapsulated photosensitizers (PS) suitable for photodynamic therapy (PDT), certain dendritic entities were prepared by surrounding the porphyrin dye structure with poly(benzyl ether) dendrons possessing peripheral ionic groups [114]. Quite remarkably, these entities spontaneously assembled into poly-ionic complex PIC-type micelles by electrostatic interactions via oppositely charged components of the dendrimer and the ionic block copolymer (Figure 19). Surprisingly, it was also found that these novel dendrimer-encapsulated porphyrin (DP) micelles containing porphyrin dye cores did not self-quench upon irradiation, but instead exhibited amazingly effective in vitro photo-cytotoxicity properties that were found to be very suitable for cancer therapy (Figure 20).

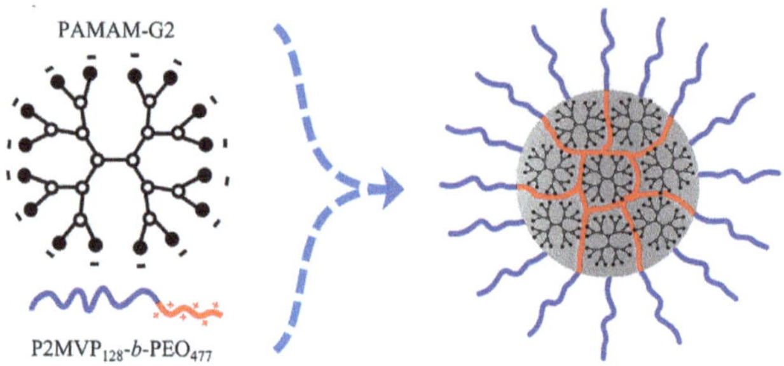

Figure 19. Charge neutralization of a G = 2 anionic surface-charged PAMAM dendrimer with a cationic di-block copolymer to form a poly(dendrimer) micelle. Reprinted with permission from Ref. [115]. Copyright 2014, The Royal Society of Chemistry.

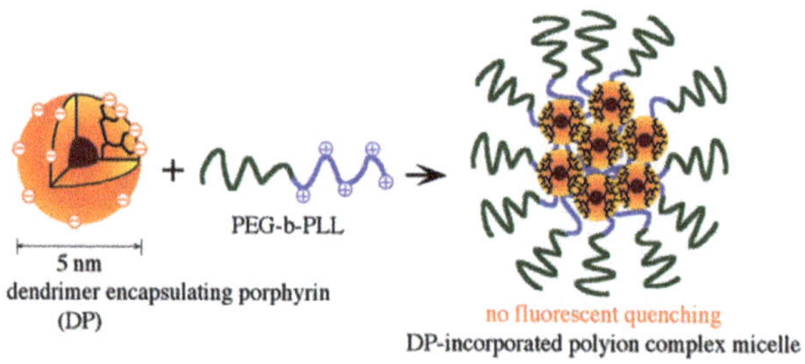

Figure 20. Charge neutralization of an anionic surface-charged PAMAM dendrimer containing an encapsulated porphyrin with a cationic di-block copolymer to form a porphyrin-containing poly(dendrimer) micelle. Reprinted with permission from Ref. [114]. Copyright 2007, The Royal Society of Chemistry.

These dendritic poly-ionic self-assemblies reported earlier by Kataoko were subsequently developed by Velders, et al. as supramolecular PAMAM assemblies and are currently referred to as dendrimicelles. They may be compared with traditional polymeric micelles, polyion complex micelles (PIC), and polymeric dendritic PIC micelles, as shown in Figure 21.

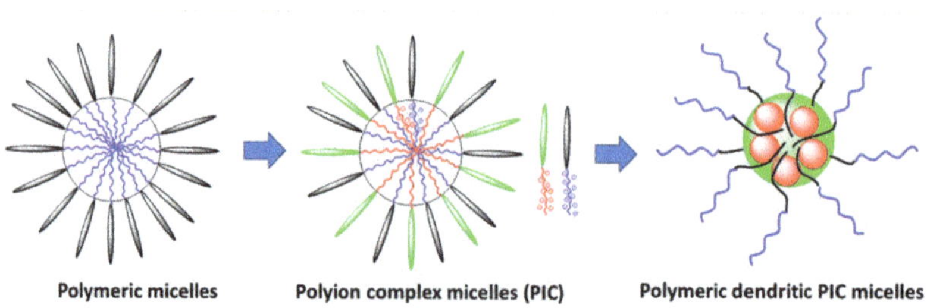

Figure 21. A comparison of polymeric micelles, their conversion into polyion complex micelles (PICs) and their integration into polymeric dendritic PIC micelles. Reprinted with permission from Ref. [116]. Copyright 2021, American Chemical Society.

These dendrimicelles are readily formed by first complexing either anionic carboxylic acid-terminated dendrimers with cationic poly(vinylpyridine)-poly(ethylene oxide) di-block copolymers or, alternatively, by combining cationic amine-terminated PAMAM dendrimers with oppositely charged anionic, poly(methacrylic acid)-poly(ethylene oxide) di-block copolymers [115,117]. These amphiphilic dendrimer complexes readily self-assemble into the corresponding dendrimicelles, wherein the aggregation number of the dendrimers in the micellar core of these dendrimicelles may be tuned by varying the dendrimer generation [115] or pH of the environment [118]. Furthermore, it was demonstrated that various metal nanoparticles (i.e., gold, etc.) [117] could be encapsulated within the individual participating PAMAM dendrimers [119–121]. This allows the use of transmission electron microscopy (TEM) to monitor the exact localization of the metal nanoparticles. More specifically, it was recently shown that dendrimer-encapsulated gold nanoparticles (AuDENs) could be systematically introduced into these dendrimicelles [117,122–124], thus providing a rational strategy for the determination of Au nanoparticle sites and the topologies of these micellar compositions [116,125,126].

Subsequently, Velders, et al. [127] reported the syntheses and isolation of discrete, covalently bridged megameric assemblies reminiscent of the original role we had proposed for dendrimers as discrete and reactive macromolecular monomers from 1979–1984. The original "Starburst Polymer" concept [31] (Figure 22) was to envision dendrimers as macromolecular monomers, which could be covalently linked via their reactive surface groups into a wide range of higher-order macromolecular architectural motifs generally referred to as "Starburst Polymers". Currently, these poly(dendrimers) or oligo (dendrimers) [27] are referred to as megamers or megameric networks, respectively. Earlier, this concept was clearly demonstrated by the syntheses of core-shell tecto (dendrimers) [45,46], as well as random megamer-type structures, as described later [27].

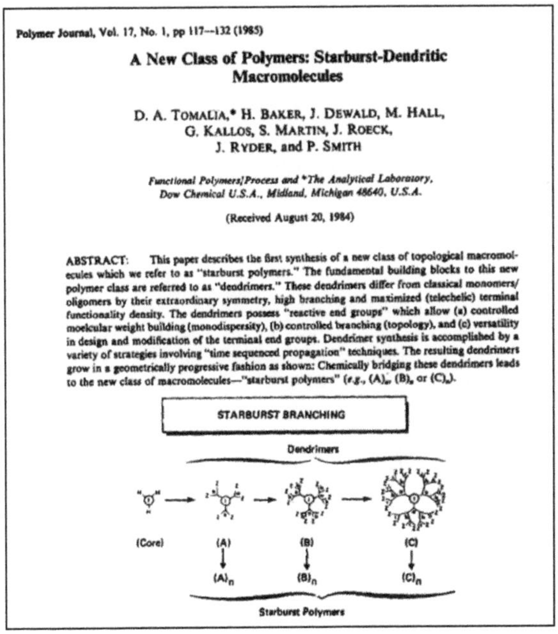
Polymer Journal, Vol. 17, No. 1, pp 117—132 (1985)

A New Class of Polymers: Starburst-Dendritic Macromolecules

D. A. TOMALIA,* H. BAKER, J. DEWALD, M. HALL, G. KALLOS, S. MARTIN, J. ROECK, J. RYDER, and P. SMITH

*Functional Polymers/Process and *The Analytical Laboratory, Dow Chemical U.S.A., Midland, Michigan 48640, U.S.A.*

(Received August 20, 1984)

ABSTRACT: This paper describes the first synthesis of a new class of topological macromolecules which we refer to as "starburst polymers." The fundamental building blocks to this new polymer class are referred to as "dendrimers." These dendrimers differ from classical monomers/oligomers by their extraordinary symmetry, high branching and maximized (telechelic) terminal functionality density. The dendrimers possess "reactive end groups" which allow (a) controlled moelcular weight building (monodispersity), (b) controlled branching (topology), and (c) versatility in design and modification of the terminal end groups. Dendrimer synthesis is accomplished by a variety of strategies involving "time sequenced propagation" techniques. The resulting dendrimers grow in a geometrically progressive fashion as shown: Chemically bridging these dendrimers leads to the new class of macromolecules—"starburst polymers" (*e.g.*, $(A)_n$, $(B)_n$ or $(C)_n$).

Figure 22. Abstract of original Tomalia, et al. (1985) [31] dendrimer publication describing the initial proposed use of dendrimers as reactive, macromolecular monomers to produce covalent, poly(dendrimer) megamers referred to as "Starburst polymers". Reprinted with permission from Refs. [15,31]. Copyright 2002, John Wiley & Sons.

More recently, innovative work by Velder, et al. [127] has advanced this original "starburst polymer concept" to a new level by attaining extraordinary control of poly(dendrimer) complexity via the formation of covalently fixed dendrimicelles. This is accomplished by the discrete labeling of specific dendrimers into Au-loaded and empty forms. This is followed by complexation with polyionic block copolymers, which organizes these selectively functionalized macromolecular, dendrimeric monomers into *dendrimicelle*-type supramolecular assemblies. Subsequent cross-linking of these supramolecular poly(dendrimers) with glutaraldehyde, followed by the release/removal of these poly-ionic block copolymers, yields the respective (a) all-empty, (b) empty-Au-functionalized, and (c) all-Au-functionalized, bridged megameric assemblies, which were each isolated, as illustrated in Figure 23.

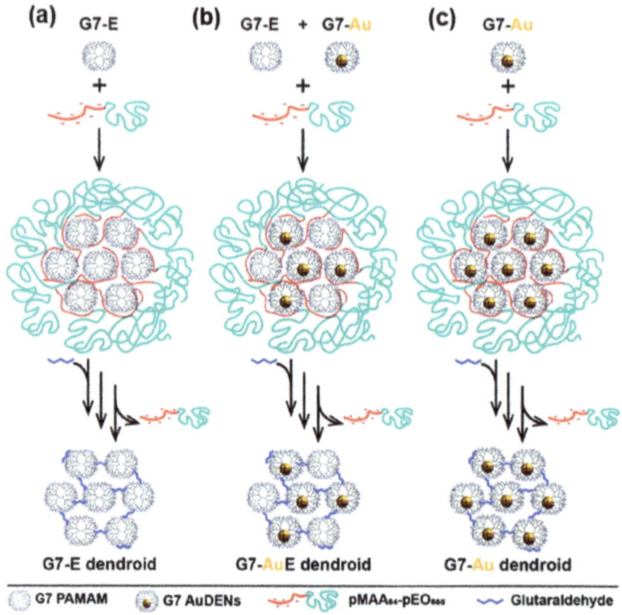

Figure 23. Self-assembly of G = 7 (empty), G = 7 (empty +Au labeled), and G = 7 (all Au labeled) dendrimers into their respective (PIC) supramolecular megamer clusters followed by cross-linking with glutaraldehyde. After removal of the polyionic copolymers, they yielded: (**a**) empty, (**b**) empty-Au-labeled, and (**c**) all Au-labeled covalent, poly(dendrimer), megamers, respectively. Reprinted with permission from Ref. [127]. Copyright 2021, American Chemical Society.

These very discretely functionalized megameric assemblies in Figure 23 should probably be referred to as selectively functionalized megamers and not be coined or referred to as dendroids, especially since the term "dendroid" was used to describe special dendritic templates for controlling or amplifying dendritic shapes, as described in earlier work [128].

2.5.4. Dendritic Supramolecular Delivery of Nucleic Acids

Historically, the first covalent dendrimer activity began in the early 1980s, whereas an analogous surge in supramolecular dendrimer development emerged in the late 1980s. The original covalent dendrimer activity was largely initiated and focused in four areas, namely by: (1) the Vögtle, low MWt = 433.6 Da; oligo-PPI dendrimer precursor, cascade structures [22] that inspired the development of enhanced processes for synthesizing macromolecule poly(propyleneimine) (PPI) dendrimers by Meijer, et al. [25] and Mülthaupt [26], (2) the Denkewalter, macromolecular (MW: ~239,000 Da) poly(L-lysine) (PLL) dendrons [129], (3) the Tomalia macromolecular (MWt: ~59,700 Da) poly(amidoamine)

(PAMAM) dendrons/dendrimers [31,130], and (4) the Newkome, non-macromolecular, lower-molecular weight (MWt: ~1300 Da) arborols [47].

The extraordinary growth in covalent and supramolecular dendrimer activity during the last decade (~2012–2024) generally parallels a quest for suitable nanoscale delivery vectors for drugs, proteins, and specific nucleic acids beyond DNA (i.e., siRNA, mRNA, etc.). Subsequently, these covalent dendrimer structures were recognized as highly effective cationic nano-vectors for gene delivery by forming charge-neutralized, supramolecular dendriplexes with nucleic acids. That activity began with PAMAM dendrimers (i.e., Szoka [131] and Tomalia/Baker [132,133] (1993–1996)), phosphorous dendrimers (i.e., Majoral/Caminade, 1999) [58,59], PPI dendrimers (Zinselmeyer, 2002) [134], carbosilane dendrimers (Munoz/Bryszewska, 2008) [135], and later with siRNA using PAMAM dendrimers (Peng, 2006) [136].

The first reported dendrimeric supramolecular activity began in the late 1980s with Tomalia/Friberg (1988) [87], as well as Percec [90,137]. It then evolved steadily with a sustained interest in drug-inclusion complexes and DNA delivery, followed by extraordinary growth during this last decade. This recent surge was driven largely by widespread interest in the delivery of smaller single- and double-stranded nucleic acids such as siRNA [138,139] and mRNA [140–142]. The siRNA and mRNA structures exhibit distinctly different physicochemical properties such as size, molecular weight, single-stranded versus double-stranded structures, and conformational flexibility. Although siRNA and mRNA are constructed from the same chemical building blocks and require delivery to the cytoplasm for activity, they are significantly different in size, overall structure (i.e., double- vs. single-stranded), and mechanism of action. That said, an effective siRNA delivery vector may not be suitable for mRNA delivery. The specific targeting and delivery of mRNA is currently an extremely active area of high interest as the result of the recent COVID-19 pandemic, as well as acute interest in the development of advanced vaccines for future pandemic urgencies. These issues are extensively reviewed elsewhere [143]. Beginning in 2016, dendrimer-based mRNA delivery vectors have been at the forefront of recent efforts to develop mRNA vaccines against SARS-CoV [144]. However, liposome-based vaccines developed by BioNTech/Pfizer and Moderna have dominated the COVID pandemic market based largely on their timely development and maturity. These current commercial mRNA delivery vectors require a complex 4-component ionizable lipid system to protect the mRNA from degradation before entering the cell. These commercial 4-component, ionizable lipid-based systems are actually second-generation, self-assembling supramolecular amphiphilic dendrons that appear to have been inspired by the earlier work of Percec et al. [109]. That said, recent breakthrough development by Percec, et al. [145,146] has produced significant advancement to a simplified one-component system based on his sequence-defined ionizable amphiphilic Janus dendrimers (IAJDs). This one-component system has exhibited substantially enhanced efficacy with controlled targeting specificity, room-temperature shelf stability, and a lower cost. The Percec IAJDs co-assemble with mRNA into dendrimersome nanoparticles (DNPs), which may be engineered/programmed to selectively target specific organs, and have been found to be vastly superior to the current four-component, lipid nanoparticle delivery vectors, which are only suitable for mRNA delivery to the liver [143].

By creating a rational library design combined with orthogonal-modular accelerated synthesis and sequence control of their hydrophilic components, Percec has synthesized IAJDs that are performing as extraordinary nano-vectors for the delivery of mRNA to specifically targeted organs. He elucidated the molecular design principles required to target IAJD-assisted mRNA delivery and identified critical functional moieties in the hydrophilic/hydrophobic components of the IAJDs that contribute to the specificity of the targeted organ [147]. This has resulted in ~6-fold enhancements in mRNA delivery levels together with the ability to specifically target key organs such as the spleen, lymph nodes, liver, or lungs [141,146–148].

Percec's discovery of IAJDs represents a significant breakthrough in the development of mRNA therapeutics. His close collaboration with Prof. Drew Weissman (i.e., the 2023

Nobel Prize Laureate for mRNA development) has enabled Percec to innovate and create a large diversity of IAJDs, many of which are described in their brilliant contribution to this current 85th special topic issue [2].

Most notable is the development of a simplified one-component, dendrimersome nanoparticle (DNP)-based IAJD system (Figure 24B) compared to the current four-component, lipid nanoparticle (LNP) commercial system, as illustrated below (Figure 24A). An abbreviated cell-transfection mechanism proposed for the (DNP)-based system is described in Figure 24C.

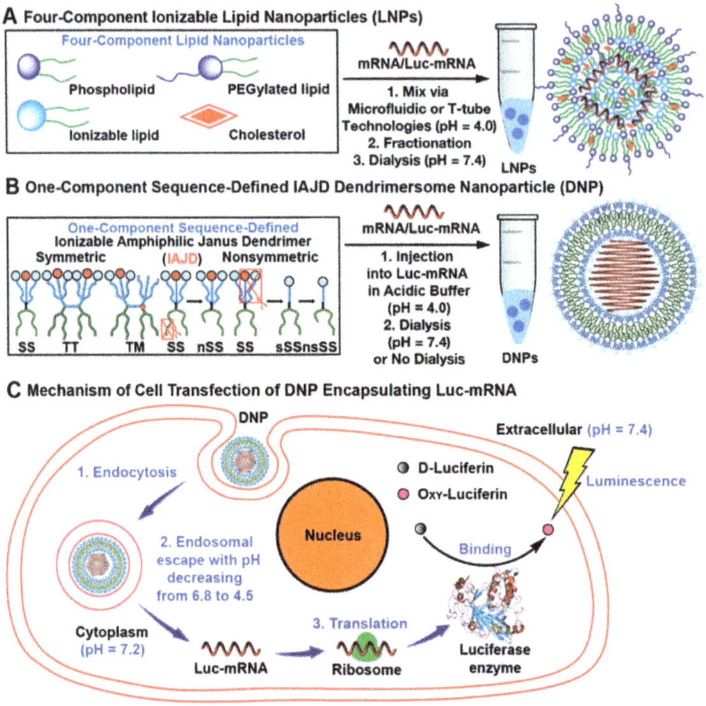

Figure 24. (**A**) A comparison of the current four-component commercial ionizable lipid nanoparticle (LNPs) system with (**B**) the new Percec-type, one-component, sequence-defined IAJD, dendrimersome nanoparticle (DNP) approach. (**C**) A comparison of specific mechanisms involved for the four-component LNP and the one-component DNP nanoparticle approaches, respectively. Reprinted with permission from Ref. [2]. Copyright 2023, MDPI.

2.6. *Expected New Application Roles in Pharmaceuticals, Nanomedicine, and Life Sciences*

An overview of DDDS advancements as a function of dendrimer complexity and commercial products (2000–2010) (Columns I-IV), as well as predicted progress during the past decade (2010–2020) (Column V) [28], is as described in Figure 25.

It is both surprising and satisfying to note that many of these 2010 predictions actually occurred, providing a list that includes Janus dendrimers, supramolecular dendrimers, non-traditional intrinsic luminescent (NTIL) dendrimers, dendrimers as specific active pharma ingredients (APIs), and targeted drug delivery, to mention a few.

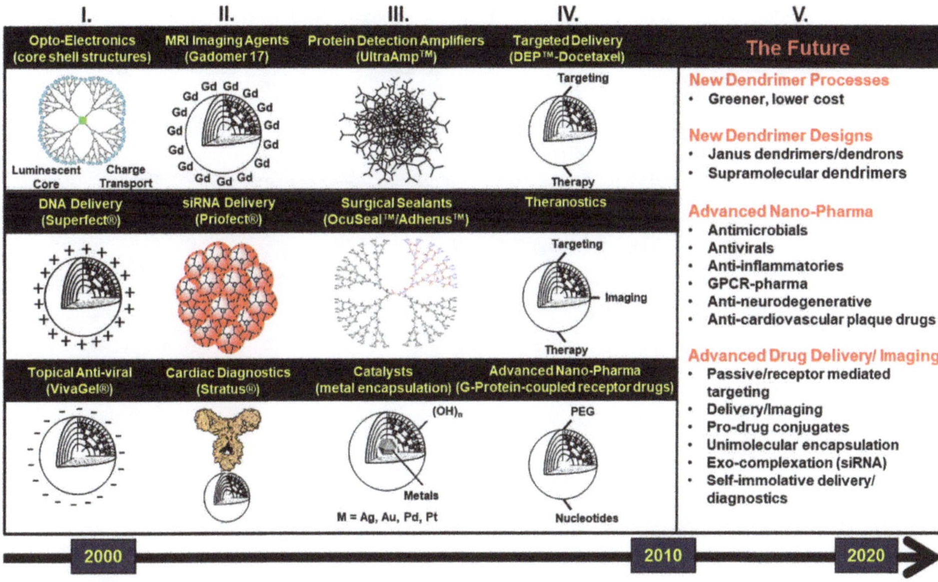

Figure 25. Increased dendrimer structure complexity required for applications defined between 2000–2010) (i.e., Columns (I)–(IV) with predictions concerning future advancements in Column (V) [149].

Based on the current literature and the excellent contributions made to this recent special topics issue, one should expect many more new and exciting application roles for dendrons, dendrimers, and the dendritic state (DDDS) in the next decade [150]. Several conservative predictions for 2024–2034 in pharmaceuticals, nanomedicine, and life sciences are described in Figure 26.

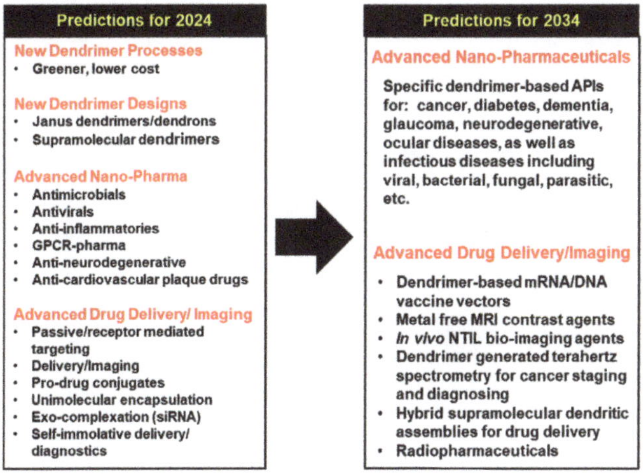

Figure 26. Predicted advancements in pharma, drug delivery, and bio-imaging in 2024 and predicted advancements for 2034.

2.7. Summary and Conclusions

The ultimate dream and hope for any major scientific discovery as significant as DDDS is that such a scientific breakthrough will evolve into a versatile and beneficial technology platform that will fulfill many unmet societal needs and will enhance the human condition (i.e., health, environmental, etc.). After viewing recent progress in the outstanding contributions to the 85th dendrimer-themed special topic issue, as well as current literature advancements, it provides me with great optimism that this dream and hope for "dendrons, dendrimers, and the dendritic state" will truly be fulfilled.

Supplementary Materials: The following supporting information can be downloaded at: https://www.mdpi.com/article/10.3390/pharmaceutics16121530/s1, Figure S1: Cascade Synthesis/Structure Reproducibility Study.

Funding: This research received no external funding.

Acknowledgments: The author is grateful to Linda S. Nixon for the critical graphics, editing, and assembly of this manuscript and many valued discussions with David M. Hedstrand and Mayank K. Singh.

Conflicts of Interest: In the interest of transparency, the intellectual property described in U.S. Patent #10,968,176B2 is currently owned by NanoSynthons LLC. Author Donald A. Tomalia is the owner/CEO of NanoSynthons LLC.

References

1. Sowinska, M.; Laskowska, A.; Guspiel, A.; Solecka, J.; Bochynska-Czyz, M.; Lipkowski, A.W.; Trzeciak, K.; Urbanczyk-Lipkowska, Z. Bioinspired amphiphilic peptide dendrimers as specific and effective compounds against drug resistant clinical isolates of *E. coli*. *Biconjugate Chem.* **2018**, *29*, 3571–3585. [CrossRef] [PubMed]
2. Lu, J.; Atochina-Vasserman, E.N.; Maurya, D.S.; Irhash Shalihin, M.; Zhang, D.; Chenna, S.S.; Adamson, J.; Liu, M.; Ur Rehman Shah, H.; Shah, H.; et al. Screening Libraries to Discover Molecular Design Principles for the Targeted Delivery of mRNA with One-Component Ionizable Amphiphilic Janus Dendrimers Derived from Plant Phenolic Acids. *Pharmaceutics* **2023**, *15*, 1572. [CrossRef] [PubMed]
3. Ornelas, C.; Astruc, D. Ferrocene-Based Drugs, Delivery Nanomaterials and Fenton Mechanism: State of the Art, Recent Developments and Prospects. *Pharmaceutics* **2023**, *15*, 2044. [CrossRef] [PubMed]
4. Caminade, A.-M.; Milewski, M.; Hey-Hawkins, E. Dendritic Structures Functionalized with Boron Clusters, in Particular Carboranes, and Their Biological Properties. *Pharmaceutics* **2023**, *15*, 2117. [CrossRef]
5. Fernanda Romero, J.; Herziger, S.; Cherri, M.; Dimde, M.; Achazi, K.; Mohammadifar, E.; Haag, R. Dendritic Glycerol-Cholesterol Amphiphiles as Drug Delivery Systems: A Comparison between Monomeric and Polymeric Structures. *Pharmaceutics* **2023**, *15*, 2452. [CrossRef]
6. Wu, T.; Liu, C.; Kannan, R.M. Systemic Dendrimer-Peptide Therapies for Wet Age-Related Macular Degeneration. *Pharmaceutics* **2023**, *15*, 2428. [CrossRef]
7. Dockery, L.T.; Daniel, M.-C. Targeted Doxorubicin-Loaded Dendronized Gold Nanoparticles. *Pharmaceutics* **2023**, *15*, 2103. [CrossRef]
8. Sztandera, K.; Rodríguez-García, J.L.; Ceña, V. In Vivo Applications of Dendrimers: A Step toward the Future of Nanoparticle-Mediated Therapeutics. *Pharmaceutics* **2024**, *16*, 439. [CrossRef]
9. Shiba, H.; Hirose, T.; Sakai, A.; Nakase, I.; Matsumoto, A.; Kojima, C. Structural Optimization of Carboxy-Terminal Phenylalanine-Modified Dendrimers for T-Cell Association and Model Drug Loading. *Pharmaceutics* **2024**, *16*, 715. [CrossRef]
10. Muñoz-Sánchez, S.; Barrios-Gumiel, A.; Javier de la Mata, F.; García-Gallego, S. Fine-Tuning the Amphiphilic Properties of Carbosilane Dendritic Networks towards High-Swelling Thermogels. *Pharmaceutics* **2024**, *16*, 495. [CrossRef]
11. Mencia, G.; Algar, S.; Lozano-Cruz, T.; Muñoz-Fernández, M.A.; Gillies, E.R.; Cano, J.; Valiente, M.; Gómez, R. Carbosilane Dendritic Amphiphiles from Cholesterol or Vitamin E for Micelle Formation. *Pharmaceutics* **2024**, *16*, 451. [CrossRef] [PubMed]
12. Cavalieri, G.; Marson, D.; Giurgevich, N.; Valeri, R.; Felluga, F.; Laurini, E.; Pricl, S. Molecular Ballet: Investigating the Complex Interaction between Self-Assembling Dendrimers and Human Serum Albumin via Computational and Experimental Methods. *Pharmaceutics* **2024**, *16*, 533. [CrossRef] [PubMed]
13. Calvo-Serrano, S.; Matamoros, E.; Céspedes, J.A.; Fernández-Santamaría, R.; Gil-Ocaña, V.; Perez-Inestrosa, E.; Frecha, C.; Montañez, M.I.; Torres, M.J. New Approaches for Basophil Activation Tests Employing Dendrimeric Antigen–Silica Nanoparticle Composites. *Pharmaceutics* **2024**, *16*, 1039. [CrossRef] [PubMed]
14. Xia, J.; Gaynor, S.G.; Matyjaszewski, K. Controlled/"Living" Radical Polymerization. Atom Transfer Radical Polymerization of Acrylates at Ambient Temperature. *Macromolecules* **1998**, *31*, 5958–5959. [CrossRef]
15. Tomalia, D.A.; Fréchet, J.M.J. Discovery of dendrimers and dendritic polymers: A brief historical perspective. *J. Polym. Sci. Part A Polym. Chem.* **2002**, *40*, 2719–2728. [CrossRef]
16. Tomalia, D.A. Birth of a new macromolecular architecture: Dendrimers as quantized building blocks for nanoscale synthetic polymer chemistry. *Prog. Polym. Sci.* **2005**, *30*, 294–324. [CrossRef]

17. Tomalia, D.A. Twenty-First Century Polymer Science After Staudinger: The Emergence of Dendrimers/Dendritic Polymers as a Fourth Major Architecture and Window to a New Nano-periodic System. In *Hierarchical Macomolecular Structures: 60 Years After the Staudinger Nobel Prize I*; Percec, V., Ed.; Springer: Berlin/Heidelberg, Germany, 2013; Volume XVI, pp. 321–389.
18. Fradet, A.; Chen, J.; Hellwich, K.-H.; Horie, K.; Kahovec, J.; Mormann, W.; Stepto, R.F.T.; Vohlidal, J.; Wilks, E.S. Nomenclature and terminology for dendrimers with regular dendrons for hyperbranched polymers (IUPAC Recommendations 2017). *Pure Appl. Chem.* **2019**, *91*, 523–561. [CrossRef]
19. Jeevanandam, J.; Tan, K.X.; Rodrigues, J. Target-specific delivery and bioavailability of pharmaceuticals via Janus and dendrimer particles. *Pharmaceutics* **2023**, *15*, 1614. [CrossRef]
20. Wang, J.; Li, B.; Qiu, L.; Qiao, X.; Yang, H. Dendrimer-based drug delivery systems: History, challenges, and latest developments. *J. Biol. Eng.* **2022**, *16*, 18. [CrossRef]
21. Nagpal, K.; Mohan, A.; Thakur, S.; Kumar, P. Dendritic platforms for biomimicry and biotechnological applications. *Artif. Cells Nanomed. Biotechnol.* **2018**, *46*, S861–S875. [CrossRef]
22. Buhleier, E.; Wehner, W.; Vögtle, F. Cascade—And nonskid-chain-like syntheses of molecular cavity topologies. *Synthesis* **1978**, *405*, 155–158. [CrossRef]
23. Denkewalter, R.G.; Kolc, J.F.; Lukasavage, W.J. Macromolecular Highly Branched Homogenous Compound Based on Lysine Units. U.S. Patent 4,289,872, 15 September 1981.
24. Mekelburger, H.-B.; Rissanen, K.; Vogtle, F. Repetitive synthesis of bulky dendrimers—A reversibly photoactive dendrimer with six azobenzene side chains. *Chem. Ber.* **1993**, *126*, 1161–1169. [CrossRef]
25. De Brabander-van den Berg, E.M.M.; Meijer, E.W. Poly(propylene imine) dendrimers: Large-scale synthesis by hetereogeneously catalyzed hydrogenations. *Angew. Chem. Int. Ed. Engl.* **1993**, *32*, 1308–1311. [CrossRef]
26. Worner, C.; Mulhaupt, R. Polynitrile and polyamine functional poly(trimethylene imine) dendrimers. *Angew. Chem. Int. Ed. Engl.* **1993**, *32*, 1306–1308. [CrossRef]
27. Tomalia, D.A.; Uppuluri, S.; Swanson, D.R.; Li, J. Dendrimers as reactive modules for the synthesis of new structure controlled, higher complexity—Megamers. *Pure Appl. Chem.* **2000**, *72*, 2343–2358. [CrossRef]
28. Tomalia, D.A.; Christensen, J.B.; Boas, U. *Dendrimers, Dendrons, and Dendritic Polymers: Discovery, Applications and the Future*; Cambridge University Press: New York, NY, USA, 2012; pp. 1–412.
29. Caminade, A.-M.; Laurent, R.; Majoral, J.-P. Characterization of dendrimers. *Adv. Drug Deliv. Rev.* **2005**, *57*, 2130–2146. [CrossRef]
30. Tomalia, D.A.; Christensen, J.B.; Boas, U. Characterization methodologies. In *Dendrimers, Dendrons, and Dendritic Polymers: Discovery, Applications and the Future*; Cambridge University Press: New York, NY, USA, 2012; pp. 162–186.
31. Tomalia, D.A.; Baker, H.; Dewald, J.; Hall, M.; Kallos, G.; Martin, S.; Roeck, J.; Ryder, J.; Smith, P. A new class of polymers: Starburst dendritic macromolecules. *Polym. J.* **1985**, *17*, 117–132.
32. Brothers II, H.M.; Piehler, L.T.; Tomalia, D.A. Slab-gel and capillary electrophoretic characterization of polyamidoamine dendrimers. *J. Chromatogr. A* **1998**, *814*, 233–246.
33. Tomalia, D.A.; Baker, H.; Dewald, J.; Hall, M.; Kallos, G.; Martin, S.; Roeck, J.; Ryder, J.; Smith, P. Dendritic macromolecules: Synthesis of Starburst dendrimers. *Macromolecules* **1986**, *19*, 2466–2468.
34. Li, J.; Swanson, D.R.; Qin, D.; Brothers II, H.M.; Piehler, L.T.; Tomalia, D.A.; Meier, D.J. Characterization of core-shell tecto(dendrimers) molecules by tapping mode atomic force microscopy. *Langmuir* **1999**, *15*, 7347–7350.
35. Li, J.; Piehler, L.T.; Qin, D.; Baker, J.R., Jr.; Tomalia, D.A. Visualization and characterization of poly(amidoamine) dendrimers by atomic force microscopy. *Langmuir* **2000**, *16*, 5613–5616. [CrossRef]
36. Prosa, T.J.; Bauer, B.J.; Amis, E.J.; Tomalia, D.A.; Scherrenberg, R. A SAXS study of the internal structure of dendritic polymer systems. *J. Polym. Sci Part B Polym. Physics* **1997**, *35*, 2913–2924. [CrossRef]
37. Tomalia, D.A.; Naylor, A.M.; Goddard III, W.A. Starburst dendrimers: Molecular level control of size, shape, surface chemistry, topology and flexibility from atoms to macroscopic matter. *Angew. Chem. Int. Ed. Engl.* **1990**, *29*, 138–175. [CrossRef]
38. Moreno-Bondi, G.; Orellana, G.; Turro, N.J.; Tomalia, D.A. Photoinduced electron transfer reaction to probe the structure of Starburst dendrimers. *Macromolecules* **1990**, *23*, 910–912. [CrossRef]
39. Miller, L.L.; Duan, R.G.; Tully, D.C.; Tomalia, D.A. Electrically conducting dendrimers. *J. Am. Chem. Soc.* **1997**, *119*, 1005–1010. [CrossRef]
40. Kallos, G.J.; Tomalia, D.A.; Hedstrand, D.M.; Lewis, S.; Zhou, J. Molecular weight determination of a polyamidoamine Starburst polymer by electrospray ionization mass spectrometry. *Rapid Commun. Mass Spectrom.* **1991**, *5*, 383–386. [CrossRef]
41. Schwartz, B.L.; Rockwood, A.L.; Smith, R.D.; Tomalia, D.A.; Spindler, R. Detection of high molecular weight Starburst dendrimers by electrospray ionization mass spectrometry. *Rapid Commun. Mass Spectrom.* **1995**, *9*, 1552–1555. [CrossRef]
42. Tolic, L.P.; Anderson, G.A.; Smith, R.D.; Brothers II, H.M.; Spindler, R.; Tomalia, D.A. Electrospray ionization fourier transform ion cyclotron resonance mass spectrometric characterization of high molecular mass starburst dendrimers. *Int. J. Mass Spectrom. Ion Process.* **1997**, *165/166*, 405–418. [CrossRef]
43. Tomalia, D.A.; Dewald, J.R. Dense Star Polymers Having Core, Core Branches, Terminal Groups. U.S. Patent 4,507,466, 26 March 1985.
44. Tomalia, D.A. Starburst Macromolecules. In Proceedings of the Flory-Pauling Macromolecular Conference (Gordon Conference)—Frontiers in Synthetic Polymer Chemistry, Santa Barbara, CA, USA, 10–14 January 1983.

45. Uppuluri, S.; Piehler, L.T.; Li, J.; Swanson, D.R.; Hagnauer, G.L.; Tomalia, D.A. Core-shell tecto(dendrimers): I. Synthesis and characterization of saturated shell models. *Adv. Mater.* **2000**, *12*, 796–800. [CrossRef]
46. Tomalia, D.A.; Brothers II, H.M.; Piehler, L.T.; Durst, H.D.; Swanson, D.R. Partial shell-filled core-shell tecto(dendrimers): A strategy to surface differentiated nano-clefts and cusps. *Proc. Natl. Acad. Sci. USA* **2002**, *99*, 5081–5087. [CrossRef]
47. Newkome, G.R.; Yao, Z.-Q.; Baker, G.R.; Gupta, V.K. Cascade molecules: A new approach to micelles. A [27]-arborol. *J. Org. Chem.* **1985**, *50*, 2003–2004. [CrossRef]
48. Ranganathan, D.; Durur, S. Synthesis of totally chiral, multiple armed, poly glu and poly asp scaffoldings on bifunctional adamantane core. *Tetrahedron Lett.* **1997**, *38*, 1265–1268. [CrossRef]
49. Tomalia, D.A.; Nixon, L.S.; Hedstrand, D.M. The Role of Branch Cell Symmetry and Other Critical Nanoscale Design Parameters in the Determination of Dendrimer Encapsulation Properties. *Biomolecules* **2020**, *10*, 642. [CrossRef] [PubMed]
50. Aharoni, S.M.; Crosby, C.R., III; Walsh, E.K. Size and Solution Properties of Globular tert-Butyloxycarbonyl-Poly(α,iε-L-Lysine). *Macromolecules* **1982**, *15*, 1093–1098. [CrossRef]
51. Fenn, J.B.; Mann, M.; Meng, C.K.; Wong, S.F.; Whitehouse, C.M. Electrospray ionization for mass spectrometry of large biomolecules. *Science* **1989**, *246*, 64–71. [CrossRef]
52. Hawker, C.J.; Frechet, J.M.J. A new convergent approach to monodisperse dendritic macromolecules. *J. Chem. Soc. Chem. Commun.* **1990**, *15*, 1010–1013. [CrossRef]
53. Hawker, C.J.; Frechet, J.M.J. Control of surface functionality in the synthesis of dendritic macromolecules using the convergent-growth approach. *Macromolecules* **1990**, *23*, 4726–4729. [CrossRef]
54. Hawker, C.J.; Fréchet, J.M.J. Preparation of polymers with controlled molecular architecture. A new convergent approach to dendritic macromolecules. *J. Am. Chem. Soc.* **1990**, *112*, 7638–7647. [CrossRef]
55. Grayson, S.; Fréchet, J.M.J. Convergent dendrons and dendrimers: From synthesis to applications. *Chem. Rev.* **2001**, *101*, 3819–3868. [CrossRef]
56. Kwock, E.W.; Neenan, T.X.; Miller, T.M. Convergent synthesis of monodisperse aryl ester dendrimers. *Chem. Mater.* **1991**, *3*, 775–777. [CrossRef]
57. Miller, T.M.; Neenan, T.X. Convergent synthesis of monodisperse dendrimers based upon 1,3,5-trisubstituted benzenes. *Chem. Mat.* **1990**, *2*, 346–349. [CrossRef]
58. Majoral, J.-P.; Caminade, A.-M. Dendrimers containing heteroatoms (Si, P, B, Ge, or Bi). *Chem. Rev.* **1999**, *99*, 845–880. [CrossRef] [PubMed]
59. Caminade, A.-M.; Turrin, C.-O.; Majoral, J.-P. *Phosphorus Dendrimers in Biology and Nanomedicine*; Pan Stanford Publishing Pte. Ltd.: Singapore, 2018; pp. 1–372.
60. Tomalia, D.A.; Berry, V.; Hall, M.; Hedstrand, D.M. Starburst dendrimers IV. Covalently fixed unimolecular assemblages reminiscent of spheroidal micelles. *Macromolecules* **1987**, *20*, 1164–1167. [CrossRef]
61. Tomalia, D.A.; Hall, M.; Hedstrand, D.M. Starburst dendrimers III. The importance of branch junction symmetry in the development of topological shell molecules. *J. Am. Chem. Soc.* **1987**, *109*, 1601–1603. [CrossRef]
62. Naylor, A.M.; Goddard III, W.A.; Keifer, G.E.; Tomalia, D.A. Starburst dendrimers 5. Molecular shape control. *J. Am. Chem. Soc.* **1989**, *111*, 2339–2341. [CrossRef]
63. Tomalia, D.A. Dendritic effects: Dependency of dendritic nano-periodic property patterns on critical nanoscale design parameters (CNDPs). *New J. Chem.* **2012**, *36*, 264–281. [CrossRef]
64. Sapra, R.; Verma, R.P.; Maurya, G.P.; Dhawan, S.; Babu, J.; Haridas, V. Designer peptide and protein dendrimers: A cross-sectional analysis. *Chem. Rev.* **2019**, *119*, 11391–11441. [CrossRef]
65. Wan, J.; Alewood, P.F. Peptide-decorated dendrimers and their bioapplications. *Angew. Chem. Int. Ed.* **2016**, *55*, 5124–5134. [CrossRef]
66. Zhong, D.; Tu, Z.; Zhang, X.; Li, Y.; Xu, X.; Gu, Z. Bioreducible peptide-dendrimeric nanogels and abundant expanded voids for efficient drug entrapment and delivery. *Biomacromolecules* **2017**, *18*, 3498–3505. [CrossRef]
67. Falanga, A.; Del Genio, V.; Galdiero, S. Peptides and Dendrimers: How to Combat Viral and Bacterial Infections. *Pharmaceutics* **2021**, *13*, 101. [CrossRef]
68. Biswaro, L.S.; da Costa Sousa, M.G.; Rezende, T.M.B.; Dias, S.C.; Franco, O.L. Antimicrobial Peptides and Nanotechnology, Recent Advances and Challenges. *Front. Microbiol.* **2018**, *9*, 855. [CrossRef] [PubMed]
69. Mahlapuu, M.; Hakansson, J.; Ringstad, L.; Bjorn, C. Antrimicrobial peptides: An emerging category of therapeutic agents. *Front. Cell. Infect. Microbiol.* **2016**, *6*, 194. [CrossRef] [PubMed]
70. Garcia-Gallego, S.; Franci, G.; Falanga, A.; Gomez, R.; Folliero, V.; Galdiero, S.; de la Mata, F.J.; Galdiero, M. Function oriented molecular design: Dendrimers as novel antimicrobial. *Molecules* **2017**, *22*, 1581. [CrossRef] [PubMed]
71. Tomalia, D.A. Dendrons/Dendrimer: Quantized, nano-element like building blocks for soft-soft and soft-hard nano-compound synthesis. *Soft Matter* **2010**, *6*, 456–474. [CrossRef]
72. Kannan, R.M.; Nance, E.; Kannan, S.; Tomalia, D.A. Emerging concepts in dendrimer-based nanomedicine: From design principles to clinical applications. *J. Intern. Med.* **2014**, *276*, 579–617. [CrossRef] [PubMed]
73. Chauhan, A.S.; Kaul, M. Engineering of "critical nanoscale design parameters" (CNDPs) in PAMAM dendrimer nanoparticles for drug delivery applications. *J. Nanopart. Res.* **2018**, *20*, 226. [CrossRef]

74. Tomalia, D.A.; Nixon, L.S.; Hedstrand, D.M. Engineering critical nanoscale design parameters (CNDPs): A strategy for developing effective nanomedicine therapies and assessing quatitative nanoscale structure-activity relationships (QNSARs). In *Pharmaceutical Applications of Dendrimers*; Chauhan, H.K.A., Ed.; Elsevier Inc.: Amsterdam, The Netherlands, 2020; pp. 1–47.
75. Moghimi, S.M.; Farhangrazi, Z.S. Nanomedicine and the complement paradigm. *Nanomedicine* **2013**, *9*, 458–460. [CrossRef]
76. Moghimi, S.M.; Wibroe, P.P.; Helvig, S.Y.; Farhangrazi, Z.S.; Hunter, A.C. Genomic perspectives in inter-individual adverse responses following nanomedicine administration: The way forward. *Adv. Drug Deliv. Rev.* **2012**, *64*, 1385–1393. [CrossRef]
77. Moghimi, S.M.; Peer, D.; Langer, R. Reshaping the future of nanopharmaceuticals: Ad Iudicium. *ACS Nano* **2011**, *5*, 8454–8458. [CrossRef]
78. Tomalia, D.A.; Hedstrand, D.M.; Nixon, L.S. Pyrrolidone Derivatives, Oligomers and Polymers. U.S. Patent 10,968,176 B2, 6 April 2021.
79. Janaszewska, A.; Gorzkiewicz, M.; Ficker, M.; Petersen, J.F.; Paolucci, V.; Christensen, J.B.; Klajnert-Maculewicz, B. Pyrrolidone modification prevents PAMAM dendrimers from activation pro-inflammatory signaling pathways in human monocytes. *Mol. Pharm.* **2018**, *15*, 12–20. [CrossRef]
80. Wu, L.-P.; Ficker, M.; Christensen, J.B.; Simberg, D.; Trohopoulos, P.N.; Moghimi, S.M. Dendrimer end-terminal motif-dependent evasion of human complement and complement activation through IgM hitchiking. *Nat. Commun.* **2021**, *12*, 4858. [CrossRef] [PubMed]
81. Shi, D.; Beasock, D.; Fessler, A.; Szebeni, J.; Ljubimova, J.Y.; Afonin, K.A. To PEGylate or not to PEGylate: Immunological properties of nanomedicine's most popular component, poly(ethyle) glycol and its alternatives. *Adv Drug Deliv. Rev.* **2022**, *180*, 114079. [CrossRef] [PubMed]
82. Kong, Y.W.; Dreaden, E.C. PEG: Will it come back to you? Polyethelyne glycol immunogencity, COVID Vaccines, and the Case for New PEG Derivatives and Alternatives. *Front. Bioeng. Biotechnol.* **2022**, *10*, 879988. [CrossRef] [PubMed]
83. Ju, Y.; Lee, W.S.; Pilkington, E.H.; Kelly, H.G.; Li, S.; Selva, K.J.; Wragg, K.M.; Subbarao, K.; Nguyen, T.H.O.; Rowntree, L.C.; et al. Anti-PEG Antibodies Boosted in Humans by SARS-CoV-2 Lipid Nanoparticle mRNA Vaccine. *ACS Nano* **2022**, *16*, 11769–11780. [CrossRef] [PubMed]
84. Singh, M.K.; Kuncha, M.; Nayak, V.L.; Sarma, A.V.S.; Kumar, M.J.M.; Chauhan, A.S.; Sistla, R. An innovative in situ method of creating hybrid dendrimer nano-assembly: An efficient next generation dendritic platorm for drug delivery. *Nanomedicine* **2019**, *21*, 102043. [CrossRef]
85. Singh, M.K.; Pooja, D.; Kulhari, H.; Jain, S.K.; Sistla, R.; Chauhan, A.S. Poly(amidoamine) dendrimer-mediated hybrid formulation for combination therapy of ramipril and hydrochlorothiazide. *Eur. J. Pharm. Sci.* **2017**, *96*, 84–92. [CrossRef]
86. Singh, M.K.; Tomalia, D.A.; Chauhan, A.S. New hybridized mult-dendrimer platforms based on the supramolecular assembly guided by systematic CNDP engineering. *Mater. Matters* **2023**, *17*, 10–18.
87. Friberg, S.E.; Podzimek, M.; Tomalia, D.A.; Hedstrand, D.M. Non-aqueous lyotropic liquid crystal with a STARBURST® dendrimer as a solvent. *Mol. Cryst. Liq. Cryst.* **1988**, *164*, 157–165. [CrossRef]
88. Sayed-Sweet, Y.; Hedstrand, D.M.; Spindler, R.; Tomalia, D.A. Hydrophobically modified poly(amidoamine) (PAMAM) dendrimers: Their properties at the air-water interface and use as nanoscopic container molecules. *J. Mater. Chem.* **1997**, *7*, 1199–1205. [CrossRef]
89. van Hest, J.C.M.; Delnoye, D.A.P.; Baars, M.W.P.L.; Van Genderen, M.H.P.; Meijer, E.W. Polystyrene-dendrimer amphiphilic block copolymers with a generation-dependent aggregation. *Science* **1995**, *268*, 1592–1595. [CrossRef]
90. Percec, V.; Chu, P.; Ungar, G.; Zhou, J. Rational design of the first nonspherical dendrimer which displays calamitic nematic and smectic thermotropic liquid crystalline phases. *J. Am. Chem. Soc.* **1995**, *117*, 11441–11454. [CrossRef]
91. Israelachvili, J.N. *Intermolecular and Surface Forces*, 2nd ed.; Academic Press: San Diego, CA, USA, 1992.
92. Zimmerman, S.C.; Zeng, F.; Reichert, E.C.; Kolotuchin, S.V. Self-Assembling Dendrimers. *Science* **1996**, *271*, 1095–1098. [CrossRef] [PubMed]
93. Kawa, M.; Fréchet, J.M.J. Self-assembled lanthanide-cored dendrimer complexes: Enhancement of the luminescence properties of lanthanide ions through site-isolation and antenna effects. *Chem. Mater.* **1998**, *10*, 286–296. [CrossRef]
94. Galeazzi, S.; Hermans, T.M.; Paolino, M.; Anzini, M.; Mennuni, L.; Giordani, A.; Caselli, G.; Makovec, F.; Meijer, E.W.; Vomero, S.; et al. Multivalent supramolecular dendrimer-based drugs. *Biomacromolecules* **2010**, *11*, 182–186. [CrossRef] [PubMed]
95. Wang, B.-B.; Zhang, W.; Jia, X.-R.; Li, Z.-C.; Ji, Y.; Wei, Y. Self-assembly of a new class of amphiphilic poly(amidoamine) dendrimers and their electrochemical properties. *J. Polym. Sci. Part A Polym. Chem.* **2005**, *43*, 5512–5519. [CrossRef]
96. Tomalia, D.A.; Majoros, I. Dendrimeric supramolecular and supramacromolecular assemblies. *J. Macromol. Sci.* **2003**, *C43*, 411–477. [CrossRef]
97. Fréchet, J.M.J. Dendrimers and supramolecular chemistry. *Proc. Natl. Acad. Sci. USA* **2002**, *99*, 4782–4787. [CrossRef]
98. Tomalia, D.A.; Pulgam, V.R.; Swanson, D.R.; Huang, B. Janus Dendrimers and Dendrons. U.S. Patent 7,977,452 B2, 12 July 2011.
99. Rudick, J.G.; Percec, V. Induced helical backbone conformations of self-oganizable dendronized polymers. *Accts. Chem. Res* **2008**, *41*, 1641–1652. [CrossRef]
100. Rosen, B.M.; Wilson, C.J.; Wilson, D.A.; Peterca, M.; Imam, M.R.; Percec, V. Dendron-mediated self-assembly, disassembly, and self-organization of complex systems. *Chem. Rev.* **2009**, *109*, 6275–6540.

101. Rosen, B.M.; Wilson, D.A.; Wilson, C.J.; Peterca, M.; Won, B.C.; Huang, C.; Lipski, L.R.; Zeng, X.; Ungar, G.; Heiney, P.A.; et al. Predicting the structure of supramolecular dendrimers via the analysis of libraries of AB_3 and constitutional isomeric AB_2 biphenylpropyl ether self-assembling dendrons. *J. Am. Chem. Soc.* **2009**, *131*, 17500–17521. [CrossRef]
102. Percec, V.; Cho, W.-D.; Ungar, G.; Yeardley, D.J.P. Increasing the diameter of cylindrical and spherical supramolecular dendrimers by decreasing the solid angle of their monodendrons via periphery functionalization. *J. Am. Chem. Soc.* **2000**, *122*, 10273–10281. [CrossRef]
103. Percec, V.; Cho, W.-D.; Mosier, P.E.; Ungar, G.; Yeardley, D.J.P. Structural analysis of cylindrical and spherical supramolecular dendrimers quantifies the concept of monodendron shape control by generation number. *J. Am. Chem. Soc.* **1998**, *120*, 11061–11070. [CrossRef]
104. Tomalia, D.A.; Khanna, S.N. In quest of a systematic framework for unifying and defining nanoscience. *Mod. Phys. Lett. B* **2014**, *28*, 1430002. [CrossRef]
105. Tomalia, D.A.; Khanna, S.N. A systematic framework and nanoparticle concept for unifying nanoscience: Hard/soft nanoelements, superatoms, meta-atoms, new emerging properties, periodic patterns, and predictive Mendeleev-like nanoperiodic tables. *Chem. Rev.* **2016**, *116*, 2705–2774. [CrossRef] [PubMed]
106. Kemsley, J. Developing superatom science. *Chem. Eng. News* **2013**, *91*, 24–25. [CrossRef]
107. Tomalia, D.A.; Huang, B.; Swanson, D.R.; Brothers II, H.M.; Klimash, J.W. Structure control within poly(amidoamine) dendrimers: Size, shape and regio-chemical mimicry of globular proteins. *Tetrahedron* **2003**, *59*, 3799–3813. [CrossRef]
108. DeMattei, C.R.; Huang, B.; Tomalia, D.A. Designed dendrimers syntheses by self-assembly of single-site, ssDNA functionalized dendrons. *Nano Lett.* **2004**, *4*, 771–777. [CrossRef]
109. Percec, V.; Wilson, D.A.; Leowanawat, P.; Wilson, C.J.; Hughes, A.D.; Kaucher, M.S.; Hammer, D.A.; Levine, D.H.; Kim, A.J.; Bates, F.S.; et al. Self-assembly of Janus dendrimers into uniform dendrimersomes and other complex architectures. *Science* **2010**, *328*, 1009–1014. [CrossRef]
110. Zhang, S.; Moussodia, R.-O.; Sun, H.-J.; Leowanawat, P.; Muncan, A.; Nusbaum, C.D.; Chelling, K.M.; Heiney, P.A.; Klein, M.L.; Andre, S.; et al. Mimicking biological membranes with programmable glycan ligands self-assembled from amphiphilic Janus glycodendrimers. *Angew. Chem. Int. Ed.* **2014**, *53*, 10899–10903. [CrossRef]
111. Percec, V.; Sahoo, D.; Adamson, J. Stimuli-responsive principles of supramolecular organizations emerging from self-assembling and self-organizable dendrons, dendrimers, and dendronized polymers. *Polymers* **2023**, *15*, 1832. [CrossRef]
112. Yu, T.; Liu, X.; Bolcato-Bellemin, A.-L.; Wang, Y.; Liu, C.; Erbacher, P.; Qu, F.; Rocchi, P.; Behr, J.-P.; Peng, L. An amphiphilic dendrimer for effective delivery of small interfering RNA and gene silencing in vitro and in vivo. *Angew. Chem. Int. Ed.* **2012**, *51*, 8478–8484. [CrossRef]
113. Chen, C.; Posocco, P.; Liu, X.; Cheng, Q.; Laurini, E.; Zhou, J.; Liu, C.; Wang, Y.; Tang, J.; Dal Col, V.; et al. Mastering Dendrimer Self-Assembly for Efficient siRNA Delivery: From Conceptual Design to In Vivo Efficient Gene Silencing. *Small* **2016**, *12*, 3667–3676. [CrossRef] [PubMed]
114. Nishiyama, N.; Jang, W.-D.; Kataoka, K. Supramolecular nanocarriers integrated with dendrimers encapsulating photosensitizers for effective photodynamic therapy and photochemical gene delivery. *New J. Chem.* **2007**, *31*, 1074–1082. [CrossRef]
115. Wang, J.; Voets, I.K.; Fokkink, R.; van der Gucht, J.; Velders, A.H. Controlling the number of dendrimer in dendrimicelle nanoconjugates from 1 to more than 100. *Soft Matter* **2014**, *10*, 7337–7345. [CrossRef] [PubMed]
116. Mignani, S.; Shi, X.; Majoral, J.-P. Dendritic macromolecular architectures: Dendrimer-based polyion complex micelles. *Biomacromolecules* **2021**, *22*, 262–274. [CrossRef] [PubMed]
117. Ten Hove, J.B.; Wang, J.; van Leeuwen, F.W.B.; Velders, A.H. Dendrimer-encapsulated nanoparticle-core micelles as a modular strategy for particle-in-a-box-in-a-box nanostructures. *Nanoscale* **2017**, *9*, 18619–18623. [CrossRef]
118. Wang, J.; Lei, L.; Voets, I.K.; Cohen, S.; Martien, A.; Velders, A.H. Dendrimicelles with pH-controlled aggregation number of core-dendrimers and stability. *Soft Matter* **2020**, *16*, 7893–7897. [CrossRef]
119. Gomez, M.V.; Guerra, J.; Myers, V.S.; Crooks, R.M.; Velders, A.H. Nanoparticle Size Determination by 1H NMR Spectroscopy. *J. Am. Chem. Soc.* **2009**, *131*, 14634–14635. [CrossRef]
120. Gomez, M.V.; Guerra, J.; Velders, A.H.; Crooks, R.M. NMR Characterization of Fourth-Generation PAMAM Dendrimers in the Presence and Absence of Palladium Dendrimer-Encapsulated Nanoparticles. *J. Am. Chem. Soc.* **2009**, *131*, 341–350. [CrossRef]
121. Zhao, M.; Sun, L.; Crooks, R.M. Preparation of Cu nanoclusters within dendrimer templates. *J. Am. Chem. Soc.* **1998**, *120*, 4877–4878. [CrossRef]
122. Ten Hove, J.B.; van Leeuwen, F.W.B.; Velders, A.H. Manipulating and monitoring nanoparticles in micellar thin film superstructures. *Nat. Commun.* **2018**, *9*, 5207. [CrossRef]
123. Ten Hove, J.B.; van Oosterom, M.N.; van Leeuwen, F.W.B.; Velders, A.H. Nanoparticles reveal extreme size-sorting and morphologies in complex coacervate superstructures. *Sci. Rep.* **2018**, *8*, 13820. [CrossRef] [PubMed]
124. Ten Hove, J.B.; Wang, J.; van Oosterom, M.N.; van Leeuwen, F.W.B.; Velders, A.H. Size-sorting and pattern formation of nanoparticle-loaded micellar superstructures in biconcave thin films. *ACS Nano* **2017**, *11*, 11225–11231. [CrossRef] [PubMed]
125. Kaup, R.; ten Hove, J.B.; Bunschoten, A.; van Leeuwen, F.W.B.; Velders, A.H. Multicompartment dendrimicelles with binary, ternary and quaternary core composition. *Nanoscale* **2021**, *13*, 15422–15430. [CrossRef] [PubMed]
126. Kaup, R.; Velders, A.H. Controlling trapping, release, and exchange dynamics of micellar core components. *ACS Nano* **2022**, *16*, 14611–14621. [CrossRef]

127. Kaup, R.; ten Hove, J.B.; Velders, A.H. Dendroids, discrete covalenty cross-linked dendrimer superstructures. *ACS Nano* **2021**, *15*, 1666–1674. [CrossRef]
128. Tang, S.; Tomalia, D.A.; Orr, B.G.; Baker, J.R., Jr.; Huang, B. Regio-specific size, shape and surface chemistry designed dendrimers based on differentiated dendroid templates. *New J. Chem.* **2013**, *37*, 690–700. [CrossRef]
129. Denkewalter, R.G.; Kolc, J.F.; Lukasavage, W.J. Macromolecular Having Highly Branched Homogenous Compounds. U.S. Patent 4,410,688, 18 October 1983.
130. Tomalia, D.A.; Dewald, J.R.; Hall, M.J.; Martin, S.J.; Smith, P.B. In Proceedings of the Preprints of the 1st SPSJ International Polymer Conference, Society of Polymer Science, Kyoto, Japan, 20–24 August 1984; p. 65.
131. Haensler, J.; Szoka, F.C., Jr. Polyamidoamine cascade polymers mediate efficient transfection of cells inculture. *Bioconjugate Chem.* **1993**, *4*, 372–379. [CrossRef]
132. Bielinska, A.; Kukowska-Latallo, J.F.; Johnson, J.; Tomalia, D.A.; Baker, J.R., Jr. Regulation of in vitro gene expression using antisense oligonucleotides or antisense expression plasmids transfected using Starburst PAMAM dendrimers. *Nucleic Acids Res.* **1996**, *24*, 2176–2182. [CrossRef]
133. Kukowska-Latallo, J.F.; Bielinska, A.U.; Johnson, J.; Spindler, R.; Tomalia, D.A.; Baker, J.R., Jr. Efficient transfer of genetic material into mammalian cells using Starburst polyamidoamine dendrimers. *Proc. Natl. Acad. Sci. USA* **1996**, *93*, 4897–4902. [CrossRef]
134. Zinselmeyer, B.H.; Mackay, S.P.; Schatzlein, A.G.; Uchegbu, I.F. The Lower-Generation Polypropylenimine Dendrimers Are Effective Gene-Transfer Agents. *Pharm. Res.* **2002**, *19*, 960–967. [CrossRef]
135. Weber, N.; Ortega, P.; Clemente, M.I.; Shcharbin, D.; Bryszewska, M.; de la Mata, F.J.; Gomez, R.; Munoz-Fernandez, M.A. Characterization of carbosilane dendrimers as effective carriers of siRNA and HIV-infected lymphocytes. *J. Control. Release* **2008**, *132*, 55–64. [CrossRef] [PubMed]
136. Zhou, J.; Wu, J.; Hafdi, N.; Behr, J.-P.; Erbacher, P.; Peng, L. PAMAM dendrimers for efficient siRNA delivery and potent gene silencing. *Chem. Commun.* **2006**, *22*, 2362–2364. [CrossRef]
137. Hudson, S.D.; Jung, H.-T.; Percec, V.; Cho, W.-D.; Johansson, G.; Ungar, G.; Balagurusamy, V.S.K. Direct Visualization of Individual Cylindrical and Spherical Supramolecular Dendrimers. *Science* **1997**, *278*, 449–452. [CrossRef]
138. Setten, R.L.; Rossi, J.J.; Han, S.-P. The current state and future directiions of RNAi-based therapeutics. *Nat. Drug Rev. Drug Disc.* **2019**, *18*, 421–446. [CrossRef] [PubMed]
139. Dzmitruk, V.; Apartsin, E.; Ihnatsyeu-Kachan, A.; Abashkin, V.; Shcharbin, D.; Bryszewska, M. Dendrimers show promise for siRNA and microRNA Therapeutics. *Pharmaceutics* **2018**, *10*, 126. [CrossRef]
140. Sahin, U.; Kariko, K.; Tureci, O. mRNA-based therapeutics—Developing a new class of drugs. *Nat. Rev. Drug Discov.* **2014**, *13*, 759–780. [CrossRef]
141. Weng, Y.; Li, C.; Yang, T.; Hu, B.; Zhang, M.; Guo, S.; Xiao, H.; Liang, X.-J.; Huang, Y. The challenge and prospect of mRNA therapeutics landscape. *Biotechnol. Adv.* **2021**, *40*, 107534. [CrossRef]
142. Xu, X.; Jian, Y.; Li, Y.; Zhang, X.; Tu, Z.; Gu, Z. Bio-Inspired Supramolecular Hybrid Dendrimers Self-Assembled from Low-Generation Peptide Dendrons for Highly Efficient Gene Delivery and Biological Tracking. *ACS Nano* **2014**, *8*, 9255–9264. [CrossRef]
143. Kisakova, L.A.; Apartsin, E.K.; Nizolenko, L.F.; Karpenko, L.I. Dendrimer-mediated delivery of DNA and RNA Vaccines. *Pharmaceutics* **2023**, *15*, 1106. [CrossRef]
144. Chahal, J.S.; Khan, O.F.; Cooper, C.L.; McPartlan, J.S.; Tsosie, J.K.; Tilley, L.D.; Sidik, S.M.; Lourido, S.; Langer, R.; Bavari, S.; et al. Dendrimer-RNA nanoparticles generate protective immunity against lethal Ebola, H1N1 influenza and Toxoplasma gondii challenges with a single dose. *Proc. Nat. Acad. Sci. USA* **2016**, *113*, E4133–E4142. [CrossRef] [PubMed]
145. Zhang, D.; Atochina-Vasserman, E.N.; Maurya, D.S.; Liu, M.; Xiao, Q.; Lu, J.; Lauri, G.; Ona, N.; Reagan, E.K.; Ni, H.; et al. Targeted delivery of mRNA with one-component ionizable amphiphilic Janus dendrimers. *J. Am. Chem. Soc.* **2021**, *143*, 17975–17982. [CrossRef] [PubMed]
146. Zhang, D.; Atochina-Vasserman, E.N.; Maurya, D.S.; Huang, N.; Xiao, Q.; Ona, N.; Liu, M.; Shahnawaz, H.; Ni, H.; Kim, K.; et al. The unexpected importance of the primary structure of the hydrophobic part of one-component ionizable amphiphilic Janus dendrimers in targeted mRNA delivery activity. *J. Am. Chem. Soc.* **2021**, *143*, 12315–12327. [CrossRef] [PubMed]
147. Sahoo, D.; Atochina-Vasserman, E.N.; Maurya, D.S.; Arshad, M.; Chenna, S.S.; Ona, N.; Vasserman, J.A.; Ni, H.; Weissman, D.; Percec, V. The constitutional isomerism of one-component ionizable amphiphilic Janus dendrimers orchestrates the total and targeted activities of mRNA delivery. *J. Am. Chem. Soc.* **2024**, *146*, 3627–3634. [CrossRef] [PubMed]
148. Lu, J.; Atochina-Vasserman, E.N.; Maurya, D.S.; Sahoo, D.; Ona, N.; Reagan, E.K.; Ni, H.; Weissman, D.; Percec, V. Targeted and equally distributed deliery of mRNA to organs with pentaerythritol-based one-component ionizable amphiphilic Janus dendrimers. *J. Am. Chem. Soc.* **2023**, *145*, 18760–18766. [CrossRef] [PubMed]
149. Tomalia, D.A.; Christensen, J.B.; Boas, U. The past, present, and future for dendrons and dendrimers. In *Dendrimers, Dendrons, and Dendritic Polymers: Discovery, Applications and the Future*; Cambridge University Press: New York, NY, USA, 2012; pp. 378–406.
150. Singh, M.K. Dendrimer Technology: Concept to Cutting-Edge Applications, 57th SPSR International Webinar on Dendrimer Technology. Available online: https://www.youtube.com/live/sAUfDi8XI64?app=desktop&feature=share (accessed on 21 July 2024).

pharmaceutics

MDPI

Article

New Approaches for Basophil Activation Tests Employing Dendrimeric Antigen–Silica Nanoparticle Composites

Silvia Calvo-Serrano [1,2,3,†], Esther Matamoros [4,5,†], Jose Antonio Céspedes [1,2], Rubén Fernández-Santamaría [1,2], Violeta Gil-Ocaña [4,5], Ezequiel Perez-Inestrosa [4,5], Cecilia Frecha [1,2], Maria I. Montañez [1,2,4,*], Yolanda Vida [4,5,*], Cristobalina Mayorga [1,2,6,‡] and Maria J. Torres [1,2,3,6,‡]

1 Allergy Research Group, Instituto de Investigación Biomédica de Málaga y Plataforma en Nanomedicina—IBIMA Plataforma Bionand, Parque Tecnológico de Andalucía, 29590 Málaga, Spain; silcalser@gmail.com (S.C.-S.); jcespedeslagos13@gmail.com (J.A.C.); rubenfernandezsantamaria@gmail.com (R.F.-S.); frechacecilia@gmail.com (C.F.); lina.mayorga@ibima.eu (C.M.); mjtorresj@uma.es (M.J.T.)
2 RICORS Red de Enfermedades Inflamatorias (REI), 28029 Madrid, Spain
3 Departamento de Medicina y Dermatología, Universidad de Málaga, 29071 Málaga, Spain
4 Departamento de Química Orgánica, Universidad de Málaga, Campus Teatinos s/n, 29071 Málaga, Spain; esthermc@uma.es (E.M.); vgil51192@gmail.com (V.G.-O.); inestrosa@uma.es (E.P.-I.)
5 Instituto de Investigación Biomédica de Málaga y Plataforma en Nanomedicina—IBIMA Plataforma Bionand, Parque Tecnológico de Andalucía, 29590 Málaga, Spain
6 Allergy Unit, Hospital Regional Universitario de Málaga-HRUM, 29010 Málaga, Spain
* Correspondence: maribelmv@uma.es (M.I.M.); yolanda.vida@uma.es (Y.V.)
† These authors contributed equally to this work and share first authorship.
‡ These authors contributed equally to this work and share last authorship.

Abstract: In vitro cell activation through specific IgE bound to high-affinity receptors on the basophil surface is a widely used strategy for the evaluation of IgE-mediated immediate hypersensitivity reactions to betalactams. Cellular activation requires drug conjugation to a protein to form a large enough structure displaying a certain distance between haptens to allow the cross-linking of two IgE antibodies bound to the basophil's surface, triggering their degranulation. However, no information about the size and composition of these conjugates is available. Routine in vitro diagnosis using the basophil activation test uses free amoxicillin, which is assumed to conjugate to a carrier present in blood. To standardize the methodology, we propose the use of well-controlled and defined nanomaterials functionalized with amoxicilloyl. Silica nanoparticles decorated with PAMAM–dendrimer–amoxicilloyl conjugates (NpDeAXO) of different sizes and amoxicilloyl densities (50–300 μmol amoxicilloyl/gram nanoparticle) have been prepared and chemically characterized. Two methods of synthesis were performed to ensure reproducibility and stability. Their functional effect on basophils was measured using an *in-house* basophil activation test (BAT) that determines $CD63^+$ or $CD203c^{high}$ activation markers. It was observed that NpDeAXO nanocomposites are not only able to specifically activate basophils but also do so in a more effective way than free amoxicillin, pointing to a translational potential diagnosis.

Keywords: PAMAM dendrimers; dendrimeric antigens; silica nanoparticles; drug allergy diagnosis; basophil activation test

1. Introduction

Nanoscale science is an exciting scientific frontier that focuses on the length scale of approximately 1−100 nm. Our growing ability to create, manipulate, and characterize at the nanoscale is contributing to the exploration and exploitation of the biomedical applications of different nanomaterials and nanostructures. Nanoparticles (Nps) and dendrimers, as well as their combination in hybrid nanocomposites, are relevant to the present study, with potential in vivo and in vitro applications [1,2]. The interaction between these nanocomposites and the immune system is an area of interest which we apply to the diagnosis of allergic reactions to drugs [3,4] with the aim of dealing with the existing limitations of established methods.

Betalactam antibiotics (BLs) are drugs of first choice for the treatment of bacterial infections, but they are also the most common cause of allergic drug reactions, with an estimated prevalence of 10%. BL allergy is most commonly induced by immunoglobulin E (IgE)-mediated mechanisms, causing symptoms varying from simple skin involvement to anaphylactic shock [5,6].

The diagnosis of antibiotic allergy is complex, most times challenging, and, due to low sensitivity of the tests, usually overestimated. In fact, currently, only less than 30% of adults and 10% of children who report "allergy" to BLs are truly confirmed after an allergological work-up [7]. Moreover, whether truly allergic to the antibiotic or not, patients are banned from the drug for life, resorting to less effective second-line antibiotics, which are associated with a higher prevalence of infections by resistant bacteria, higher costs, longer hospitalizations, and increased readmission rates [7,8]; this is the reason why accurate diagnostic tests are needed.

BL allergy diagnosis involves clinical history, followed by in vivo methods consisting of a skin test (ST) and DPT (drug provocation test). Since clinical history may not always be accurate and the sensitivity of STs is not optimal, the final diagnosis usually relies on DPTs, which, due to patient risk, are contraindicated in severe reactions [9]. Given the described limitations of in vivo tests, in vitro tests can represent good alternatives for diagnosis. Indeed, the basophil activation test (BAT) and the quantification of serum-specific IgE (sIgE) are being used as complementary methods in combination with STs to avoid DPT despite their current suboptimal sensitivity [10–12].

The BAT is a flow-cytometry-based technique that has gained importance as a diagnostic tool for sIgE-mediated drug allergy [9] as it attempts to mimic in vivo IgE-mediated cell activation and mediator release during an allergic response. This test identifies basophils (anti-IgE, CCR3, CRTH2, and CD203c) and quantifies activation markers (CD63 and CD203c) expressed on their surface after stimulation with the suspected drug. BAT sensitivity depends on the drug involved; in the case of penicillins, it ranges from 22% to 55% [10]. If we focus on amoxicillin (AX), the most frequently consumed BL responsible for drug allergy, the sensitivity of the BAT is around 50%. Such a low sensitivity can be associated with the low level of sIgE on basophils, common in drug allergy and which limits its activation and consequent degranulation in the assay. Another limitation could lie in the nature of AX since it is a small molecule that cannot induce an allergic reaction alone. However, in blood, this drug reacts to proteins, forming covalent amoxicilloyl(AXO)–protein conjugates that feature both efficient antigen presentation and sufficient size to accomplish the minimal structural requirements for basophil activation [11]. Requirements refer to immunological recognition by at least two adjacent IgE antibodies that are bound to their high-affinity receptor (FcεRI) on the cell surface, which leads to the IgE cross-linking process and subsequent activation and degranulation with the release of inflammatory mediators that characterize an allergic reaction [13,14].

Research focused on understanding these triggering conjugates has described the identification of AX target proteins and modification sites, as well as their in vitro immunological recognition at the sIgE level [15,16], but none at the basophil level. As a consequence, the only thing we can assume about the BAT assay is that free AX binds to proteins in fresh blood samples. Although the nature and chemical composition of the conjugates that induce cell activation are not known and include inter-assay variability between subjects, it seems clear that the process is influenced by their size and multivalency of the drug–protein conjugates.

To gain insight into the structural requirements needed for optimal interaction between the drug moieties and sIgE on the basophil surface, we propose the use of nanoscale-size customized synthetic materials that can effectively interact with sIgE bound to receptors on the cell surface. Nanotechnology can handle existing problems with natural protein conjugates, such as low density of drug determinants and low reproducibility, and achieve effective diagnostic outcomes by controlling conjugate size and increasing the multivalence and the availability of peripheral drug antigenic determinants. Additionally, the use of homogeneous well-defined and characterized materials facilitates the standardization of the test and the interpretation of results.

We previously designed dendrimeric antigen (DeAn) conjugates, in which the dendrimer plays the role of a synthetic protein and is decorated with multiple units of drug antigenic determinant, with potential uses for sIgE quantification [17–19]. Another study demonstrated that DeAns participate effectively in the intramolecular cross-linking of sIgE bound to FcεRI on basophils [20]. Specifically, two-generation PAMAM dendrimers (G2 and G4) decorated with AXO resulted in DeAXO conjugates, which showed higher stimulation rates for the larger conjugates in BATs performed with samples of BL-allergic patients [20].

In line with these results, other studies focusing on the process of membrane antibody–receptor (IgE-FcεRI) binding and cross-linking reported that larger conjugates lead to higher degranulation degrees on rat basophilic leukemia cells [21,22]. Bidendron antigens (BiAns) based on multivalent AXO dendrons spaced by flexible polyethyleneglycol (PEG) linkers of different lengths (600–12,000 Da) showed, in the cellular assays sensitized with antibodies from sera of AX-allergic patients (AX-AP), activation responses only with the longer structures (containing PEG 6000–12,000 Da) involving an estimated distance of 13–20 nm between AXO determinants [22]. To achieve bigger nanomaterials, another study used gold Nps as a solid support for the covalent immobilization of a synthetic hapten ligand at high density, observing that 20 and 50 nm Nps elicited the greatest cellular response. However, a reduced hapten density inhibited degranulation [21]. Moreover, other parameters have been reported to influence efficient cross-linking, such as the density of ligand epitopes (or valency) [23], the proximity of the ligand epitopes and steric hindrance [24], three-dimensional structure, flexibility, or rigidity [13].

This study aims to develop nanomaterials to efficiently activate basophils in the context of AX allergy. Nanosystems were designed inspired by the optimal nano-size described for cell activation, as well as by previous studies of sIgE recognition of DeAns, and taking into account the advantages of Nps as platforms in bioapplications, such as robustness, high surface-to-volume ratio, size similar to biomolecules, and chemically tuneable surface. Silica Nps were chosen as an inert scaffold to increase the size of the DeAXO conjugates and to present the antigenic determinant disposed in a manner that allows simultaneous attachment to IgEs on cell receptors. In addition, the selection of silica was encouraged by our experience in the use of DeAn–silica particle composites (DeAn@SiO_2; Φ = 500 nm) in immunoassays for the effective determination of sIgE from BLs from sample subjects [25,26].

Herein, different silica Nps decorated with DeAXO have been designed to evaluate the influence of both conjugate size and antigenic determinant density on the basophil activation mechanism. For this purpose, Nps of different sizes (20, 30, and 50 nm) have been prepared, and, by tuning the chemical modification protocols, different ligand (antigenic determinant) densities in their surface have been obtained. We further analyzed the effect of the different Nps and compared it with those produced by free AX in an *in-house* BAT based on a consensus protocol [27] in samples of AX-AP.

2. Materials and Methods

2.1. Nps Chemical Studies

Standard chemicals were obtained from Aldrich or VWR and used without further purification. PAMAM dendrimers were purchased from Aldrich. Milli-Q™ water was obtained by using the ultrapure Millipore® Direct-Q® 3. Phosphate-buffered saline (PBS) and 4 M lithium acetate buffer of pH 5.3 were prepared as described [28]. Macrosep® Advance centrifugal devices with 100 K MWCO from Pall Lab were used for the Np dispersions.

2.1.1. Np Synthesis

- **20dNps**

Silica particles were prepared adapting previously reported procedures [29,30]. Aqueous NH_3 (25%, 0.75 mL) was added over a methanol/butanol (4:1) mixture (60 mL) and the mixture was stirred for 15 min. Then, tetraethyl orthosilicate (TEOS, 2.5 mmol) was added and the mixture was stirred at room temperature for 16 h to obtain the silica nanospheres. The particle dispersion was centrifuged (25 min, 3500 rpm; centrifugal devices with 100 K MWCO) and washed with HCl 1 M and Milli-Q™ water. A colloidal dispersion (300 mL) of Nps (20 nm of diameter; **20dNps**) in water was obtained.

- **30dNps**

Silica particles were prepared adapting previously reported procedures [29,30]. Absolute ethanol (500 mL) was added over a Tween-20/1-butylamine (1:1.1) mixture (2.1 g) and the mixture was stirred for 15 min. Then, tetraethyl orthosilicate (TEOS, 2.5 mmol) was added and the mixture was stirred at room temperature for 16 h to obtain the silica nanospheres. The particle dispersion was centrifuged (25 min, 3500 rpm; centrifugal devices with 100 K MWCO) and washed with HCl 1 M and Milli-Q™ water. A colloidal dispersion (300 mL) of Nps (30 nm of diameter; **30dNps**) in water was obtained.

- **50dNps**

Silica particles were prepared adapting previously reported procedures [31]. Aqueous NH_3 (25%, 0.16 mL) was added over a water/ethanol (1:20) mixture (100 mL) and the mixture was stirred for 15 min. Then, tetraethyl orthosilicate (TEOS, 31.25 mmol) was added and the mixture was stirred at room temperature for 16 h to obtain the silica nanospheres. The particle dispersion was centrifuged (25 min, 3500 rpm; centrifugal devices with 100 K MWCO) and washed with HCl 1 M and Milli-Q™ water, and 300 mL of a colloidal dispersion of Nps (50 nm of diameter; **50dNps**) in water was obtained.

- **50Nps**

Silica particles were prepared adapting previously reported procedures [32]. Aqueous NH_3 (25%, 7.12 mL) was added over ethanol (114 mL) and the mixture was stirred at 50 °C for 6 h. Then, tetraethyl orthosilicate (TEOS, 20 mmol) was added and the mixture was stirred at 30 °C for 6 days to obtain the silica nanospheres. The particles were centrifuged (40 min, 6500 rpm) and washed with HCl 1 M and Milli-Q™ water, and 800 mg of Nps (50 nm of diameter; **50Nps**) were obtained as a colorless solid after lyophilization.

2.1.2. Np Surface Modification

- **20dNpNH$_2$**, **30dNpNH$_2$**, and **50dNpNH$_2$**

A colloidal dispersion of Nps (**20dNps**, **30dNps**, and **50dNps**) in water (120 mL) was placed in a centrifugal device with 100 K MWCO. Toluene (120 mL × 3 times) was added and the mixture centrifuged (20 min, 6500 rpm) to change the solvent. Finally, toluene (300 mL) was added and the Nps dispersion was sonicated for 15 min. Then, 3-(aminopropyl)-triethoxysilane (APTES, 5 mmol) was added and mixture was sonicated for 1 h. The solution was refluxed under stirring overnight after the addition of 4.2 mmol of extra APTES. The particle dispersion was centrifuged (20 min, 6500 rpm; centrifugal devices with 100 K MWCO) and washed with toluene (×3 times) and Milli-Q™ water (×3 times). A colloidal dispersion of Nps in water was obtained.

- **50NpNH$_2$**, **50Np$^{0.1}$NH$_2$** and **50Np$^{0.01}$NH$_2$**

50Nps were suspended in toluene (30 mL/100 mg of Nps) and sonicated for 15 min. Then, 3-(aminopropyl)-triethoxysilane (APTES) was added (see Supplementary Materials) and the mixture was sonicated for 1 h, after which it was refluxed under stirring overnight. The obtained particles were centrifuged (40 min, 6500 rpm), washed with toluene (×3 times) and Milli-Q™ water (×3 times), and finally lyophilized to obtain the desired amino-functionalized particles.

- **20dNpCO$_2$H, 30dNpCO$_2$H**, and **50dNpCO$_2$H**

A colloidal dispersion of Nps (**20dNpNH$_2$, 30dNpNH$_2$** and **50dNpNH$_2$**) in water (100 mL) was placed in a centrifugal device with 100 K MWCO. Dimethylformamide (DMF, 120 mL × 3 times) was added and the mixture centrifuged (20 min, 6500 rpm) to change the solvent. Finally, DMF (35 mL) was added and the Np dispersion was sonicated for 15 min. Then, succinic anhydride (8 mmol) in 15 mL of DMF was added to the previous mixture and sonicated for additional 15 min. Triethylamine (TEA, 0.8 mmol) was then added and the solution stirred at room temperature overnight. The particle dispersion was centrifuged (20 min, 6500 rpm; centrifugal devices with 100 K MWCO) and washed with DMF (×3 times) and Milli-Q™ water (×3 times). A colloidal dispersion of Nps in water was obtained.

- **50NpCO$_2$H, 50Np$^{0.1NH2}$CO$_2$H**, or **50Np$^{0.01NH2}$CO$_2$H**

Nps (**50NpNH$_2$, 50Np$^{0.1}$NH$_2$** and **50Np$^{0.01}$NH$_2$**) were suspended in DMF (2.5 mL/100 mg of Nps) and sonicated for 15 min. Then, succinic anhydride was added to the previous mixture and sonicated for an additional 15 min. Triethylamine (TEA) was then added and the solution stirred at room temperature overnight. The obtained particles were centrifuged (40 min, 6500 rpm), washed with DMF (×3 times) and Milli-Q™ water (×3 times), and finally lyophilized to obtain the desired carboxy-functionalized particles (see Supplementary Materials).

- **20dNpDe, 30dNpDe**, and **50dNpDe**

A colloidal dispersion of Nps (**20dNpCO$_2$H, 30dNpCO$_2$H**, and **50dNpCO$_2$H)** in water (100 mL) was placed in a centrifugal device with 100 K MWCO. DMF (100 mL × 3 times) was added and the mixture centrifuged (20 min, 6500 rpm) to change the solvent. Finally, anhydrous DMF (100 mL) was added and the solution kept under argon pressure. Then, 1-(3-(dimethylamino) propyl)-3-ethylcarbodiimide hydrochloride (EDCI, 0.4 mmol) and *N*-hydroxisuccinimide (NHS, 0.7 mmol) in 10 mL of anhydrous DMF were added and the Np dispersion was sonicated for 15 min. Then, PAMAM-G2 dendrimers (1.7×10^{-3} mmol) in 10 mL of anhydrous DMF were added to the previous mixture and sonicated for an additional 15 min, after which the solution was stirred at room temperature overnight. The particle dispersion was centrifuged (20 min, 6500 rpm; centrifugal devices with 100 K MWCO) and washed with DMF (×3 times) and Milli-Q™ water (×3 times). A colloidal dispersion of Nps in water was obtained.

- **50NpDe, 50Np$^{0.1}$De, 50Np$^{0.01}$De, 50Np$^{0.1NH2}$De**, or **50Np$^{0.01NH2}$De**

Nps (**50NpCO$_2$H, 50Np$^{0.1NH2}$CO$_2$H**, and **50Np$^{0.01NH2}$CO$_2$H)**, EDCI, and NHS were suspended in anhydrous DMF (1.5 mL/100 mg of Nps) and sonicated for 15 min. Then, PAMAM-G2 dendrimers in anhydrous DMF (1.5 mL/100 mg of Nps) were added to the previous mixture and sonicated for additional 15 min after which the solution was stirred at room temperature overnight. The obtained particles were centrifuged (40 min, 6500 rpm), washed with DMF (×3 times) and Milli-Q™ water (×3 times), and finally lyophilized to obtain the desired dendrimer-functionalized particles see Supplementary Materials).

- **20dNpDeAXO, 30dNpDeAXO**, and **50dNpDeAXO**

A colloidal dispersion of Nps (**20dNpDe, 30dNpDe**, and **50dNpDe**) in water (60 mL) was placed in a centrifugal device with 100 K MWCO. A 0.05 M $Na_2CO_3/NaHCO_3$ aqueous buffer at pH 10.2 (60 mL × 3 times) was added and the mixture centrifuged (20 min, 6500 rpm) to change the solvent. Finally, 0.05 M $Na_2CO_3/NaHCO_3$ aqueous buffer at pH 10.2 (60 mL) was added and the Np dispersion was sonicated for 15 min. Then, 4 mL of a freshly prepared solution of amoxicillin (AX) 10 mg/mL in 0.05 M $Na_2CO_3/NaHCO_3$ aqueous buffer at pH 10.2 was added to the previous mixture and sonicated for an additional 15 min, after which the suspension was stirred at 4 °C for 7 days. During this period, 10 mg of AX was added at approximately 24 h intervals. The particle dispersion was centrifuged

(20 min, 6500 rpm; centrifugal devices with 100 K MWCO) and washed with PBS (×3 times) and Milli-Q™ water (×3 times). A colloidal dispersion of Nps in water was obtained.

- **50NpDeAXO**, **50Np$^{0.1De}$DeAXO**, **50Np$^{0.01De}$DeAXO**, **50Np$^{0.1NH2}$DeAXO**, or **50Np$^{0.01NH2}$DeAXO**

Nps were treated following previously reported procedures [25,26] to obtain the desired functionalized particles.

2.1.3. Np Characterization

Dynamics light scattering (DLS)

The hydrodynamic diameter of the particles has been determined following previously reported procedures [25,26] using a Malvern Zetasizer Nano ZS90 instrument ("red laser" (λ = 633 nm) with a detection angle of 90°).

Transmission electron microscopy (TEM)

TEM images were recorded following previously reported procedures [25,26] in a PHILIPS CM-200 instrument.

Z Potential measurements

Z potential measurements were carried out following previously reported procedures [25,26] in a Malvern Zetasizer Nano ZS90 instrument.

Fourier-transformed infrared (FTIR) spectroscopy

FTIR measurements were carried out following previously reported procedures [25,26] in a Nicolet Nexus spectrometer (Thermo Fisher Scientific, Waltham, USA) with a Smart Golden Gate attenuated total reflectance (ATR) accessory.

Quantification of free primary amino groups

The quantification of free primary amino groups on the Np surface was carried out following a previously described procedure [25,33] using a VARIAN CARY 100BIO UV-Visible spectrophotometer. For Nps in dispersion, 1 mL of the corresponding colloidal dispersion was dried and weighed. This solid residue was dispersed in 1 mL of Milli-Q™ water and the suspension used in the test. Values were normalized to the obtained Np mass. For solid Nps, 1 mL of the corresponding Np suspension (1.5mg Nps/mL Milli-Q™ water) was used.

^{1}H-NMR spectra of **50NpDeAXO**

^{1}H HRMAS-NMR (High-Resolution Magic Angle Spinning Nuclear Magnetic Resonance) spectra were recorded at room temperature in an AVANCEIII HD 600 (Bruker AXS, Billerica, USA) spectrometer using a double-resonance probe of 4 mm at a spinning rate of 5 kHz. The magnetic field was 14.1 T corresponding to a ^{1}H resonance frequency of 600.09 MHz. The ^{1}H chemical shifts are referenced to D_2O. ^{1}H HRMAS-NMR spectra were recorded with a 4.6 us 90° pulse and 5 s delay and summing 300 scans.

2.2. Patients Selection and Allergological Work Up

Patients with a clinical history of immediate hypersensitivity reactions to AX (AX-APs) and tolerant healthy controls (HCs) were diagnosed according to European Academy of Allergy and Clinical Immunology guidelines [10,34] with a detailed clinical history, followed by a positive STs (SPT and/or IDT), and if negative, DPT with AX. Patients were classified according to the severity of the reactions as grade I (urticaria/angioedema), grade II (anaphylaxis), grade III (shock), and grade IV (ARREST) following the Ring and Messmer classification [35].

A skin prick test (SPT) and, if negative, intradermal test (IDT) were carried out as previously described [34] using solutions prepared daily from DAP Penicillin® test Kit (Diater S.A, Madrid, Spain) at maximum concentrations of 0.04 and 0.5 mg/mL of major (benzylpenicilloyl-octa-L-lysine (BP-OL) and minor determinants (sodium benzylpenilloate), respectively, and with 20 mg/mL for AX and for clavulanic acid. Readings were taken after 20 min. If the ST was negative, DPT was performed firstly with penicillin V (Laboratorios ERN S.A., Barcelona, Spain) and, if negative, a second time with AX (GlaxoSmithKline, Madrid, Spain) [34]. DPT was developed by oral route in a single-blind placebo-controlled procedure at incremental doses, starting with lower doses and with a minimum 30 min interval between each until the total cumulative therapeutic dose [36]. Patients were monitored during DPT and for 2 h after the last dose.

2.3. Cell Viability Measurement

Basophil viability after stimulation with the different Nps was assessed using 7-aminoactinomycin D (7-AAD, (Invitrogen, Carlsbad, CA, USA), which is passively taken up by cells with loss of membrane integrity, like non-viable basophils. Briefly, cells were incubated with the different Nps for 25 min, lysed, washed, and incubated with 7-AAD. The percentage of cell viability was recorded in the region of low 7-AAD signal, in the basophil gate ($CCR3^+/CD203c^+$), with a minimum acquisition of 500 basophils per sample. The following conditions were compared: no stimulus, anti-IgE, N-Formylmethionyl-leucyl-phenylalanine (fMLP), AX, and Nps.

2.4. Basophil Activation Test (BAT) with Different Nanoparticles (Nps)

An *in-house* BAT based on a recent consensus protocol was performed [27] on AX-APs and HCs. The drug-containing stimulus solutions, either the free AX or Nps that have been preserved in the solid state, were prepared just prior to the assay. In the case of Nps prepared as suspension, this fresh preparation was not possible. Briefly, heparinized blood samples were exposed to 100 µL of 2.5, 1.25, and 0.25 mg/mL AX (Alpha Aesar, Heysham, UK) [27] or **NpDeAXO** at a concentration range of 0.005 to 300 µM of AXO units, depending to the Np used. Anti-human IgE (Becton-Dickinson, East Rutherford, New Jersey, USA) antibody at 0.01 mg/mL and fMLP at 4 µM were used as positive controls, while stimulation buffer was used as negative control. Then, basophils were stained with APC-anti-human CCR3, FITC-anti-human CD63, and PE-anti-human CD203c monoclonal antibodies (Biolegend, San Diego, CA, USA). Stained cells were analyzed by FACSCalibur flow-cytometer (Becton-Dickinson Bioscience, San Jose, CA, USA) by acquiring more than 500 basophils per sample, identified as $SSC^{low}/CCR3^+$ [37]. Their level of activation was analyzed by the expression of CD63 or the upregulation of CD203c ($CD203c^{high}$) markers using FlowJo® software v.8.2 (FlowJo LLC, Becton Dickinson, Ashland, OR, USA).

2.5. Statistical Analyses

Normality was assessed by the Kolmogorov–Smirnov test. Quantitative variables without normal distribution were compared with Mann–Whitney U and Kruskall–Wallis tests and qualitative variables with X^2 test. Receiver operating characteristic (ROC) curves were performed to calculate the cut-offs for each of the NPs. Figures were made with GraphPad Prism 7 (GraphPad Software Inc, San Diego, CA, USA) and statistical analyses were performed using the SPSS program version 25.

3. Results and Discussion

3.1. Synthesis and Characterization of Nps

A series of SiO_2 Nps of different sizes ranging from 20 to 50 nm were prepared and characterized. All Nps were prepared using the Stöber methodology [38,39]. However, it has been described that the preparation of Nps with a uniform size of below 50 nm is rather difficult. Thus, the water-in-oil microemulsion process was adapted depending on the desired final particle size to obtain **20dNps**, **30dNps**, and **50dNps** [39]. Based on reported methodologies [29,30], the molar ratio of TEOS/aqueous NH_3 (25%)/organic solvent was modified until observing the desired size NPs. Nanoparticle size and distribution were determined by dynamic light scattering (DLS) experiments, and those were consistent with the observed TEM images (Figures S1 and S2, Supplementary Materials). From the TEM images, the diameter of the particles is about 20, 30, and 50 nm (**20dNps**, **30dNps**, **50dNps**, respectively). The average particle diameters in solution determined by DSL are 28, 37, and 52 nm, respectively. Those values agree with the TEM observation and indicate a rather good monodispersity of the particles. However, thermodynamically, Nps tend to agglomerate to reduce high surface energy, a process that occurs more frequently in the case of smaller Nps [39]. As a result, we observed that **20dNps**, **30dNps**, and **50dNps** are sufficiently stable in diluted solution but, when centrifuged to obtain a solid (or a concentrated solution), they agglomerate and do not disperse well again in solution, forming aggregates of various sizes that cannot be controlled. This makes the manipulation of the Nps difficult for the chemical modification of their surface, the consequent chemical characterization, and the performance of diagnostic tests. Moreover, it is a major handicap for their application in hospitals.

Therefore, great effort was invested to obtain Nps of these sizes which could be handled in the solid state and, when added to aqueous media, would disperse easily without forming aggregates. Adapting previously reported procedures [32], **50Nps** were obtained as a colorless solid, easy to manipulate and easily dispersible in aqueous media. From the TEM images, we can observe that the prepared nanoparticles were highly monodispersed spheres about 50 nm in outer diameter. The average particle diameter in solution determined by DSL is 60 nm (Figures S1 and S2, Supplementary Materials).

For the covalent immobilization of the dendrimeric antigen (DeAXO) on the Np surface, we used our previously described procedure (Figure 1) [25,26]. First, Nps were treated with APTES to introduce amino terminal groups to the particles surface. These groups were then treated with succinic anhydride to attach the carboxylic moiety. Generation-2 PAMAM dendrimers were covalently anchored through the formation of an amide bond between carboxylic moiety on the particle surface and the amino terminal groups of the PAMAM dendrimers. Finally, AX was reacted with the free amino groups of the dendrimers to generate the dendrimeric antigen DeAXO on the Np surfaces through the opening of the antibiotic β-lactam ring.

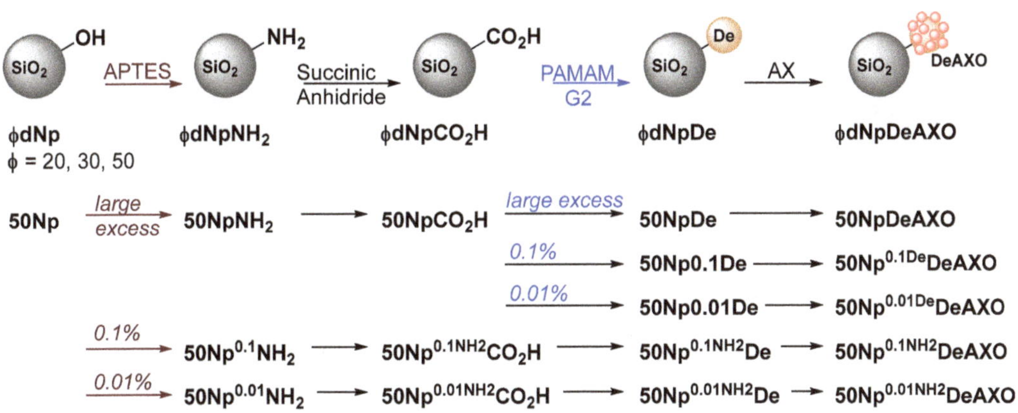

Figure 1. General procedure for the chemical modification of **ϕdNp** dispersions and **50Nps** with different DeAXO densities in their surface.

As previously mentioned, the chemical functionalization of **20dNps**, **30dNps**, and **50dNps** was carried out always maintaining low concentration dispersions of Nps. For this purpose, centrifugal devices with a 100 K cut-off filtration membrane were used, allowing us to exchange solvents for the different reactions as well as to purify the obtained modified Np dispersions. A large excess of the reagents was always used to achieve the maximum surface modification at all times.

The obtained Nps dispersions were analyzed with Zeta potential (ξ) measurements and evaluations of the amount of free primary amino groups present on the Np surface using a ninhydrin test (see Table S1, Supplementary Materials). Zeta potential (ξ) measurements were used to monitor the chemical modifications performed on the Np surfaces, since modification of their chemical nature was expected to alter its charge. The ξ values obtained from PBS dispersions (solvent that mimics physiological pH 7.4) agree with the expected surface charge [25,26]. Negative values were observed for Nps with negatively charged terminal functional groups in PBS (-OH for **ϕdNp** or -COOH for **ϕdNpCO$_2$H**, see Figure 1). On the other hand, ξ positive values have been observed for Nps where positively charged groups are present (-NH$_2$ for **ϕdNpNH$_2$** and **ϕdNpDe**). It should be noted that the values observed for Nps with dendrimers (**ϕdNpDe**) practically double those observed for **ϕdNpNH$_2$**, and this is is consistent with the introduction of 15 amino groups per dendrimer [33]. The reaction with AX caused a shift in the using of the zeta potential to values around $\xi = -8$ mV for **ϕdNpDeAXO**, which is in perfect agreement with the data obtained in our previous works [25,26].

Ninhydrin test values are very useful to evaluate the degree of amino functionalization of the Nps (see Table S1, Supplementary Materials). An almost complete coverage of the particle surfaces with the dendrimers has been observed [25,26]. Considering that all the amino groups of the dendrimers reacted [17], we can then assume that the amounts of AXO units are approximately 290 μmol per gram of **20dNpDeAXO** and 270 μmol per gram of **30dNpDeAXO** or **30dNpDeAXO** (Table 1). As expected, the smallest particles have the highest number of AXO groups per gram since they have the highest surface area/mass ratio. No significant differences were found into the amount of AXO/gram between Nps of 30 and 50 nm of diameter.

Table 1. Chemical properties of the prepared Nps.

Nps	Aspect	Diameter (nm)	AXO (μmolAXO/gNps) [1]
20dNpDeAXO	Suspension	20	290
30dNpDeAXO	Suspension	30	270 [2]
50dNpDeAXO	Suspension	50	270 [2]
50NpDeAXO	Solid	50	300
50Np$^{0.1De}$DeAXO	Solid	50	130
50Np$^{0.01De}$DeAXO	Solid	50	80
50Np$^{0.1NH2}$DeAXO	Solid	50	100
50Np$^{0.01NH2}$DeAXO	Solid	50	50

[1] Approximated value from ninhydrin test results (see Tables S1 and S2 of Supplementary Materials). [2] No significant differences have been observed between those values.

The chemical functionalization of **50Nps** was carried out following our previously described procedures working with the solid dried Nps [25,26]. In a first modification, a large excess of the reagents was always used to achieve the maximum surface modification, obtaining **50NpDeAXO**. Two approaches have been used to achieve different DeAXO densities on the particle surface in a reproducible way. In the first one, the amount of APTES used in the first step of the chemical procedure was reduced 0.1% and 0.01% to obtain **50Np0.1NH$_2$** and **50Np0.01NH$_2$**, respectively (marked in red in Figure 1). In the second one, the amount of PAMAM-G2 dendrimers added was reduced by the same proportion to obtain **50Np0.1De** and **50Np0.01De**, respectively (marked in blue in Figure 1). Thus, four more different Nps decorated with dendrimers on their surface have been obtained, which, after AX treatment, have given rise to Nps with different degrees of surface functionalization.

Zeta potential (ξ) values show the same trend as in the case of the previous Nps and are consistent with the chemical modifications that the Nps undergo on their surface throughout the process (see Table S2, Supplementary Materials). In this case, the estimation of the degree of functionalization of the Nps and therefore of the DeAXO density on their surface is determined by the values obtained from the ninhydrin test. The number of AXO units that we can assume were incorporated into the Nps, expressed as μmol of AXO per gram of Nps, are shown in Table 1

^{1}H-NMR spectra of **50NpDeAXO** were recorded (Figure 2). No signals are observed around 5.5 ppm, indicating the absence of closed β-lactam rings. The rest of the signals confirm the presence of the PAMAM dendrimers (between 3.7 and 2.0 ppm) and the AXO units (between 6.75 and 7.5 ppm) in the Nps [19].

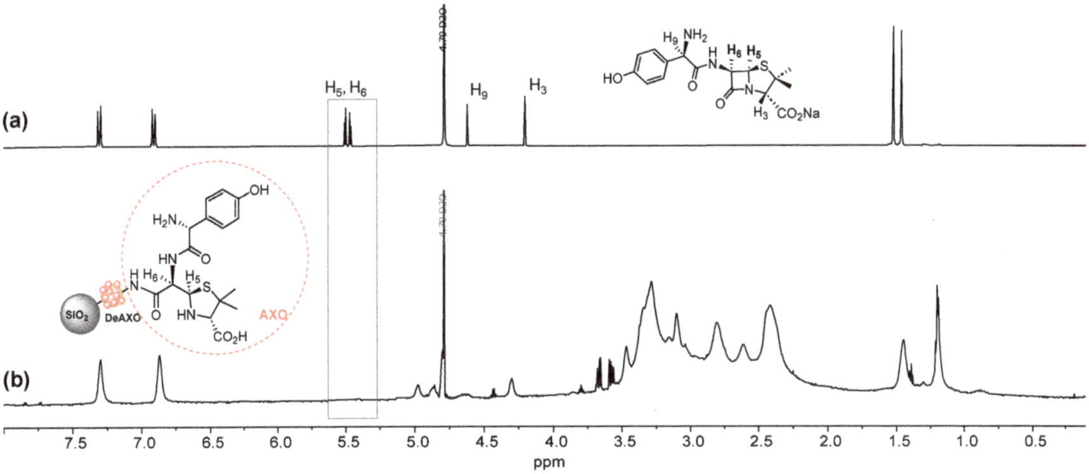

Figure 2. NMR spectra of (**a**) AX in basic D_2O and (**b**) **50NpDeAXO** in D_2O suspensions.

Stability of **50NpDeAXO** (stored as solids) were checked with DLS measurements of freshly prepared dispersions in distilled water at different time-points (0, 1, 2, 3, 4 and 5 h after preparation, more than enough time to perform the BAT assay). The results of DLS showed no aggregates. This is an indication that the preparation of dispersions without aggregates is feasible after resuspension of the stored Nps (as a solid at 5 °C, at least for a 6-month period of storage) (Figures S2–S7 in Supplementary Materials).

3.2. *Evaluation of Basophil Activation Capacity of Nanoparticles:* ***20dNpDeAXO, 30dNpDeAXO, 50dNpDeAXO,*** *and* ***50NpDeAXO***

DeAXO-functionalized Nps obtained as colloidal dispersions, including those of 20nm (**20dNpDeAXO**), 30nm (**30dNpDeAXO**), and 50 nm (**50dNpDeAXO**), were evaluated for their ability to activate basophils by BAT in samples from 10 AX-APs and 10 HCs. Clinical features of the AX-AP cohort can be found in Table S3. Results indicate that **20dNpDeAXO** and **30dNpDeAXO** did not produce any remarkable basophil activation (below 5%) in AX-APs or HCs at all concentrations used, measured either by CD63 or CD203c^{high} activation markers (Figure 3A–D). Interestingly, **50dNpDeAXO** triggered basophil activation, showing a higher percentage of CD63$^+$basophils in AX-APs compared to HCs (Figure 3E). Conversely, when using the CD203c^{high} marker, despite a dose–response activation, discrimination between AX-APs and HCs was not significant (Figure 3F).

To perform more accurate studies about the effect on basophils of DeAXO-decorated Nps, we prepared Nps with an improved methodology to isolate them in a solid state (**50NpDeAXO**), which allows a more precise control of the DeAXO display compared to Nps obtained as dispersions and offers an increased reproducibility in the preparation of dispersions for the BAT assay and consequently in its result. In addition, in view of a potential use of the **50NpDeAXO** as a platform for downstream applications involving whole blood, toxicity must be excluded. Therefore, the viability of basophils treated with **50NpDeAXO** was investigated by incubating samples with the different AX or Np concentrations, followed by 7-AAD viability staining. We observed high levels of viability with **50NpDeAXO**, like the ones obtained with free AX (Figure S8).

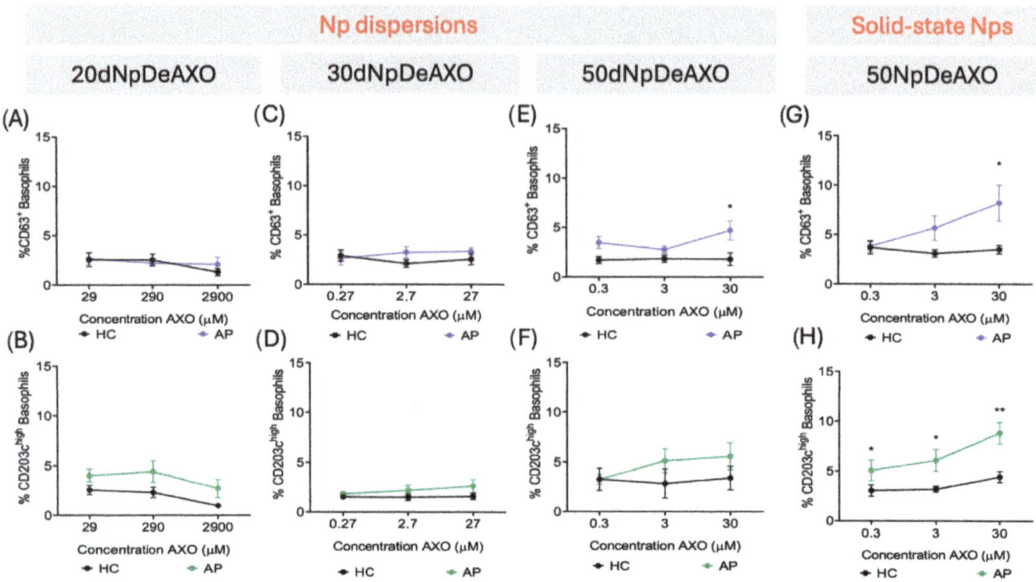

Figure 3. Basophil activation test (BAT) dose–response curves of **NpDeAXO** of different sizes: 20 nm (**A**,**B**), 30 nm (**C**,**D**), and 50 nm (**E**,**F**) and (**G**,**H**). *Np dispersions* or *solid-state Nps* labels at the top of the figure only indicate the synthetic methodology used for Np preparation. Black lines represent healthy controls (HCs), and blue and green lines represent allergic patients (APs). Size sample included HCs (N = 10) and APs (N = 10) for Nps synthesized as dispersions (**A–F**), while HCs (N = 45) and APs (N = 54) were included in the study for the Nps synthesized as a solid state. * $p < 0.05$, ** $p < 0.01$.

The selected **50NpDeAXO**, because of the optimal Np size, 50 nm, and the improved synthetic method, which allows for greater stability and reproducibility in the measurements, were evaluated for their ability to activate basophils, by BAT, in samples from 54 AX-APs and 45 HCs. Further on, although both 50nm Nps (**50dNpDeAXO** and **50NpDeAXO)** allowed a clear discrimination of AX-APs and HCs, comparative analysis revealed that **50NpDeAXO**, at 30 μM, showed a higher ability to activate basophils in AX-APs, either through CD63 or CD203c^{high} activation markers (8.2% and 8.8%, respectively) compared to **50dNpDeAXO** (4.7% and 5.6%, respectively; Figure 3E–H).

A different sample size has been evaluated with each of the Nps of the same 50 nm size, dispersed or in solid state, which may partly explain the difference in the results between Figure 3E,G. However, being able to more accurately measure/weigh the amount of AXO units supported on the Nps put into the assay when using **50NpDeAXO**, compared to dispersed **50dNpDeAXO**, should imply a higher reproducibility and precision in the results obtained and may mainly explain these improved results obtained with **50NpDeAXO**. The later results confirmed that controlling the exact amount of amoxicilloyl supported in the Nps that are evaluated in the cell assay is very important to obtain accurate results. In fact, when we compare the two synthesis methods, we observe that obtaining particles of the same size (50 nm) in a more controlled manner also improves and provides better results. The evaluation of precise **NpDeAn** in the BAT, in which the size of the Nps is crucial for activation, indicated, due to controlled nano-size, the optimal distance of 50 nm for obtaining maximal activation in this assay. These findings underscore the importance of considering the Np size and synthesis method in the design of nanomaterials for biomedical applications, at least in the allergy field.

In agreement with these results, other studies on the cell activation process via membrane antibody–receptor (IgE-FcεRI) binding and cross-linking have described that larger synthetic immunogens lead to higher degranulation degrees on rat basophilic leukemia cells [21,22]. Flexible BiAns based on multivalent AXO dendrons showed activation responses only with the longer structures presenting an estimated distance of 13–20 nm between AXO determinants [22]. Another study involving rigid supports, as herein, reports that gold Nps fully decorated with a synthetic hapten ligand of sizes larger than 19.8 nm and up to 50 nm exhibit more efficient cell activation [21].

3.3. *Effect of AXO Density on the Np Basophil Activation Capacity*

Given the substantial potential of DeAXO-decorated Nps, it was critical to undertake a comprehensive study of the influence of the degree of functionalization with AXO on the Nps to activate basophils from AX-APs in a specific way (Figure 4). For this purpose, a series of **50NpDeAXO** with different surface DeAXO densities was obtained, namely **50NpDeAXO**, **50Np$^{0.1De}$DeAXO**, **50Np$^{0.1NH2}$DeAXO**, **50Np$^{0.01De}$DeAXO**, and **50Np$^{0.01NH2}$DeAXO** containing between 300 and 50µmolAXO/gNp (Figure 1 and Table 1). The capacity of all these **50NpDeAXO** derivatives to activate basophils was tested in AX-APs (N = 4) and HCs (N = 6).

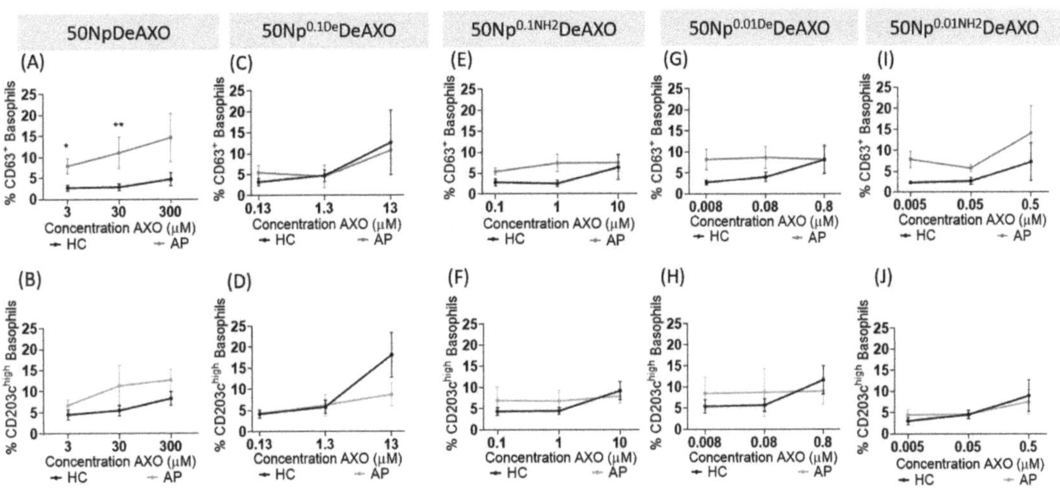

Figure 4. BAT dose–response curves of Nps with different DeAXO surface densities: 300 µmol AXO/gNp (**A**,**B**); 130 µmolAXO/gNp (**C**,**D**); 100 µmol AXO/gNp (**E**,**F**); 80 µmol AXO/gNp (**G**,**H**); 50 µmol AXO/gNp (**I**,**J**). Black lines represent healthy controls (HCs), and blue and green lines represent allergic patients (APs). Size sample included HCs (N = 6) and APs (N = 4) (**A**–**J**). * $p < 0.05$, ** $p < 0.01$.

BAT dose–response curves were constructed to evaluate the relationship between the concentration of Np-surface-displayed AXO and immune activation (Figure 4). Of all Nps tested, **50NpDeAXO** (300 µmol AXO/g Np) was the only one that induced basophil activation in a dose-dependent manner (Figure 4A,B). Consistently, Nps with the higher AXO content on their surface exhibited an enhanced discriminatory capacity between AX-APs and HCs ($p = 0.019$ and 0.0095, at 3 µM and 30 µM, respectively) when evaluating the expression of CD63 activation markers (Figure 4A).

In contrast, the rest of the Nps, displaying lower densities of AXO, showed null capacity to discriminate AX-APs from HCs (Figure 4C–J). Interestingly, the different treatments of the Nps to chemically modify them in order to have less DeAXO coating did not seem to influence their efficacy through any of the activation markers tested (CD63 or CD203c^{high}) (Figure 4E,F,I,J).

For this BAT application, allergens may contain at least two epitopes and the distance between epitopes is crucial for activation. Nps with the higher surface coverage of DeAn seem particularly efficient in cross-linking sIgE on basophils. By decreasing the AXO surface coverage, activation decreases, probably due to increased spacing between each AXO molecule.

It is likely that the multivalency of the dendrimers in NpDeAXO favors the IgE interaction via a dendritic or synergistic effect and thus degranulation. This is consistent with cell activation induced by other multivalent systems: bigger dendrimer-derived structures [20,22,23] or Np rigid systems displaying the higher valence of ligands (antigenic determinants) induced increased degranulation in antigen-study interactions [21]. However, a reduced hapten density inhibited degranulation [21].

To sum up, the biggest Nps with the highest density of AXO were the best performer in terms of patient basophil activation, most probably through a specific AXO recognition. However, as it can be seen in Figure 4A, at the maximum concentration of Nps in the assay, expressed in terms of an AXO unit concentration as 300 μM, the cellular response was highly variable, resulting in a high deviation. We believe that the dispersion at this high concentration of Nps is relatively unstable; furthermore, it is difficult for the operator to handle and we cannot assume that the dispersions tested are always homogeneous. Consequently, dispersions obtained at such high Np concentrations influence the variation in the BAT results.

3.4. AXO Displayed in Nps is more Potent Than Free AX in Inducing Specific Basophil Activation

We wanted to compare the efficiency of sIgE bridging depending on the way AX is presented, free AX or at the surface of the Nps, by analyzing the basophil activation levels in terms of AX concentrations (Figure 5). Due to the intrinsic characteristic of insolubility of the nanoparticles, they could not be evaluated at the same high concentration as the free AX. It was only possible to evaluate up to the concentration of the Np dispersions obtained that were stable. In fact, the Np concentration of 300 μM of AXO was discarded because in cytometry it generated a lot of debris and hindered the selection of the study population and a correct analysis. Unfortunately, Np concentration could not be increased beyond 30 μM AXO due to a compromise of Np solubility that impaired flow-cytometer data acquisition (Supplementary Figure S9). Samples from 54 AX-APs and 45 HCs were analyzed by BAT using free AX at 6800 μM, 3400 μM, and 680 μM and **50NpDeAXO** at 30 μM, 3 μM, and 0.3 μM of AXO, represented in Figure 5. Data showed that **50NpDeAXO** at the highest concentration of AXO (30 μM) induced similar basophil activation levels to free AX at 680 μM, indicating that **50NpDeAXO** is 23 times more potent in activating basophils from AX-APs than free AX, either by CD63 or CD203c^{high} activation markers.

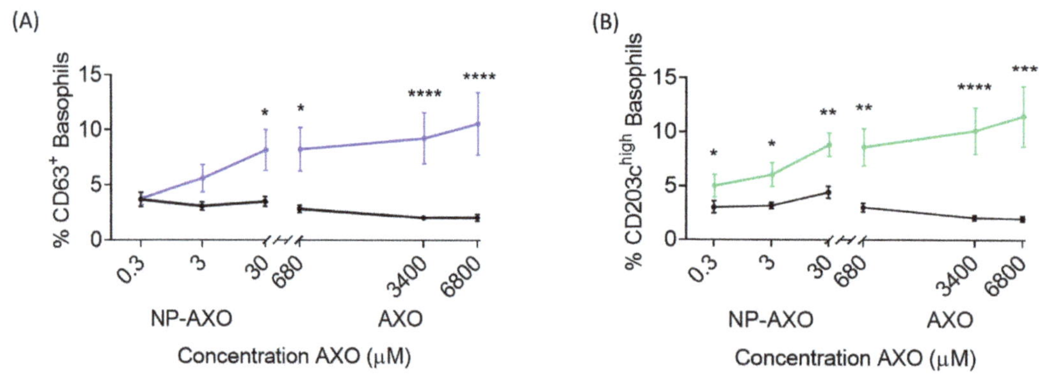

Figure 5. BAT dose–response curves using **50NpDeAXO** and free AX at three different concentrations. APs (N = 54) are depicted by blue or green lines and HCs (N = 45) are depicted by black lines. * $p < 0.05$, ** $p < 0.01$, *** $p < 0.001$, **** $p < 0.0001$.

These results indicate that AX is better recognized and more effective for activation when it is supported on the NpDe compared to the use of free AX. The selected NpDeAXO of 50 nm size interacts with effector cells through more effective multivalent binding of antigenic determinants facilitating the formation of large sIgE-FcεRI clusters, which in turn induce high levels of cell degranulation and serve as a predictive marker of IgE-mediated AX allergy.

3.5. Evaluation of the Discrimination Capacity of Allergic Patients and Healthy Controls by ***50NpDeAXO***

To delineate the clinical utility of our Np-based detection system, ROC curves were built to calculate the optimal cut-off and the AUC (Figure S10, Supplementary Materials). Results indicated that **50NpDeAXO** at 30 and 3 μM allowed the detection of 25.9% and 22.2% of positive cases, respectively, through CD63 markers (Figure 6A) and 25.9% and 24.4% at 30 and 3 μM, respectively, through CD203c^{high} markers (Figure 6B). The achieved specificity of NpDeAXO was 94.7% at 30 μM and 95.56% at 3 μM for both markers (Table S4, Supplementary Materials), similar to the values obtained for free AX at 680 μM. The availability of AXO units in the DeAn supported on Nps seems suitable, mimicking its availability in conjugates with natural proteins for recognition by sIgE on basophils and subsequent activation, which would have great potential in clinical application.

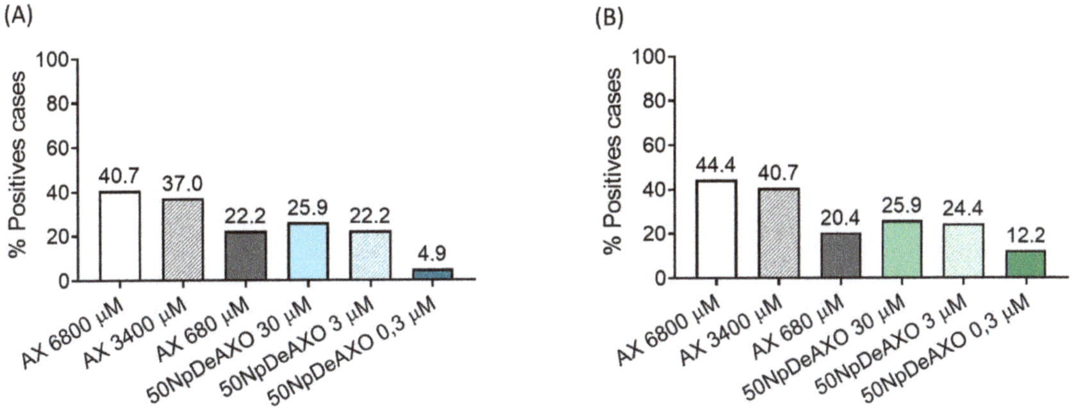

Figure 6. Percentage of positive cases in allergic patients (N = 54) in BAT using CD63 (**A**) and CD203c^{high} (**B**) as basophil activation markers. Positive cases were obtained after using the cut-offs described in Table S4 for AX and **50NpDeAXO** at the different concentrations with both CD63 and CD203c.

4. Conclusions

The accurate in vitro diagnosis of BL allergy is a continuing challenge affecting both outpatient and hospital care. By employing a combination of Nps with DeAns instead of the free drug as stimulus, a novel approach to perform the BAT has been developed and studied for first time on human samples. Our results have established that DeAXO-decorated Nps (**NpDeAXO**) of 50 nm in size are effective triggers of basophils from patients with allergy to AX. Moreover, a fully covered surface with DeAXO on Nps is relevant for the spacing between any two AXO moieties to be optimal for the sIgE cross-linking on the basophil surface.

Through this proof-of-concept study, we have demonstrated that **NpDeAXO** Nps are able to induce a more efficient basophil activation than the free AX molecule, as a more than 20-fold lower concentration induces equal or higher levels of basophil activation. This means that AX in the context of the Np system, in comparison with free AX, is better recognized in a more effective way. This indicates that both the availability and the distribution of the AXO antigenic determinants in the dendrimers supported on the Nps is optimal for the efficient immune recognition that takes place in the assay. This demonstrates that Nps can be precise platforms for investigating the suitable size for successful basophil activation and degranulation. Moreover, we have also confirmed that another critical factor in increasing basophil reactivity is the number of AXO units covering the Np. Since the maximum functionalization of the Np surface has already been achieved, the only strategy to increase this hapten density could lie in increasing the number of Nps in the assay (Np concentration). However, the high concentration of Nps affects the stability of the Np dispersions, limiting flow-cytometry measurements. Therefore, further work is needed to overcome the only limitation presented in this study by the nanoparticles: the possibility of increasing the concentration of either Nps or AXO determinants in the assay to achieve more stable dispersions capable of accurate flow-cytometry, which would undoubtedly increase the sensitivity of the test. This work constitutes a starting point for this new approach to BAT-type assays, which, however, requires further optimization of the system for application in clinical practice.

Supplementary Materials: The following supporting information can be downloaded at: https://www.mdpi.com/article/10.3390/pharmaceutics16081039/s1, Figure S1: TEM images and size distribution (determined by DLS; bottom line) of the obtained Nps: (a) **20dNp**; (b) **30dNp**; (c) **50dNp**; (d) **50Np**; Figure S2: FSC vs. SSC FACS dot plots of samples treated with free AX at 6800, 3400, and 680 μM and **50NpDeAXO** at 300, 30, and 3 μM of AXO. The debris smear observed at the highest concentration of Nps tested is depicted by a red ellipse. NS: non-stimulated, fMLP: N-Formylmethionyl-leucyl-phenylalanine, aIgE: anti-immunoglobulin E antibody; Figure S3. Viability of AX and **50NpDeAXO**-treated basophils. HC and AP samples were treated with free AX or **50NpDeAXO** at the concentrations used in the BAT and stained with L/D viability fluorescent dye and analyzed by FACS. (**A**) Representative plots of gating strategy and analysis. (B) % Viability of the low signal region of the plots (mean +/− SD). NS: non-stimulated, fMLP: N-Formylmethionyl-leucyl-phenylalanine, aIgE: anti-immunoglobulin E antibody; Figure S4: CD63 and CD203c^{high} ROC curves of free AX and **50NpDeAXO** at three different concentrations; Figure S5: DLS spectrum of a dispersion of **50NpDeAXO** 3 hours after its preparation; Figure S6: DLS spectrum of a dispersion of **50NpDeAXO** 4 hours after its preparation; Figure S7: DLS spectrum of a dispersion of **50NpDeAXO** 5 hours after its preparation; Figure S8: FSC *vs* SSC FACS dot plots of samples treated with free AX at 6800, 3400 and 680 μM and **50NpDeAXO** at at 300, 30 and 3 μM of AXO. The debris smear observed at the highest concentration of Nps tested is depicted by a red ellipse. NS: non-stimulated, fMLP: N-Formylmethionyl-leucyl-phenylalanine, aIgE: anti-Immunoglobulin E antibody; Figure S9: Viability of AX and **50NpDeAXO**-treated basophils. HC and AP samples were treated with free AX or **50NpDeAXO** at the concentrations used in the BAT and stained with L/D viability fluorescent dye, and analysed by FACS. A) representative plots of gating strategy and analysis, B) % Viability of the low signal region of the plots (mean +/- SD). NS: non-stimulated, fMLP: N-Formylmethionyl-leucyl-phenylalanine, aIgE: anti-Immunoglobulin E antibody; Figure S10: CD63 and CD203chigh ROC curves of free AX and **50NpDeAXO** at three different concentrations; Table S1: Chemical properties of the prepared Nps in dispersion; Table S2: Chemical properties of the prepared solid Nps; Table S3: Characteristics of the AX-allergic cohort; Table S4: AUC, cut-off, sensitivity, specificity with the corresponding 95% CI and the *p*-value of (**A**) free AX and (B) 50NpDeAXO at three different concentrations, using CD63 or CD203^{c}high basophil activation markers. * $p < 0.05$, ** $p < 0.01$.

Author Contributions: Y.V. and M.I.M. conceived and designed the experiments; E.M. and V.G.-O. performed the chemical synthesis, characterization and analysis of the nanoparticles (both in dispersion and solid state); S.C.-S., J.A.C., R.F.-S., and C.F. performed cellular tests and analyzed BAT data (determination of optimal concentrations, cell viability measurements and statistical analysis); M.J.T. evaluated and selected patients and controls; Y.V., M.I.M., C.F., and C.M. analyzed all the data and wrote the paper with input from E.P.-I. and M.J.T. All authors have read and agreed to the published version of the manuscript.

Funding: This work was supported by the Spanish Ministerio de Ciencia e Innovación (Proyectos de I+D+I «Programación Conjunta Internacional», EuroNanoMed 2019 (PCI2019-111825-2), Ministerio de Ciencia e Innovación (PID2022-136705NB-I00, CNS2022-136144), Instituto de Salud Carlos III

(ISCIII) (through projects co-funded by the European Union: AC19/00082, PI21/00329, PI20/01734, PI23/00620, RETICS ARADYAL RD16/0006/0001 and RD16/0006/0012, RICORS Red de Enfermedades Inflamatorias RD21/0002/0008); Junta de Andalucía (ProyExcel00971 and PE-0172-2018, all co-funded by the European Union). C.M. holds "Nicolas Monardes" research contract by Andalusian Regional Ministry Health (Grant No. RC-0004-2021). This project has received funding from the European Union's Horizon 2020 research and innovation programme under the Marie Sklodowska-Curie grant agreement No 101027955. S.C.-S. holds a grant from the Ministry of Economic Transformation, Industry, Knowledge, and Universities of the Andalusian Regional Government under the predoctoral contract with reference PREDOC_01545.

Institutional Review Board Statement: This study was conducted in accordance with the Declaration of Helsinki and approved by the Provincial Ethics Committee of Malaga (AC19/00082, 26/03/2020).

Informed Consent Statement: All subjects included were informed and signed the informed consent to participate in the study.

Data Availability Statement: Data is contained within the article or Supplementary Material.

Acknowledgments: NMR experiments have been performed in the ICTS "NANBIOSIS", more specifically by the U28 Unit at the Instituto de Investigación Biomédica de Málaga y Plataforma en Nanomedicina—IBIMA, Plataforma Bionand.

Conflicts of Interest: The authors declare no conflicts of interest.

References

1. Brunetti, V.; Bouchet, L.M.; Strumia, M.C. Nanoparticle-Cored Dendrimers: Functional Hybrid Nanocomposites as a New Platform for Drug Delivery Systems. *Nanoscale* **2015**, *7*, 3808–3816. [CrossRef]
2. Shen, M.; Shi, X. Dendrimer-Based Organic/Inorganic Hybrid Nanoparticles in Biomedical Applications. *Nanoscale* **2010**, *2*, 1596–1610. [CrossRef] [PubMed]
3. Mayorga, C.; Perez-Inestrosa, E.; Molina, N.; Montañez, M.I. Development of Nanostructures in the Diagnosis of Drug Hypersensitivity Reactions. *Curr. Opin. Allergy Clin. Immunol.* **2016**, *16*, 300–307. [CrossRef] [PubMed]
4. Mayorga, C.; Perez-Inestrosa, E.; Rojo, J.; Ferrer, M.; Montañez, M.I. Role of Nanostructures in Allergy: Diagnostics, Treatments and Safety. *Allergy* **2021**, *76*, 3292–3306. [CrossRef]
5. Uetrecht, J. Immune-Mediated Adverse Drug Reactions. *Chem. Res. Toxicol.* **2009**, *22*, 24–34. [CrossRef]
6. Uetrecht, J. Idiosyncratic Drug Reactions: Past, Present, and Future. *Chem. Res. Toxicol.* **2008**, *21*, 84–92. [CrossRef] [PubMed]
7. Doña, I.; Labella, M.; Bogas, G.; Sáenz de Santa María, R.; Salas, M.; Ariza, A.; Torres, M.J. Antibiotic Allergy De-Labeling: A Pathway against Antibiotic Resistance. *Antibiotics* **2022**, *11*, 1055. [CrossRef]
8. Macy, E.; Contreras, R. Health Care Use and Serious Infection Prevalence Associated with Penicillin "Allergy" in Hospitalized Patients: A Cohort Study. *J. Allergy Clin. Immunol.* **2014**, *133*, 790–796. [CrossRef]
9. Doña, I.; Torres, M.J.; Montañez, M.I.; Fernández, T.D. In Vitro Diagnostic Testing for Antibiotic Allergy. *Allergy. Asthma Immunol. Res.* **2017**, *9*, 288–298. [CrossRef]
10. Mayorga, C.; Celik, G.; Rouzaire, P.; Whitaker, P.; Bonadonna, P.; Rodrigues-Cernadas, J.; Vultaggio, A.; Brockow, K.; Caubet, J.C.; Makowska, J.; et al. In Vitro Tests for Drug Hypersensitivity Reactions: An ENDA/EAACI Drug Allergy Interest Group Position Paper. *Allergy* **2016**, *71*, 1103–1134. [CrossRef]
11. Ebo, D.G.; Bridts, C.H.; Mertens, C.H.; Sabato, V. Principles, Potential, and Limitations of Ex Vivo Basophil Activation by Flow Cytometry in Allergology: A Narrative Review. *J. Allergy Clin. Immunol.* **2021**, *147*, 1143–1153. [CrossRef] [PubMed]
12. Santos, A.F.; Alpan, O.; Hoffmann, H.J. Basophil Activation Test: Mechanisms and Considerations for Use in Clinical Trials and Clinical Practice. *Allergy* **2021**, *76*, 2420–2432. [CrossRef] [PubMed]
13. Paar, J.M.; Harris, N.T.; Holowka, D.; Baird, B. Bivalent Ligands with Rigid Double-Stranded DNA Spacers Reveal Structural Constraints on Signaling by FcεRI. *J. Immunol.* **2002**, *169*, 856–864. [CrossRef]
14. Miyake, K.; Shibata, S.; Yoshikawa, S.; Karasuyama, H. Basophils and Their Effector Molecules in Allergic Disorders. *Allergy* **2021**, *76*, 1693–1706. [CrossRef] [PubMed]
15. Ariza, A.; Collado, D.; Vida, Y.; Montañez, M.I.; Pérez-Inestrosa, E.; Blanca, M.; Torres, M.J.; Cañada, F.J.; Pérez-Sala, D. Study of Protein Haptenation by Amoxicillin Through the Use of a Biotinylated Antibiotic. *PLoS ONE* **2014**, *9*, e90891. [CrossRef]
16. Torres, M.J.; Montañez, M.I.; Ariza, A.; Salas, M.; Fernandez, T.D.; Barbero, N.; Mayorga, C.; Blanca, M. The Role of IgE Recognition in Allergic Reactions to Amoxicillin and Clavulanic Acid. *Clin. Exp. Allergy* **2016**, *46*, 264–274. [CrossRef]
17. Montañez, M.I.; Perez-Inestrosa, E.; Suau, R.; Mayorga, C.; Torres, M.J.; Blanca, M. Dendrimerized Cellulose as a Scaffold for Artificial Antigens with Applications in Drug Allergy Diagnosis. *Biomacromolecules* **2008**, *9*, 1461–1466. [CrossRef]
18. Montañez, M.I.; Najera, F.; Perez-Inestrosa, E. NMR Studies and Molecular Dynamic Simulation of Synthetic Dendritic Antigens. *Polymers* **2011**, *3*, 1533–1553. [CrossRef]

19. Montañez, M.I.; Najera, F.; Mayorga, C.; Ruiz-Sanchez, A.J.; Vida, Y.; Collado, D.; Blanca, M.; Torres, M.J.; Perez-Inestrosa, E. Recognition of Multiepitope Dendrimeric Antigens by Human Immunoglobulin E. *Nanomed. Nanotechnol. Biol. Med.* **2015**, *11*, 579–588. [CrossRef]
20. Molina, N.; Martin-Serrano, A.; Fernandez, T.D.; Tesfaye, A.; Najera, F.; Torres, M.J.; Mayorga, C.; Vida, Y.; Montanez, M.I.; Perez-Inestrosa, E. Dendrimeric Antigens for Drug Allergy Diagnosis: A New Approach for Basophil Activation Tests. *Molecules* **2018**, *23*, 997. [CrossRef]
21. Huang, Y.F.; Liu, H.; Xiong, X.; Chen, Y.; Tan, W. Nanoparticle-Mediated IgE-Receptor Aggregation and Signaling in RBL Mast Cells. *J. Am. Chem. Soc.* **2009**, *131*, 17328–17334. [CrossRef] [PubMed]
22. Tesfaye, A.; Rodríguez-Nogales, A.; Benedé, S.; Fernández, T.D.; Paris, J.L.; Rodriguez, M.J.; Jiménez-Sánchez, I.M.; Bogas, G.; Mayorga, C.; Torres, M.J.; et al. Nanoarchitectures for Efficient IgE Cross-Linking on Effector Cells to Study Amoxicillin Allergy. *Allergy* **2021**, *76*, 3183–3193. [CrossRef] [PubMed]
23. Baird, E.J.; Holowka, D.; Coates, G.W.; Baird, B. Highly Effective Poly(Ethylene Glycol) Architectures for Specific Inhibition of Immune Receptor Activation. *Biochemistry* **2003**, *42*, 12739–12748. [CrossRef] [PubMed]
24. Gieras, A.; Linhart, B.; Roux, K.H.; Dutta, M.; Khodoun, M.; Zafred, D.; Cabauatan, C.R.; Lupinek, C.; Weber, M.; Focke-Tejkl, M.; et al. IgE Epitope Proximity Determines Immune Complex Shape and Effector Cell Activation Capacity. *J. Allergy Clin. Immunol.* **2016**, *137*, 1557–1565. [CrossRef] [PubMed]
25. Gil-Ocaña, V.; Jimenez, I.M.; Mayorga, C.; Doña, I.; Céspedes, J.A.; Montañez, M.I.; Vida, Y.; Torres, M.J.; Perez-Inestrosa, E. Multiepitope Dendrimeric Antigen-Silica Particle Composites as Nano-Based Platforms for Specific Recognition of IgEs. *Front. Immunol.* **2021**, *12*, 750109. [CrossRef]
26. Vida, Y.; Montañez, M.I.; Collado, D.; Najera, F.; Ariza, A.; Blanca, M.; Torres, M.J.; Mayorga, C.; Perez-Inestrosa, E. Dendrimeric Antigen–Silica Particle Composites: An Innovative Approach for IgE Quantification. *J. Mater. Chem. B* **2013**, *1*, 3044–3050. [CrossRef] [PubMed]
27. Pascal, M.; Edelman, S.M.; Nopp, A.; Möbs, C.; Geilenkeuser, W.J.; Knol, E.F.; Ebo, D.G.; Mertens, C.; Shamji, M.H.; Santos, A.F.; et al. EAACI Task Force Report: A Consensus Protocol for the Basophil Activation Test for Collaboration and External Quality Assurance. *Allergy* **2024**, *79*, 290–293. [CrossRef] [PubMed]
28. Moore, S. Amino Acid Analysis: Aqueous Dimethyl Sulfoxide as Solvent for the Ninhydrin Reaction. *J. Biol. Chem.* **1968**, *243*, 6281–6283. [CrossRef]
29. Riccò, R.; Nizzero, S.; Penna, E.; Meneghello, A.; Cretaio, E.; Enrichi, F. Ultra-Small Dye-Doped Silica Nanoparticles via Modified Sol-Gel Technique. *J. Nanoparticle Res.* **2018**, *20*, 117. [CrossRef]
30. Cornejo-Monroy, D.; Sánchez-Ramírez, J.F.; Pescador Rojas, J.A.; Herrera-Pérez, J.L.; González- Araoz, M.P.; Guarneros, C. Nanoesferas Monodispersas de SiO2: Síntesis Controlada y Caracterización. *Superf. y Vacío* **2009**, *22*, 44–48.
31. Jafarzadeh, M.; Rahman, I.A.; Sipaut, C.S. Synthesis of Silica Nanoparticles by Modified Sol-Gel Process: The Effect of Mixing Modes of the Reactants and Drying Techniques. *J. Sol-Gel Sci. Technol.* **2009**, *50*, 328–336. [CrossRef]
32. Jia, G.; Ji, Z.; Wang, H.; Chen, R. Preparation and Properties of Five-Layer Graded-Refractive-Index Antireflection Coating Nanostructured by Solid and Hollow Silica Particles. *Thin Solid Films* **2017**, *642*, 174–181. [CrossRef]
33. Ruiz-Sanchez, A.J.; Montañez, M.I.; Mayorga, C.; Torres, M.J.; Kehr, N.S.; Vida, Y.; Collado, D.; Najera, F.; De Cola, L.; Perez-Inestrosa, E. Dendrimer-Modified Solid Supports: Nanostructured Materials with Potential Drug Allergy Diagnostic Applications. *Curr. Med. Chem.* **2012**, *19*, 4942–4954. [CrossRef] [PubMed]
34. Romano, A.; Atanaskovic-Markovic, M.; Barbaud, A.; Bircher, A.J.; Brockow, K.; Caubet, J.C.; Celik, G.; Cernadas, J.; Chiriac, A.M.; Demoly, P.; et al. Towards a More Precise Diagnosis of Hypersensitivity to Beta-Lactams—An EAACI Position Paper. *Allergy* **2020**, *75*, 1300–1315. [CrossRef]
35. Brown, S.G.A. Clinical Features and Severity Grading of Anaphylaxis. *J. Allergy Clin. Immunol.* **2004**, *114*, 371–376. [CrossRef] [PubMed]
36. Aberer, W.; Bircher, A.; Romano, A.; Blanca, M.; Campi, P.; Fernandez, J.; Brockow, K.; Pichler, W.J.; Demoly, P. Drug Provocation Testing in the Diagnosis of Drug Hypersensitivity Reactions: General Considerations. *Allergy* **2003**, *58*, 854–863. [CrossRef] [PubMed]
37. Sonder, S.U.; Plassmeyer, M.; Loizou, D.; Alpan, O. Towards Standardizing Basophil Identification by Flow Cytometry. *Front. Allergy* **2023**, *4*, 1133378. [CrossRef] [PubMed]
38. Stöber, W.; Fink, A.; Bohn, E. Controlled Growth of Monodisperse Silica Spheres in the Micron Size Range. *J. Colloid Interface Sci.* **1968**, *26*, 62–69. [CrossRef]
39. Tadanaga, K.; Morita, K.; Mori, K.; Tatsumisago, M. Synthesis of Monodispersed Silica Nanoparticles with High Concentration by the Stöber Process. *J. Sol-Gel Sci. Technol.* **2013**, *68*, 341–345. [CrossRef]

pharmaceutics

MDPI

Article

Structural Optimization of Carboxy-Terminal Phenylalanine-Modified Dendrimers for T-Cell Association and Model Drug Loading

Hiroya Shiba [1], Tomoka Hirose [1], Akinobu Sakai [1], Ikuhiko Nakase [2], Akikazu Matsumoto [1] and Chie Kojima [1,*,†]

1 Department of Applied Chemistry, Graduate School of Engineering, Osaka Metropolitan University, 1-1 Gakuen-cho, Naka-ku, Sakai 599-8531, Osaka, Japan

2 Department of Biological Science, Graduate School of Science, Osaka Metropolitan University, 1-1 Gakuen-cho, Naka-ku, Sakai 599-8531, Osaka, Japan

* Correspondence: kojima.c.ac@m.titech.ac.jp

† Current address: Department of Materials Science and Engineering, School of Materials and Chemical Technology, Tokyo Institute of Technology, 4259 Nagatsuta-cho, Midori-ku, Yokohama 226-8503, Kanagawa, Japan.

Abstract: Dendrimers are potent nanocarriers in drug delivery systems because their structure can be precisely controlled. We previously reported that polyamidoamine (PAMAM) dendrimers that were modified with 1,2-cyclohexanedicarboxylic acid (CHex) and phenylalanine (Phe), PAMAM-CHex-Phe, exhibited an effective association with various immune cells, including T-cells. In this study, we synthesized various carboxy-terminal Phe-modified dendrimers with different linkers using phthalic acid and linear dicarboxylic acids to determine the association of these dendrimers with Jurkat cells, a T-cell model. PAMAM-*n*-hexyl-Phe demonstrated the highest association with Jurkat T-cells. In addition, dendri-graft polylysine (DGL) with CHex and Phe, DGL-CHex-Phe, was synthesized, and its association with Jurkat cells was investigated. The association of DGL-CHex-Phe with T-cells was higher than that of PAMAM-CHex-Phe. However, it was insoluble in water and thus it is unsuitable as a drug carrier. Model drugs, such as protoporphyrin IX and paclitaxel, were loaded onto these dendrimers, and the most model drug molecules could be loaded into PAMAM-CHex-Phe. PTX-loaded PAMAM-CHex-Phe exhibited cytotoxicity against Jurkat cells at a similar level to free PTX. These results suggest that PAMAM-CHex-Phe exhibited both efficient T-cell association and drug loading properties.

Keywords: dendrimer; drug delivery system; encapsulation; phenylalanine; T-cells

1. Introduction

The design of nanocarriers is important in drug delivery systems (DDSs). Precisely designed nanocarriers deliver bioactive compounds to target T-cells to enhance pharmacological effects and reduce side effects [1–3]. Various nanocarriers have been studied [4–6], and dendrimers are promising nano-sized materials. Because dendrimers are produced through stepwise reactions, their molecular weight, particle size, and surface charge can be controlled [7,8]. Dendrimers can also incorporate or modify various bioactive compounds within their internal space or at their surface [9,10]. Thus, dendrimers have been extensively studied as potential DDS nanocarriers. There are many kinds of dendrimers, such as polyamidoamine (PAMAM), polypropyleneimine, and polyester dendrimers [11–13]. Polylysine dendrimers and dendri-graft polylysines (DGLs) are also dendritic polymers, and because these are composed of lysine, they are useful as biomaterials with excellent biocompatibility [14,15]. PAMAM dendrimers and DGLs are commercially available, and PAMAM dendrimers have been extensively studied for anticancer drug and gene delivery [16,17].

T-cells play a vital role in our immune system, which determines the quantity and quality of the immune response against foreign invading substances or pathogens. Thus, the regulation of T-cell functions is important for the treatment and prevention of various diseases, which is attractive for immunotherapy [18–21]. For example, immune checkpoint inhibitors are used to enhance T-cell responses to diseased cells [22,23], and chimeric antigen receptor (CAR)-T-cells, which are genetically engineered T-cells, have been developed [24,25]. T-cell lymphocytic leukemia is one of the target diseased cells that should receive treatment. Thus, the establishment of a DDS for therapeutic materials to T-cells is required. Although antibodies and viruses have been studied for the delivery of therapeutic materials to T-cells, it remains challenging to efficiently deliver them inside the T-cells using nonviral materials [26].

Previously, we reported that PAMAM dendrimers with different anionic terminals containing carboxylate, sulfonate, or phosphate were highly accumulated in lymph nodes [27]. Although carboxy- and sulfo-terminal dendrimers did not efficiently associate with any immune cells, the dendrimers with both 1,2-cyclohexanedicarboxylic acid (CHex) and phenylalanine (Phe) at the termini (PAMAM-CHex-Phe and PAMAM-Phe-CHex) were highly associated with immune cells, including T-cells and their subsets [27,28]. We further revealed that these dendrimers were suitable for delivering protoporphyrin IX (PpIX) and plasmid DNA to T-cells [29,30]. It was previously reported that the Phe residues of the dendrimers influenced the association with T-cells, and it was determined that the highest T-cell association was at a 75% Phe density [29]. In this study, we attempted to optimize the dendrimer structure for the association with T-cells and model drug loading. Aromatic phthalic acid (Ph) and linear dicarboxylic acids with different lengths were used as the linker instead of CHex to evaluate the effect of the linker structure on the interaction with T-cells. We also synthesized DGLs modified with CHex and Phe to investigate the interaction with T-cells and elucidate the effect of the core structure (Figure 1). Furthermore, PpIX and paclitaxel (PTX) were used as model drugs, and the drug loading ability of these dendrimers was investigated.

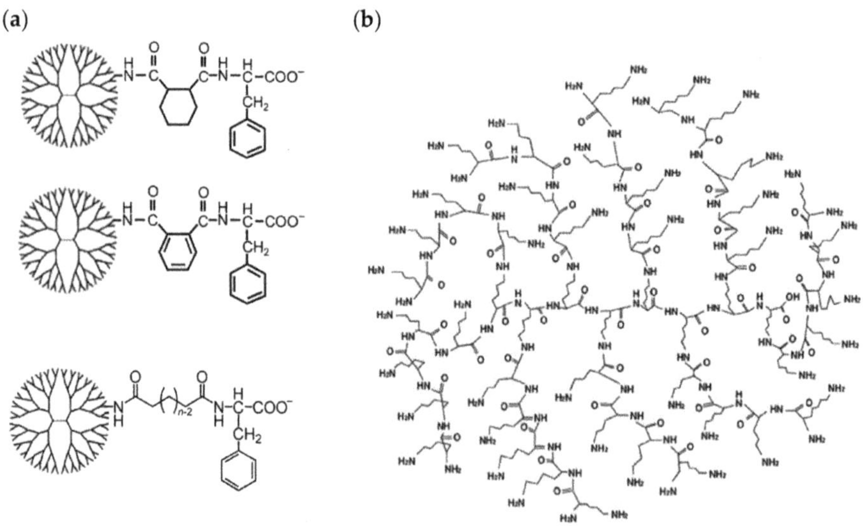

Figure 1. Structures of (**a**) carboxy-terminal phenylalanine (Phe)-modified PAMAM dendrimers used in this study and (**b**) DGL of G2.

2. Materials and Methods

2.1. Synthesis

PAMAM-CHex-Phe synthesized in our previous study was used [29]. PAMAM-Ph-Phe was synthesized, as shown in our previous report [31]. Briefly, 170 mg (12.0 μmol) of amino-functional ethylenediamine core PAMAM dendrimer of G4 (Sigma-Aldrich Co., St.

Louis, MO, USA) was dissolved in dimethyl sulfoxide (DMSO)/*N*,*N*-dimethyl formamide (DMF) mixture (4 mL, 5/1 in vol ratio) and then excess phthalic anhydride (FUJIFILM Wako Pure Chemical Co., Osaka, Japan, 1.0 g, 6.8 mmol) and triethylamine (TEA, 600 μL, 4.3 mmol) were added to the solution. The mixture was stirred overnight at ambient temperature (approximately 25 °C), and the reaction mixture was dialyzed (MWCO 2k) in DMSO and then water for purification. PAMAM-Ph was obtained after lyophilization, whose yield was
198 mg (64%). Then, PAMAM-Ph (100 mg, 3.9 μmol) was dissolved in 5 mL of DMSO, and then 0.24 g (0.56 mmol) of L-Phe methyl ester hydrochloride (Phe-OMe·HCl, Nacalai Tesque, Inc., Kyoto, Japan), 0.20 g (0.53 mmol) of [benzotriazol-1-yloxy(dimethylamino)methylidene]-dimethylazanium hexafluorophosphate (HBTU, Watanabe Chemical Industries, Ltd., Hiroshima, Japan), and 70 μL (0.50 mmol) of TEA were added to the dendrimer solution and stirred for 4 days at ambient temperature. The dendrimer was dialyzed in DMSO and then methanol. PAMAM-Ph-Phe-OMe was obtained after lyophilization, whose yield was 123 mg (98%). Then, deprotection was performed, as follows. PAMAM-Ph-Phe-OMe (123 mg, 3.8 μmol) was dissolved in 4 mL of methanol, and 0.5 mL of 4 M NaOH methanol solution was added. After stirring for 3 h in an ice bath, the reaction mixture was dialyzed in water for purification. PAMAM-Ph-Phe was obtained after lyophilization, whose yield was 87 mg (71%).

PAMAM-C_6-Phe was synthesized, as follows. An amount of 40 mg (2.8 μmol) of amino-terminal G4 PAMAM dendrimer was dissolved in DMSO, and about 140 equivalents of monomethyl suberate (Tokyo Chemical Industry Co., Ltd., Toyo, Japan), 100 equivalents of HBTU, and 100 equivalents of TEA were added to the dendrimer solution and stirred for 4 days at ambient temperature. The dendrimer solution was dialyzed in methanol for purification and lyophilized to obtain PAMAM-C_6-OMe, whose yield was 71 mg (89%). Then, the deprotection of PAMAM-C_6-OMe was performed, as described above. PAMAM-C_6 was obtained after lyophilization, whose yield was 61 mg (92%). Then, PAMAM-C_6 (55 mg, 2.1 μmol) was dissolved in 5 mL of DMSO and L-Phe benzyl ester 4-toluenesulfonate salt (Phe-OBzl·Tos, Peptide Institute, Inc., Osaka, Japan, 0.14 g, 0.35 mmol), HBTU (0.1 g, 0.27 mmol), and TEA (45 μL, 0.32 mmol) were added to the dendrimer solution and stirred for 4 days at ambient temperature. The dendrimer solution was dialyzed in methanol. Lyophilization was carried out to obtain PAMAM-C_6-Phe-OBzl, whose yield was 78 mg (76%). Then, the deprotection of PAMAM-C_6-Phe-OBzl was performed, as described above. PAMAM-C_6-Phe was obtained after lyophilization (64.3 mg, 62%). PAMAM-C_4-Phe and PAMAM-C_8-Phe were synthesized in accordance with the procedure of PAMAM-C_6-Phe by replacing monomethyl suberate with monomethyl adipate (Tokyo Chemical Industry) and monomethyl sebacate (Tokyo Chemical Industry), respectively. The yields of PAMAM-C_4-Phe-OBzl, PAMAM-C_8-Phe-OBzl, PAMAM-C_4-Phe and PAMAM-C_8-Phe were 66 mg (67%), 61 mg (57%), 59 mg (59%) and 49 mg (45%), respectively.

DGL-CHex-Phe was synthesized, as follows. An amount of 100 mg (11.6 μmol) of generation 2 (G2) of DGL (COLCOM, Montarnaud, France) was dissolved in 5 mL of 125 mM $NaHCO_3$ aqueous solution, and then about 150 equivalents of cis-1,2-cyclohexanedicarboxylic anhydride (Tokyo Chemical Industry) were added. The pH of the DGL solution was adjusted to about 9 using 4 M NaOH aqueous solution. After stirring for 1 day at ambient temperature, the DGL solution was dialyzed in 125 mM $NaHCO_3$ aqueous solution and then water. DGL-CHex was obtained after lyophilization (133.8 mg, 68%). Then, DGL-CHex (96.5 mg, 5.7 μmol) was dispersed in DMSO for 1 day and Phe-OBzl·Tos (176.4 mg, 0.41 mmol), HBTU (171.1 mg, 0.45 mmol), and TEA (113 μL, 0.82 mmol) were added to the DGL solution and stirred for 2 days at room temperature. DGL-CHex-Phe-OBzl was precipitated by adding HCl aqueous solution. After drying under vacuum conditions, DGL-CHex-Phe-OBzl was obtained, whose yield was 126 mg (81%). Then, deprotection of DGL-CHex-Phe-OBzl was performed, as described above. DGL-CHex-Phe was obtained after lyophilization (116 mg, 85%).

Fluorescein isothiocyanate (FITC, Tokyo Chemical Industry)-labeled PAMAM-CHex and PAMAM-CHex-Phe synthesized in our previous reports were used [29]. Other dendrimers were labeled with FITC in the same procedure as our previous report [29]. Briefly, 5–10 mg of dendrimers was dissolved in 0.5 mL of 100 mM $NaHCO_3$ aqueous solution, and 6–10 equivalents of *N*-(2-aminoethyl) carbamic acid *tert*-butyl ester (Tokyo Chemical Industry) and 6 equivalents of 4-(4,6-dimethoxy-1,3,5-triazin-2-yl)-4-methylmorpholinium chloride (DMT-MM, FUJIFILM Wako Pure Chemical) were added to the dendrimer solutions and stirred overnight at ambient temperature. The dendrimer solutions were ultrafiltrated for purification by Amicon®Ultra (MWCO 3 kDa, Merck Millipore, Darmstadt, Germany) using 125 mM $NaHCO_3$ aqueous solution and water. Then, the deprotection of *tert*-butoxycarbonyl (Boc) group by the treatment with 1 mL of trifluoroacetic acid (TFA, FUJIFILM Wako Pure Chemical) for 3 h in an ice bath was performed. After the removal of TFA and drying under vacuum conditions, these dendrimers were dissolved in 1 mL of DMSO. An amount of 15 equivalents of FITC to the dendrimer and excess TEA were added to the dendrimer solution. After stirring for two days at ambient temperature, the reaction mixtures were diluted with water until the concentration of DMSO was less than 2.5%. After purification by ultrafiltration (MWCO 3 kDa) and the following lyophilization, FITC-labeled dendrimers were obtained.

2.2. Characterization

Proton nuclear magnetic resonance (^{1}H-NMR) spectra were recorded on a JNM-ECX (JEOL Ltd., Tokyo, Japan) spectrometer at a resonance frequency of 400 MHz at ambient temperature in glass tubes to estimate the bound numbers of Phe and the linker compound to the dendrimer. The UV–Vis spectra were measured by using a Jasco Model V630 UV/Vis spectrophotometer (JASCO Inc., Tokyo, Japan) to estimate the bound number of FITC to the dendrimer from the calibration curve and the absorbance at 513 nm in the spectra. The Log p (octanol/water partition coefficient) value was calculated by using ChemDraw (PerkinElmer Inc., Shelton, CT, USA).

2.3. Association of Dendrimers with Jurkat Cells

The association of dendrimers synthesized in this report with Jurkat cells was investigated by using GUAVA® InCyte™ (Luminex, Austin, TX, USA), according to our previous report [29]. Briefly, each FITC-labeled PAMAM-CHex, PAMAM-CHex-Phe and PAMAM-Ph-Phe, PAMAM-C_4-Phe, PAMAM-C_6-Phe, PAMAM-C_8-Phe, DGL-CHex, and DGL-CHex-Phe was added to RPMI (FITC 5 μM). Because DGL-CHex-Phe was not soluble in water, 500 μM of DGL-CHex-Phe-containing DMSO solution was prepared and diluted with RPMI. The dendrimer solutions were added to 1×10^5 Jurkat cells and incubated for 3 h at 37 °C. Then, phosphate-buffered saline (PBS) was added to the cell suspension and centrifuged to collect the cells. After washing with PBS (400 μL) once, fluorescence-activated cell sorting (FACS) was performed to measure the mean green fluorescence intensity.

2.4. Adsorption of Dendrimers onto Liposomes

The adsorption of dendrimers onto liposomes was performed according to the method, as we previously reported [29]. Briefly, hydrogenated soy phosphatidylcholine (HSPC, NOF Corp., Tokyo, Japan, 10 mg/mL) dispersed in chloroform solution was dried overnight under vacuum conditions. Then, the dried solid was dissolved in 0.1 M 4-(2-hydroxyethyl)-1-piperazineethanesulfonic acid (HEPES) buffer (pH 7.4) and sonicated for 2 min using a bath sonicator (ASU-6, AS ONE Corp., Osaka, Japan) to obtain the dispersed liposomes (HSPC, 1.6 mg/mL). Then, 25 μL of the FITC-labeled PAMAM dendrimer-containing aqueous solutions (100 μM FITC) was mixed with 475 μL of the liposome solution and incubated for 3 h at 37 °C. The centrifugation (11,000 rpm for 15 min at 37 °C) was carried out to precipitate liposomes, and liposomes were washed with HEPES buffer. Then, chloroform/methanol (1/1, 0.5 mL) was added and shaken for 20 min at 37 °C to dissolve liposomes. The fluorescence intensity was measured to estimate the adsorption of these dendrimers to liposomes by using an FP-6200 spectrofluorometer (JASCO Inc.). The excitation and emission wavelengths were measured at 495 nm and 520 nm, respectively. The adsorption ratio of dendrimer to liposomes was calculated from the fluorescence intensity ratio of the solution before and after liposome treatment.

2.5. Model Structure of the Dendrimers

The molecular structure of the 4-terminal PAMAM dendrimers with Phe and linkers, such as CHex, Ph, and C_6, in water was calculated using Spartan 08 (Wavefunction Inc., Irvine, CA, USA).

2.6. Encapsulation of Model Drugs in PAMAM Dendrimers

The loading of PpIX in dendrimers was performed according to the method described in our previous report [29]. Briefly, PpIX (Sigma-Aldrich) and each dendrimer were dissolved in DMF, and mixed to adjust the mole ratio of PpIX/dendrimer at 10/1. The solution was then evaporated, dried under vacuum conditions, and dissolved in water (dendrimer 0.1 mM). The loaded PpIX in the dendrimer was collected from the supernatant after centrifugation, because free PpIX was insoluble in water. The UV–Vis spectrum of each supernatant was measured to estimate the amount of encapsulated PpIX. The amount of loaded PpIX was calculated from the calibration curve and absorbance at 406 nm.

The loading of PTX in the dendrimers was performed according to the method described in our previous report [32]. Briefly, PTX (Tokyo Chemical Industry) and each dendrimer were dissolved in methanol at a 5:1 mol ratio of PTX:dendrimer. The solution was then evaporated, dried under vacuum conditions, and dissolved in water (dendrimer 0.1 mM). PTX loaded in the dendrimer was collected from the supernatant after centrifugation. The amount of encapsulated PTX was estimated by HPLC analysis using the calibration curve. The same experiment was carried out by replacing water used after drying with saline as a solvent. After the incubation at room temperature (approximately at 25 °C) for 24 h, the supernatant was collected to measure the retained PTX in the solution.

2.7. Cytotoxicity of the PTX-Loaded Dendrimer

The cytotoxicity of the PTX-loaded PAMAM-CHex-Phe was examined, according to our previous report [30]. Briefly, free PTX and the PTX-loaded PAMAM-CHex-Phe prepared in Section 2.6 were added to 1×10^4 Jurkat cells in 100 μL of RPMI medium at a PTX concentration of 10 nM. After incubation for 48 h, cells were washed with PBS. Then, 5 mg/mL of 3-(4,5-dimethylthiazol-2-yl)-2,5-diphenyl-2H-tetrazolium bromide (MTT)-containing PBS solution (10 μL) and RPMI (90 μL) was added to the cells and incubated for 3 h. After centrifugation at 3000 rpm for 5 min, the supernatant was removed, and 0.1 M HCl-containing isopropyl alcohol (200 μL) was added to dissolve cells. The absorbance at 570 nm was measured to estimate the amount of cell viability. The cell viability (%) was calculated from the percentage of the absorbance of cells treated with the sample to that of intact cells. The cytotoxicity of Jurkat cells treated with 10 μM of the dendrimer without PTX for 24 h was also examined.

3. Results and Discussion

3.1. Synthesis of Carboxy-Terminal Phe-Modified Dendrimers

Firstly, carboxy-terminal Phe-modified PAMAM dendrimers with different linkers, such as CHex, Ph, C_4, C_6, and C_8, and DGL-CHex-Phe were synthesized (Figure 2). The amino-terminal PAMAM G4 dendrimer was reacted with an excess of acid anhydrides (CHex and Ph) or linear dicarboxylic acid monoesters (C_4, C_6, and C_8) to conjugate the different linkers. The hydrolysis of the ester group was carried out for dendrimers reacted with linear dicarboxylic acid monoesters. Then, Phe with a protective group at the carboxy-terminal was conjugated to the carboxy-termini of the dendrimers. The subsequent deprotection of the ester group was performed. DGL-CHex-Phe was synthesized using the same procedure as for PAMAM-CHex-Phe by replacing PAMAM with DGL. For comparison, carboxyl-terminal dendrimers without Phe, PAMAM-CHex, and DGL-CHex were also synthesized. The synthesized dendrimers were characterized by ^{1}H NMR spectroscopy. The average bound numbers of CHex, Ph, C_4, C_6, and C_8 were evaluated from the integral ratios of the signals at around 1.1–1.9 ppm for CHex, 7.2–7.8 ppm for Ph, 1.5–2.2 ppm for C_4–C_8, 4.2 ppm for Phe, 2.2 ppm for PAMAM dendrimer, and 4.1 ppm for DGL (Figures S1–S4), which are listed in Table 1. The terminal numbers of PAMAM G4 and DGL G2 were 64 and 48, respectively. The linker compounds and Phe were conjugated to the dendrimer at all termini. The dendrimers were then labeled with a green fluorescent dye, FITC. Two to nine FITC molecules were conjugated to each dendrimer after introducing small amounts of amino groups to the dendrimer according to the method described in our previous report (Table 1) [29]. These FITC-labeled dendrimers were used to investigate the associations with the cells and liposomes. The molecular weights of these dendrimers are also listed in Table 1. The molecular weights of the dendrimers increased after the Phe modification. The Phe-modified PAMAM dendrimers were similar, regardless of the linker compounds. The DGLs were smaller than the PAMAM dendrimers.

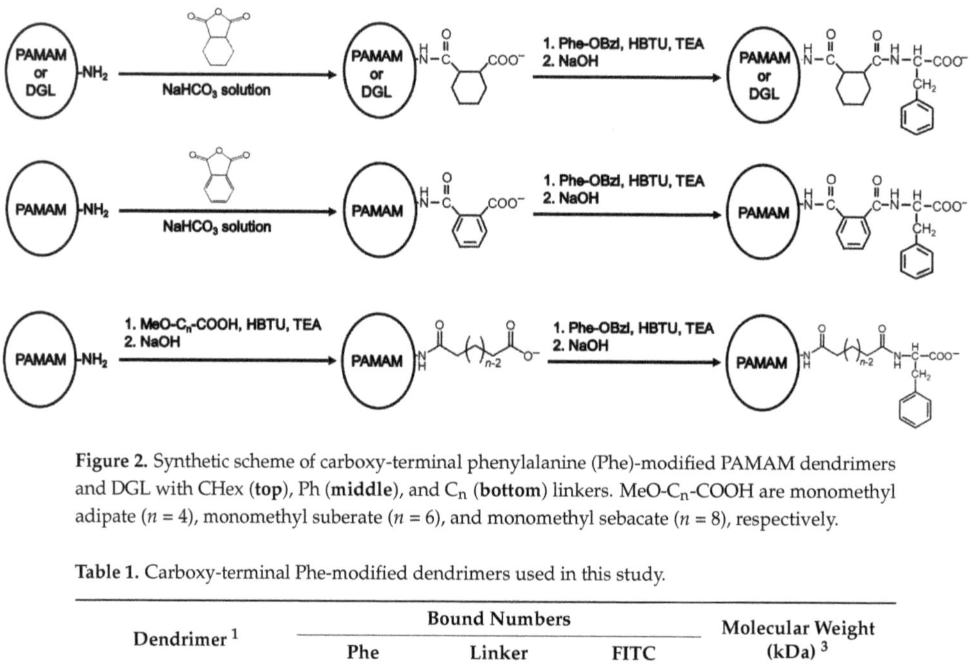

Figure 2. Synthetic scheme of carboxy-terminal phenylalanine (Phe)-modified PAMAM dendrimers and DGL with CHex (**top**), Ph (**middle**), and C_n (**bottom**) linkers. MeO-C_n-COOH are monomethyl adipate (n = 4), monomethyl suberate (n = 6), and monomethyl sebacate (n = 8), respectively.

Table 1. Carboxy-terminal Phe-modified dendrimers used in this study.

Dendrimer [1]	Bound Numbers			Molecular Weight (kDa) [3]
	Phe	Linker	FITC	
PAMAM-CHex [2]	0	64 (CHex)	4.0	24.0
PAMAM-CHex-Phe [2]	64	64 (CHex)	7.0	33.5
PAMAM-Ph-Phe	59	64 (Ph)	3.7	32.4
PAMAM-C_4-Phe	64	64 (C_4)	2.0	31.7
PAMAM-C_6-Phe	64	64 (C_6)	8.0	33.5
PAMAM-C_8-Phe	64	64 (C_8)	7.0	35.3
DGL-CHex	0	48 (CHex)	9.3	17.0
DGL-CHex-Phe	48	48 (CHex)	4.5	24.1

[1] The numbers of terminal groups of PAMAM and DGL are 64 and 48, respectively. [2] Refer to our previous reports [29]. [3] Calculated molecular weight of each dendrimer without FITC.

3.2. Association of Carboxy-Terminal Phe-Modified Dendrimers with Jurkat Cells

The association of dendrimers with Jurkat cells, as a T-cell model, was examined. The mean fluorescence intensity of the Jurkat cells treated with FITC-labeled PAMAM dendrimers was measured by FACS. Figure 3a shows that the mean fluorescence intensity of the carboxy-terminal Phe-modified PAMAM dendrimers containing linear C_4, C_6, and C_8 was higher than that of PAMAM-CHex-Phe and PAMAM-Ph-Phe. This indicates that the linear dicarboxylic acid-containing dendrimers associate with Jurkat cells more efficiently than PAMAM-CHex-Phe and PAMAM-Ph-Phe. PAMAM-C_6-Phe exhibited the highest fluorescence intensity. Our previous results indicate that PAMAM-CHex-Phe was internalized into Jurkat cells, which were observed by confocal microscopy [28]. Thus, it is possible that these dendrimers were also internalized into Jurkat cells. Linear linkers were effective in inducing an association with T-cells, although our previous reports indicate that PAMAM-C_2-Phe (PAMAM-Suc-Phe) was not associated with Jurkat cells [28]. Therefore, T-cell association can be optimized by adjusting the length of the alkyl chain at the dendrimer termini. The linkers of PAMAM-CHex-Phe, PAMAM-Ph-Phe, and PAMAM-C_6-Phe have the same number of carbons. The Log p values of PAMAM-CHex-Phe, PAMAM-Ph-Phe, and PAMAM-C_6-Phe, whose dendrimer contains four termini, were calculated as a model and were estimated as 6.8, −0.8, and 4.1, respectively. This indicates that the hydrophobicity of PAMAM-CHex-Phe and PAMAM-C_6-Phe was similar, which was more hydrophobic than PAMAM-Ph-Phe. The association of PAMAM-Ph-Phe and PAMAM-CHex-Phe with Jurkat cells was similar despite the difference in Log p values. PAMAM-C_6-Phe exhibited a greater association with Jurkat cells than PAMAM-CHex-Phe despite having similar Log p values. These indicate that the Log p values are not the main factor involved in the association with T-cells. Ishii et al. reported that the modification of nanoparticle surfaces with polyethylene glycol (PEGs) of different lengths enhanced ligand mobility and target recognition [33]. In our previous report, we demonstrated that the Phe density at the dendrimer terminus affects the cellular interactions in PAMAM-CHex-Phe [29]. The most stable molecular structures of PAMAM-CHex-Phe, PAMAM-Ph-Phe, and PAMAM-C_6-Phe, whose dendrimer contains four termini, were calculated and presented in Figure 4. PAMAM-C_6-Phe has a more spread structure than the others, which suggests that the Phe residues of PAMAM-C_6-Phe readily interact with Jurkat cells. The interaction of these dendrimers with the cellular membranes was investigated using liposomes as a model (Figure 5). Although adsorption to the liposomes was slightly increased by adding Phe and changing the linkers, it was less than 10%. Thus, it is likely that these dendrimers did not directly interact with the lipid membranes. Further investigation is required to elucidate the cell association mechanism of these dendrimers.

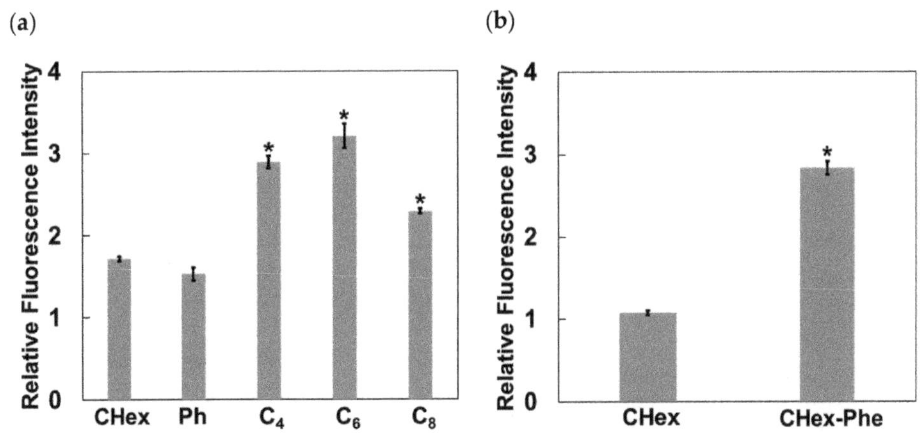

Figure 3. Association of dendrimers with Jurkat cells. (**a**) Fluorescence intensity of PAMAM-R-Phe normalized to PAMAM-CHex. R means CHex, Ph and C_n linkers. (**b**) Fluorescence intensity of DGL-CHex and DGL-CHex-Phe normalized to PAMAM-CHex. * $p < 0.05$ vs. PAMAM-CHex.

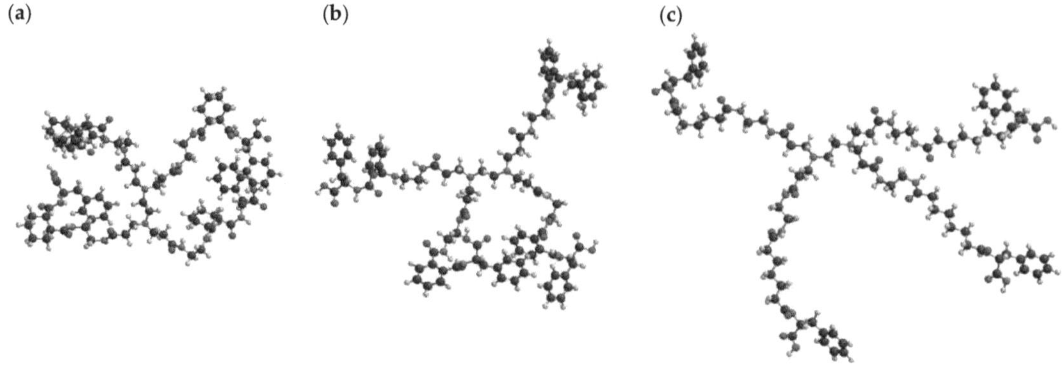

Figure 4. Structure of carboxy-terminal phenylalanine (Phe)-modified PAMAM dendrimers via different linkers with four termini. (**a**) PAMAM-CHex-Phe, (**b**) PAMAM-Ph-Phe, and (**c**) PAMAM-C_6-Phe. White, black, blue, and red balls correspond to hydrogen, carbon, nitrogen, and oxygen atoms, respectively.

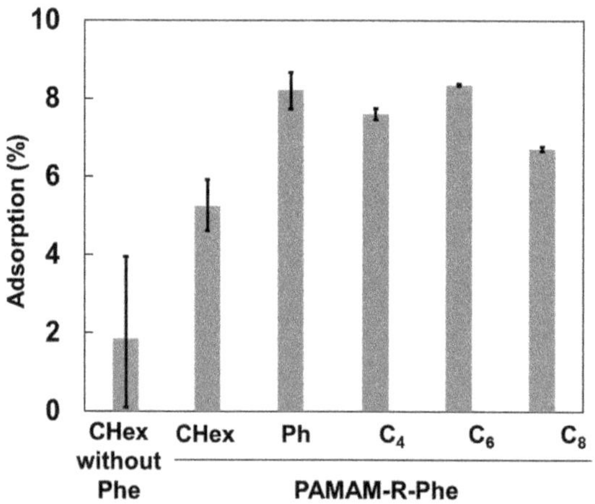

Figure 5. Adsorption of carboxy-terminal phenylalanine (Phe)-modified dendrimers to liposomes via different linkers after the 3 h-incubation.

Figure 3b shows the mean fluorescence intensity of DGL-CHex and DGL-CHex-Phe. The fluorescence intensity of DGL-CHex without Phe was similar to that of PAMAM-CHex without Phe. The fluorescence intensity of DGL-CHex-Phe was higher than that of PAMAM-CHex-Phe. Although DGL-CHex-Phe exhibited excellent cell association properties, it was not soluble in water. Thus, DGL-CHex-Phe was unsuitable as a drug carrier.

3.3. Model Drug Loading Using Carboxy-Terminal Phe-Modified Dendrimers with Various Linkers

The drug loading ability of nanocarriers as a DDS is important. PpIX and PTX were used as model drugs in this study (Figure 6). PpIX is a water-insoluble photosensitizer that is beneficial for photodynamic therapy [29]. PTX is a water-insoluble anticancer agent [32]. It was recently reported that PTX exhibited some immune-modulating effects [34]. Thus, the delivery of these drugs into T-cells is useful for the treatment of T-cell leukemia as well as immunotherapy. The drug loading ability of PAMAM-CHex-Phe, PAMAM-Ph-Phe, and PAMAM-C_6-Phe was examined in water, as previously reported [29,32]. When 10 equivalents of PpIX were added to each dendrimer, 3.9, 1.8, and 0.3 molecules of PpIX were loaded into PAMAM-CHex-Phe, PAMAM-Ph-Phe, and PAMAM-C_6-Phe, respectively (Figure 7a). When five equivalents of PTX were added to each dendrimer, 0.78, 0, and 0.10 molecules of PTX were loaded into PAMAM-CHex-Phe, PAMAM-Ph-Phe, and PAMAM-C_6-Phe, respectively (Figure 7b). PAMAM-CHex-Phe could encapsulate more PpIX and PTX than the other dendrimers, which suggests that the linker also affected the drug loading ability. Although PAMAM-C_6-Phe was efficiently associated with cells, the drug loading ability was low. In our previous report, we revealed that the encapsulation of guest molecules into PAMAM dendrimers was based on electrostatic and hydrophobic interactions [29]. Because PAMAM-Ph-Phe is more hydrophilic than PAMAM-CHex-Phe and PAMAM-C_6-Phe, as estimated from their Log p values, the interaction of PAMAM-Ph-Phe with the hydrophobic drug molecules was possibly suppressed. It is likely that the spread-out structure of PAMAM-C_6-Phe, as shown in Figure 4, suppressed the interaction with drug molecules. More PpIX was encapsulated in these dendrimers than PTX because PpIX has a carboxy group that can interact with the inner tertiary amines of these dendrimers. The water solubility of these molecules was greatly enhanced when bound to the dendrimers. In particular, the water solubility of PTX was extremely low (reported as 0.35 μM) [35]. However, the water solubility of PTX was 78 μM in the aqueous solution of PAMAM-CHex-Phe, which is an increase of about 200 times. Thus, PAMAM-CHex-Phe not only enhanced the water solubility of hydrophobic molecules but was also associated with T-cells, which are the most useful properties for delivering small drug molecules to T cells.

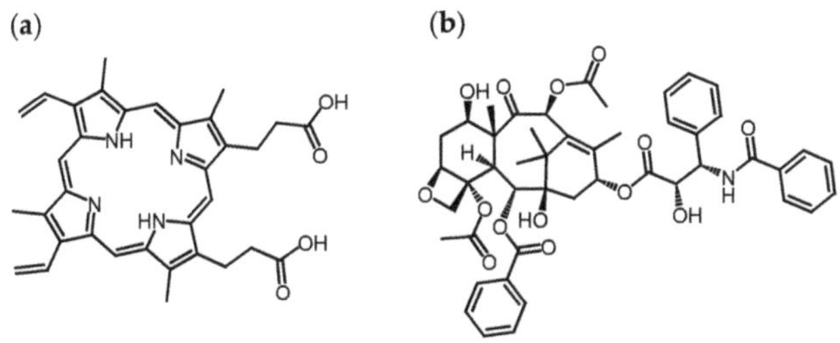

Figure 6. Chemical structure of (**a**) PpIX and (**b**) PTX.

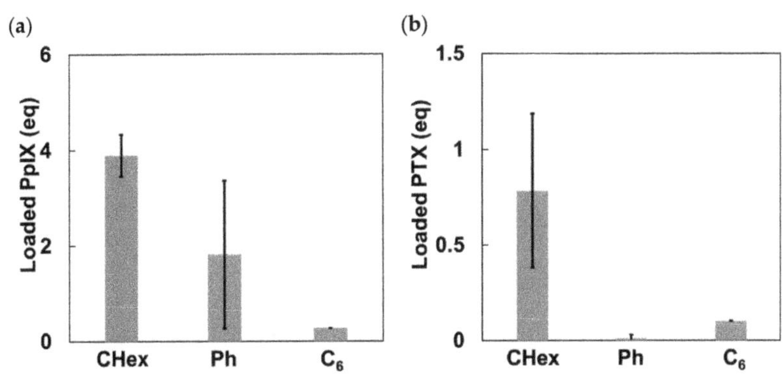

Figure 7. Loading of (**a**) PpIX and (**b**) PTX into PAMAM-CHex-Phe, PAMAM-Ph-Phe, and PAMAM-C_6-Phe in water.

3.4. Drug Action of PTX-Loaded PAMAM-CHex-Phe

We examined the drug action of the PTX-loaded PAMAM-CHex-Phe, the most promising drug–dendrimer complex, to Jurkat cells by the MTT cytotoxicity assay. The cytotoxicity of free PTX and PAMAM-CHex-Phe without PTX against Jurkat cells was also examined. Table 2 shows that the cell viability of Jurkat cells treated with PTX-loaded PAMAM-CHex-Phe was 28%, which was similar to that of free PTX. The cell viability of 10 μM

PAMAM-CHex-Phe without PTX was 90%, although the dendrimer concentration was much higher than the PTX-loaded PAMAM-CHex-Phe. This indicates that PAMAM-CHex-Phe itself is essentially not cytotoxic. These suggest that PTX loaded in PAMAM-CHex-Phe worked as a similar drug action to free PTX. The retention of PTX in the dendrimer was also investigated. Before and after 24 h incubation in saline, the PTX concentration in the supernatant was measured. The PTX loaded in the dendrimer in saline was almost the same in water. Only 20% of PTX was retained in the supernatant after 24 h, but the concentration of PAMAM-CHex-Phe in the supernatant was almost unchanged. These suggest that the drug was released from the dendrimer. Our results suggest that PAMAM-CHex-Phe has potential as a small drug nanocarrier for direct delivery to T-cells.

Table 2. Cell viability of free PTX, PTX-loaded PAMAM-CHex-Phe, and PAMAM-CHex-Phe.

Compound	Concentration		Incubation Time	Cell Viability (%)
	PTX	Dendrimer		
free PTX	10 nM	-	48 h	23 ± 14%
PTX-loaded PAMAM-CHex-Phe	10 nM	13 nM	48 h	28 ± 2%
PAMAM-CHex-Phe	-	10,000 nM	24 h	91 ± 20%

4. Conclusions

We synthesized and characterized carboxy-terminal Phe-modified dendrimers with different linkers and cores to investigate the effect of the dendrimer structure to the association with Jurkat cells and model drug loading. PAMAM dendrimers with linear linkers exhibited a higher association with T-cells than dendrimers with cyclic linkers. DGL-CHex-Phe demonstrated a higher association with T-cells than PAMAM-CHex-Phe. This indicates that the linker and core structure of the dendrimer are factors involved in the association with T-cells. In addition, the dendrimer structure also affected the drug loading ability. PAMAM-CHex-Phe exhibited the greatest drug loading ability for PpIX and PTX, whose water solubility was drastically improved. PTX-loaded PAMAM-CHex-Phe exhibited similar cytotoxicity against Jurkat cells to free PTX, but PAMAM-CHex-Phe itself did not exhibit any significant cytotoxicity. These results suggest that PAMAM-CHex-Phe showed efficient cell association and drug loading properties, thus making it a potent small molecular drug carrier for direct drug delivery to T-cells. Recently, PTX has shown immune-modulating effects as well as anticancer effects [34]. PTX-loaded PAMAM-CHex-Phe may be used to stimulate immune cells as well as for the treatment of T-cell leukemia. Our previous papers indicated that carboxy-terminal Phe-modified dendrimers were associated with various kinds of immune cells [27–29]. The targeting property is required for the applications to DDS, which remains to be investigated.

Supplementary Materials: The following supporting information can be downloaded at: https://www.mdpi.com/article/10.3390/pharmaceutics16060715/s1, Figure S1: ^{1}H NMR spectra of (a) PAMAM-C_8-Phe, (b) PAMAM-C_6-Phe, (c) PAMAM-C_4-Phe in D_2O containing NaOD; Figure S2: ^{1}H NMR spectrum of PAMAM-CHex-Phe in D_2O containing NaOD; Figure S3: ^{1}H NMR spectrum of PAMAM-Ph-Phe in D_2O containing NaOD; Figure S4: ^{1}H NMR spectra of (a) DGL-CHex-Phe and (b) DGL-CHex in D_2O containing NaOD.

Author Contributions: Conceptualization, H.S.; investigation, H.S., T.H., and A.S.; data curation, T.H. and A.S.; validation, I.N., A.M., and C.K.; writing—original draft preparation, H.S.; writing—review and editing, H.S. and C.K.; resources, I.N. and C.K.; supervision, A.M.; project administration, C.K.; funding acquisition, C.K. All authors have read and agreed to the published version of the manuscript.

Funding: This work was supported by JSPS KAKENHI, grant numbers JP20H05232, JP22H04556, and JP19H05714 (Grant-in-Aid for Scientific Research on Innovative Areas: Aquatic Functional Materials) and JP24K01558 (Grant-in-Aid for Scientific Research (B)). This work was also supported by the 2022 and 2023 Osaka Metropolitan University (OMU) Strategic Research Promotion Project (Priority Research).

Institutional Review Board Statement: Not applicable.

Informed Consent Statement: Not applicable.

Data Availability Statement: Data supporting the findings of this study are available from the corresponding author upon reasonable request.

Conflicts of Interest: H.S. is an employee of Kao Co., Ltd. The remaining authors declare that the research was conducted in the absence of any commercial or financial relationships that could be construed as a potential conflict of interest.

References

1. Allen, T.M.; Cullis, P.R. Drug delivery systems: Entering the mainstream. *Science* **2004**, *303*, 1818–1822. [CrossRef] [PubMed]
2. Riehemann, K.; Schneider, S.W.; Luger, T.A.; Godin, B.; Ferrari, M.; Fuchs, H. Nanomedicine—Challenge and perspectives. *Angew. Chem. Int. Ed.* **2009**, *48*, 872–897. [CrossRef] [PubMed]
3. Blanco, E.; Shen, H.; Ferrari, M. Principles of nanoparticle design for overcoming biological barriers to drug delivery. *Nat. Biotechnol.* **2015**, *33*, 941–951. [CrossRef] [PubMed]
4. Wilczewska, A.Z.; Niemirowicz, K.; Markiewicz, K.H.; Car, H. Nanoparticles as drug delivery systems. *Pharmacol. Rep.* **2012**, *64*, 1020–1037. [CrossRef] [PubMed]
5. Svenson, S.; Tomalia, D.A. Dendrimers in biomedical applications—Reflections on the field. *Adv. Drug Deliv. Rev.* **2005**, *57*, 2106–2129. [CrossRef]
6. Khandare, J.; Calderón, M.; Dagia, N.M.; Haag, R. Multifunctional dendritic polymers in nanomedicine: Opportunities and challenges. *Chem. Soc. Rev.* **2012**, *41*, 2824–2848. [CrossRef] [PubMed]
7. Mignani, S.; Rodrigues, J.; Tomas, H.; Zablocka, M.; Shi, X.; Caminade, A.M.; Majoral, J.P. Dendrimers in combination with natural products and analogues as anti-cancer agents. *Chem. Soc. Rev.* **2018**, *47*, 514–532. [CrossRef]
8. Sherje, A.P.; Jadhav, M.; Dravyakar, B.R.; Kadam, D. Dendrimers: A versatile nanocarrier for drug delivery and targeting. *Int. J. Pharm.* **2018**, *548*, 707–720. [CrossRef]
9. Lee, C.C.; MacKay, J.A.; Fréchet, J.M.J.; Szoka, F.C. Designing dendrimers for biological applications. *Nat. Biotechnol.* **2005**, *23*, 1517–1526. [CrossRef]
10. Menjoge, A.R.; Kannan, R.M.; Tomalia, D.A. Dendrimer-based drug and imaging conjugates: Design considerations for nanomedical applications. *Drug Discov.* **2010**, *15*, 171–185. [CrossRef]
11. Esfand, R.; Tomalia, D.A. Poly(amidoamine) (PAMAM) dendrimers: From biomimicry to drug delivery and biomedical applications. *Drug Discov. Today* **2001**, *6*, 427–436. [CrossRef] [PubMed]
12. Taratula, O.; Garbuzenko, O.B.; Kirkpatrick, P.; Pandya, I.; Savla, R.; Pozharov, V.P.; He, H.; Minko, T. Surface-engineered targeted PPI efficient intracellular and intratumoral siRNA delivery. *J. Control. Release* **2009**, *140*, 284–293. [CrossRef]
13. Padilla De Jesús, O.L.; Ihre, H.R.; Gagne, L.; Fréchet, J.M.J.; Szoka, F.C., Jr. Polyester dendritics systems for drug delivery applications: In vitro and in vivo evaluation. *Bioconjug. Chem.* **2002**, *13*, 453–461. [CrossRef]
14. Leong, N.J.; Mehta, D.; McLeod, V.M.; Kelly, B.D.; Pathak, R.; Owen, D.J.; Porter, C.J.H.; Kaminskas, L.M. Doxorubicin Conjugation and Drug Linker Chemistry Alter the Intravenous and Pulmonary Pharmacokinetics of a PEGylated Generation 4 Polylysine Dendrimer in Rats. *J. Pharm. Sci.* **2018**, *107*, 2509–2513. [CrossRef]
15. Ohsaki, M.; Okuda, T.; Wada, A.; Hirayama, T.; Niidome, T.; Aoyagi, H. In vitro gene transfection using dendritic poly(L-lysine). *Bioconjug. Chem.* **2002**, *13*, 510–517. [CrossRef]
16. Haensler, J.; Szoka, F.C. Polyamidoamine cascade polymers mediate efficient transfection of cells in culture. *Bioconjug. Chem.* **1993**, *4*, 372–379. [CrossRef] [PubMed]
17. Ke, W.; Shao, K.; Huang, R.; Han, L.; Liu, Y.; Li., J.; Kuang, Y.; Ye, L.; Lou, J.; Jiang, C. Gene delivery targeted to the brain using an Angiopep–conjugated polyethylenenglycol–modified polyamidoamine dendrimer. *Biomaterials* **2009**, *30*, 6976–6985. [CrossRef] [PubMed]
18. Cevaal, P.M.; Ali, A.; Czuba-Wojnilowicz, E.; Symons, J.; Lewin, S.R.; Cortez-Jugo, C.; Caruso, F. In Vivo T Cell-Targeting Nanoparticle Drug Delivery Systems: Considerations for Rational Design. *ACS Nano* **2021**, *15*, 3736–3753. [CrossRef]
19. Gong, N.; Sheppard, N.C.; Billingsley, M.M.; June, C.H.; Mitchell, M.J. Nanomaterials for T-cell cancer immunotherapy. *Nat. Nanotechnol.* **2021**, *16*, 25–36. [CrossRef]
20. Zheng, Y.; Tang, L.; Mabardi, L.; Kumari, S.; Irvine, D.J. Enhancing adoptive cell therapy of cancer through targeted delivery of small molecule immunomodulators to internalizing or noninternalizing receptors. *ACS Nano* **2017**, *11*, 3089–3100. [CrossRef]

21. Schmid, D.; Park, C.G.; Hartl, C.A.; Subedi, N.; Cartwright, A.N.; Puerto, R.B.; Zheng, Y.; Maiarana, J.; Freeman, G.J.; Wucherpfennig, K.W.; et al. T cell-targeting nanoparticles focus delivery of immunotherapy to improve antitumor immunity. *Nat. Commun.* **2017**, *8*, 1747. [CrossRef]
22. Fu, Z.; Zhang, X.; Gao, Y.; Fan, J.; Gao, Q. Enhancing the anticancer immune response with the assistance of drug repurposing and delivery systems. *Clin. Transl. Med.* **2023**, *13*, 1320–1354. [CrossRef]
23. Ou, W.; Thapa, R.K.; Jiang, L.; Soe, Z.C.; Gautam, M.; Chang, J.H.; Jeong, J.H.; Ku, S.K.; Choi, H.G.; Yong, C.S.; et al. Regulatory T cell-targeted hybrid nanoparticles combined with immune-checkpoint blockage for cancer immunotherapy. *J. Control. Release* **2018**, *281*, 84–96. [CrossRef]
24. Li, R.; Chen, Z.; Li, J.; Dai, Z.; Yu, Y. Nano-drug delivery systems for T cell-based immunotherapy. *Nano Today* **2022**, *46*, 101621–101636. [CrossRef]
25. Siriwon, N.; Kim, Y.J.; Siegler, E.; Chen, X.; Rohrs, J.A.; Liu, Y.; Wang, P. CAR-T Cells Surface-Engineered with Drug-Encapsulated Nanoparticles Can Ameliorate Intratumoral T-cell Hypofunction. *Cancer Immunol. Res.* **2018**, *6*, 812–824. [CrossRef] [PubMed]
26. Riley, R.S.; June, C.H.; Langer, R.; Mitchell, M.J. Delivery technologies for cancer immunotherapy. *Nat. Rev. Drug Discov.* **2019**, *18*, 175–196. [CrossRef] [PubMed]
27. Nishimoto, Y.; Nagashima, S.; Nakajima, K.; Ohira, T.; Sato, T.; Izawa, T.; Yamate, J.; Higashikawa, K.; Kuge, Y.; Ogawa, M.; et al. Carboxyl-, sulfonyl-, and phosphate-terminal dendrimers as a nanoplatform with lymph node targeting. *Int. J. Pharm.* **2020**, *576*, 119021. [CrossRef]
28. Shiba, H.; Nishio, M.; Sawada, M.; Tamaki, M.; Michigami, M.; Nakai, S.; Nakase, I.; Fujii, I.; Matsumoto, A.; Kojima, C. Carboxy-terminal dendrimers with phenylalanine for a pH-sensitive delivery system into immune cells including T cells. *J. Mater. Chem. B* **2022**, *10*, 2463–2470. [CrossRef]
29. Shiba, H.; Hirose, T.; Fu, Y.; Michigami, M.; Fujii, I.; Nakase, I.; Matsumoto, A.; Kojima, C. T Cell-Association of Car-boxy-Terminal Dendrimers with Different Bound Numbers of Phenylalanine and Their Application to Drug Delivery. *Pharmaceutics* **2023**, *15*, 888. [CrossRef]
30. Kojima, C.; Sawada, M.; Nakase, I.; Matsumoto, A. Gene Delivery into T-Cells Using Ternary Complexes of DNA, Lipofec-tamine, and Carboxy-Terminal Phenylalanine-Modified Dendrimers. *Macromol. Biosci.* **2023**, *23*, 2300139–2300145. [CrossRef] [PubMed]
31. Tamaki, M.; Fukushima, D.; Kojima, C. Dual pH-sensitive and UCST-type thermosensitive dendrimers: Phenylala-nine-modified polyamidoamine dendrimers with carboxyl termini. *RSC Adv.* **2018**, *8*, 28147–28151. [CrossRef] [PubMed]
32. Kojima, C.; Hirose, T.; Katayama, R.; Matsumoto, A. Solubilization of Paclitaxel by Self-Assembled Amphiphilic Phospho-lipid-Mimetic Polymers with Varied Hydrophobicity. *Polymers* **2021**, *13*, 2805. [CrossRef]
33. Ishii, T.; Miyata, K.; Anraku, Y.; Naito, M.; Yi, Y.; Jinbo, T.; Takae, S.; Fukusato, Y.; Hori, M.; Osada, K.; et al. Enhanced target recognition of nanoparticles by cocktail PEGylation with chains of varying lengths. *Chem. Commun.* **2016**, *52*, 1517–1519. [CrossRef] [PubMed]
34. Manspeaker, M.P.; Thomas, S.N. Lymphatic immunomodulation using engineered drug delivery systems for cancer immunotherapy. *Adv. Drug Deliv. Rev.* **2020**, *160*, 19–35. [CrossRef]
35. Ezrahi, S.; Aserin, A.; Garti, N. Basic principles of drug delivery systems-the case of paclitaxel. *Adv. Colloid Interface Sci.* **2019**, *263*, 95–130. [CrossRef]

pharmaceutics

MDPI

Article

Molecular Ballet: Investigating the Complex Interaction between Self-Assembling Dendrimers and Human Serum Albumin via Computational and Experimental Methods

Gabriele Cavalieri [1,†], Domenico Marson [1,†], Nicoletta Giurgevich [1], Rachele Valeri [1], Fulvia Felluga [2], Erik Laurini [1,*,‡] and Sabrina Pricl [1,3,‡]

1 Molecular Biology and Nanotechnology Laboratory (MolBNL@UniTS), DEA, University of Trieste, Piazzale Europa 1, 34127 Trieste, Italy; gabriele.cavalieri@phd.units.it (G.C.); domenico.marson@dia.units.it (D.M.); nicoletta.giurgevich@studenti.units.it (N.G.); rachela_valeri@yahoo.it (R.V.); sabrina.pricl@dia.units.it (S.P.)

2 Department of Chemical and Pharmaceutical Sciences, DSCF, University of Trieste, Via Giorgieri 1, 34127 Trieste, Italy; ffelluga@units.it

3 Department of General Biophysics, Faculty of Biology and Environmental Protection, University of Lodz, ul. Pomorska 141/143, 90-236 Łódź, Poland

* Correspondence: erik.laurini@dia.units.it

† These authors contributed equally to this work.

‡ Senior co-authors.

Abstract: Dendrimers, intricate macromolecules with highly branched nanostructures, offer unique attributes including precise control over size, shape, and functionality, making them promising candidates for a wide range of biomedical applications. The exploration of their interaction with biological environments, particularly human serum albumin (HSA), holds significant importance for biomedical utilization. In this study, the interaction between HSA and a recently developed self-assembling amphiphilic dendrimer (AD) was investigated using various experimental techniques. Fluorescence spectroscopy and isothermal titration calorimetry revealed moderate interactions between the protein and the AD nanomicelles (NMs), primarily attributed to favorable enthalpic contributions arising from electrostatic interactions and hydrogen bonding. Structural analysis indicated minimal changes in HSA upon complexation with the AD NMs, which was further supported by computational simulations demonstrating stable interactions at the atomistic level. These findings provide valuable insights into the binding mechanisms and thermodynamic parameters governing HSA/AD NM interactions, thereby contributing to the understanding of their potential biomedical applications.

Keywords: human serum albumin; amphiphilic dendrimer; isothermal titration calorimetry; spectroscopy; HPC molecular simulations

1. Introduction

Dendrimers represent a class of highly branched macromolecules with unique nanostructures. Their distinctive architecture, characterized by successive layers of branching emanating from a central core, imparts remarkable chemical and physical properties, distinguishing them from traditional linear polymers. Unlike linear polymers, dendrimers exhibit well-defined and uniform structures, resembling miniature trees with precise control over their size, shape, and functionality. This precise architecture grants dendrimers numerous advantages, including high surface-to-volume ratios, monodispersity, and the ability to encapsulate guest molecules within their internal void spaces. The structure of dendrimers typically comprises three fundamental components: a central core featuring multiple reactive sites, branches that extend from the core in a radially symmetric manner, and terminal functional groups decorating the outermost layer. This dendritic topology enables dendrimers to possess a high degree of molecular uniformity, with each generation exhibiting a defined number of branches emanating from the core. Furthermore, the stepwise synthetic approach employed in dendrimer synthesis facilitates precise control over the size and functionalization of dendrimers, offering unparalleled versatility in tailoring their properties for specific applications [1–4].

The unique characteristics of dendrimers have led to their widespread exploration and utilization across various scientific disciplines and industrial sectors. In particular, dendrimers have found extensive applications in fields such as drug delivery, gene therapy, diagnostics, materials science, and nanotechnology [5,6]. Their ability to encapsulate and deliver therapeutic agents with precision and efficiency has positioned dendrimers as promising candidates for the development of next-generation drug delivery systems. Additionally, their tunable surface chemistry enables the design of dendrimer-based materials for targeted imaging, sensing, and diagnostic applications [7,8].

The advantages associated with dendrimers employed in medical and healthcare applications primarily fall within the purview of therapeutic delivery. Leveraging tailored drug delivery systems effectively mitigates concerns inherent to free drug administration. These concerns include short half-lives, aqueous insolubility, aberrations in biodistribution, and pharmacokinetic deviations of the administered therapeutics. The precise targeting of different anatomical locales or tissue types serves to curtail toxicity, uphold therapeutic thresholds through controlled release kinetics, and enhance therapy bioavailability by preventing premature degradation and increasing absorptive efficiency, exemplifying the realm of controlled drug delivery [9].

Among the most extensively explored dendrimer families is the poly(amidoamine) (PAMAM) dendrimer. However, their translation into clinical settings requires the ready availability of high-quality consistent quantities. Regrettably, the iterative nature of dendrimer synthesis poses significant challenges, with structural anomalies escalating with generation number. These defective dendrimers closely resemble their intact counterparts in chemical composition and physical attributes, complicating purification endeavors. This crucial limitation contributed to the failure of a preclinical trial involving dendrimer-mediated delivery of an anticancer agent [10,11].

To address these challenges, recent emphasis has shifted toward the self-assembly strategy for constructing noncovalent supramolecular dendrimers. Small amphiphilic dendrimers featuring hydrophobic alkyl chains and hydrophilic PAMAM dendrons offer a promising avenue. Synthesis of these molecules in large quantities with high purity is achievable through divergent, convergent, or hybrid methodologies. Taking advantage of their amphipathic character, amphiphilic dendrimers exploit hydrophobic interactions in their core and hydrogen bonds within dendron shells to spontaneously form stable supramolecular dendrimers. Tailoring the length and composition of hydrophobic chains and PAMAM dendron generations, alongside modifying terminal functionalities, imparts unparalleled structural versatility for diverse biomedical applications.

Among the myriad of newly engineered and synthesized molecules capable of self-assembly, our team has recently proposed and investigated the amphiphilic dendrimer (AD). Comprising two lipid-like C_{18} chains and a PAMAM dendron head (Figure 1), this dendrimer spontaneously organizes into nearly spherical nanomicelles (NMs), characterized by a micellar diameter of approximately 10 nm, a critical micellar concentration (CMC) ranging from 3.2 to 5.7 μM, and an aggregation number (N_{agg}) of 17 AD monomers per micelle, as determined through small-angle X-ray scattering (SAXS), nuclear magnetic resonance (NMR), and isothermal titration calorimetry (ITC). These AD NMs have shown promise as nanovectors (NVs) for gene therapy [12] and the delivery of poorly soluble antitumoral drugs [13]. For example, in a recent study, AD NMs were used to encapsulate Vemurafenib (VEM) and Dabrafenib (DAB), two clinically used anticancer drugs for melanoma, aiming to mitigate major side effects and enhance drug effectiveness. This led to the formation of well-defined core–shell NMs (with high encapsulation efficiency (∼70% for DAB and ∼60% for VEM) and drug loading capacity (∼27% and ∼24% for DAB and

VEM, respectively). Importantly, in vitro testing of AD NMs loaded with DAB and VEM in four melanoma cell lines revealed enhanced responses compared to free drug treatment.

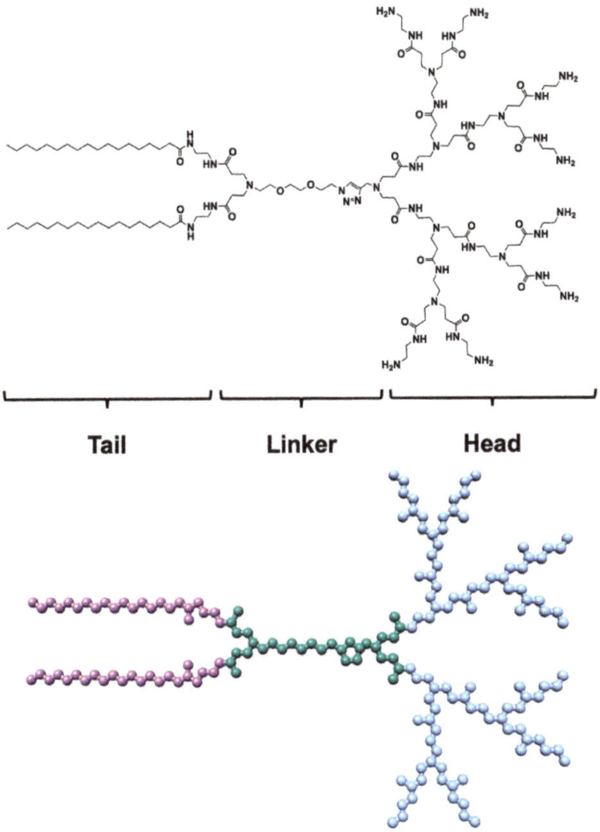

Figure 1. (**Upper panel**) 2D chemical structure of the AD monomer. (**Lower panel**) Atomistic representation of the AD monomer. The atoms are represented as spheres and colored by the corresponding region as follows: hydrophobic tails, purple; linker, teal; polar head, sky blue. For clarity, hydrogen atoms are missing.

An important issue common to all NVs arises from their uncertain behavior in vivo due to the emergence of a protein corona (PC) upon interaction with biological settings [14–17]. When these systems encounter biological fluids, they promptly acquire a layer of biomolecules, predominantly proteins, leading to PC formation. This protein coat surrounding the NVs poses significant challenges for the biomedical application of nanomaterials, particularly regarding biodistribution and toxicity. Today, the connection between the surface attributes of the NVs and the characteristics/composition of the PC remains elusive. For example, studies indicate that NV traits such as surface charge, chemical nature of the terminal groups, and size (among others) significantly influence the nature of the protein corona. Additionally, PC molecular attributes and composition do affect the cellular uptake of the NVs; for instance, while, occasionally, the PC acts as a barrier, protecting the NVs and limiting their direct interaction with biological systems, certain proteins in the corona may, on the other hand, facilitate processes such as adhesion and adsorption onto cell membranes, enhancing the biological activity of the nanodelivery system. Accordingly, specific and thorough investigations are needed to understand the direct correlation between the structure and the ensuing effects.

To further complicate the issue, various proteins exhibit distinct binding affinities to NVs, dictating their sequence of adsorption onto the nanocarrier surface. Proteins with stronger affinities form the so-called hard corona, binding tightly to the surface compared to those forming the soft corona, which are endowed with lower affinities. Initially, the most abundant proteins adhere to the surface, replaced over time by higher-affinity proteins, a process termed the Vroman effect [18]. This phenomenon impacts NV biodistribution which, in turn, is crucial for in vivo applications. Among the most abundant components of almost every PC is human serum albumin (HSA). Due to its abundance in the bloodstream, HSA plays a crucial role in the pharmacokinetics of virtually all drugs, affecting their effectiveness, delivery rate, and toxicity [19]. Importantly, HSA emerges as a dominant protein that adheres to nanocarrier surfaces, a process typically viewed as benign or even advantageous, as it can not only reduce opsonization or inflammation but also prolong the circulation time of NVs, since the HSA corona can reduce the cellular uptake of NVs by macrophages [20–23].

In this perspective, understanding the interaction of HSA with our AD NMs is a crucial initial step for elucidating how these carriers are coated upon exposure to physiological environments, thus shedding further light on their fate, function, and potential biomedical applications. Accordingly, the formation of the HSA protein corona on the AD NMs was investigated through morphological, spectroscopic, calorimetric, and in silico techniques.

2. Materials and Methods

2.1. Reagents and Chemicals

Globulin- and fatty acid-free human serum albumin (product number A1887) was purchased from Sigma-Aldrich Inc. (Saint Louis, MO, USA). AD amphiphiles were synthesized and characterized as described in detail in our previous work [13].

2.2. Sample Preparation and Analytical Procedures

HSA stock solutions were prepared by dissolving a specific amount of protein in phosphate-buffered saline 1× (PBS, pH = 7.4). The protein concentration was determined via ultraviolet (UV) spectroscopy at a wavelength λ = 280 nm. AD nanocarrier stock solutions were prepared in PBS buffer at a final concentration of 2 mM.

2.3. Far-UV Circular Dichroism Spectroscopy

Far-ultraviolet circular dichroism (CD) spectra were recorded from 200 to 260 nm at a scan rate of 20 nm/min using a J-1500 spectropolarimeter (Jasco, Tokyo, Japan). The path length of the cell was 0.2 cm, with step size and bandwidth set to 0.5 and 1 nm, respectively. The resultant CD spectra represent the averaged data from three accumulations. The fractional composition of secondary structural elements within HSA, both in the presence and absence of AD, was determined using the CD Multivariate SEE program employing standard calibration models. The concentration of HSA was kept fixed at 2 μM, while AD concentration was varied in the range of 1–25 μM.

2.4. Steady-State and 3D Fluorescence Spectroscopy

All fluorescence spectroscopy (FS) measurements were carried out using a FP-8350 spectrofluorometer (Jasco, Tokyo, Japan) in a 1.0 cm quartz cell. The excitation wavelength (λ_{exc}) was set to 280 nm, and the fluorescence spectra were recorded in the range of 300−450 nm at 298 K using 5 and 10 nm slit widths for the emission and the excitation bandwidth, respectively. During all fluorescence quenching titrations, the concentration of HSA was kept fixed at 2 μM, while AD concentration was varied in the range of 2–20 μM. Each dendrimer/protein solution was allowed to incubate for 2 h before recording the corresponding fluorescence spectrum. Additionally, 3D fluorescence spectroscopy was performed following the aforementioned protocol, with an excitation wavelength ranging from 220 to 350 nm and recording the spectrum in the range between 220 to 500 nm at 298 K.

2.5. Isothermal Titration Calorimetry Studies

Isothermal titration calorimetry experiments were performed with a MicroCal PEAQ-ITC calorimeter (Malvern Panalytical, Malvern, UK) at 298 K (cell volume = 208 μL). The thermodynamics associated with HSA/AD complex formation were investigated in PBS-buffered solutions. Specifically, a solution of HSA (30 μM, sample cell) was subjected to 19 step-by-step injections of 2 μL volume of AD (900 μM, syringe). In this way, it was ensured that AD was always found at a concentration above the CMC throughout the titration, as described in our previous works [24–26]. Prior to each experiment, the solutions and buffer were degassed for 30 min at room temperature under stirring at 700 rpm. Control experiments were performed to measure nonspecific heats, which were subsequently subtracted from the relevant dataset to obtain corrected integrated data. The experimental data acquired from the ITC experiment were analyzed using the "one set of sites" model. Subsequently, the fitted data were graphically depicted, with the *y*-axis denoting the heat generated in each injection and the *x*-axis representing the molar ratio between the concentration of albumin and the concentration of AD nanomicelles during titration within the sample cell. The concentration of AD nanomicelles was determined by employing the mass conservation principle, as outlined by the following equation [27,28]:

$$[AD_{tot}] = [AD_{mon}] + N_{agg} \times [AD_{mic}]. \quad (1)$$

where $[AD_{tot}]$ is the total concentration of AD in the sample cell during the ITC experiment, $[AD_{mon}]$ is the concentration in its monomeric state, N_{agg} corresponds to the micellar aggregation number and $[AD_{mic}]$ is the concentration in its fully n-meric state. All experiments were conducted in triplicate.

2.6. Dynamic Light Scattering and Zeta Potential Measurements

All measurements of nanomicelle size and zeta (ζ)-potential were performed by dynamic light scattering (DLS) on a Zetasizer Nano-ZS (Malvern, UK) at 25 °C. AD NMs and HSA were dissolved in PBS and the measurements were performed using a 5 mV He-Ne laser (operating wavelength $\lambda = 633$ nm, scattering angle $\theta = 173°$).

2.7. Transmission Electron Microscopy

The morphology of the HAS/AD complex was examined using transmission electron microscopy (TEM). Briefly, a 5 mL volume of the complex solution was deposited onto a carbon grid and allowed to dry for 1 h. Subsequently, the grid was stained with uranyl acetate and imaged using a Philips EM 208 (Philips, Eindhoven, The Netherlands) electron microscope operating at 100 kV. The imaging system was equipped with a Quemesa camera from Olympus Soft Imaging Solutions (Hamburg, Germany) and utilized the RADIUS 2.3 software for image acquisition.

2.8. Molecular Simulations

To characterize both the isolated form and the self-assembled state of the AD amphiphile, a well-established procedure described in our prior work was adopted [13,29]. Accordingly, gaff2 atom types were assigned and partial charges were determined via the RESP method using the RED server [30–32]. The structure of HSA was obtained from the protein data bank (PDB, entry 4k2c) and parameterized with the AMBER ff14SB force-field [33]. The Delphi 8.5 software was exploited to assess the distribution of electrostatic potential around the HSA surface, aiding in the appropriate orientation of the protein molecules to the charged nanomicelles. Parameters such as internal dielectric, scale, perfil, and ionic strength were set to the values of 4, 2.0, 70.0, and 0.15 M, respectively. By employing the same set of parameters and by setting the surfpot parameter to 4.0 Å, Delphi 8.5 was used for the calculation of the (ζ)-potential of the systems in the presence of explicit ions. The resulting AD/HSA molecular system was then solvated in a TIP3P water box extending at least 15 Å from each solute molecule [34]. Sodium and chlorine atoms were added to achieve a physiological concentration of 0.15 M. The complete protocol details can be found in our previous publications [13,29]. In brief, each system underwent energy minimization followed by gradual heating to 300 K at a pressure of 1 atm. Subsequently, a series of 5 simulations with gradually lowered positional restraints applied to the heavy atoms of the solute were performed in the isobaric–isothermal (NPT) ensemble. Unrestrained molecular dynamics (MD) simulations in the NPT ensemble were next conducted for 1 μs, with data collected from the last 100 ns of simulation where a stable complex was achieved. The energetic analysis was performed using the Molecular Mechanics/Poisson-Boltzmann Surface Area (MM/PBSA) approach implemented in the MMPBSA.py module of the AMBER22 suite, with an internal dielectric constant of 16 to accurately represent the highly charged environment at the binding interface [35–37]. Structural investigations were carried out using the AMBER22 main program CPPTRAJ and in-house developed Python scripts [38]. All simulations were executed with AMBER 22 running on our own GPU/CPU hybrid cluster and the pre-exascale Tier-0 EuroHPC Leonardo supercomputer (CINECA, Bologna, Italy) [37,39].

3. Results and Discussion

3.1. Experimental Binding Analysis of the HSA/AD Complex

3.1.1. Fluorescence Spectra and Binding Constants of the HSA/AD Complexes

Human serum albumin is composed of a single chain containing 585 amino acids, with a unique tryptophan residue (W214) located within subdomain II A. The emission from W214 primarily dictates the fluorescence spectra of HSA in the UV range. Upon interaction with other molecules, alterations in tryptophan fluorescence may arise, influenced either by conformational changes in the protein or direct quenching effects. Accordingly, changes in HSA fluorescence were monitored to investigate the binding of HSA with the AD nanomicelles, as shown in Figure 2A. The most notable change observed in the fluorescence spectrum upon addition of AD was the quenching in fluorescence intensity (Figure 2A). Increasing concentrations of AD in the experiment led to a linear decrease in tryptophan fluorescence. Therefore, the quenching behavior could be analyzed using the Stern–Volmer equation as follows:

$$F_0/F = 1 + K_{SV} \times [Q]. \quad (2)$$

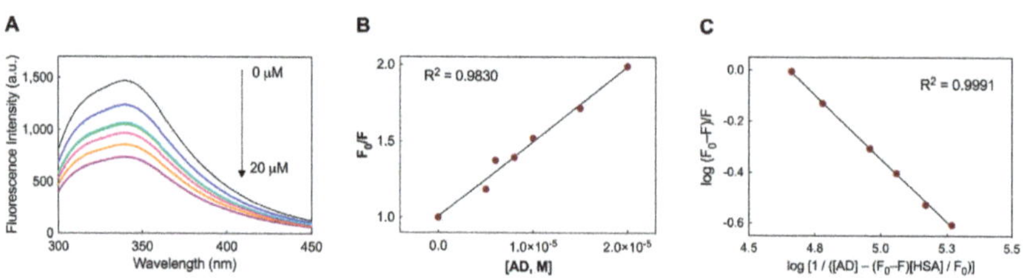

Figure 2. (**A**) Fluorescence emission spectra recorded for the HSA/AD NM systems. The spectra include measurements for free HSA (2 μM, black) and HSA at 2 μM with varying concentrations of AD NMs (5 μM in blue, 6 μM in cyan, 8 μM in magenta, 10 μM in orange, and 20 μM in purple). (**B**) Stern-Volmer plot illustrating the fluorescence quenching of HSA induced by the AD NMs (R^2 = 0.9830). (**C**) Plots of $\log(F_0 - F)/F$ vs. $\log[1/([AD)] - (F_0 - F)[HSA]/(F_0)])$ for HSA fluorescence quenching by AD NMs (R^2 = 0.9991).

In the equation above, F_0 represents the fluorescence intensity without the quencher, while F denotes the intensity with the quencher present. K_{SV} stands for the Stern–Volmer quenching constant, and [Q] indicates the concentration of the quencher. The equation assumes a linear relationship between F_0/F and [Q] (see insert in Figure 2A), with the slope representing the value of K_{SV}. In the present case, the calculated value of K_{SV} for AD is $4.9\ (\pm 0.2) \times 10^4\ M^{-1}$.

Under the assumption that HSA and AD interact via an independent binding site within the protein structure, the binding constant (K_D) values can be estimated from the plot in Figure 2B by using the following modified version of the Stern-Volmer equation [40]:

$$\log(F_0 - F)/F = \log(1/K_D) - \log[1/([AD] - (F_0 - F)[HSA]/F_0)]. \quad (3)$$

where F_0 and F represent the fluorescence intensities as in the classic Stern-Volmer equation, [AD] denotes the increasing concentrations of the nanovector utilized in the experiment, while [HSA] is the fixed protein concentration of HSA (2 μM) adopted in the quenching assay. The K_D value was determined by assessing the linear correlation between the two logarithmic terms in the modified Stern-Volmer equation. This analysis resulted in an affinity value of 22.9 ± 4.2 μM, indicative of a moderate interaction between the nanomicelles and the serum protein [41,42].

3.1.2. Isothermal Titration Calorimetry Binding Analysis

An isothermal titration calorimetry study was conducted to describe and quantify the interactions between the self-assembling AD nanocarrier and HSA in aqueous solutions at physiological pH (7.4). Various ITC conditions were explored to accurately determine the thermodynamic binding parameters between HSA and AD, aiming to unveil the interaction mechanisms between these two entities. This comprehensive analysis involved not only the assessment of binding affinity, expressed through the dissociation constant (K_b) and the relevant Gibbs free energy (ΔG), but also the enthalpic (ΔH) and entropic ($-T\Delta S$) components, which characterize the interaction mechanism. Upon examination of the raw thermogram (Figure 3, upper panel insert), it is evident that each injection of AD, administered in discrete amounts, correlates with a negative heat flow peak, indicating an exothermic reaction between the protein and the nanocarrier. The determination of K_b values can be directly inferred from the sigmoidal profile of the integrated ITC data (Figure 3, upper panel), specifically from the slope at the inflection point. The binding strength obtained, represented by a mean affinity value of 13.4 ± 3.1 μM, indicates a moderate binding interaction between the serum macromolecule and the AD nanomicelles. Remarkably, the values obtained from the ITC experiments are quantitatively consistent with the results obtained from the fluorescence assay for the HSA/AD complexes.

The analysis of the complete binding thermodynamics (Figure 3, bottom panel) allowed for a detailed understanding of the interaction mechanism between the AD nanocarriers and HSA. Notably, the primary outcome of this analysis reveals the binding of the AD/HSA complex to be thermodynamically spontaneous, as indicated by the negative value of ΔG (−6.65 ± 0.26 kcal/mol, Figure 3). Subsequently, by integrating the obtained findings with the distinctive molecular determinants within the HSA/AD complex, the main interaction mechanisms between the AD nanovector and HSA could be delineated as follows:

1. robust electrostatic interactions are established between the positively charged terminal groups of the AD NMs and the side chains of some aspartic and glutamic acid residues within HSA;
2. a limited network of hydrogen bonds (HBs) forms between the internal groups of the AD molecules and specific amino acid residues of the serum protein, facilitating the exposure of side chains that serve as counterparts for the formation of proton bridges. Notably, within the AD dendron, the oxygens of the internal amide groups serve a hydrogen bond acceptor, with the -NH moieties of the same groups acting as HB donors;
3. these two types of interactions are mainly enthalpic in nature, as indicated by the favorable ΔH value obtained from the titrations (−4.02 ± 0.12 kcal/mol, Figure 3).

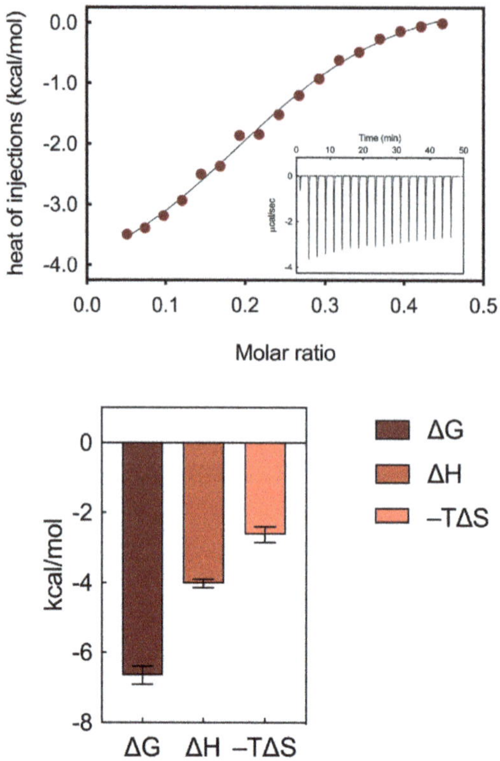

Figure 3. (**Upper panel**) ITC plot for the titration of HSA with AD nanomicelles (inset shows the measured heat power vs. time elapsed during HSA/AD binding). (**Bottom panel**) Summary of thermodynamic data extracted from ITC for the binding of AD nanosystems to HSA.

A couple of other not negligible interactions can be taken into account to complete the thermodynamics scenario. In particular, the following:

1. weak hydrophobic interactions occur between the hydrocarbon/aliphatic components of the nanocarrier heads and the side chain of hydrophobic amino acids of HSA;
2. secondary hydrophobic alterations occur due to bond formation at the respective surfaces, leading to the release of water molecules, ions and counterions. The latter two interactions contribute to favorable entropic changes, enhancing the stability of the interaction between the protein and the NMs, as demonstrated by the value of $-T\Delta S = -2.63 \pm 0.22$ kcal/mol (Figure 3).

3.2. Structural and Thermal Perturbation of HSA upon AD Binding

3.2.1. Determination of the HSA Secondary Structure and Melting Temperature through Circular Dichroism Spectroscopy

Circular dichroism spectroscopy is a valuable technique for elucidating protein structures and examining conformational changes induced by ligand interactions [43]. In the far-UV CD spectra of HSA, two negative bands are observed at 208 (π-π^*) and 220 nm (n-π^*), indicative of an α-helix-rich protein secondary structure. To ascertain the impact of AD nanovector binding on the secondary structure of HSA, CD spectra of free HSA and its AD complexes (Figure 4A) were recorded. These experiments were conducted to compare the percentage of α-helix content in free HSA and in the presence of the nanovector, at concentrations below (monomer form) or above (nanomicelles) its critical micelle concentration (CMC), with CD spectra values recorded between 200 and 260 nm at 25 °C.

The percentage α-helicity of HSA was estimated from the Mean Residue Ellipticity (MRE) values at 208 nm using the following equation:

$$MRE_{208} = (\text{observed CD (mdeg)})/(10C_p nl) \quad (4)$$

$$\alpha\text{-helix}\ (\%) = [(-MRE_{208} - 4000)/(33000 - 4000)] \times 100. \quad (5)$$

in which MRE is the value of the mean residue ellipticity at λ = 208 nm (expressed in deg cm^2 $dmol^{-1}$), C_p is the molar concentration of HSA (2 μM), n denotes the number of amino acids in the protein primary sequence (585 for HSA), l is the path length of the CD cell (0.1 cm), while 33,000 and 4000 (in deg cm^2 $dmol^{-1}$) correspond to the MRE_{208} values of pure α-helical and β-sheet/random coil structures, respectively. The findings of this analysis are depicted in Figure 4B. The CD spectra yielded a percentage of α-helix of 59.3 for the unbound HSA, aligning with previous studies reported in the literature [44].

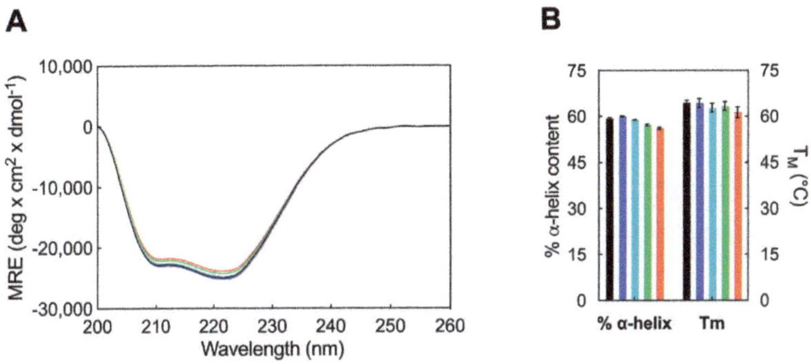

Figure 4. (**A**) Far-UV CD spectra of HSA alone (black line) and in the presence of AD in concentration of 1 μM (blue line), 5 μM (cyan line), 10 μM (green line) and 25 μM (red line). CD experiments were carried out in PBS buffer solution at 25 °C, with [HSA] maintained at 2 μM. (**B**) The α-helical content (left *y*-axis) and melting temperature (right *y*-axis) of HSA are depicted in the absence (black columns) and presence of AD at concentrations of 1 μM (blue columns), 5 μM (cyan columns), 10 μM (green columns), and 25 μM (red columns).

The results of the CD experiments indicate that the secondary structure of HSA remains unaffected by the interaction with AD at concentrations below its CMC (e.g., 1 μM), revealing that AD in its monomeric form does not induce significant conformational changes in the secondary structural motifs of the protein. Upon increasing AD concentration above its CMC, a slight decreasing trend is observed, resulting in a final α-helix percentage of 56.1% (Figure 4A), measured at the maximum AD concentration of 25 μM.

Furthermore, temperature-dependent CD spectroscopy was employed to investigate the potential impact of AD on altering the melting temperature (T_M) of HSA. T_M values were determined by recording CD spectra at 222 nm across a temperature range of 25 °C to 95 °C, with the addition of nanocarriers below and above their CMC. The obtained results are presented in Figure 4B. Consequently, the assessment of HSA thermal stability, based on T_M estimation, yielded consistent findings with the standard CD spectra. In fact, there were no significant fluctuations observed in the T_M value of HSA in the presence of AD monomers or at lower molar ratios of HSA/AD nanomicelles (Figure 4B). However, at higher concentrations, AD NMs were capable of reducing the albumin T_M by approximately 3 °C. Thus, it is only in the presence of a large quantity of AD amphiphiles in their self-assembled form that HSA exhibits a slight decrease in thermal stability, aligning with the modest reduction observed in α-helical content (Figure 4B).

In summary, the interaction between serum albumin and AD nanomicelles did not induce any substantial structural alterations within the protein structure. This observation is consistent with the moderate binding strength of the HSA/AD complexes, as elucidated previously through fluorescence spectroscopy and ITC analysis.

3.2.2. Three-Dimensional Fluorescence Spectroscopy

3D fluorescence spectroscopy serves as a further, valuable tool for probing changes in HSA conformation. The fluorescence intensity of the primary peak in the 3D FS spectrum is associated with the polarity of the microenvironment and the secondary structure of the protein. Notably, the peak ($\lambda_{ex}/\lambda_{em}$ = 280/343 nm/nm) predominantly reflects the spectral characteristics of W214 of HSA, while the other peaks correspond to the first-order Rayleigh scattering peak ($\lambda_{ex} = \lambda_{em}$) [19]. To corroborate the findings obtained from CD spectroscopy, 3D FS spectra (Figure 5) were recorded.

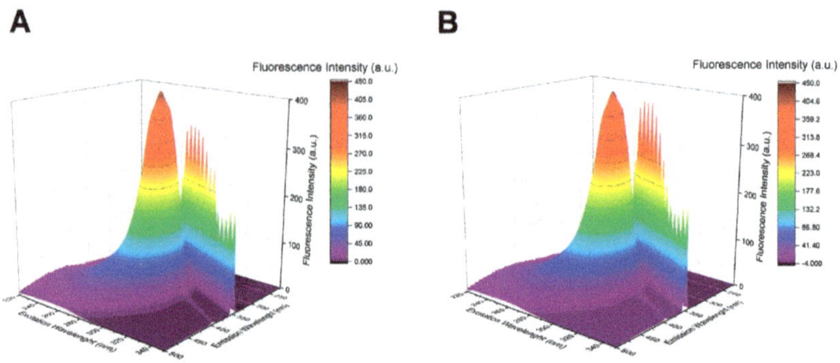

Figure 5. 3D fluorescence spectra of HSA in absence (**A**) and in presence (**B**) of AD nanomicelles (10 μM).

As seen in Figure 5, no significant shifts in the peaks of HSA are observed in the analysis of the 3D FS spectra in the presence of AD nanomicelles. These results suggest that there are no notable alterations in the structure of HSA around the tryptophan residue located at position 214 following interaction with AD. Consequently, it can be inferred that the binding between HSA and the NVs likely occurs predominantly at the external surface of the proteins, particularly with the charged surface of the nanomicelles.

3.2.3. Transmission Electron Microscopy and Dynamic Light Scattering Analysis

Transmission electron microscopy (TEM) analysis of the HSA/AD NM systems revealed the formation of a molecular complex exhibiting a diameter approximately 20 nm with a spherical morphology (Figure 6A). Dynamic light scattering (DLS) experiments conducted in aqueous solution provided measurements of the hydrodynamic diameter (d) and the ζ-potential (ζ), yielding values of 17.6 ± 0.3 nm (Figure 6B) and +8.3 mV, respectively. In our previous work [13], the ζ-potential for pristine AD NMs was recorded as +27 mV, while literature data suggests that pure HSA typically exhibits negative ζ values around −15 mV [45]. This suggests that although the positively charged AD NMs primarily interacts with the negative residues of HSA, each HSA molecule within the complex aligns in a manner where its more positively charged areas are exposed to the surrounding solvent. This evidence, along with the calculated N_{agg} for the AD NMs [13] and the molar ratio detected from the ITC experiments, supports a plausible composition of six serum proteins around a single AD nanoassembly, consistent with experimental results obtained in similar systems [46].

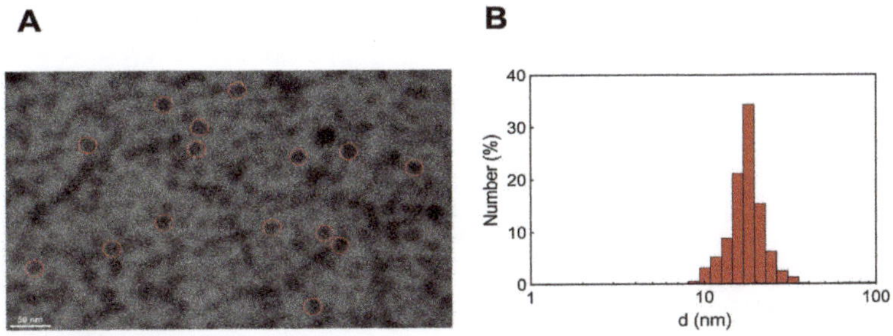

Figure 6. (**A**) TEM images of HSA/AD complexes. Red circles highlight three representative HSA/AD NM structures in each TEM ensemble. (**B**) Hydrodynamic diameter (d) of HSA/AD complexes at 25 °C as measured by DLS.

3.3. Computational Studies

3.3.1. Binding Analysis of the HSA/AD Complex

Based on the experimental findings, it is likely that HSA and the AD NMs primarily interact through surface interactions involving the polar external amino acid residues of the protein and the hydrophilic, positively charged heads of the NVs. To elucidate the interactions between these two molecular entities at the atomistic level, an investigation was initiated by examining the electrostatic potential surrounding the serum protein using Delphi 8.5 [47] in conjunction with UCSF Chimera 1.17.3 [48]. While the serum protein typically exhibits an abundance of negatively charged amino acids under physiological conditions, the analysis revealed that these residues are not uniformly distributed on its surface. Nonetheless, a distinct surface with a notable overall negative potential was identified, particularly over the IA, IIA, and IIB domains of HSA (Figure S1), thus indicating a preferential site for binding with the positively charged AD nanomicelle. This facilitated the formation of the initial complex between HSA molecules and the AD nanomicelle. Consistent with our experimental evidence and literature data on a similar system [46], the complex is composed of six protein molecules making up the PC around one self-assembled AD NM. The determination of the surface electrostatic potential enabled us to validate the 6:1 stoichiometry of the HSA/AD complex. Specifically, the ratio between the solvent accessible surface area (SASA) of the AD nanomicelle (35,618 Å^2) and the SASA corresponding to the region of HSA exhibiting the most negative potential distribution (Figure S1, 5835 Å^2) within a single protein yielded a value of 6.1, closely resembling the experimentally determined HSA/AD ratio. Consequently, after establishing the appropriate orientation of HSA molecules relative to AD nanomicelle, six HSA molecules were manually positioned in proximity to the AD nanomicelle. Each HSA molecule was placed at a minimum distance of 10 Å from the AD nanomicelle, with the protein molecules evenly distributed on the surface of the AD nanomicelle (Figure 7).

Focusing on the primary interactions at the atomic level between HSA and the AD NM, the initial phase involved assessing the contacts between the micelle's atoms and the residues of the protein along the corresponding equilibrated MD trajectory. Essentially, this process entailed determining the closest distance between every amino acid on the HSA molecules and any atom within the micelle for each snapshot of the MD simulation (Figure S2). Initial observations unveiled a consistent interaction pattern, where the HSAs making up the protein corona appeared to contact the NM at very similar regions and amino acids. Subsequently, the frequency of protein nm contacts was calculated by defining a contact as a scenario where the minimum distance between two interacting atoms (belonging to the protein and the NM, respectively), was less than 6.5 Å in any given MD frame. This approach resulted in the generation of a more detailed fingerprint of the interactions between each protein and the AD NM, as illustrated in Figure 8.

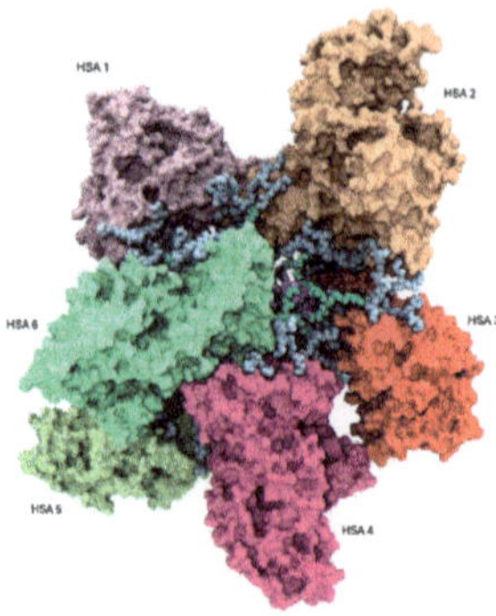

Figure 7. Atomistic representation of the HSA/AD (6/1) complex. Each protein structure is depicted as a colored surface, while the atoms of the AD nanomicelle are represented as spheres colored according to the scheme adopted in Figure 1.

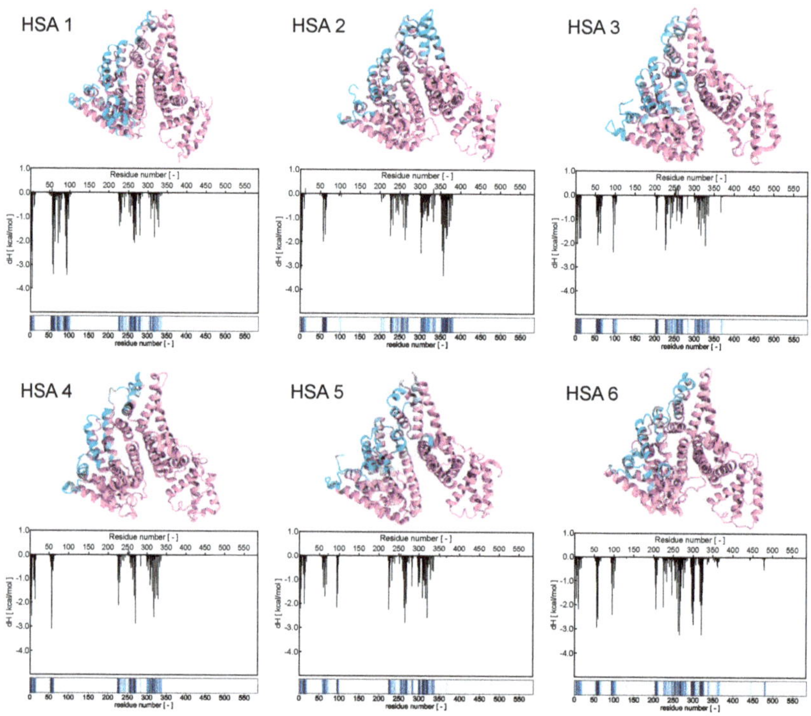

Figure 8. The six panels represent each HSA bound to the AD micelle in Figure 7. (**top panels**) HSA protein is represented by its secondary structure, and the aminoacid residues are colored in pink (no contact) or cyan (consistent contacts). (**middle panels**) the enthalpic free energy decomposition for each HSA residue as obtained from the MM/PBSA analysis. (**bottom panels**) The interaction fingerprint is based on the frequency of interaction of each HSA residue with the AD micelle. Fingerprints are colored based on the contact frequency with shades of blue: white representing 0 contact frequency while dark blue representing a constant contact throughout the MD trajectory.

Examination of these binding fingerprints revealed consistent interaction patterns across all HSA molecules (Figure 8, bottom panels). To quantitatively characterize these patterns in terms of energy, a MM/PBSA analysis was conducted. This analysis allowed for the deconvolution of the enthalpic binding energy into individual contributions from each amino acid within the protein. Subsequently, comparison between the interaction fingerprints (Figure 8, bottom panels) and the energy contributions of each amino acid (Figure 8, middle panels and Table S1) revealed a significant correlation between the energy profiles and the structural data.

For a deeper understanding of the interaction between HSA and the AD NV, the number of charged AD groups involved in stable salt bridges (SBs) with the protein's residues. These SBs were deemed significant if they persisted for at least 50% of the MD simulation duration. Results revealed that approximately 72.8% of the charged terminals on the AD NM formed stable SBs with negatively charged (i.e., aspartic and glutamic acid) residues on HSA. While salt bridges play a pivotal role in binding and represent a significant portion of the interactions identified through contact and energy analysis, they are not the sole contributors. Hydrogen bonds and van der Waals forces also contribute to the stabilization of the macromolecular complexes as represented in Figure S3. Although the interaction sites are distributed widely across the protein's surface (Figure 8, upper panels), two regions of HSA appear particularly crucial for binding with the positively charged branches of the AD NM. These regions include the helix containing residues E252, D255, D256, D259, E266, and D269, as well as the small loop containing residues E60 and D63. These regions form highly stable salt bridges with the nanomicelle terminal nitrogen in each HSA molecule comprising the protein corona (Figure 8).

3.3.2. Binding Analysis of the HSA/AD Complex

Further analysis of the atomistic MD data for the HSA/AD NM complex revealed that the overall sizes of both the HSA chains and the AD NM remain unchanged upon the formation of the protein corona, as evidenced by the corresponding value of the radius of gyrations (R_g). This parameter serves as an indicator of the compactness of a given molecular (super)structure and directly reflects its size in solution. As illustrated in Figure 9A, there is virtually no alteration in the micelle's R_g upon formation of the HSA PC, with R_g values of 30.82 $\pm$ 0.62 Å for the AD NM alone and 30.98 $\pm$ 0.32 Å within the HSA complex.

As previously documented by SAXS experiments [13], the AD NMs exhibit a triaxial ellipsoid shape in solution. Accordingly, the analysis of the gyration tensor's principal components performed in the present work provided further insights into the overall geometry of the HSA/AD complex. The square roots of the gyration tensor's eigenvalues represent the characteristic semi-axis lengths of the ellipsoid characterizing both the AD NM and its complex with HSA. Remarkably, upon complexation, the AD micelle maintains its triaxial ellipsoid configuration (with semi-axis lengths of 45.8 $\pm$ 0.4 Å, 39.78 $\pm$ 0.3 Å, and 37.18 $\pm$ 0.3 Å), indicating that its interaction with serum proteins does not induce structural alterations in the AD nanostructure, despite protein distribution across its surface. Notably, when examining the overall 6:1 HSA/AD complex, its shape resembles that of an oblate spheroid, featuring a discernible minor axis (with semi-axis lengths of 81.8 $\pm$ 0.5 Å, 80.2 $\pm$ 0.3 Å, and 71.4 $\pm$ 0.7 Å).

From the perspective of the protein, its interaction with the micelles does not seem to notably perturb its overall structure. As demonstrated in Figure 9A, the size of each protein when bound to the AD micelle (as indicated by the R_g value) remains largely unchanged upon complex formation. In fact, the calculated R_g values for different HSA chains range from 26.98 to 27.35 Å, with a maximum standard deviation of 0.18 Å.

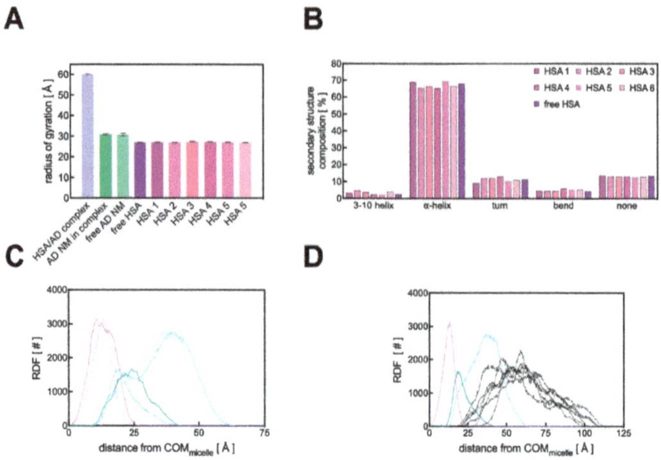

Figure 9. (**A**) Comparison of the radius of gyration (R_g) values for the HSA/AD complex, the AD NM within the complex, a free AD NM, a free HSA molecule, and each of the 6 HSA chains within the HSA/AD assembly. (**B**) Comparison of the secondary structure composition for the 6 HSA molecules in the AD complex and an isolated HSA chain. (**C**) Radial distribution functions of the AD NM atoms (tail in purple, linker in aquamarine, head in cyan), showing variations between unbound and complexed states. Dotted lines represent the RDF values for the unbound AD NM, while the solid lines represent the values for the AD NM in complex with HSA. (**D**) RDF of the complete HSA/AD complex relative to the center of mass of the AD NM. The RDF of the protein atoms are represented as black lines.

These values align with the R_g value computed for a single HSA under similar conditions (27.01 ± 0.16 Å) and are consistent with previously reported literature data on HSA [49]. To delve deeper into the potential impacts of AD nanomicelle binding on the internal structure of HSA, the secondary structure content of the proteins, both free and bound to the AD NM, was analyzed using the DSSP algorithm [50], which assigns secondary structures to amino acids based on their 3D coordinates. The secondary structure of a single HSA simulated under similar conditions predominantly comprises α-helices (68.0%), along with some turns (11.5%), and no β-sheets, consistent with existing literature [44]. In complex with the AD NM, the α-helix percentages vary between 65.3 and 69.4%, and the turns between 9.2 and 13.2%, with no β-sheet formation observed. These findings suggest that the interaction between the HSA chains and the AD NV does not significantly alter the arrangement of protein secondary structure, as evidenced in Figure 9B. Furthermore, considering again the 6:1 full HSA/AD NM complex, the relevant computed R_g is 60.01 ± 0.27 Å (Figure 9A). This value implies that the proteins and the AD NM do not interact as rigid objects, for which a higher R_g value would be expected.

The surface-averaged electrostatic potential (SAEP) was next calculated to estimate the ζ-potential potential of the HSA/AD NM complex. Initially, the ζ-potential of the pure HSA protein was determined to be −11.5 mV, while the value for the AD NM alone was calculated to be 30.48 mV. Upon complexation with HSA, the overall positive ζ-potential of the complex decreased to 10.2 mV. This suggests that although the positively charged AD NM could be largely neutralized by the negative residues of HSA, each HSA molecule in the complex is oriented with its more positively charged regions (Figure S1, right panel) facing the solvent. This unique orientation of HSA thus contributes to the observed positive ζ-potential value of the supramolecular assembly.

Finally, to complete the investigation of the structure of the HSA/AD complex and the relevant interactions, the radial distribution function (RDF) analysis was performed. This method involves selecting a reference point, typically the center of mass (COM) of a large molecule or a specific residue, and then calculating the distribution of atoms from another molecular entity as the distance from this reference point increases. Initially, this technique was employed to examine the arrangement of each AD amphiphile within the nanomicelle itself and to determine whether the adsorption of the HSA proteins onto the NV altered its internal organization (see Figure 1 for details). As shown in Figure 9C, the internal distribution of the AD NM atoms remains largely unchanged upon complexation with HSA, consistent with the previously described results. By plotting the RDF of HSA atoms around the COM of the AD nanomicelle (Figure 9D), it becomes evident that there is a high degree of interpenetration between the proteins and the NV, which supports the previously described R_g value estimated for the complex. Furthermore, upon observing the distribution of HSA atoms relative to the different components of the NV, a strong interpenetration of the proteins within the polar heads of the AD nanomicelle is observed, aligning with the overall binding mechanism underlying the HSA/AD complex.

4. Conclusions

Dendrimers, which are complex compounds with highly branched nanostructures, offer precise control over their size, shape, and functionality, making them unique macromolecules. Their uniform architecture provides several advantages, such as high surface-to-volume ratios and monodispersity, which are crucial for their applications in drug delivery and diagnostics. However, challenges arise due to structural anomalies during dendrimer synthesis, which can affect their clinical translation. Recent research efforts have focused on self-assembly strategies to address these limitations. One promising approach involves the use of amphiphilic dendrimers, which form stable nanomicelles suitable for drug delivery. However, understanding how these dendrimers interact with biological environments, particularly with human serum albumin, is essential for realizing their biomedical potential.

Accordingly, in the present effort the interaction between HSA and the recently designed self-assembling, amphiphilic dendrimer AD was investigated using various experimental techniques. Fluorescence spectroscopy revealed a linear decrease in tryptophan fluorescence of HSA upon binding to AD nanomicelles, indicating quenching behavior, which was analyzed using the Stern–Volmer equation. The calculated Stern–Volmer quenching constant (K_{SV}) for the AD NMs was determined to be 4.9×10^4 M^{-1}, while the affinity value obtained from the modified Stern–Volmer equation was equal to 22.9 ± 4.2 μM, indicating a moderate affinity between the protein and the nanovector. Additionally, isothermal titration calorimetry confirmed the moderate entity of the interaction between HSA and the AD NMs, with a mean affinity value of 13.4 ± 3.1 μM. Thermodynamic analysis indicated thermodynamically spontaneous binding with favorable enthalpic contributions primarily from electrostatic interactions and hydrogen bonding. Circular dichroism spectroscopy showed no significant structural changes in HSA upon interaction with AD below its critical micellar concentration, with only slight decreases in α-helical content and thermal stability observed at higher AD concentrations. Three-dimensional fluorescence spectroscopy further supported these findings, indicating no significant alterations in HSA structure around the HSA tryptophan residue W214 upon AD binding. Computational analysis of the HSA/AD complex binding revealed surface interactions between polar amino acid residues of HSA and the hydrophilic, positively charged heads of the nanovector. Delving into atomistic details, electrostatic potential around HSA was analyzed, revealing a predominantly negative potential over specific domains, ideal for binding with AD nanomicelles. Moreover, molecular dynamics simulations unveiled consistent interaction patterns between HSA and the AD NV at the atomistic level. Further energetic analysis elucidated enthalpic contributions, with stable salt bridges playing a pivotal role. Finally, structural analysis indicated minimal alteration in the overall structure of HSA upon complexation with AD micelles, corroborated by radial distribution functions and zeta potential measurements. Overall, this study sheds light on the binding mechanisms and thermodynamic parameters governing the interaction between HSA and the self-assembled AD nanovector, offering valuable insights into their potential biomedical applications.

In a broader context, the observed moderate binding pattern between HSA and the AD nanomicelles holds considerable implications for pharmaceutical research, especially within the realm of drug delivery. Understanding the nature of the interactions between these entities is paramount for refining drug delivery systems and enhancing their efficacy. In the domain of drug delivery, a moderate binding pattern can be construed as advantageous, as it fosters three primary beneficial outcomes [19,51]:

(i) mitigated carrier-induced toxicity, since an excessive binding affinity between any drug vector and HSA can perturb normal protein functions. A moderate binding pattern serves to alleviate such risks, thus increasing the safety of the drug delivery system;

(ii) enhanced circulation stability, since moderate binding ensures a stable interaction between the drug carrier and HAS, and this, in turn, can enhance the circulation time of the drug delivery system in the bloodstream. This prolonged circulation time improves drug bioavailability and increases the likelihood of reaching target tissues;

(iii) diminished immunogenicity since nanovector binding to HSA may mitigate the recognition of the drug delivery system as foreign by the immune system. This effect could potentially decrease immune responses, such as clearance by the reticuloendothelial system or the initiation of inflammatory reactions.

Finally, understanding the binding mechanisms and thermodynamic parameters empowers researchers to engineer nanocarriers with customized properties, optimizing drug loading, circulation stability, and targeted drug release, thereby advancing therapeutic outcomes in pharmaceutical applications [52].

Supplementary Materials: The following supporting information can be downloaded at: https://www.mdpi.com/article/10.3390/pharmaceutics16040533/s1, Figure S1: Solvent-accessible surface of HSA; Figure S2: Average minimum distances.; Figure S3: Representative interactions between AD and HSA. Table S1: enthalpic free energy decomposition data; HSA_AD_complex.pdb: atomistic coordinates of the HSA/AD complex.

Author Contributions: Conceptualization, E.L. and S.P.; methodology, G.C., E.L., F.F., D.M. and S.P.; software, D.M.; formal analysis, G.C., N.G., R.V., E.L., D.M. and S.P.; investigation, N.G., G.C., R.V., F.F. and D.M.; data curation, N.G., R.V., G.C. and D.M.; writing—original draft preparation, N.G., R.V., G.C., D.M. and E.L.; writing—review and editing, E.L., F.F., D.M., G.C. and S.P.; supervision, E.L., F.F. and S.P.; project administration, E.L. and S.P.; funding acquisition, E.L. and S.P. All authors have read and agreed to the published version of the manuscript.

Funding: This research was funded by ICSC-Centro Nazionale di Ricerca in high-performance computing, big data, and quantum computing (Spoke 7, WP4 (Pilot applications), T.2.8 (Development and optimization of HPC-based integrated workflows based on flagship codes for personalized (nano)medicine) to E.L. and S.P.). The authors wish also to acknowledge the generous financial support from the Italian Association for Cancer Research (AIRC, grant "Novel hot-spot mutations in BCR-ABL1: role in resistance to CML target therapy–IG17413" to S.P.), and the Fondazione Cassa di Risparmio di Trieste (Fondazione CRTrieste, grant "Far-UV CD spectroscopy in translational medicine" to S.P.).

Institutional Review Board Statement: Not applicable.

Informed Consent Statement: Not applicable.

Data Availability Statement: The original contributions presented in the study are included in the article/Supplementary Materials, further inquiries can be directed to the corresponding authors.

Acknowledgments: We acknowledge CINECA (ISCRA-B project NoOneOut-HP10BPK7ZX to D.M.). The authors wish also to express warm gratitude to Susanna Bosi and Roberta Bortul for their technical support during the TEM measurements at the CIMA (Interdepartmental Center of Advanced Microscopy) of the University of Trieste.

Conflicts of Interest: The authors declare no conflicts of interest.

References

1. Astruc, D.; Boisselier, E.; Ornelas, C. Dendrimers designed for functions: From physical, photophysical, and supramolecular properties to applications in sensing, catalysis, molecular electronics, photonics, and nanomedicine. *Chem. Rev.* **2010**, *110*, 1857–1959. [CrossRef] [PubMed]
2. Tomalia, D.A.; Khanna, S.N. A Systematic Framework and Nanoperiodic Concept for Unifying Nanoscience: Hard/Soft Nanoelements, Superatoms, Meta-Atoms, New Emerging Properties, Periodic Property Patterns, and Predictive Mendeleev-like Nanoperiodic Tables. *Chem. Rev.* **2016**, *116*, 2705–2774. [CrossRef] [PubMed]
3. Sandoval-Yañez, C.; Rodriguez, C.C. Dendrimers: Amazing Platforms for Bioactive Molecule Delivery Systems. *Materials* **2020**, *13*, 570. [CrossRef] [PubMed]
4. Pérez-Ferreiro, M.; Abelairas, A.M.; Criado, A.; Gómez, I.J.; Mosquera, J. Dendrimers: Exploring Their Wide Structural Variety and Applications. *Polymers* **2023**, *15*, 22. [CrossRef] [PubMed]
5. Wu, L.-P.; Ficker, M.; Christensen, J.B.; Trohopoulos, P.N.; Moghimi, S.M. Dendrimers in Medicine: Therapeutic Concepts and Pharmaceutical Challenges. *Bioconjug. Chem.* **2015**, *26*, 1198–1211. [CrossRef] [PubMed]
6. Seidi, F.; Jenjob, R.; Crespy, D. Designing Smart Polymer Conjugates for Controlled Release of Payloads. *Chem. Rev.* **2018**, *118*, 3965–4036. [CrossRef] [PubMed]
7. Saluja, V.; Mishra, Y.; Mishra, V.; Giri, N.; Nayak, P. Dendrimers based cancer nanotheranostics: An overview. *Int. J. Pharm.* **2021**, *600*, 120485. [CrossRef]
8. Cruz, A.; Barbosa, J.; Antunes, P.; Bonifácio, V.D.B.; Pinto, S.N. A Glimpse into Dendrimers Integration in Cancer Imaging and Theranostics. *Int. J. Mol. Sci.* **2023**, *24*, 5430. [CrossRef] [PubMed]
9. Tewabe, A.; Abate, A.; Tamrie, M.; Seyfu, A.; Siraj, E.A. Targeted Drug Delivery—From Magic Bullet to Nanomedicine: Principles, Challenges, and Future Perspectives. *J. Multidiscip. Healthc.* **2021**, *14*, 1711–1724. [CrossRef] [PubMed]
10. Tarach, P.; Janaszewska, A. Recent Advances in Preclinical Research Using PAMAM Dendrimers for Cancer Gene Therapy. *Int. J. Mol. Sci.* **2021**, *22*, 2912. [CrossRef]
11. Kheraldine, H.; Rachid, O.; Habib, A.M.; Al Moustafa, A.-E.; Benter, I.F.; Akhtar, S. Emerging innate biological properties of nano-drug delivery systems: A focus on PAMAM dendrimers and their clinical potential. *Adv. Drug Deliv. Rev.* **2021**, *178*, 113908. [CrossRef] [PubMed]
12. Wei, T.; Chen, C.; Liu, J.; Liu, C.; Posocco, P.; Liu, X.; Cheng, Q.; Huo, S.; Liang, Z.; Fermeglia, M.; et al. Anticancer drug nanomicelles formed by self-assembling amphiphilic dendrimer to combat cancer drug resistance. *Proc. Natl. Acad. Sci. USA* **2015**, *112*, 2978–2983. [CrossRef] [PubMed]
13. Russi, M.; Valeri, R.; Marson, D.; Danielli, C.; Felluga, F.; Tintaru, A.; Skoko, N.; Aulic, S.; Laurini, E.; Pricl, S. Some things old, new and borrowed: Delivery of dabrafenib and vemurafenib to melanoma cells via self-assembled nanomicelles based on an amphiphilic dendrimer. *Eur. J. Pharm. Sci. Off. J. Eur. Fed. Pharm. Sci.* **2023**, *180*, 106311. [CrossRef]
14. Mahmoudi, M.; Landry, M.P.; Moore, A.; Coreas, R. The protein corona from nanomedicine to environmental science. *Nat. Rev. Mater. Mar.* **2023**, *8*, 422–438. [CrossRef] [PubMed]
15. Bashiri, G.; Padilla, M.S.; Swingle, K.L.; Shepherd, S.J.; Mitchell, M.J.; Wang, K. Nanoparticle protein corona: From structure and function to therapeutic targeting. *Lab. Chip.* **2023**, *23*, 1432–1466. [CrossRef] [PubMed]
16. García-Álvarez, R.; Vallet-Regí, M. Hard and Soft Protein Corona of Nanomaterials: Analysis and Relevance. *Nanomaterials* **2021**, *11*, 888. [CrossRef]
17. Kopac, T. Protein corona, understanding the nanoparticle-protein interactions and future perspectives: A critical review. *Int. J. Biol. Macromol.* **2021**, *169*, 290–301. [CrossRef] [PubMed]
18. Vroman, L.; Adams, A.L.; Fischer, G.C.; Munoz, P.C. Interaction of high molecular weight kininogen, factor XII, and fibrinogen in plasma at interfaces. *Blood* **1980**, *55*, 156–159. [CrossRef] [PubMed]
19. Yang, F.; Zhang, Y.; Liang, H. Interactive association of drugs binding to human serum albumin. *Int. J. Mol. Sci.* **2014**, *15*, 3580–3595. [CrossRef] [PubMed]
20. Sen, T.; Mandal, S.; Haldar, S.; Chattopadhyay, K.; Patra, A. Interaction of Gold Nanoparticle with Human Serum Albumin (HSA) Protein Using Surface Energy Transfer. *J. Phys. Chem. C* **2011**, *115*, 24037–24044. [CrossRef]
21. Peng, Q.; Zhang, S.; Yang, Q.; Zhang, T.; Wei, X.-Q.; Jiang, L.; Zhang, C.-L.; Chen, Q.-M.; Zhang, Z.-R.; Lin, Y.-F. Preformed albumin corona, a protective coating for nanoparticles based drug delivery system. *Biomaterials* **2013**, *34*, 8521–8530. [CrossRef] [PubMed]
22. Cai, R.; Chen, C. The Crown and the Scepter: Roles of the Protein Corona in Nanomedicine. *Adv. Mater.* **2019**, *31*, 1805740. [CrossRef] [PubMed]
23. Vincent, M.P.; Bobbala, S.; Karabin, N.B.; Frey, M.; Liu, Y.; Navidzadeh, J.O.; Stack, T.; Scott, E.A. Surface chemistry-mediated modulation of adsorbed albumin folding state specifies nanocarrier clearance by distinct macrophage subsets. *Nat. Commun.* **2021**, *12*, 648. [CrossRef] [PubMed]

24. Chan, C.W.; Laurini, E.; Posocco, P.; Pricl, S.; Smith, D.K. Chiral recognition at self-assembled multivalent (SAMul) nanoscale interfaces—Enantioselectivity in polyanion binding. *Chem. Commun.* **2016**, *52*, 10540–10543. [CrossRef] [PubMed]
25. Rodrigo, A.C.; Bromfield, S.M.; Laurini, E.; Posocco, P.; Pricl, S.; Smith, D.K. Morphological control of self-assembled multivalent (SAMul) heparin binding in highly competitive media. *Chem. Commun.* **2017**, *53*, 6335–6338. [CrossRef] [PubMed]
26. Thornalley, K.A.; Laurini, E.; Pricl, S.; Smith, D.K. Enantiomeric and Diastereomeric Self-Assembled Multivalent Nanostructures: Understanding the Effects of Chirality on Binding to Polyanionic Heparin and DNA. *Angew. Chem. Int. Ed. Engl.* **2018**, *57*, 8530–8534. [CrossRef] [PubMed]
27. Olesen, N.E.; Holm, R.; Westh, P. Determination of the aggregation number for micelles by isothermal titration calorimetry. *Thermochim. Acta* **2014**, *588*, 28–37. [CrossRef]
28. Laurini, E.; Aulic, S.; Skoko, N.; Marson, D.; Fermeglia, M.; Pricl, S. ITC for Characterization of Self-Assembly Process of Cationic Dendrons for siRNA Delivery. *Methods Mol. Biol.* **2021**, *2282*, 245–266. [CrossRef] [PubMed]
29. Dhumal, D.; Maron, B.; Malach, E.; Lyu, Z.; Ding, L.; Marson, D.; Laurini, E.; Tintaru, A.; Ralahy, B.; Giorgio, S.; et al. Dynamic self-assembling supramolecular dendrimer nanosystems as potent antibacterial candidates against drug-resistant bacteria and biofilms. *Nanoscale* **2022**, *14*, 9286–9296. [CrossRef] [PubMed]
30. Wang, J.; Wolf, R.M.; Caldwell, J.W.; Kollman, P.A.; Case, D.A. Development and testing of a general amber force field. *J. Comput. Chem.* **2004**, *25*, 1157–1174. [CrossRef] [PubMed]
31. Bayly, C.I.; Cieplak, P.; Cornell, W.; Kollman, P.A. A well-behaved electrostatic potential based method using charge restraints for deriving atomic charges: The RESP model. *J. Phys. Chem.* **1993**, *97*, 10269–10280. [CrossRef]
32. Vanquelef, E.; Simon, S.; Marquant, G.; Garcia, E.; Klimerak, G.; Delepine, J.C.; Cieplak, P.; Dupradeau, F.-Y. R.E.D. Server: A web service for deriving RESP and ESP charges and building force field libraries for new molecules and molecular fragments. *Nucleic Acids Res.* **2011**, *39* (Suppl. 2), W511–W517. [CrossRef] [PubMed]
33. Maier, J.A.; Martinez, C.; Kasavajhala, K.; Wickstrom, L.; Hauser, K.E.; Simmerling, C. ff14SB: Improving the Accuracy of Protein Side Chain and Backbone Parameters from ff99SB. *J. Chem. Theory Comput.* **2015**, *11*, 3696–3713. [CrossRef] [PubMed]
34. Jorgensen, W.L.; Chandrasekhar, J.; Madura, J.D.; Impey, R.W.; Klein, M.L. Comparison of simple potential functions for simulating liquid water. *J. Chem. Phys.* **1983**, *79*, 926–935. [CrossRef]
35. Wang, E.; Sun, H.; Wang, J.; Wang, Z.; Liu, H.; Zhang, J.Z.H.; Hou, T. End-Point Binding Free Energy Calculation with MM/PBSA and MM/GBSA: Strategies and Applications in Drug Design. *Chem. Rev.* **2019**, *119*, 9478–9508. [CrossRef]
36. Miller, B.R.I.; McGee, T.D., Jr.; Swails, J.M.; Homeyer, N.; Gohlke, H.; Roitberg, A.E. MMPBSA.py: An Efficient Program for End-State Free Energy Calculations. *J. Chem. Theory Comput.* **2012**, *8*, 3314–3321. [CrossRef] [PubMed]
37. Case, D.A.; Aktulga, H.M.; Belfon, K.; Ben-Shalom, I.Y.; Berryman, J.T.; Brozell, S.R.; Cerutti, D.S.; Cheatham, T.E., III; Cisneros, G.A.; Cruzeiro, V.W.D.; et al. *Amber 2023*; University of California: San Francisco, CA, USA, 2023.
38. Roe, D.R.; Cheatham, T.E.I. PTRAJ and CPPTRAJ: Software for Processing and Analysis of Molecular Dynamics Trajectory Data. *J. Chem. Theory Comput.* **2013**, *9*, 3084–3095. [CrossRef] [PubMed]
39. Amber22.pdf. Available online: https://ambermd.org/doc12/Amber22.pdf (accessed on 13 March 2024).
40. Bi, S.; Ding, L.; Tian, Y.; Song, D.; Zhou, X.; Liu, X.; Zhang, H. Investigation of the interaction between flavonoids and human serum albumin. *J. Mol. Struct.* **2004**, *703*, 37–45. [CrossRef]
41. Chaves, O.A.; Oliveira, C.H.d.S.; Ferreira, R.C.; Ferreira, V.F.; Ferreira, S.B.; Serpa, C.; Cesarin-Sobrinho, D.; Silva, F.d.A.d.; Netto-Ferreira, J.C. Spectroscopic and in silico evaluation on the interactive behavior between substituted β-2,3-dihydrofuran naphthoquinones and human serum albumin. *Chem. Phys. Impact* **2024**, *8*, 100465. [CrossRef]
42. Naveenraj, S.; Anandan, S. Binding of serum albumins with bioactive substances—Nanoparticles to drugs. *J. Photochem. Photobiol. C Photochem. Rev.* **2013**, *14*, 53–71. [CrossRef]
43. Miles, A.J.; Janes, R.W.; Wallace, B.A. Tools and methods for circular dichroism spectroscopy of proteins: A tutorial review. *Chem. Soc. Rev.* **2021**, *50*, 8400–8413. [CrossRef] [PubMed]
44. Mishra, V.; Heath, R.J. Structural and Biochemical Features of Human Serum Albumin Essential for Eukaryotic Cell Culture. *Int. J. Mol. Sci.* **2021**, *22*, 8411. [CrossRef] [PubMed]
45. Hosainzadeh, A.; Gharanfoli, M.; Saberi, M.; Chamani, J. Probing the interaction of human serum albumin with bilirubin in the presence of aspirin by multi-spectroscopic, molecular modeling and zeta potential techniques: Insight on binary and ternary systems. *J. Biomol. Struct. Dyn.* **2012**, *29*, 1013–1050. [CrossRef] [PubMed]
46. Cedervall, T.; Lynch, I.; Lindman, S.; Berggard, T.; Thulin, E.; Nilsson, H.; Dawson, K.A.; Linse, S. Understanding the nanoparticle–protein corona using methods to quantify exchange rates and affinities of proteins for nanoparticles. *Proc. Natl. Acad. Sci. USA* **2007**, *104*, 2050–2055. [CrossRef] [PubMed]
47. Rocchia, W.; Alexov, E.; Honig, B. Extending the Applicability of the Nonlinear Poisson−Boltzmann Equation: Multiple Dielectric Constants and Multivalent Ions. *J. Phys. Chem. B* **2001**, *105*, 6507–6514. [CrossRef]
48. Pettersen, E.F.; Goddard, T.D.; Huang, C.C.; Couch, G.S.; Greenblatt, D.M.; Meng, E.C.; Ferrin, T.E. UCSF Chimera—A visualization system for exploratory research and analysis. *J. Comput. Chem.* **2004**, *25*, 1605–1612. [CrossRef]
49. Lyu, X.; Zhang, Q.; Liang, D.; Huang, Y. Interaction between human serum albumin and cholesterol-grafted polyglutamate as the potential carriers of protein drugs. *Acta Pharm. Sin. B* **2019**, *9*, 186–193. [CrossRef]
50. Kabsch, W.; Sander, C. Dictionary of protein secondary structure: Pattern recognition of hydrogen-bonded and geometrical features. *Biopolymers* **1983**, *22*, 2577–2637. [CrossRef] [PubMed]

51. Li, C.; Zhang, D.; Pan, Y.; Chen, B. Human Serum Albumin Based Nanodrug Delivery Systems: Recent Advances and Future Perspective. *Polymers* **2023**, *15*, 16. [CrossRef]
52. Shen, Z.; Xiang, Y.; Vergara, S.; Chen, A.; Xiao, Z.; Santiago, U.; Jin, C.; Sang, Z.; Luo, J.; Chen, K.; et al. A resource of high-quality and versatile nanobodies for drug delivery. *iScience* **2021**, *24*, 103014. [CrossRef] [PubMed]

pharmaceutics

MDPI

Article

Fine-Tuning the Amphiphilic Properties of Carbosilane Dendritic Networks towards High-Swelling Thermogels

Silvia Muñoz-Sánchez [1,†], Andrea Barrios-Gumiel [1,†], Francisco Javier de la Mata [1,2,3] and Sandra García-Gallego [1,2,3,*]

[1] University of Alcala, Faculty of Sciences, Department of Organic and Inorganic Chemistry, and Research Institute in Chemistry "Andrés M. Del Río" (IQAR), 28805 Madrid, Spain; silvia.munoz@uah.es (S.M.-S.); andrea.barrios@edu.uah.es (A.B.-G.); javier.delamata@uah.es (F.J.d.l.M.)
[2] Networking Research Center on Bioengineering, Biomaterials and Nanomedicine (CIBER-BBN), 28029 Madrid, Spain
[3] Institute Ramón y Cajal for Health Research (IRYCIS), 28034 Madrid, Spain
[*] Correspondence: sandra.garciagallego@uah.es
[†] These authors contributed equally to the work.

Abstract: Dendritic hydrogels based on carbosilane crosslinkers are promising drug delivery systems, as their amphiphilic nature improves the compatibility with poorly water-soluble drugs. In this work, we explored the impact of the complementary polymer on the amphiphilic properties of the dendritic network. Different polymers were selected as precursors, from the highly lipophilic propylene glycol (PPG) to the hydrophilic polyethylene glycol (PEG), including amphiphilic Pluronics L31, L35 and L61. The dithiol polymers reacted with carbosilane crosslinkers through UV-initiated thiol–ene coupling (TEC), and the resultant materials were classified as non-swelling networks (for PPG, PLU_{L31} and PLU_{L61}) and high-swelling hydrogels (for PEG and PLU_{L35}). The hydrogels exhibited thermo-responsive properties, shrinking at higher temperatures, and exhibited an intriguing drug release pattern due to internal nanostructuring. Furthermore, we fine-tuned the dendritic crosslinker, including hydroxyl and azide pendant groups in the focal point, generating functional networks that can be modified through degradable (ester) and non-degradable (triazol) bonds. Overall, this work highlighted the crucial role of the amphiphilic balance in the design of dendritic hydrogels with thermo-responsive behavior and confirmed their potential as functional networks for biomedical applications.

Keywords: hydrogel; thermogel; network; polymer; dendrimer; dendron; thermo-responsive; drug delivery

1. Introduction

In recent years, there has been intense research in the design of polymer networks, driven by the multiple materials accomplished like elastomers, gels and porous crystalline materials [1]. These networks, which are formed by linear polymers connected by multifunctional junctions, are highly versatile. The components (strands and junctions) can be flexible or rigid, and the connections can be covalent or non-covalent. Importantly, polymer networks represent an outstanding opportunity to control the material's macroscopic properties at a molecular level [2]. Among polymer networks, hydrogels stand out due to their high biocompatibility, high porosity and ability to absorb large amounts of water [3,4]. They can be classified as "permanent" hydrogels, which are chemically stable and formed by covalent bonds, and "reversible" hydrogels if ionic, hydrophobic or hydrogen bonding are the main interactions within the network. Additionally, some hydrogels can exhibit stimuli-responsive properties, which are highly valuable in biomedical applications like tissue repair and drug delivery [5]. These hydrogels modify their properties in response to external stimuli like temperature. A wide variety of physical thermogels are described in the literature, based on polymers such as poly(*N*,*N*-diethylacrylamide) (PDEAAm), poly(*N*-vinylcaprolactam) (PVCL), poly[2-(dimethylamino)ethyl methacrylate] (PDMAEMA), poly(ethylene glycol) (PEG), Pluronic, and isopropylacrylamide (PNIPAM) [6]. For example, Wang and co-workers developed a dual pH/temperature-responsive hydrogel using Pluronic F127, *N*,*N*,*N*-trimethyl chitosan (TMC) and PEG-modified hyaluronic acid (PEG-HA) for their potential application in transdermal therapy [7]. The authors described an improvement in the rheological parameters in the hydrogel due to strong inter-micellar interactions. In another example, Lu et al. successfully fabricated thermo-responsive PNIPAM gels and encapsulated an antibacterial peptide, producing a sustained and controlled release over time [8]. However, most thermogels are reversible physical networks with weak bonds, so they have very poor mechanical properties and are more prone to degrade over time than covalent hydrogels [9,10].

Among the multifunctional junctions that can generate polymer networks, dendrimers are outstanding molecules due to their multivalency and monodispersity. Dendritic networks exhibit a higher control of their structure and, thus, a better structure-to-property understanding [11]. The seminal work by Gitsov and Zhu on the synthesis of amphiphilic dendritic hydrogels based on PEG and dendritic poly(benzyl ethers) [12] led to the design of many other dendritic networks based on PAMAM, PAMAM-OS, PPI, Poly-L-lysine, glycerol or polyester (bis-MPA). These include covalent networks [13], physical networks [14] and mixed inter-penetrating networks (IPN) [15].

Recently, carbosilane dendrimers have also been employed to generate dendritic hydrogels with amphiphilic properties [16,17]. The preparation of these hydrogels was carried out by click chemistry through the highly efficient thiol–ene coupling reaction (TEC). Vinyl-decorated carbosilane dendrimers reacted with a dithiol molecule in the presence of a photoinitiator and UV light, providing dendritic hydrogels that loaded and released bioactive molecules. These hydrogels were especially useful for cargoes with poor water-solubility, which lack compatibility with hydrophilic hydrogels. These studies offered some hints about the impact of the non-dendritic component. In the work by Recio-Ruiz et al. [16], DTT (a short dithiol molecule) was used, which generated low-swelling networks with an SD in the range of 6–16%. In the work by Muñoz-Sánchez et al. [17], PEG1k(SH)$_2$ was used and high-swelling networks were obtained, with an SD in the range of 150–225% for traditional SiGnV$_m$ dendrimers or 163–300% for the new amphiphilic dendrimers with the *N*,*N*′-bis(2-hydroxyethyl) ethylenediamine core.

Interested in fine-tuning the amphiphilic properties of carbosilane dendritic hydrogels, in this work, we explored the impact of the linear polymer in the generation of dendritic networks. Different polymers were selected as precursors, from the highly lipophilic propylene glycol (PPG) to the hydrophilic polyethylene glycol (PEG), including the amphiphilic Pluronics L31, L35 and L61. Pluronics are a family of block copolymers (X-Y-X) formed by polyethylene glycol (PEG) and propylene glycol (PPG). These amphiphilic copolymers are highly versatile and commercially available in a broad range of molecular weights and hydrophilic–lipophilic balance (HLB) values [18]. These polymers show remarkable property changes in response to temperature, making them very promising for biomedical applications and as a possible drug delivery vehicle due to their excellent biocompatibility and environmental sensitivity [19]. Using a similar approach through UV-initiated TEC crosslinking with carbosilane dendrimers, we accomplished either non-swelling networks or high-swelling hydrogels with thermo-responsive properties. The impact of the polymer, the pendant groups on the dendritic crosslinker and the temperature were evaluated regarding properties like the swelling degree, the drug release and the mechanical properties, as described below.

2. Materials and Methods

2.1. Materials

Reagents and solvents were purchased from commercial sources and used as received. The Pluronics L31, L35 and L61, PEG1k and PPG1k, and 3-mercaptopropionic acid and p-toluenesulfonic acid monohydrate were purchased from Sigma Aldrich (St. Louis, MO, USA). 2,2-dimethoxy-2-phenylacetophenone (DMPA) was purchased from Acros Organics (Geel, Belgium). Toluene was purchased from PanReac (Barcelona, Spain). Chloroform was purchased from J.T. Baker (Phillipsburg, NJ, USA). Acetone, tetrahydrofuran, caffeic acid and methanol were purchased from Sigma Aldrich with the HPLC grade. Sulfuric acid was purchased from Hanssell (Madrid, Spain). Vinyl-decorated dendrimer Si-G1V$_8$ (**D1**) and dendrons N$_3$-G3V$_8$ (**D2**) and HO-G3V$_8$ (**D3**) were synthesized as previously reported [20,21].

Synthesis of Linear Polymers P(SH)$_2$

General protocol: The precursor polymer P(OH)$_2$ was suspended or dissolved in toluene. Two drops of concentrated H_2SO_4 were added, and the solution was heated to 100 °C with stirring to obtain a clear, homogeneous solution. To this solution, 3-mercaptopropionic acid was added, and the solution was refluxed under Dean–Stark conditions for 20 h. The solvent was removed in vacuo and the polymer was isolated through different strategies.

PEG$_{1k}$(SH)$_2$ (**P1**): The polymer was prepared through the general protocol using the following reagents: PEG (1000 g/mol, 10.1 g, 10.1 mmol), toluene (100 mL), and 3-mercaptopropionic acid (3.5 mL, 40 mmol). The resultant oil was precipitated in ether, and the product was isolated as a white gel (7.4 g, 62% yield). ^{1}H-NMR (CDCl$_3$): δ 4.2 (t, -CH_2OCO-), 3.6 (m, -O(CH_2)$_2$O-), 2.7 (m, -OC$CH_2$$CH_2$SH), 1.6 (t, -S*H*). The NMR signals matched the ones previously described in the literature [22].

PPG$_{1k}$(SH)$_2$ (**P2**): The polymer was prepared through the general protocol using the following reagents: PPG (1000 g/mol, 10.1 g, 10.1 mmol) and 3-mercaptopropionic acid (3.5 mL, 40 mmol). The resultant oil was dissolved in CH_2Cl_2 and washed with saturated $NaHCO_3$ and NaCl. The organic phase was dried with $MgSO_4$ and filtered and evaporated, obtaining the product as a yellow oil (10.5 g, 88% yield). ^{1}H-NMR (CDCl$_3$): δ 5.1 (t, -CH_2OCO-), 3.5 (m, -O$CH_2$$CH$(CH$_3$)O-), 2.6 (m, C$CH_2$$CH_2$SH), 1.6 (t, -SH), 1.1 (d, -OCH$_2$CH(CH_3)O-).

PLU$_{L31}$(SH)$_2$ (**P3**): The polymer was prepared through the general protocol using the following reagents: Pluronic L31 (1100 g/mol, 11.7 g, 10.6 mmol) and 3-mercaptopropionic acid (3.70 mL, 42 mmol). The resultant oil was dialyzed in toluene to eliminate the impurities, obtaining the product as a yellow oil (6.0 g, 44%). ^{1}H-NMR (CDCl$_3$): δ 4.2 (t, -CH_2OCO-), 3.6 (m, -O(CH_2)$_2$O-), 3.5 (m, -O$CH_2$$CH$(CH$_3$)O-), 2.6 (m, OC$CH_2$$CH_2$SH), 1.6 (t, -SH), 1.1 (d, -OCH$_2$CH(CH_3)O-).

PLU$_{L61}$(SH)$_2$ (**P4**): The polymer was prepared through the general protocol using the following reagents: Pluronic L61 (2000 g/mol, 10.3 g, 5.15 mmol) and 3-mercaptopropionic acid (1.85 mL, 21 mmol). The resultant oil was dissolved in Et$_2$O and washed with saturated $NaHCO_3$ and NaCl. The organic phase was dried with $MgSO_4$ and evaporated, obtaining the product as a yellow oil (5.3 g, 47% yield). ^{1}H-NMR (CDCl$_3$): δ 4.2 (t, -CH$_2$OCO-), 3.6 (m, -O(CH_2)$_2$O-), 3.5 (m, -O$CH_2$$CH$(CH$_3$)O-), 2.6 (m, OC$CH_2$$CH_2$SH), 1.6 (t, -SH), 1.1 (d, -OCH$_2$CH(CH_3)O-).

PLU$_{L35}$(SH)$_2$ (**P5**): The polymer was prepared through the general protocol using the following reagents: Pluronic L35 (1900 g/mol, 10.9 g, 5.75 mmol) and 3-mercaptopropionic acid (1.83 mL, 21 mmol). The resultant oil was dialyzed in toluene to eliminate the impurities, obtaining the product as a yellow oil (6.3 g, 58%). ^{1}H-NMR (CDCl$_3$): δ 4.23 (4 H, m, -CH_2OCO-), 3.67 (4H, m, CO$_2$CH$_2$$CH_2$O), 3.60 (72H, s, -O($CH_2$)$_2$O-), 3.50 (16H, m, -OCH$_2$$CH$(CH$_3$)O-), 3.46 (32H, m, -O$CH_2$CH(CH$_3$)O-), 2.71 (4H, m, -OC$CH_2CH_2$SH), 2.62 (4H, m, -OCCH$_2$$CH_2$SH), 1.65 (2H, m, -SH), 1.10 (48H, d, -OCH$_2$CH(CH_3)O-). ^{13}C-RMN (400 MHz CDCl$_3$): δ 171.0 (CO$_2$), 75.5 (O-CH-CH$_3$), 75.2–73.0 (O-CH$_2$-CH), 70.4 (O-CH$_2$CH$_2$-O), 38.9 (COO-CH$_2$CH$_2$-O), 63.5 (COO-CH$_2$CH$_2$-O), 38.5 (HS-CH$_2$CH$_2$-COO), 19.6 (HS-CH$_2$CH$_2$-COO), 17.5 (CH$_3$-CH).

2.2. General Methods

NMR spectroscopy. NMR spectra were acquired at CAIQ-UAH, using the Varian NMR System-500 (Varian, Inc., Palo Alto, CA, USA), Varian Mercury Plus-300 and Bruker AVANCE Neo 400 instruments (Bruker, Billerica, MA, USA) at room temperature and using $CDCl_3$ as the solvent. The chemical shifts are expressed in ppm using the solvent as an internal reference in ^{1}H-NMR ($CDCl_3$ δ (H) = 7.24 ppm) and in ^{13}C-NMR ($CDCl_3$ δ (C) = 77.0 ppm). HSQC was also carried out under these conditions.

Mass spectrometry. A MALDI-TOF/TOF, model ULTRAFLEX III of BRUKER, was used. The sample was dissolved in dichloromethane (2 mg/mL). The sample was mixed with the DCTB matrix (8 mg/mL in DCM) and NaI (2 mg/mL in acetone). The detection was performed in reflector mode with the detection of positive ions in the range of 500–5000 Da.

High-Performance Liquid Chromatography (HPLC). Drug release studies were performed at CAIQ-UAH on Agilent 1200 HPLC equipment (Agilent, Santa Clara, CA, USA), using an ACE Excel 5 C18 250 × 4.6 mm column and a mobile phase of 2% acetic acid and acetonitrile (50:50), with an injection volume of 10 μL. The drug was detected at a wavelength of 254 nm.

Rheometer. The viscoelastic properties of hydrogels were measured using a Discovery Hybrid Rheometer 10 (DHR-10) from TA Instruments (New Castle, DE, USA) at 25 °C and 37 °C using parallel-plate geometry (8 mm diameter). An amplitude sweep (0.1–100% strain at 1 Hz), a frequency sweep (0.1–10 Hz at 1% strain) and ramp temperature (20–40 °C at 1 Hz and 1% strain) assays were performed.

2.3. Synthesis of Dendritic Hydrogels

2.3.1. Synthesis of Dendritic Hydrogels

$P(SH)_2$ (4 eq.) was dissolved in a THF:MeOH mixture (1:2, 150 μL), and subsequently, the dendrimer/dendron (1 eq.) and DMPA (5 mol% of vinyl groups) were added. The resulting mixture was argon bubbled for a few seconds and introduced into several Teflon plugs with a capacity of around 200 μL before exposure to UV light for 4–6 h. A UV darkroom Vilber CN-15.LC was used (Vilber, Eberhardzell, Germany), with a total intensity of 30 W at 365 nm. Finally, the hydrogels were washed several times with acetone until the DMPA was eliminated, as confirmed by TLC (hexane:ethyl acetate, 80:20).

2.3.2. Post-Functionalization of Dendritic Hydrogels

Esterification of Rhodamine B to *Hy*[(HO-G3V_8)x($PLU_{L61}(SH)_2$)]. Rhodamine B (1.2 eq.) was dissolved in dichloromethane (4 mL) and was reacted with EDCI·HCl (1.2 eq.). The mixture was stirred for 30 min, and DMAP (0.2 eq.) was added. Subsequently, the hydrogel (70 mg) was immersed in the solution and maintained with slight stirring (150 rpm). After 20 h, the hydrogel was thoroughly washed with dichloromethane to remove non-bound dye, and was dried, obtaining a pink hydrogel.

CuAAC covalent attachment of Rhodamine B to *Hy*[(N_3-G3V_8)x($PLU_{L61}(SH)_2$)]. Rhodamine B isothiocyanate (50 mg, 0.093 mmol) was reacted with propargylamine (6 μL, 0.093 mmol) to generate the alkyne derivative of Rhodamine B. Subsequently, an aqueous solution of the alkyne derivative of Rhodamine (1.2 eq) was prepared. Copper sulfate (1.2 eq., 2.8 mg, 0.011 mmol) and sodium ascorbate (2.4 eq., 4.5 mg, 0.0226 mmol) were added. The hydrogel was immersed in the solution and maintained at 50 °C, with slight stirring (150 rpm) for 20 h. The hydrogel was thoroughly washed with water and acetone to remove non-bound dye, and was dried, obtaining a pink hydrogel.

2.4. Characterization of Hydrogels

2.4.1. Swelling Degree (SD%)

The hydrogels were immersed in distilled water for several days. Periodically, they were removed, and their size and weight were measured. All gels were tested in duplicate. The SD is calculated with the following equation:

$$SD\% = ((W - W_D)/W) \times 100$$

where W is the weight of the swollen gel, and W_D is the dry gel mass after purification.

2.4.2. Crosslinking Degree (CD%)

The crosslinking percentage was calculated using the following equation:

$$CD(\%) = (1 - (M_{UV} - M_W)/M_{UV}) \times 100$$

where W_{UV} is the dry mass after the UV reaction, and M_W is the dry mass after purification. All measurements were performed in duplicate.

2.4.3. Caffeic Acid Loading and Release Assay

The drug loading was performed by immersing the dry hydrogel (~60 mg) in a solution of caffeic acid (50 mg in 1 mL ethanol) for 60 h at 37 °C. Then, the hydrogel was extracted from the solution and dried to remove all embedded solvents. The remaining caffeic acid in the ethanol solution was quantified through HPLC.

For the release assay, the CA-encapsulated hydrogel was immersed in 1 mL of water solution at either 25 °C or 37 °C. Small aliquots (50 μL) were collected over time to quantify the CA release through HPLC. The solvent volume was kept constant by adding 50 μL of water after each extraction, so a small dilution effect (5% decrease in concentration) must be considered.

3. Results

Dendritic hydrogels based on carbosilane crosslinkers are promising materials as drug delivery systems. In our previous studies, different vinyl-decorated dendrimers were reacted with DTT or $PEG(SH)_2$ (**P1**) through TEC click chemistry, delivering amphiphilic networks that improved compatibility with lipophilic drugs. Additionally, we demonstrated their versatility and the ability to respond to certain stimuli like pH and temperature. In this work, we explored the impact of the linear polymer on the design of amphiphilic hydrogels.

3.1. Synthesis of Linear Polymers

In the design of the amphiphilic hydrogels, we used a lipophilic carbosilane crosslinker and a complementary hydrophilic polymer. To analyze the required hydrophilic-lipophilic balance to generate adequate hydrogels, we synthesized a library of different polymers $P(SH)_2$ from different precursors: PEG_{1k}, PPG_{1k}, PLU_{L31}, PLU_{L35} and PLU_{L61}. We adapted the protocol previously described for **P1** by Macdougall et al. [18]. The dithiol polymers (**P1–P5**) were prepared from the commercial precursors through esterification with 2-mercaptopropionic acid at 100° C in toluene. Depending on the nature of the polymer, different isolation protocols were employed, which impacted the final yield. Moderate yields were achieved in the range of 45–90%, being higher for the most lipophilic polymer. The final polymers were characterized through NMR, confirming the presence of the new -SH groups required for the crosslinking (Figures S1–S4). The polymers presented different HLB values, from the highly hydrophilic **P1** (HLB 18) to the highly hydrophobic **P2** (HLB 10.78).

The characterization of **P5** is discussed as an example. The HSQC spectrum is presented in Figure 1, while the individual ^1H and ^{13}C spectra are included in Figure S1. Compared to the precursor polymer, **P5** showed three new multiplets in the ^1H-NMR spectrum at 1.65, 2.62 and 2.71 ppm from the -$CO(CH_2)_2SH$ fragment (signals a, b and c in Figure 1). Furthermore, the methylene group closer to the new ester bond (signal d) shifted to 4.2 ppm. The methylene groups from the ethylene glycol (EG) units (labeled as *, e) and those from the propylene glycol (PG) units (labeled as f, g, h) exhibit much less shifting. In ^{13}C-NMR, a signal around 171.0 ppm is observed, assigned to the carbonyl group. This polymer was also studied through MALDI-TOF. A Gaussian curve is observed between 700 and 3500 Da, centered around 2200 Da (Figure S5). Despite the complexity of the spectra, due to the variable number of EG and PG units, it confirmed the correct attachment of both terminal thiol units.

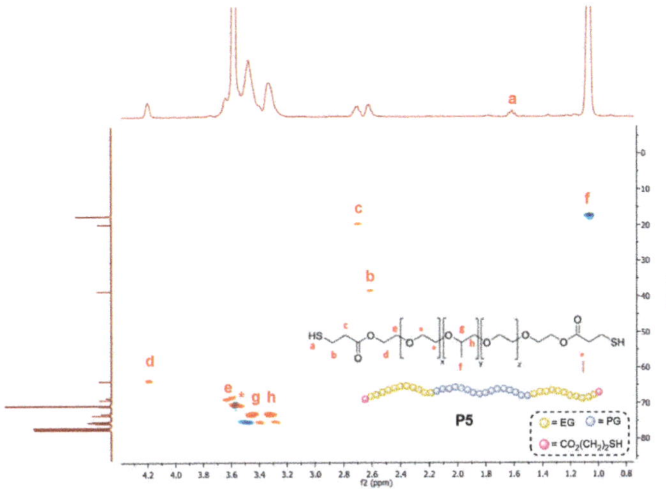

Figure 1. HSQC{^1H-^{13}C} spectrum of $PLU_{L35}(SH)_2$ (**P5**) in $CDCl_3$, confirming the presence of the -$CO(CH_2)_2SH$ fragment in the terminals of the polymer. ^1H-NMR spectrum is shown on the top, and ^{13}C-NMR is shown on the left of the figure.

3.2. *Synthesis and Characterization of Dendritic Hydrogels*

For the synthesis of the dendritic hydrogels, we followed the recently reported protocol using a vinyl-decorated carbosilane dendritic crosslinker and a dithiol linear polymer; Figure 2 [16,17]. Photoinitiated thiol–ene coupling (TEC) was used as the main tool. In a general protocol, the dendritic crosslinker and the polymer were dissolved in a THF:MeOH mixture. Subsequently, DMPA (5 mol% alkene) was added, and the mixture was exposed to UV light (365 nm) until the hydrogel was fully cured. Finally, the hydrogel was washed with acetone until complete removal of the photoinitiator and other impurities was achieved. All the hydrogels were characterized by studying their crosslinking degree (CD%) and swelling degree (SD%) in water.

3.2.1. Impact of the Linear Polymer $P(SH)_2$

In the first experiment, we performed a screening of the different linear polymers $P(SH)_2$ to evaluate the impact on the swelling properties of the dendritic networks. For comparative purposes, we used dendrimer Si-G1V$_8$ (**D1**) for the synthesis of all networks and studied their swelling degree at 25 °C (Figure 3). As expected, the network prepared with the hydrophobic PPG did not swell, and the one prepared from the hydrophilic PEG swelled up to 275% (at 25 °C); for the amphiphilic Pluronics, with intermediate properties between PPG and PEG, a different behavior was found. PLU_{L31} and PLU_{L61} are short polymers (M_n 1100 and 2000, respectively) with only 10% PEG. The crosslinking with the highly lipophilic dendrimer **D1** generates a network incapable of swelling in water (Figure 3A). However, for PLU_{L35} (M_n 1900 and 50% PEG), the hydrogel swells up to 190%.

These results highlight the impact of the hydrophilic–lipophilic balance within the network to accomplish an effective swelling.

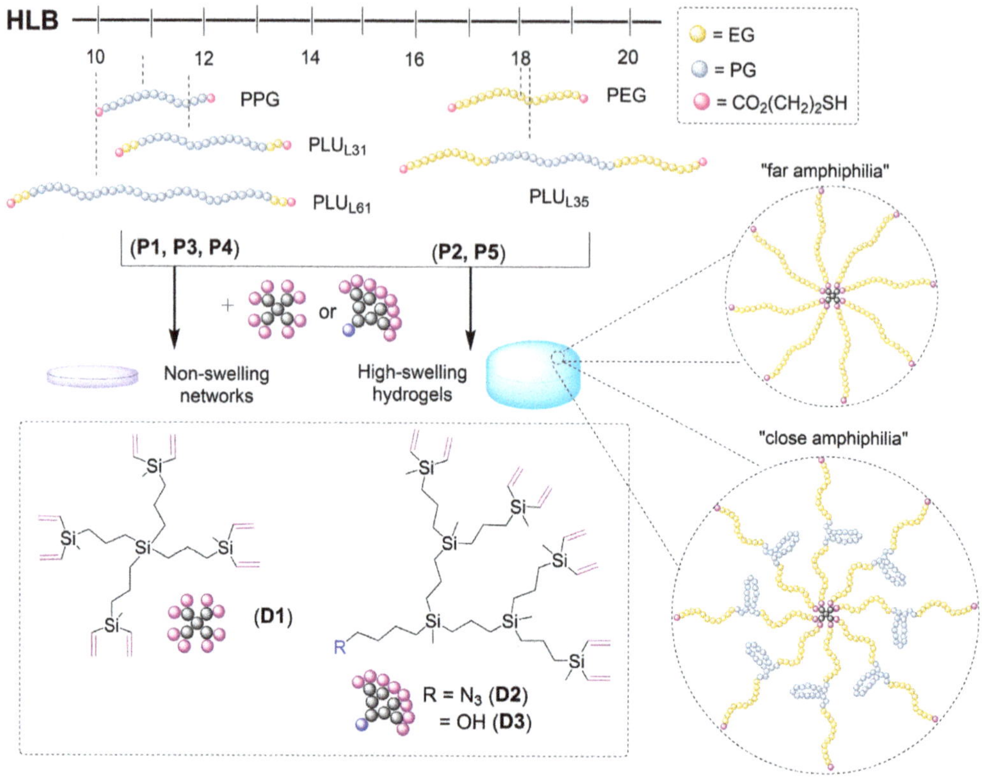

Figure 2. Schematic overview of the synthesis of the dendritic networks. Top: Polymer precursors **P1–P5**, including their HLB. Bottom: Dendritic precursors **D1–D3**. Middle: Resultant networks and hydrogels, including representation of their nanostructuring in water. In "far" amphiphilia, the hydrophobic and hydrophilic sections are provided by different components (dendrimer and PEG, respectively), so the hydrophobic pockets are located more distantly in the hydrogel. In "close" amphiphilia, the polymer is intrinsically amphiphilic (Pluronic L35), and the hydrophobic pockets caused by the dendrimer and the PPG sections are found closer.

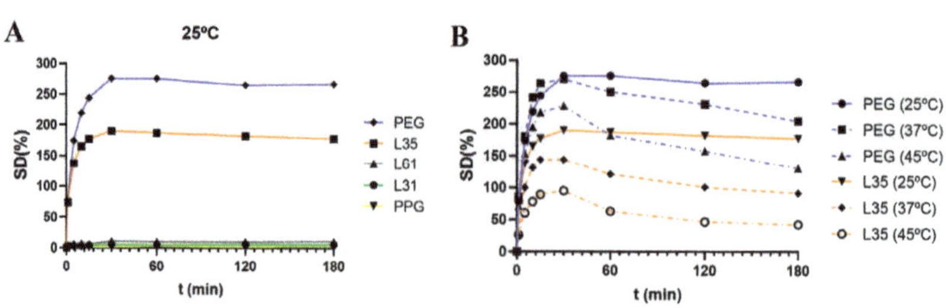

Figure 3. (**A**) Comparative swelling degree at 25 °C of hydrogels *Hy*[(Si-G1V$_8$)x(PX)], prepared from carbosilane dendrimer **D1** and the different polymers. (**B**) Comparative swelling degree at 25, 37 and 45 °C of hydrogels based on PEG$_{1k}$ and PLU$_{L35}$.

Overall, we found two dendritic hydrogels with an adequate amphiphilic balance to swell in water: *Hy*[(Si-G1V$_8$)x(P1)] (**H1Si**), with "far amphiphilia", as the lipophilic and the hydrophilic properties are provided by different entities, and thus the hydrophobic pockets are located more distantly in the hydrogel; and *Hy*[(Si-G1V$_8$)x(P5)] (**H5Si**), with "close amphiphilia", due to the presence of an intrinsically amphiphilic polymer in the network, and then the hydrophobic pockets caused by the dendrimer and the PPG fragments are found closer. The swelling behavior of these two hydrogels was further explored at different temperatures (Figure 3B). A similar pattern is observed: a fast swelling in the first 30 min to reach a maximum, then a progressive decrease until reaching a plateau around 2 h. In both cases, the swelling decreased when increasing the temperature. At higher temperatures, the higher mobility of the polymer chains enables a collapse of the lipophilic sections and expels the molecules of water from the pores of the network.

3.2.2. Impact of the Dendritic Crosslinker

In the second round of experiments, we selected two polymers with similar lengths but very different natures: the hydrophobic PLU$_{L61}$(SH)$_2$ (**P4**) and the hydrophilic PLU$_{L35}$(SH)$_2$ (**P5**); and we also modified the dendritic crosslinker: Si-G1V$_8$ (**D1**), N$_3$-G3V$_8$ (**D2**) and HO-G3V$_8$ (**D3**). The crosslinkers presented the same number of alkene groups available for crosslinking but had a different topology, having azide or hydroxyl groups in the focal points of the dendrons. This assay provided information about the impact of topology and pendant groups in two different types of dendritic networks: non-swelling (using **P4**) and high-swelling (using **P5**). The polymers (4 eq.) were crosslinked with **D1–D3** (1 eq.) to generate the corresponding networks *Hy*[(X-GnV$_8$)x(P4)] and *Hy*[(X-GnV$_8$)x(P5)] (Table 1).

Table 1. Overview of the different linear polymers and the derived dendritic hydrogels, including relevant parameters.

Polymer	M$_n$ [a] (g/mol)	%PEG	HLB [b]	Dendritic Hydrogel	CD (%)	SD (%) [c] 25/37 °C
PEG$_{1k}$(SH)$_2$ (**P1**)	1000	100	18	*Hy*[(Si-G1V$_8$)x(P1)] (**H1Si**)	91 (3 h)	276/271
PPG$_{1k}$(SH)$_2$ (**P2**)	1000	0	10.78	*Hy*[(Si-G1V$_8$)x(P2)] (**H2Si**)	94 (3 h)	2/3
PLU$_{L31}$(SH)$_2$ (**P3**)	1100	10	11.80	*Hy*[(Si-G1V$_8$)x(P3)] (**H3Si**)	94 (3 h)	6/5
PLU$_{L61}$(SH)$_2$ (**P4**)	2000	10	10.05	*Hy*[(Si-G1V$_8$)x(P4)] (**H4Si**)	71 (3 h)	11/9
				Hy[(N$_3$-G3V$_8$)x(P4)] (**H4N$_3$**)	92 (3 h)	[d]
				Hy[(HO-G3V$_8$)x(P4)] (**H4OH**)	92 (3 h)	[d]
PLU$_{L35}$(SH)$_2$ (**P5**)	1900	50	18.10	*Hy*[(Si-G1V$_8$)x(P5)] (**H5Si**)	90 (4 h)	216/112
				Hy[(N$_3$-G3V$_8$)x(P5)] (**H5N$_3$**)	76 (4 h)	198/95
				Hy[(HO-G3V$_8$)x(P5)] (**H5OH**)	81 (4 h)	222/120

[a] Calculated M$_n$ of precursor polymer. [b] Calculated through Davies method (ChemAxon). [c] Maximum swelling degree. [d] Not measured.

As expected, none of the PLU$_{L61}$ networks swelled in water. For PLU$_{L35}$ hydrogels, the SD% increased with a decreasing temperature, following the same pattern in both tests (25 and 37 °C); Figure 4A. The non-functional and the HO-functional hydrogels (with **D1** and **D3** crosslinkers, respectively) showed a similar SD of 200–220% at 25 °C, which substantially decreased to 95–120% at 37 °C. Both have a higher swelling than the N$_3$-functional hydrogel (with **D2** crosslinker) despite having a higher CD%. This fact highlights the impact of the pendant group on the ability to swell in water.

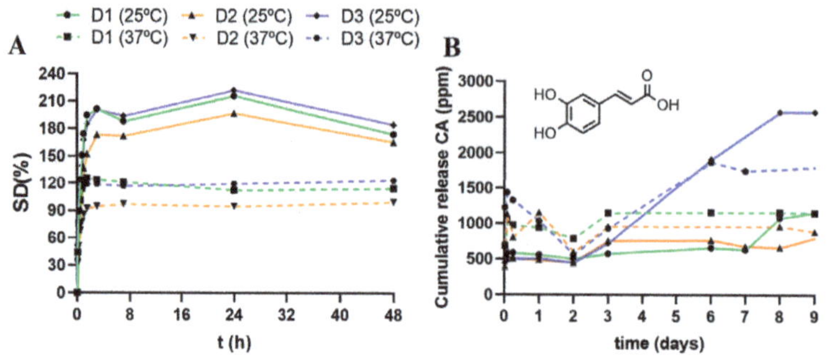

Figure 4. Comparative swelling degree (**A**) and cumulative release of caffeic acid (**B**) at 25 and 37 °C of *Hy*[(X-GnV$_8$)x(PLU$_{L35}$)] hydrogels, with Si-G1V$_8$ (**D1**), N$_3$-G3V$_8$ (**D2**) and HO-G3V$_8$ (**D3**).

The impact of the dendritic crosslinker was also studied regarding the drug loading and release of hydrophobic cargo. As a proof-of-concept, caffeic acid was loaded in the hydrogels, and the release was studied over time at 25 and 37 °C. The loading was performed by immersing the dry hydrogels in a solution of caffeic acid (50 mg in 1 mL of ethanol) for 60 h at 37 °C. These conditions were selected to maximize the loaded cargo. Then, the hydrogels were removed from the solution and dried to remove all embedded solvents. The remaining caffeic acid on the ethanol solution was quantified through HPLC, showing that the hydrogels loaded 25.5 ± 0.9 mg, 23.9 ± 3.4 mg and 19.3 ± 1.4 mg for **H5OH**, **H5N$_3$** and **H5Si**, respectively. Accordingly, the loading efficiency is in the range of 39–51%, which is positively influenced by the presence of the pendant groups.

CA-encapsulated hydrogels were then immersed in a water solution at 25 °C or 37 °C. Small aliquots (50 µL) were collected over time to quantify the CA release through HPLC. The results are represented in Figure 4B. At 25 °C, the three hydrogels behaved similarly for the first 48 h, showing no release. However, after 48 h, relevant differences appeared, showing a release that follows the trend Si (**D1**) < N$_3$ (**D2**) << OH (**D3**). At 37 °C, a higher release was observed compared to 25 °C. **H5Si** follows a similar pattern at both temperatures but duplicates the amount of released CA. The maximum released amount was accomplished around day 3 at 37 °C, but required 9 days at 25 °C to reach the same amount. **H5N$_3$** exhibited a burst release during the first hours, but the cargo was re-encapsulated during the first 2 days. Then, a sustained release started, reaching a maximum amount around day 3, which continued until day 8. **H5OH** also exhibited a burst release and a re-encapsulation of cargo during the first 2 days and then a subsequent sustained release until day 6. This assay confirmed the impact of both the pendant groups and the temperature to modulate the drug release.

This initial drug resorption had already been observed in other carbosilane dendritic hydrogels [12]. The hydrogel prepared with the traditional dendrimer Si-G1V$_8$ exhibited a burst release of ibuprofen and then a sustained release during the first 4 days. However, the hydrogels prepared with the aromatic-core dendrimer ArG2V$_{12}$ exhibited a resorption of the drug during the first 3 days and then a subsequent sustained release. When immersed in water, the hydrogel underwent a redistribution of its nanostructure, with a potent "sponge effect", which later acted as a reservoir of the aromatic drug. In the present work, the CA resorption occurs during the first 2 days, probably related to the rearrangement of PLU$_{L35}$ chains in water. The change of solvent from the loading step (ethanol) to the release step (water) requires some time to equilibrate the encapsulated cargo in the hydrogels. This resorption is especially relevant in the presence of azide and hydroxyl pendant groups, which aid in CA capture.

3.3. Mechanical Characterization of Dendritic Hydrogels

Rheology provides quantitative information on the viscoelasticity of the hydrogels. We herein explored hydrogels *Hy*[(X-GnV$_8$)x(PLU$_{L35}$)] with **D1** (X = Si), **D2** (X = N$_3$) and **D3** (X = OH) to evaluate the impact of the pendant groups in a non-swelling state. Two main parameters were studied: the storage modulus (G′), which measures the elasticity, and the loss modulus (G″), which represents the viscous part of a material and has the ability to dissipate energy in the form of heat. If G′ > G″, the material can be considered mainly elastic.

The measurements must be performed within the linear viscoelastic region (LVR), where the material can be deformed without losing its microstructural properties. We calculated the LVR through an amplitude sweep assay at 25 and 37 °C, keeping the frequency at 1 Hz and varying the oscillatory strain from 0.1% to 100%. A sudden drop in G′ that ultimately intersects with G″ indicates the critical strain, where the material microstructure is altered and, therefore, its viscoelastic properties. As depicted in Figure 5, the temperature is crucial for the critical deformation. At higher temperatures, the hydrogel can tolerate higher strains before being permanently deformed. For **H5Si**, the critical strain switches from 10% (25 °C) to 25% (at 37 °C). For **H5N$_3$**, it changes from 12% to 27%, and for **H5OH**, from 17% to 45%. Accordingly, we selected 1% OS as the optimum.

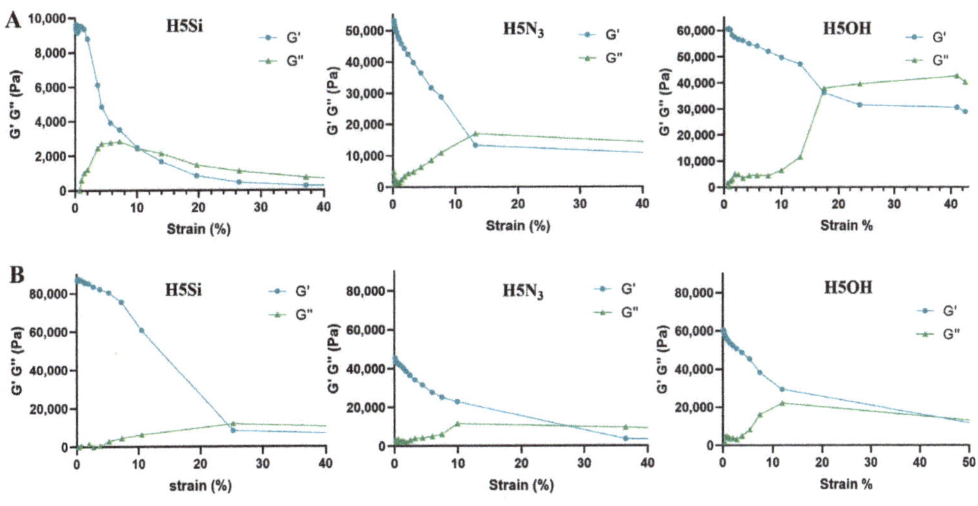

Figure 5. Amplitude sweeps at 25 °C (**A**) and 37 °C (**B**) for each hydrogel **H5X**.

Once the LVR was established, the hydrogels were studied through a frequency sweep assay. The assay was performed in the range of 0.1–10 Hz with the OS at 1% at 25 and 37 °C; Figure 6A. This assay provides more information about the behavior of the material (solid, liquid or gel). Due to the gel nature of our materials, they present a phase angle (δ) independent of the frequency and, therefore, a horizontal linearity. The storage moduli are substantially higher than the loss moduli, confirming the elastic (solid-state) nature of the hydrogels. At both temperatures, all hydrogels were stable, as G′ and G″ were not affected by the increase in frequency. Commonly, the storage modulus increases with the crosslinking degree of the hydrogel. However, we herein observed that the storage moduli decreased **D2** (N$_3$) > **D3** (OH) > **D1** (Si), in an opposite trend to the CD%. These results highlight the impact of the pendant groups, which reinforce the elasticity of the network.

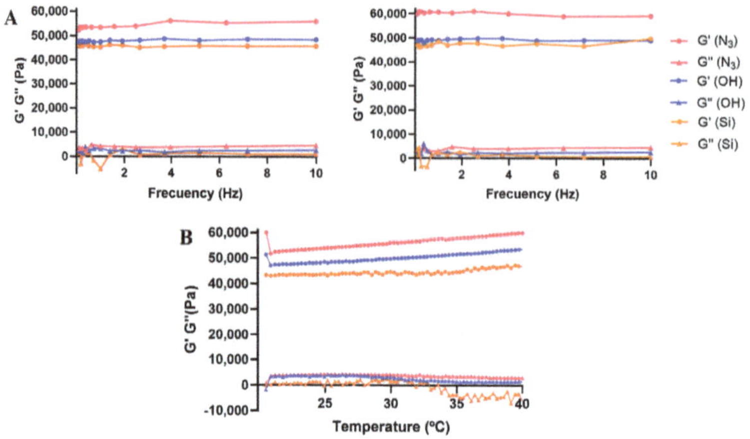

Figure 6. Storage (G′) and loss (G″) moduli in (**A**) frequency sweeps at 25 °C (**left**) and 37 °C (**right**), with OS 1%; (**B**) temperature sweep, from 20 to 40 °C, at 1 Hz and 1% strain; for hydrogels *Hy*[(X-GnV$_8$)x(P5)].

In a final assay, we performed a temperature sweep in the range of 20–40 °C at a constant frequency and deformation (1 Hz and 1% strain). As shown in Figure 6B, all hydrogels followed a similar trend, slightly increasing the storage modulus (G′) with the temperature and visibly decreasing the loss modulus (G″) above 35 °C, especially in **D1**. This indicates that the hydrogels are rheologically stable in the range of 20–40 °C and that the solid-state behavior is reinforced at higher temperatures.

3.4. Post-Functionalization of Dendritic Networks

The dendritic networks prepared with crosslinkers **D2** and **D3** present available azide and hydroxyl groups for further post-functionalization. As a proof-of-concept, we studied the covalent attachment of the fluorescent tag rhodamine through degradable and non-degradable bonds. In this case, we used the non-swelling networks *Hy*[(HO-G3V$_8$)x(PLU$_{L61}$(SH)$_2$)] (**H4OH**) and *Hy*[(N$_3$-G3V$_8$)x(PLU$_{L61}$(SH)$_2$)] (**H4N$_3$**) as precursors to explore the accessibility of the reactants in non-swelling situations.

On the one hand, we performed the esterification of Rhodamine B with EDCI·HCl in dichloromethane for 20 h at r.t. After thorough washings with dichloromethane to remove any unreacted compound, we visually confirmed the attachment of rhodamine (Figure 7). On the other hand, we performed a CuAAC click reaction on the azide bonds to generate permanent triazol bonds in the network. We first modified the Rhodamine B isothiocyanate with propargylamine. Then, we performed the CuAAC reaction in water in the presence of $CuSO_4$ and sodium ascorbate for 20 h at 50 °C. Again, after thorough washings with water and acetone, we visually confirmed the attachment of rhodamine. This result supports the ability of the dendritic networks to undergo post-modification with relevant moieties, like fluorescent tags, drugs or other bioactive molecules.

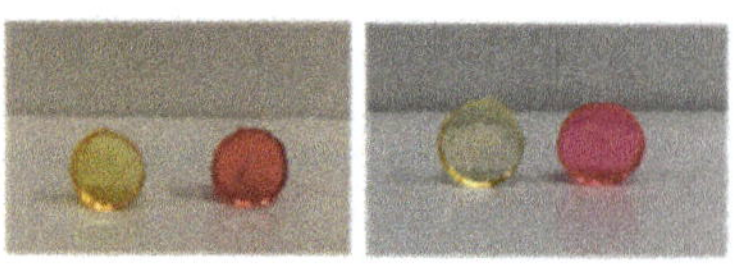

Figure 7. Image depicting hydrogels Hy[(HO-G3V$_8$)x(PLU$_{L61}$(SH)$_2$)] (**H4OH**) and Hy[(N$_3$-G3V$_8$)x(PLU$_{L61}$(SH)$_2$)] (**H4N$_3$**) before (yellow color) and after (pink color) covalent attachment of Rhodamine B.

4. Discussion

The field of polymer networks pursues a key target: to control the material's macroscopic properties at a molecular level. In this work, we contribute to this target by addressing three relevant elements: linear polymers, multifunctional junctions and crosslinking reactions.

Dendritic crosslinkers can be seen as a relevant tool due to their multivalent but defined structure that improves structural control. Additionally, their nature, size and functionalities can be fine-tuned, being highly versatile. In particular, we herein demonstrated that carbosilane dendrimers offer unique properties as multifunctional crosslinkers arising from their monodisperse, highly stable and lipophilic properties. Unlike other dendrimers employed in dendritic networks, with a main hydrophilic nature, carbosilane systems are especially interesting for the design of amphiphilic hydrogels for drug delivery purposes, as they increase the compatibility with poorly water-soluble drugs. Additionally, they can be precisely defined to incorporate pendant groups in the networks using heterofunctional dendrons like N_3-G3V_8 (**D2**) and HO-G3V_8 (**D3**).

Regarding the linear polymers, in this work, we demonstrated the crucial impact of the amphiphilic balance by switching the nature of the linear polymer. An adequate amphiphilic balance delivered high-swelling hydrogels, while a mainly hydrophobic framework generated non-swelling networks. Two different types of hydrogels were accomplished as follows: with "far" amphiphilia, where the hydrophobic and hydrophilic sections are provided by different components (dendrimer and PEG, respectively), or with "close" amphiphilia, as the used polymer is intrinsically amphiphilic (Pluronic L35). Despite the fact that PLU_{L35} is longer than PEG_{1k}, the PEG hydrogels exhibited higher swelling, confirming the impact of the linear counterpart. The modification of Pluronic polymers with terminal hydrophobic units affects their sol–gel transition. Qian et al. designed a thermosensitive hydrogel based on PCL-PLU_{L35}-PCL [23]. This polymer exhibited a special gel–sol transition arising from the hydrophobic interactions and partial crystallization. However, if the molecular weight of the PCL portion reaches an excessive value, it becomes too hydrophobic for thermo-reversible gelation. This example also supports the impact of amphiphilic balance on the design of polymer networks.

Finally, the use of highly efficient crosslinking reactions like thiol–ene chemistry (TEC) can facilitate the structural control of the networks. TEC has been previously employed to generate different dendritic networks, through a fast and robust approach [24,25]. In our case, TEC generated a high CD% (70–95%), which also depended on the lipophilicity of the polymer and the dendritic pendant groups. The more lipophilic network, the higher the crosslinking degree was observed. Other photo-cross-linkable hydrogels have been described in the literature, mainly relying on modified polymers [26]. For example, Pluronic F127 was di-acrylated and crosslinked upon exposure to UV light in the absence and presence of vinyl-functional hyaluronic acid, which acted as a multifunctional crosslinker [27]. The chemical crosslinking resulted in a micellar hydrogel network structure. Similarly to our studies, the authors demonstrated that at higher temperatures (37 °C vs. 13 °C), swelling ratios substantially decreased. They also observed that the SD% continuously decreases with increasing temperature until a sharper decrease around 20 °C [28]. This indicated that the local micellization of the Pluronic component had occurred, which was induced by rising temperature, and played a critical role in the de-swelling of the HA/Pluronic hydrogels. The hydrophobic PPG middle block of Pluronic self-associated and reduced the mesh size in the hydrogels at higher temperatures. Nevertheless, the authors also described the mass erosion of these hydrogels. The micelles slowly degraded due to the hydrolytic scission of the ester linkage between the Pluronic and acrylate groups. Accordingly, the use of thiol–ene chemistry as herein reported, offers a higher stability to the covalently crosslinked Pluronic hydrogels.

These three components, linear polymer, dendritic crosslinker and the TEC reaction, clearly affected the design of the networks as well as their properties, like swelling, drug release and mechanical properties. The swelling was mainly determined by the amphiphilic balance, requiring overcoming a certain barrier to jump from a non-swelling network to a high-swelling hydrogel. The PEG_{1k} and PLU_{L35} polymers enabled us to overcome this barrier. Subsequently, the type of amphiphilia ("far" or "close") fine-tuned the swelling behavior of the network, as well as the thermo-responsive behavior of the hydrogel. These hydrogels showed a lower swelling at 37 °C than at 25 °C due to the rearrangement of the hydrophobic sections in the network and the nanostructuring that expelled the water molecules from the hydrogel. The nanostructuring of hydrogels has been extensively described in the literature. For example, amphiphilic block copolymers and peptide oligomers with specific sequences can go through self-assembly to form a nanostructured hydrogel under physiological conditions [27]. Composite hydrogels have also been described, which include metal nanoparticles, carbon nanotubes, nano-cellulose or MOFs [29]. These embedded nanomaterials can modulate the biological response. The drug release, herein exemplified with caffeic acid, is closely connected to the swelling. At 37 °C, the drug release is higher. This behavior can also be modulated by the presence of pendant groups: the hydroxyl groups substantially improve the release. Furthermore, a peculiar pattern was found at 37 °C, exhibiting a burst release, then drug resorption for the first 48 h, and a subsequent sustained release. These hydrogels showed a restructuring of the nanostructure upon exposure to water, which acted as a drug reservoir.

The mechanical properties of our hydrogels, with $G' >> G''$ over the entire frequency range, are in agreement with an extremely soft viscoelastic solid. This behavior has already been seen for other photo-crosslinked Pluronic hydrogels, with G' values in the range of 1000–10,000 Pa [27,30,31]. For our hydrogels, much stiffer networks were obtained above 45,000 Pa. All these examples confirmed that G' and G'' were much higher than that of the physical Pluronic hydrogels produced by simply increasing the temperature [32]. For physical Pluronic hydrogels, with the temperature rise, the hydrophobic interactions inside the Pluronic increased and determined the micelles and polymicelles formation, which further generated a physical network. After the transition point, G' becomes higher than G'', suggesting network formation. With our hydrogels, we also confirmed that the storage modulus was clearly affected by the pendant groups, showing the following trend: **D2** (N_3) > **D3** (OH) > **D1** (Si). Surprisingly, this was an inverse trend to the CD%. This fact revealed the potential reinforcement of the covalent network with additional crosslinking points due to, for example, H-bonding.

5. Conclusions

Carbosilane-based dendritic hydrogels enable good control of the material macroscopic properties at a molecular level. The use of versatile linear polymers, monodisperse multifunctional crosslinkers and a highly efficient crosslinking reaction like TEC improve the control over the design of the network. The precise design enables the achievement of on-demand properties, like adequate hydrophilic–lipophilic balance, to obtain high-swelling hydrogels with thermo-responsive properties. These networks can be designed with "far" or "close" amphiphilia, which impacts the hydrogel nanostructuring and thus fine-tunes their properties like swelling and drug release. Furthermore, they can present pendant groups that can be post-functionalized to provide additional properties. This opens new avenues for different biomedical applications that require permanent activity on the network or even a more controlled release of a molecule through covalent bond cleavage. Overall, this work highlighted the potential of carbosilane dendritic hydrogels with thermo-responsive behavior in the biomedical field.

6. Patents

Some of the results of this article are included in the patent "Hidrogeles con dominios dendríticos de naturaleza carbosilano, su preparación y sus usos", PCT/ES2022/070728.

Supplementary Materials: The following supporting information can be downloaded at: https://www.mdpi.com/article/10.3390/pharmaceutics16040495/s1, Figures S1–S4: ^{1}H, ^{13}C-NMR of polymers P2–P5; Figure S5: MALDI-TOF spectra of polymer P5.

Author Contributions: Conceptualization, S.G.-G.; formal analysis, S.M.-S., S.G.-G. and A.B.-G.; investigation, S.M.-S. and A.B.-G.; data curation, S.M.-S. and A.B.-G.; writing—original draft preparation, S.M.-S. and S.G.-G.; writing—review and editing, S.G.-G. and F.J.d.l.M.; supervision, S.G.-G. and F.J.d.l.M.; funding acquisition, S.G.-G. and F.J.d.l.M. All authors have read and agreed to the published version of the manuscript.

Funding: The authors acknowledge the funding received from Ministerio de Ciencia e Innovación (PID2020112924RB-100), Comunidad de Madrid and University of Alcalá (projects CM/JIN/2021-003 and CM/BG/2021-01) and Junta de Comunidades de Castilla–la Mancha (Project SBPLY/19/180501/000269). The authors also acknowledge funding from the DISCOVER-UAH-CM Project (ref. REACT UE-CM2021-01), cofounded by the Community of Madrid (CAM) and the European Union (UE) through the European Regional Development Fund (ERDF) and supported as part of the EU's response to the COVID-19 pandemic. S.G.-G. gives thanks to the Ministry of Universities for a Beatriz Galindo research grant (BG20/00231). CIBER-BBN is an initiative funded by the VI National R&D&i Plan 2008-2011, Iniciativa Ingenio 2010, Consolider Program, CIBER Actions, and is financed by the Instituto de Salud Carlos III with assistance from the European Regional Development Fund.

Institutional Review Board Statement: Not applicable.

Informed Consent Statement: Not applicable.

Data Availability Statement: The data presented in this study are available in this article (and Supplementary Material).

Conflicts of Interest: The authors declare no conflicts of interest. The funders had no role in the design of the study, in the collection, analyses, or interpretation of data, in the writing of the manuscript, or in the decision to publish the results.

References

1. Gu, Y.; Zhao, J.; Johnson, J.A. Polymer networks: From plastics and gels to porous frameworks. *Angew. Chem. Int. Ed.* **2019**, *59*, 5022–5049. [CrossRef]
2. Danielsen, S.P.O.; Beech, H.K.; Wang, S.; El-Zaatari, B.M.; Wang, X.; Sapir, L.; Ouchi, T.; Wang, Z.; Johnson, P.N.; Hu, Y.; et al. Molecular characterization of polymer networks. *Chem. Rev.* **2021**, *121*, 5042–5092. [CrossRef] [PubMed]
3. Caló, E.; Khutoryanskiy, V.V. Biomedical applications of hydrogels: A review of patents and commercial products. *Eur. Polym. J.* **2015**, *65*, 252–267. [CrossRef]
4. Thang, N.H.; Chien, T.B.; Cuong, D.X. Polymer-based hydrogels applied in drug delivery: An overview. *Gels* **2023**, *9*, 523. [CrossRef]
5. Stuart, M.A.C.; Huck, W.T.; Genzer, J.; Müller, M.; Ober, C.; Stamm, M.; Sukhorukov, G.B.; Szleifer, I.; Tsukruk, V.V.; Urban, M.; et al. Emerging applications of stimuli-responsive polymer materials. *Nat. Mater.* **2010**, *9*, 101–113. [CrossRef] [PubMed]
6. Zhang, K.; Xue, K.; Loh, X.J. Thermo-responsive hydrogels: From recent progress to biomedical applications. *Gels* **2021**, *7*, 77. [CrossRef]
7. Chatterjee, S.; Hui, P.C.-l.; Kan, C.-w.; Wang, W. Dual-responsive (pH/temperature) Pluronic F-127 hydrogel drug delivery system for textile-based transdermal therapy. *Sci. Rep.* **2019**, *9*, 11658. [CrossRef]
8. Cao, M.; Wang, Y.; Hu, X.; Gong, H.; Li, R.; Cox, H.; Zhang, J.; Waigh, T.A.; Xu, H.; Lu, J.R. Reversible thermoresponsive peptide–PNIPAM hydrogels for controlled drug delivery. *Biomacromolecules* **2019**, *20*, 3601–3610. [CrossRef] [PubMed]
9. Yeh, M.-Y.; Zhao, J.-Y.; Hsieh, Y.-R.; Lin, J.-H.; Chen, F.-Y.; Chakravarthy, R.D.; Chung, P.-C.; Lin, H.-C.; Hung, S.-C. Reverse thermo-responsive hydrogels prepared from Pluronic F127 and gelatin composite materials. *RSC Adv.* **2017**, *7*, 21252–21257. [CrossRef]
10. Constantinou, A.P.; Georgiou, T.K. Pre-clinical and clinical applications of thermoreversible hydrogels in biomedical engineering: A review. *Polym. Int.* **2021**, *70*, 1433–1448. [CrossRef]
11. Olofsson, K.; Andrén, O.C.J.; Malkoch, M. Recent advances on crosslinked dendritic networks. *J. Appl. Polym. Sci.* **2013**, *131*, 39876. [CrossRef]
12. Gitsov, I.; Zhu, C. Amphiphilic hydrogels constructed by Poly(ethylene glycol) and shape-persistent dendritic fragments. *Macromolecules* **2002**, *35*, 8418–8427. [CrossRef]
13. Mongkhontreerat, S.; Andrén, O.C.J.; Boujemaoui, A.; Malkoch, M. Dendritic hydrogels: From exploring various crosslinking chemistries to introducing functions and naturally abundant resources. *J. Polym. Sci. A* **2015**, *53*, 2431–2439. [CrossRef]
14. Apartsin, E.; Caminade, A.-M. Single-component physical hydrogels of dendritic molecules. *J. Compos. Sci.* **2023**, *7*, 26. [CrossRef]

15. Kabanov, V.A.; Zezin, A.B.; Rogacheva, V.B.; Panova, T.V.; Bykova, E.V.; Joosten, J.G.H.; Brackman, J. Self-organization of cationic dendrimers in polyanionic hydrogels. *J. Faraday Discuss.* **2005**, *128*, 341. [CrossRef] [PubMed]
16. Recio-Ruiz, J.; Carloni, R.; Ranganathan, S.; Muñoz-Moreno, L.; Carmena, M.J.; Ottaviani, M.F.; de la Mata, F.J.; García-Gallego, S. Amphiphilic dendritic hydrogels with carbosilane nanodomains: Preparation and characterization as drug delivery systems. *Chem. Mater.* **2023**, *35*, 2797–2807. [CrossRef] [PubMed]
17. Muñoz-Sánchez, S.; Heredero-Bermejo, I.; de la Mata, F.J.; García-Gallego, S. Bifunctional carbosilane dendrimers for the design of multipurpose hydrogels with antibacterial action. *Chem. Mater.* **2024**, *36*, 266–274. [CrossRef]
18. Naharros-Molinero, A.; Caballo-González, M.A.; de la Mata, F.J.; García-Gallego, S. Direct and reverse Pluronic micelles: Design and characterization of promising drug delivery nanosystems. *Pharmaceutics* **2022**, *14*, 2628. [CrossRef] [PubMed]
19. Elluru, M.; Ma, H.; Hadjiargyrou, M.; Hsiao, B.S.; Chu, B. Synthesis and characterization of biocompatible hydrogel using Pluronics-based block copolymers. *Polymer* **2013**, *54*, 2088–2095. [CrossRef]
20. Strašák, T.; Čermák, J.; Sýkora, J.; Horský, J.; Walterová, Z.; Jaroschik, F.; Harakat, D. Carbosilane metallodendrimers with titanocene dichloride end groups. *Organometallics* **2012**, *31*, 6779–6786. [CrossRef]
21. Mencia, G.; Lozano-Cruz, T.; Valiente, M.; de la Mata, F.J.; Cano, J.; Gómez, R. New ionic carbosilane dendrons possessing fluorinated tails at different locations on the skeleton. *Molecules* **2020**, *25*, 807. [CrossRef] [PubMed]
22. Macdougall, L.J.; Pérez-Madrigal, M.M.; Arno, M.C.; Dove, A.P. Nonswelling Thiol–Yne Cross-Linked Hydrogel Materials as Cytocompatible Soft Tissue Scaffolds. *Biomacromolecules* **2018**, *19*, 1378–1388. [CrossRef] [PubMed]
23. Liu, C.; Gong, C.; Pan, Y.; Zhang, Y.; Wang, J.; Huang, M.; Wang, Y.; Wang, K.; Gou, M.; Tu, M.; et al. Synthesis and characterization of a thermosensitive hydrogel based on biodegradable amphiphilic PCL-Pluronic (L35)-PCL block copolymers. *Colloid Surf. A* **2007**, *302*, 430–438. [CrossRef]
24. Mongkhontreerat, S.; Öberg, K.; Erixon, L.; Löwenhielm, P.; Hult, A.; Malkoch, M. UV initiated thiol–ene chemistry: A facile and modular synthetic methodology for the construction of functional 3D networks with tunable properties. *J. Mater. Chem. A* **2013**, *1*, 13732–13737. [CrossRef]
25. Granskog, V.; García-Gallego, S.; von Kieseritzky, J.; Rosendahl, J.; Stenlund, P.; Zhang, Y.; Petronis, S.; Lyvén, B.; Arner, M.; Håkansson, J.; et al. High-performance Thiol–Ene composites unveil a new era of adhesives suited for bone repair. *Adv. Funct. Mater.* **2018**, *28*, 1800372. [CrossRef]
26. Chung, H.J.; Park, T.G. Self-assembled and nanostructured hydrogels for drug delivery and tissue engineering. *NanoToday* **2009**, *4*, 429–437. [CrossRef]
27. Chun, K.W.; Lee, J.B.; Kim, S.H.; Park, T.G. Controlled release of plasmid DNA from photo-cross-linked pluronic hydrogels. *Biomaterials* **2005**, *26*, 3319–3326. [CrossRef]
28. Kim, M.R.; Park, T.G. Temperature-responsive and degradable hyaluronic acid/Pluronic composite hydrogels for controlled release of human growth hormone. *J. Control Release* **2002**, *80*, 69–77. [CrossRef]
29. Cabrera-Munguía, D.A.; Caldera-Villalobos, M.; Flores-Guía, T.E.; Cano-Salazar, L.F.; Claudio-Rizo, J.A. Composites in hydrogel state with nanostructured components for biomedical applications. In *Nanotechnology for Biomedical Applications*; Materials horizons: From nature to nanomaterials; Gopi, S., Balakrishnan, P., Mubarak, N.M., Eds.; Springer: Singapore, 2022.
30. Lee, J.B.; Yoon, J.J.; Lee, D.S.; Park, T.G. Photo-crosslinkable, thermo-sensitive and biodegradable pluronic hydrogels for sustained release of protein. *J. Biomater. Sci. Polym. Ed.* **2004**, *15*, 1571–1583. [CrossRef]
31. Yoo, H.S. Photo-cross-linkable and thermo-responsive hydrogels containing chitosan and Pluronic for sustained release of human growth hormone (hGH). *J. Biomater. Sci. Polym. Ed.* **2007**, *18*, 1429–1441. [CrossRef]
32. Lupu, A.; Gradinaru, L.M.; Rusu, D.; Bercea, M. Self-healing of Pluronic® F127 hydrogels in the presence of various polysaccharides. *Gels* **2023**, *9*, 719. [CrossRef] [PubMed]

pharmaceutics

MDPI

Article

Carbosilane Dendritic Amphiphiles from Cholesterol or Vitamin E for Micelle Formation

Gabriel Mencia [1,2,3], Sergio Algar [1,2], Tania Lozano-Cruz [1,2,3], Mª Ángeles Muñoz-Fernández [2,4,5], Elizabeth R. Gillies [6], Jesús Cano [1,2,3], Mercedes Valiente [7,*] and Rafael Gómez [1,2,3,*]

1 Department of Organic and Inorganic Chemistry, Research Institute in Chemistry "Andrés M. Del Río" (IQAR), University of Alcalá, 28805 Madrid, Spain; gabi.men.ber@gmail.com (G.M.); sergioalgar@ucm.es (S.A.); tania.lozano@uah.es (T.L.-C.); jesus.cano@uah.es (J.C.)
2 Networking Research Center on Bioengineering, Biomaterials and Nanomedicine (CIBER-BBN), 28029 Madrid, Spain; mmunoz.hgugm@gmail.com
3 Ramón y Cajal Health Research Institute (IRYCIS), 28034 Madrid, Spain
4 Laboratory Platform (Immunology), General Universitary Hospital Gregorio Marañón (HGUGM), 28007 Madrid, Spain
5 Spanish HIV HGM BioBank, Health Research Institute Gregorio Marañón (HGUGM), 28007 Madrid, Spain
6 Department of Chemistry and Chemical and Biochemical Engineering, School of Biomedical Engineering, University of Western Ontario, London, ON N6G1Z1, Canada; egillie@uwo.ca
7 Department of Analytical Chemistry, Physical Chemistry and Chemical Engineering, Research Institute in Chemistry "Andrés M. Del Río" (IQAR), University of Alcalá, 28805 Madrid, Spain
* Correspondence: mercedes.valiente@uah.es (M.V.); rafael.gomez@uah.es (R.G.); Tel.: +34-91-8854670 (M.V.); +34-91-8854685 (R.G.)

Abstract: Cationic dendritic amphiphiles were prepared through the linkage of interesting hydrophobic molecules such as cholesterol or vitamin E to the focal point of carbosilane dendrons. These new dendritic systems self-assembled in saline, producing micellar aggregates with hydrodynamic diameters ranging from 6.5 to 9.2 nm, and critical micelle concentrations of approximately 5 and 10 μM for second- and third-generation systems, respectively. The assemblies were able to encapsulate drugs of different charges (anionic, neutral, and cationic). Surprisingly, a 92% encapsulation efficiency for diclofenac was achieved in micelles prepared from second-generation dendrons. Toxicity measurements on peripheral blood mononuclear cells indicated different behavior depending on the generation, corresponding to the micellar regime. In contrast to the third-generation system, the second-generation system was non-toxic up to 20 μM, opening a window for its use in a micellar regimen, thereby operating as a drug delivery system for different biomedical applications.

Keywords: carbosilane; dendron; cholesterol; tocopherol; micelle; drug encapsulation

1. Introduction

Classical surfactants are substances formed using a hydrocarbon chain attached to an ionic polar group. Of these, the oldest used are fatty acids which are biomolecules that make up the main components of fats and consist of a carboxylic acid group attached to a hydrocarbon chain that can be of different lengths and degrees of saturation. However, other naturally occurring compounds are able to form amphiphilic systems, and, therefore, its aggregates are cholesterol and vitamin E.

Cholesterol is an essential steroid lipid in the cytoplasmic membrane, where it fulfills a very important structural function, giving rise to the final physical–chemical properties of the membrane. In addition, it is involved in biosynthetic hormone processes, such as those of testosterone and progesterone, as well as vitamin D. In the field of micellar aggregates, Haberland and Reynolds demonstrated in the 1970s that cholesterol was an amphiphilic molecule capable of forming micelles at concentrations in the order of nanomolars [1]. Therefore, in recent years, many amphiphilic structures derived from cholesterol have emerged by modifying its polar zone to improve its solubility and offer new features depending on the desired application (gene therapy, drug encapsulation, antitumor therapy, etc.) [2–4]. In addition, in the last decade, so-called quatsomes have been developed, where cholesterol plays a fundamental role in helping other surfactants to form more complex systems [5]. In particular, cholesterol interacts with the hydrocarbon tail of the surfactant cetyltrimethylammonium bromide (CTAB) through hydrophobic interactions. This interaction causes the non-covalent association of the two molecules to behave as a single unit, resulting in geometry changes from conical to cylindrical and favoring the formation of vesicles. Therefore, the addition of different proportions of cholesterol causes a change from classical spherical micelles of CTAB to vesicles.

Although the number of amphiphilic systems that contain cholesterol is extensive, there are only a few examples of its use to generate classic amphiphilic head/tail dendritic systems. For instance, bis-MPA dendrons were reported, which were capable of micelle formation at *c.a.* 5 µM with diameters of approximately 7 and 15 nm for a second-generation system, depending on whether they had one or two cholesterol groups at the focal point (tail), respectively [6–8]. Another example involved poly(amidoamine) (PAMAM)-type dendrons, with a critical micellar concentration (CMC) of 20 µM, and micelle diameters of about 115–130 nm [9,10]. In both cases, the dendritic skeletons had relatively hydrophilic characteristics, and the studies were focused on the delivery of nucleic acids with cationic micelles. In both cases, interaction with DNA occurred, which allowed these systems to be used as gene therapy carriers.

Vitamin E is a generic term that includes a total of eight biologically active compounds with similar functions. All of these compounds contain a chromanol ring and differ in their degree of methylation of the aromatic ring and in the saturation of the side chain, giving rise to the derivatives α-, β-, γ- and Δ-tocopherol and -tocotrienol. These molecules, encompassed under the name vitamin E, are the most abundant liposoluble antioxidants in cells, and their main function is to break the chain of reactions that gives rise to the oxidation of lipids [11,12]. Among them, α-tocopherol has the greatest bioavailability and activity. Numerous scientific studies in which d-α-tocopherol was used in the synthesis of amphiphilic molecules, as a lipophilic component for the generation of micelles, have been reported [13–16]. These amphiphilic systems almost always presented poly(ethylene glycol) (PEG) as the hydrophilic unit [17–20]. Another example was that formed with inulin polysaccharide as a hydrophilic part [21]. These systems with CMCs between 3 and 75 µM were able to successfully encapsulate curcumin and celecoxib with efficiencies of 37 and 52%, respectively.

Regarding its use in dendritic systems, d-α-tocopherol covalently linked to the periphery of PAMAM dendrons was reported for different biomedical applications [22–24]. In the specific field of dendritic micelles, d-α-tocopherol as a hydrophobic component, was bound to the periphery of poly-lysine type hydrophilic dendrons with PEG at the focal point [25,26]. These dendrons had CMCs between 1.3 and 1.5 µM, and their micelles diameters ranged from 10 to 20 nm. In addition, these micelles were able to encapsulate proteins for biomolecular transport applications. However, no amphiphilic dendrons have been reported in the literature with the classical head/tail structure where the periphery of the dendron served as the hydrophilic head group, and the tail composed of a d-α-tocopherol molecule was attached to the focal point.

In general terms, dendritic micelles have been shown to exhibit advantages compared to those composed of conventional surfactants. For instance, they can exhibit better stability in solution and lower CMCs, in addition to their multivalency that allows enhanced interactions with biological systems compared to individual small molecules [27–30]. In this sense, we have recently reported the design of new amphiphilic carbosilane dendrons with pH-dependent behavior based on the presence of carboxylate groups at the periphery and a fatty acid in the focal point to encapsulate hydrophilic and hydrophobic drugs [31]. Here, we present our results concerning the formation of carbosilane dendritic micelles using cholesterol or vitamin E (d-α-tocopherol) as the hydrophobic tail at the focal point of the dendritic scaffold and hydrophilic ammonium groups at the periphery, along with their viability for drug encapsulation.

2. Materials and Methods

2.1. Materials

Reagents were purchased from commercial suppliers and used without further purification. Solvents were dried and distilled under an argon prior to use, unless specified otherwise. The dendron precursors NH2Gn(SNMe2)m (n = 1, m = 2 (i); n = 2, m = 4 (ii); n = 3, m = 8 (iii)), BrGn(V)m (n = 1, m = 2 (iv); n = 2, m = 4 (v); n = 3, m = 8 (vi)) [32] were synthesized as previously reported. *Click* reactions (thiol-ene addition) were carried out employing a HPK 125 W mercury lamp (Heraeus Noblelight; λ_{max} = 365 nm). Hydrophilic drugs including ibuprofen, procaine and lidocaine (the latter in its neutral form), as well as diclofenac as a hydrophobic drug, were purchased from commercial sources (Figure 1).

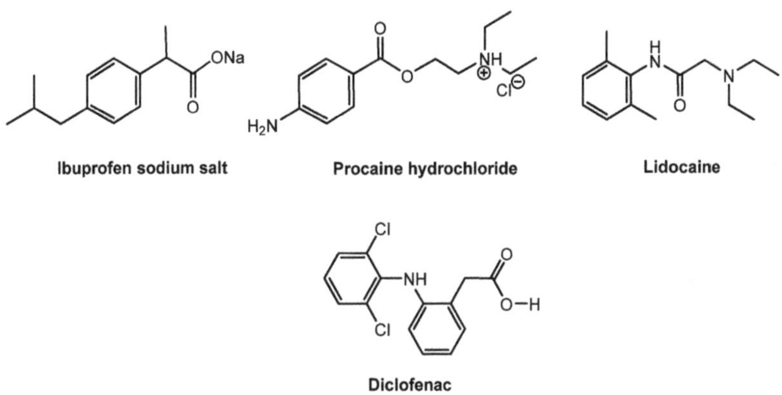

Figure 1. Molecular structures of selected drugs.

2.2. Analytical and Spectroscopic Techniques

NMR spectroscopy. NMR spectra were recorded with a Varian Unity-300, Varian Mercury-300 or Bruker 400 Ultrashield spectrometer. All chemical shifts were determined using the residual solvent signal.

Mass spectrometry. The measurements were conducted employing an Agilent 6210 TOF LC-ESI-MS system. Methanol (1% formic acid) served as eluent solvent for the positive mode while methanol/water was utilized for the negative mode.

Elemental analysis. Elemental analyses of C, H, and S were obtained on a LECO CHNS-932 microanalyzer.

Surface tension measurements. The measurements were carried using the ring method in a Lauda TE 2/3 tensiometer. The optimized NaI concentration was determined in aqueous solutions containing 1 mM of dendron with a salt concentration ranging from 0 to 30 mM. The critical micellar concentration (CMC) was determined using aqueous solutions of dendrons ranging from 1 to 100 µM with NaI at 40 mM.

Dynamic light scattering. The assembly diameters were determined utilizing a Nano ZS zetasizer from Malvern Instruments Ltd, Malvern, United Kingdom. All measurements were carried out at 25 °C in non-reusable plastic cells. The data are presented as the mean ± standard deviation of three separate experiments.

UV-Vis spectroscopy. Spectroscopic measurements were performed in a UVIKON 941 Plus spectrophotometer at 25 °C with quartz cells.

High-performance liquid chromatography (HPLC). HPLC analyses were performed with an Agilent 1200 HPLC with DAD detector (Model G1315D).

2.3. Protocols for Drug Encapsulation

Hydrophilic drug encapsulation. Encapsulation was determined quantitatively via absorbance measurements of saline aqueous solutions (NaI 40 mM) at 1.5 mM of ibuprofen sodium salt, 1.5 mM of lidocaine, and 10 μM of procaine hydrochloride in the presence of dendrons in the range of 0.5–50 μM.

Hydrophobic drug encapsulation. Drug encapsulation efficiency was determined by analyzing samples of the micellar formulations as follows. Briefly, **5** or **17** (0.5–5.5 mM) and diclofenac (1 mM) were co-dissolved in 100 μL of methanol. After 4 h of stirring, 2 mL of aqueous saline solution (NaI 40 mM) was added. The mixture was stirred for 24 h at room temperature to allow for the evaporation of the organic solvent. The suspension was then filtered (0.2 μm CA filter), and the filter was washed with methanol (3 mL) to determinate non-encapsulated diclofenac. Both the micellar solution and the non-encapsulated diclofenac were analyzed using HPLC. The drug encapsulation efficiency was calculated using the following equation:

$$\text{Encapsulation Efficiency (EE,\%)} = \text{Weight of loaded drug/Weight of drug initially added} \times 100$$

In vitro release profile. In vitro release of diclofenac from the diclofenac-loaded micelles (**5** + diclofenac) was studied using the dialysis bag method. Briefly, 1 mL of drug-micelle solution in phosphate-buffered saline (PBS, 10 mM, pH = 7.4) was placed in a regenerated cellulose dialysis bag (MWCO: 1 kDa), which was incubated in 250 mL of PBS at 37 °C. At predetermined time points, 100 μL of the dialysis bag was taken with buffer replacement to maintain the constant volume. The samples were analyzed using HPLC. A control experiment to determine the release of the free drug in 1 mL of acetonitrile-water (1:3) was also carried out as described above.

2.4. Biological Experiments

Viability studies. MTT assay was performed in the selected cell line to evaluate the biocompatibility of the dendrons. The assays were carried out on peripheral blood mononuclear cells (PBMCs), which were treated at concentrations ranging from 0.5 to 50 μM of the cationic dendron families and grown in PRMI medium supplemented with 10% of FBS. The cells were plated in a p96 multiwell plate and exposed to dendrons at concentrations ranging from 0.5 to 50 μM for 48 hours. Cells were treated after incubation with 0.5 mg/mL of MTT for 2 h, and crystals were dissolved in DMSO. Absorbance was measured at 570/690 nm, and viability was expressed relative to untreated cells. DMSO was used as a death control and untreated cells as the cell viability control. Data are presented as mean ± SD of three single experiments performed in triplicate. GraphPad software Prism v.5.0 (GraphPad Software, San Diego, CA, USA) was used for the statistical analysis of the results. Data with three replicates are displayed as bars ±SD. A p-value of ≤0.05 was considered to be statistically significant (* $p < 0.05$; ** $p < 0.01$; *** $p < 0.001$).

2.5. Synthesis and Characterization

A selection of the synthetic procedures based on first-generation dendrons are reported in this section. For the synthesis of the second and third generations and other compounds, see the Supporting Information.

Synthesis of $ChG_1(NMe_2)_2$ (1).

An aqueous solution (3 mL) of cholesteryl chloroformate (0.772 g; 1.72 mmol) was added dropwise to a methanolic solution (2 mL) of dendron $NH_2G_1(SNMe_2)_2$ (**i**) (1.5 g; 1.72 mmol) [32] and NEt_3 (0.28 mL; 2.0 mmol) under vigorous stirring. A total of 30 min later, volatiles were removed, and CH_2Cl_2/H_2O extraction was carried out. The organic phase was evaporated and the crude product was purified using size-exclusion chromatography in acetone, yielding the desired dendron **1** as a yellowish oil (53%).

^{1}H-NMR ($CDCl_3$): δ (ppm) -0.03 (s, 3H, -Si(CH_3)-), 0.49–0.55 (m, 6H, -$NCH_2CH_2CH_2CH_2$Si-, -SiCH_2CH_2S-), 0.62 (s, 3H, CH_3C-, cholesterol), 0.81 (d, 6H, CH_3CH-, cholesterol), 0.86 (d, 3H,

CH$_3$CH-, cholesterol), 0.95 (s, 3H, *CH*$_3$C-, cholesterol), 0.84–2.00 (m, 32H, -*CH*$_2$-, -*CH*-, cholesterol, -NCH$_2$*CH*$_2$*CH*$_2$CH$_2$Si-), 2.20 (m, 12H, -N(*CH*$_3$)$_2$), 2.50 (m, 12H, -SiCH$_2$*CH*$_2$S-, -S*CH*$_2$CH$_2$N-, -SCH$_2$*CH*$_2$N-), 3.10 (m, 2H, -N*CH*$_2$CH$_2$CH$_2$CH$_2$Si-), 4.42 (m, 1H, -*CH*CONH-), 4.81 (m, 1H, -CON*H*-), 5.30 (m, 1H, -C=*CH*CH$_2$-, cholesterol). ^{13}C-NMR (CDCl$_3$): δ (ppm) -5.32 (-Si(CH$_3$)-), 13.3 (-NCH$_2$CH$_2$CH$_2$CH$_2$Si-), 14.5 (-SiCH$_2$CH$_2$S-), 11.8, 18.7, 19.3, 21.0, 22.5, 22.8, 23,8, 24.2, 27.9, 28.2, 31.8, 35.7, 36.1, 36.5, 36.9, 38,5, 39.4, 39.7, 42.2, 49.9, 56.0, 56.6 (CH$_3$-, -CH$_2$-, -CH-, -C-, cholesterol), 20.9 (-NCH$_2$CH$_2$CH$_2$CH$_2$Si-), 27.6 (-SiCH$_2$CH$_2$S-), 29.7 (-SCH$_2$CH$_2$N-), 33.8 (-NCH$_2$CH$_2$CH$_2$CH$_2$Si-), 40.4 (-NCH$_2$CH$_2$CH$_2$CH$_2$Si-), 45.3 (-N(CH$_3$)$_2$), 59.2 (-SCH$_2$CH$_2$N-), 74.0 (-CHCONH-), 122.2 (-C=CHCH$_2$-, cholesterol), 139.6 (-C=CHCH$_2$-, cholesterol), 155.9 (-CONH-). Mass spectrometry: [M+H]$^+$ = 792.5918 Da (calcd. = 792.5925 Da.). Elemental analysis $C_{45}H_{85}N_3O_2S_2Si$ (792.40 g/mol): calcd. = C, 68.21; H, 10.81; N, 5.30; O, 4.04; S, 8.09; Si, 3.54. Found = C, 67.79; H, 10.62; N, 4.41; S, 8.21.

Synthesis of ChG1(NMe3I)2 (4).

Iodomethane (0.10 mL, 1.61 mmol) was added dropwise to a solution of dendron ChG$_1$(NMe$_2$)$_2$ (**1**) (0.50 g, 0.63 mmol) in 100 mL of THF. The reaction was stirred at room temperature for 4 h, and then the solvent was evaporated, and the product was washed with Et$_2$O (3x10 mL). The desired dendron was obtained as a yellow solid (94%).

^{1}H-NMR (CD$_3$OD): δ (ppm) 0.15 (s, 3H, -Si(*CH*$_3$)-), 0.62–0.74 (m, 6H, -NCH$_2$CH$_2$CH$_2$*CH*$_2$Si-, -Si*CH*$_2$CH$_2$S-), 0.76 (s, 3H, *CH*$_3$C- cholesterol), 0.92 (d, 6H, *CH*$_3$CH-, cholesterol), 0.98 (d, 3H, *CH*$_3$CH-, cholesterol), 1.08 (s, 3H, *CH*$_3$C-, cholesterol), 0.95–2.43 (m, 32H, -*CH*$_2$-, -*CH*-, cholesterol, -NCH$_2$*CH*$_2$*CH*$_2$CH$_2$Si-), 2.78 (m, 4H, -SiCH$_2$*CH*$_2$S-), 3.02 (m, 4H, -S*CH*$_2$CH$_2$N-), 3.13 (m, 2H, -N*CH*$_2$CH$_2$CH$_2$CH$_2$Si-), 3.23 (s, 18H, -N(*CH*$_3$)$_3$), 3.66 (m, 4H, -SCH$_2$*CH*$_2$N-), 4.40 (m, 1H, -*CH*CONH-), 5.42 (m, 1H, -C=*CH*CH$_2$-, cholesterol). ^{13}C-RMN (CD$_3$OD): δ (ppm) -4.90 (-Si(CH$_3$)-), 14.1 (-NCH$_2$CH$_2$CH$_2$CH$_2$Si-), 15.6 (-SiCH$_2$CH$_2$S-), 12.4, 19.3, 22.3, 23.0, 23.2, 25.0, 25.4, 28.9, 29.1, 29.3, 33.0, 33.2, 37.1, 37.4, 37.8, 38.3, 39.8, 40.7, 43.5, 51.6, 57.5, 58.1 (CH$_3$-, -CH$_2$-, -CH-, -C-, cholesterol), 22.0 (-NCH$_2$CH$_2$CH$_2$CH$_2$Si-), 32.3 (-SiCH$_2$CH$_2$S-), 34.7 (-NCH$_2$CH$_2$CH$_2$CH$_2$Si-), 38.5 (-SCH$_2$CH$_2$N-), 41.1 (-NCH$_2$CH$_2$CH$_2$CH$_2$Si-), 53.9 (-N(CH$_3$)$_3$), 67.1 (-SCH$_2$CH$_2$N-), 75.4 (-CHCONH-), 122.4 (-C=CHCH$_2$-, cholesterol), 141.3 (-C=CHCH$_2$-, cholesterol), 158.7 (-CONH-). Mass spectrometry: [M-I]$^+$ = 948.5323 Da (calcd. = 948.5367 Da). Elemental analysis $C_{47}H_{91}I_2N_3O_2S_2Si$ (1076.28 g/mol): calcd. = C, 52.45; H, 8.52; I, 23.58; N, 3.90; O, 2.97; S, 5.96; Si, 2.61. Found. = C, 52.11; H, 7.79; N, 3.52; S, 5.54.

Synthesis of EG$_1$(V)$_2$ (7).

A mixture of BrG$_1$(V)$_2$ (**iv**) [32] (1.0 g; 4.29 mmol), d-α-tocopherol (1.85 g; 4.29 mmol) in 50 mL of acetone and then K$_2$CO$_3$ (1.20 g; 8.68 mmol) and 18-crown-6 (0.092 g; 0.35 mmol) were added and stirred at 90 °C for 48 h. Then, the solvent was removed under a vacuum, and the purification was carried out through H$_2$O/Et$_2$O extraction. The organic fraction was dried with MgSO$_4$ before the solvent was removed. Dendron **7** was obtained as an orange oil (87%).

^{1}H-NMR (CDCl$_3$): δ (ppm) 0.18 (s, 3H, -Si(*CH*$_3$)-), 0.75 (m, 2H, -OCH$_2$CH$_2$CH$_2$*CH*$_2$Si-), 0.88 (m, 12H, *CH*$_3$CH-), 1.00–1.68 (m, 23H, -*CH*$_2$-, -*CH*-, tocopherol, -OCH$_2$CH$_2$*CH*$_2$CH$_2$Si-), 1.25 (s, 3H, -CH$_2$C(*CH*$_3$)OC$_{Ar}$-), 1.83 (m, 4H, -*CH*$_2$C(CH$_3$)OC$_{Ar}$-, -OCH$_2$*CH*$_2$CH$_2$CH$_2$Si-), 2.10 (s, 3H, *CH*$_3$C$_{Ar}$-), 2.13 (s, 3H, *CH*$_3$C$_{Ar}$-), 2.17 (s, 3H, *CH*$_3$C$_{Ar}$-), 2.58 (t, 2H, -C$_{Ar}$*CH*$_2$CH$_2$-), 3.64 (t, 2H, -O*CH*$_2$CH$_2$CH$_2$CH$_2$Si-), 5.73 (m, 2H, -Si*CH*=CH$_2$), 6.08 (m, 4H, -SiCH=*CH*$_2$). ^{13}C-NMR (CDCl$_3$): δ (ppm) -5.22 (-Si(CH$_3$)-), 11.9, 12.0, 12.8 (CH$_3$C$_{Ar}$-), 14.1 (-OCH$_2$CH$_2$CH$_2$CH$_2$Si-), 19.7, 19.8, 20.5, 21.1, 22.7, 22.8, 23.9, 24.5, 24.9, 28.0, 31.4, 32.7, 32.8, 37.3, 37.5, 39.4, 40.1 (-CH$_3$-, -CH$_2$-, -CH-, tocopherol), 30.0 (-OCH$_2$CH$_2$CH$_2$CH$_2$Si-), 34.0 (-OCH$_2$CH$_2$CH$_2$CH$_2$Si-), 72.6 (-OCH$_2$CH$_2$CH$_2$CH$_2$Si-), 74.6 (-CH$_2$(CH$_3$)COC$_{Ar}$-), 117.3 (-*C$_{Ar}$*CH$_2$CH$_2$-), 122.6, 125.6, 127.6 (CH$_3$*C$_{Ar}$*-), 132.7 (-SiCH=CH$_2$), 136.7 (-SiCH=CH$_2$), 147.4 (-*C$_{Ar}$*OC-), 148.2 ((-*C$_{Ar}$*OCH$_2$-). Mass spectrometry: [M+H]$^+$ = 583.4937 Da (calcd. = 583.4905 Da). Elemental analysis$C_{38}H_{66}O_2Si$ (583.03 g/mol): calcd. = C, 78.28; H, 11.41; O, 5.49; Si, 4.82. Found = C, 77.92; H, 11.05.

Synthesis of EG$_1$(SNMe$_2$·HCl)$_2$ (10).

Following a similar procedure described for the starting material **i** [32], dendron **10** was obtained as a white solid (95%) using $EG_1(V)_2$ (**7**) (1.0 g; 1.72 mmol), $SH(CH_2)_2SNMe_2 \cdot HCl$ (0.511 g; 3.61 mmol), DMPA (0.052 g; 0.20 mmol).

^{1}H-NMR (CD_3OD): δ (ppm) 0.14 (s, 3H, -Si(CH_3)-), 0.64–0.80 (m, 6H, -$OCH_2CH_2CH_2CH_2Si$-, -$SiCH_2CH_2S$-), 0.88 (m, 12H, CH_3CH-), 0.95–1.65 (m, 23H, -CH_2-, -CH-, tocopherol, -$OCH_2CH_2CH_2CH_2Si$-), 1.21 (s, 3H, -$CH_2C(CH_3)OC_{Ar}$-), 1.79 (m, 4H, -$CH_2C(CH_3)OC_{Ar}$-, -$OCH_2CH_2CH_2CH_2Si$-), 1.94–2.19 (m, 9H, CH_3C_{Ar}-), 2.56 (t, 2H, -$C_{Ar}CH_2CH_2$-), 2.75 (m, 4H, -$SiCH_2CH_2S$-), 2.94 (m, 12H, -N$(CH_3)_2$HCl), 2.99 (m, 4H, -SCH_2CH_2N-), 3.39 (m, 4H, -SCH_2CH_2N-), 3.62 (t, 2H, -$OCH_2CH_2CH_2CH_2Si$-).

Synthesis of $EG_1(SNMe_2)_2$ (13).

Following the procedure described for **1**, dendron **13** was obtained as a yellow oil (49%) using $EG_1(SNMe_2.HCl)_2$ (**10**) (1.5 g; 1.72 mmol) and Na_2CO_3 (0.532 g; 5.02 mmol).

^{1}H-NMR ($CDCl_3$): δ (ppm) 0.03 (s, 3H, -Si(CH_3)-), 0.63 (m, 2H, -$OCH_2CH_2CH_2CH_2Si$-), 0.88 (m, 12H, CH_3CH-), 0.92 (m, 4H, -$SiCH_2CH_2S$-), 0.97–1.62 (m, 23H, -CH_2-, -CH-, tocopherol, -$OCH_2CH_2CH_2CH_2Si$-), 1.20 (s, 3H, -$CH_2C(CH_3)OC_{Ar}$-), 1.77 (m, 4H, -$CH_2C(CH_3)OC_{Ar}$-, -$OCH_2CH_2CH_2CH_2Si$-), 2.05 (s, 3H, CH_3C_{Ar}-), 2.09 (s, 3H, CH_3C_{Ar}-), 2,.13 (s, 3H, CH_3C_{Ar}-), 2.22 (m, 12H, -N$(CH_3)_2$), 2.41–2.68 (m, 14H, -$C_{Ar}CH_2CH_2$-, -$SiCH_2CH_2S$-, -SCH_2CH_2N-, -SCH_2CH_2N-, 3.60 (t, 2H, -$OCH_2CH_2CH_2CH_2Si$-). ^{13}C-NMR ($CDCl_3$): δ (ppm) -5.55 (-Si(CH_3)-), 11.6, 11.7, 12.6 (CH_3C_{Ar}-), 14.2–14.5 (-$SiCH_2$-), 19.5, 19.6, 20.4, 20.8, 22.5, 22.6, 23.7, 24.2, 24.6, 27.8, 31.1, 32.5, 32.6, 37.1, 37.3, 39.2, 39.8 (-CH_3-, -CH_2-, -CH-, tocopherol), 27.5 (-$SiCH_2CH_2S$-), 29.6 (-SCH_2CH_2N-), 29.8 (-$OCH_2CH_2CH_2CH_2Si$-), 33.9 (-$OCH_2CH_2CH_2CH_2Si$-), 49.2 (-N$(CH_3)_2$), 59.1 (-SCH_2CH_2N-), 72.2 (-$OCH_2CH_2CH_2CH_2Si$-), 74.5 (-$CH_2(CH_3)COC_{Ar}$-), 117.2 (-$C_{Ar}CH_2CH_2$-), 122.5, 125.5, 127.5 (CH_3C_{Ar}-), 147.4 (-$C_{Ar}OC$-), 148.1 (-$C_{Ar}OCH_2$-). Mass spectrometry: $[M+H]^+$ = 793.6105 Da (calcd. = 793.6129 Da). Elemental analysis $C_{46}H_{88}N_2O_2S_2Si$ (793.43 g/mol): calcd. = C, 69.64; H, 11.18; N, 3.53; O, 4.03; S, 8.08; Si, 3.54. Found. = C, 69.84; H, 10.73; N, 3.04; S, 7.61.

Synthesisof $EG_1(NMe_3I)_2$ (16).

Following the procedure described for **4**, dendron **16** was obtained as a yellow solid (96%) using $EG_1(NMe_2)_2$ (**13**) (0.50 g, 0.63 mmol) and MeI (0.10 mL, 1.61 mmol).

^{1}H-NMR (CD_3OD): δ (ppm) 0.18 (s, 3H, -Si(CH_3)-), 0.81 (m, 2H, -$OCH_2CH_2CH_2CH_2Si$-), 0.91 (m, 12H, CH_3CH-), 1.06 (m, 4H, -$SiCH_2CH_2S$-), 1.09–1.74 (m, 23H, -CH_2-, -CH-, tocopherol, -$OCH_2CH_2CH_2CH_2Si$-), 1.27 (s, 3H, -$CH_2C(CH_3)OC_{Ar}$-), 1.84 (m, 4H, -$CH_2C(CH_3)OC_{Ar}$-, -$OCH_2CH_2CH_2CH_2Si$-), 2.09 (m, 3H, CH_3C_{Ar}-), 2.16 (m, 3H, CH_3C_{Ar}-), 2.19 (m, 3H, CH_3C_{Ar}-), 2.63 (t, 2H, -$C_{Ar}CH_2CH_2$-), 2.81 (m, 4H, -$SiCH_2CH_2S$-), 3.02 (m, 4H, -SCH_2CH_2N-), 3.21 (m, 18H, -N$(CH_3)_3$), 3.68 (m, 6H, -$OCH_2CH_2CH_2CH_2Si$-, -SCH_2CH_2N-). ^{13}C-NMR (CD_3OD): δ (ppm) -4,75 (-Si(CH_3)-), 12.1, 12.3, 13.2 (CH_3C_{Ar}-), 14.5 (-$OCH_2CH_2CH_2CH_2Si$-), 15.7 (-$SiCH_2CH_2S$-), 20.3, 21.6, 21.7, 21.9, 23.1, 23.2, 23.3, 24.3, 25.4, 28.9, 32.7, 33.7, 33.9, 37.0, 38.3, 38.4, 38.5, 40.5 (-CH_3-, -CH_2-, -CH-, tocopherol), 25.9 (-$SiCH_2CH_2S$-), 29.1 (-SCH_2CH_2N-), 31.7 (-$OCH_2CH_2CH_2CH_2Si$-), 35.2 (-$OCH_2CH_2CH_2CH_2Si$-), 53.9 (-N$(CH_3)_3$), 67.2 (-SCH_2CH_2N-), 73.6 (-$OCH_2CH_2CH_2CH_2Si$-), 75.8 (-$CH_2(CH_3)COC_{Ar}$-), 118.9 (-$C_{Ar}CH_2CH_2$-), 123.7, 126.8, 127.9 (CH_3C_{Ar}-), 148.9 (-$C_{Ar}OC$-), 149.5 (-$C_{Ar}OCH_2$-). Mass spectrometry: $[M-I]^+$ = 949.5547 Da (calcd. = 949.5571 Da). Elemental analysisistal $C_{48}H_{94}I_2N_2O_2S_2Si$ (1077.31 g/mol): calcd. = C, 53.52; H, 8.80; I, 23.56; N, 2.60; O, 2.97; S, 5.95; Si, 2.61. Found= C, 53.14; H, 8.27; N, 2.20; S, 5.46.3.

3. Results and Discussion

3.1. Synthesis of Amphiphilic Dendrons

Amphiphilic dendrons with different functional groups at their peripheries and focal points were prepared using protocols developed in our research group for analogous dendritic systems [32]. Hydrophobic molecules with self-assembly inducing capabilities, including cholesterol or d-α-tocopherol, were incorporated at the focal points. Then, nucleophilic acyl substitution reactions were used to functionalize the dendrimer peripheries with hydrophilic trimethylammonium groups which would exhibit cationic charge regardless of the pH.

3.1.1. Cationic Dendrons with Cholesterol at the Focal Point

The conjugation of the cholesterol molecule at the focal point using a carbamate linkage was performed by employing a chloroformate derivative of cholesterol (Scheme 1). The reactions with the chloroformate were carried out using primary amine-containing dendrons $NH_2G_n(SNMe_2)_m$ (n = 1, m = 2 (**i**); n = 2, m = 4 (**ii**); n = 3, m = 8 (**iii**)), previously prepared in good yields, following Gabriel and thiol-ene reactions [32]. After a typical extraction workup, the desired cholesterol-modified dendrons $ChG_n(NMe_2)_m$ (n = 1, m = 2 (**1**); n = 2, m = 4 (**2**); n = 3, m = 8 (**3**)) were obtained as colorless oils with good yields (70–80%). The reactions were monitored using ^{1}H-NMR spectroscopy (Figure S1) where signals at 3.13 ppm corresponding to the methylene group attached to the nitrogen atom, confirmed bond formation. In addition, resonances attributed to the cholesterol fragment were observed at 5.34 ppm (-C=CH-) and 4.47 ppm (-CH(O)-). The peak corresponding to the proton in the carbamate N-H appeared at 4.59 ppm but exhibited slight concentration-dependent shifting. In the ^{13}C-NMR spectrum (Figure S2), the resonances ascribed to the same units were observed at 40.6 ppm ($-CH_2N-$), 74.1 ppm (-CH(O)-), and 139.7 and 122.3 ppm (-C=CH-). In addition, the characteristic signal of the carbonyl group was seen at 155.9 ppm.

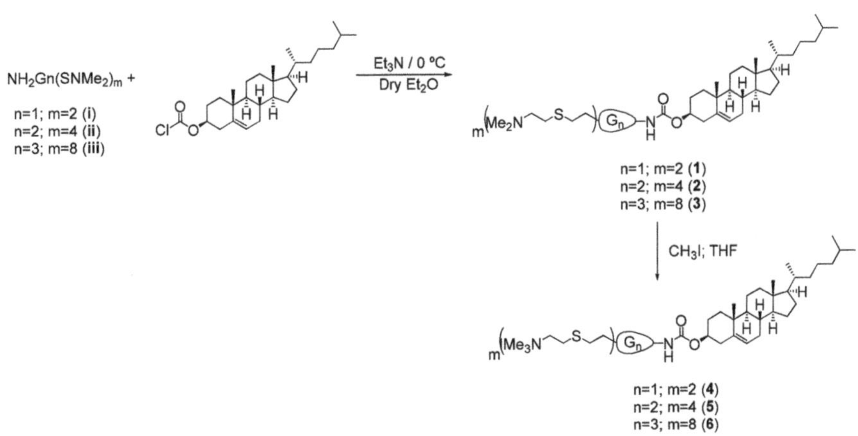

Scheme 1. Synthesis of ammonium-terminated dendrons with cholesterol at the focal point.

Finally, the preparation of ammonium-terminated dendrons was achieved through the reaction of **1–3** with an excess of MeI in dry THF (Scheme 1). Amphiphilic dendrons with cholesterol at the focal point $ChG_n(NMe_3I)_m$ (n = 1, m = 2 (**4**); n = 2, m = 4 (**5**); n = 3, m = 8 (**6**)) were obtained as yellow solids with excellent yield (>90%). ^{1}H-NMR spectroscopic evaluation supported the correct formation of the desired compounds based on the visualization of the deshielding effect observed for moieties adjacent to the nitrogen atom (Figure S3). After the reaction, the resonances appeared at 2.78, 3.02, and 3.66 ppm for methylene groups in $-SiCH_2CH_2S-$, $-SCH_2CH_2N-$, and $-SCH_2CH_2N-$, respectively. In addition, the methyl unit was observed at 3.23 ppm as a singlet. In the ^{13}C-NMR spectrum (Figure S4), the same methylene fragments were observed at 32.3 ($-SiCH_2CH_2S-$), 38.5 ($-SCH_2CH_2N-$), and 67.1 ($-SCH_2CH_2N-$) ppm, while the carbon atom in the methyl moiety ($-NMe_3I$) was deshielded and appeared at 53.9 ppm. Figure 2A shows the full structures of amphiphilic cationic compounds **4–6**.

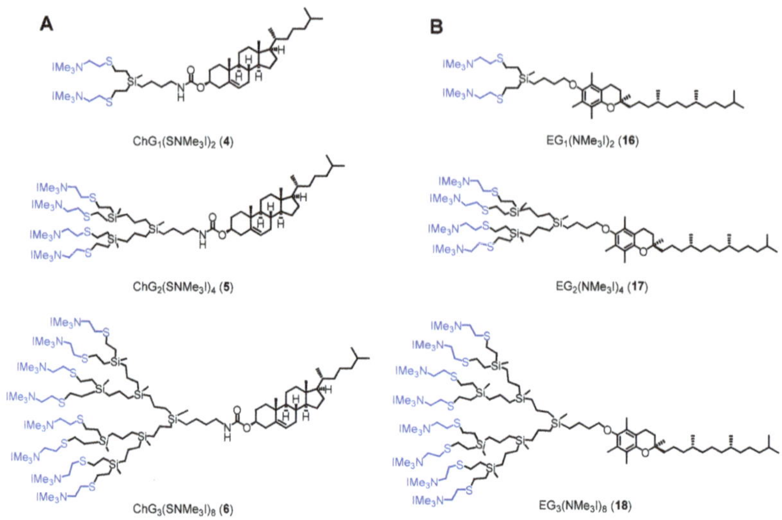

Figure 2. Amphiphilic ammonium-terminated dendrons with cholesterol (**4–6**; (**A**)) or d-α-tocopherol (**16–18**; (**B**)) at the focal point.

3.1.2. Cationic Dendrons with d-α-Tocopherol at the Periphery

The d-α-tocopherol, also called vitamin E, was incorporated at the dendron focal points through ether linkages. First, dendrons with a bromine atom at the focal point $BrG_n(V)_m$ (n = 1, m = 2 (**iv**); n = 2, m = 4 (**v**); n = 3, m = 8 (**vi**)) were selected as precursors [32]. Then, following a previously reported protocol, a solution of dendrons **iv-vi**, d-α-tocopherol, K_2CO_3, and crown ether (18-crown-6) was stirred at 90 °C (Scheme 2) [32]. The desired compounds $EG_n(V)_m$ (n = 1, m = 2 (**7**); n = 2, m = 4 (**8**); n = 3, m = 8 (**9**)) were obtained as viscous oils with very good yields (85–95%). In the ^{1}H-NMR spectra, the disappearance of the resonance corresponding to the hydroxyl group in free d-α-tocopherol and the shifting of the peak corresponding to the adjacent methylene group up to 3.64 ppm confirmed the conjugation (Figure S5). In addition, the chemical shifts of the peaks corresponding to the methyl groups on the aromatic ring of d-α-tocopherol were affected by the ether bond formation, appearing at 2.09, 2.13, and 2.17 ppm. In the ^{13}C-NMR spectra (Figure S6), the most characteristic signals corresponded to the methylene group in the dendron (72.6 ppm) and the aromatic carbon atom (148.2 ppm) of d-α-tocopherol, both of which were directly bonded to the oxygen atom of the ether, and were consequently deshielded.

The next step was the functionalization of the peripheral vinyl groups of the dendrons via click chemistry (Scheme 2). A methanolic solution of thiol derivative 2-(dimethylamino) ethanethiol hydrochloride ($SH(CH_2)_2NMe_2{\cdot}HCl$) and DMPA photoinitiator was added in two portions to a solution of compounds **7–9** in THF. Irradiation with UV light after each addition for 2 h resulted in the cationic compounds $EG_n(NMe_2{\cdot}HCl)_m$ (n = 1, m = 2 (**10**); n = 2, m = 4 (**11**); n = 3, m = 8 (**12**)) as orange solids soluble in MeOH without further purification. The reaction was monitored by loss of alkenyl resonances. The new signals corresponding to -$SiCH_2CH_2S$-, -SCH_2CH_2N-, and -$CH_2NMe_2{\cdot}HCl$ were observed around 2.75, 2.99, and 3.39 ppm in ^{1}H-NMR spectra (Figure S7). The methyl unit -$N(CH_3)_2{\cdot}HCl$ appeared as a singlet at 2.94 ppm, overlapping with the methylene group in -SCH_2CH_2N-.

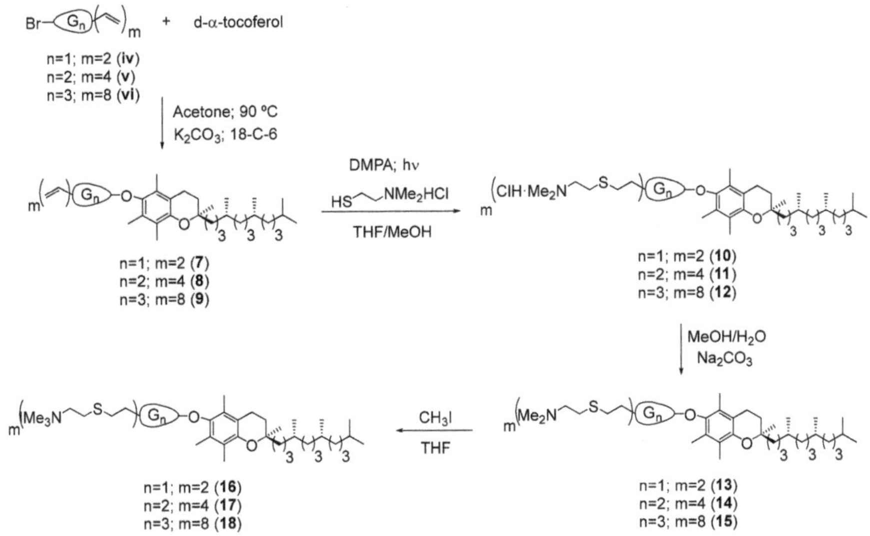

Scheme 2. Synthesis of ammonium-terminated dendrons with d-α-tocopherol at the focal point.

Then, to prepare the corresponding quaternary ammonium-functionalized dendrons, neutralization, and subsequent quaternization of $-NMe_2{\cdot}HCl$ moieties were necessary. The first step was carried out in MeOH using aqueous aliquots of $NaCO_3$ as a base (Scheme 2). Size-exclusion chromatography in acetone was selected as the purification method. Thus, dendrons $EG_n(NMe_2)_m$ (n = 1, m = 2 (**13**); n = 2, m = 4 (**14**); n = 3, m = 8 (**15**)) were obtained as orange oils in size-dependent yields (50–80%). In the ^{1}H-NMR spectra (Figure S8), all characteristic signals described for **10–12** were further shielded, showing that the peaks corresponding to the methylene groups overlapped around 2.50 ppm ($-SiCH_2CH_2S-$ and $-SCH_2CH_2N-$) and that of the methyl unit ($-NMe_2$) was observed at 2.22 ppm. In ^{13}C-NMR spectra (Figure S9), the key peaks appeared at 27.5 ($-SiCH_2CH_2S-$), 29.6 ($-SCH_2CH_2N-$), 45.2 ($-NMe_2$), and 59.1 ($-SCH_2CH_2N-$) ppm.

Lastly, the quaternization of amino groups ($-NMe_2$) with MeI in dry THF led to the final amphiphilic cationic dendrons with vitamin E at the focal point $EG_n(NMe_3I)_m$ (n = 1, m = 2 (**16**); n = 2, m = 4 (**17**); n = 3, m = 8 (**18**)) as orange solids with excellent yields (>90%). Compounds **16–18** were characterized using NMR spectroscopy. In the ^{1}H NMR spectra (Figure S10), the resonances attributed to methylene groups close to the nitrogen atom were observed distinctly at 2.81 ($-SiCH_2CH_2S-$), 3.02 ($-SCH_2CH_2N-$), and 3.68 ($-SCH_2CH_2N-$) ppm. In addition, peaks corresponding to the methyl units ($-NMe_3I$) appeared at 3.21 ppm. Analogously, resonances were shifted in the ^{13}C-NMR spectra (Figure S11) with peaks corresponding to the carbon atoms in methylene and methyl fragments attached to nitrogen nuclei detected at 53.9 ppm for $-NMe_3I$ and 67.2 ppm for $-CH_2N-$, while those bound to sulfur atoms appeared at 25.9 ppm in $-SiCH_2CH_2S$ and 29.1 ppm in $-SCH_2CH_2N-$. Figure 2B shows the full structures of the amphiphilic cationic compounds **16–18**.

3.2. *Micelle Formation*

Our previous studies with amphiphilic carbosilane dendrons showed that the carbosilane scaffold plays an important role in the self-assembly process [33]. Specifically, the higher generation favors the micellization process. The critical micellar concentration (CMC) of amphiphilic compounds was evaluated for second- and third-generation ammonium-containing dendrons (**5–6** and **17–18**) using surface tension measurements. Due to the ionic charge of the dendrons, CMC is strongly affected by the presence of salts in the medium (see Figure S12). Salt addition decreases the repulsive electrostatic forces between headgroups and favors micelle formation. Without salt addition, data showed that no micelle formation took place below 10 mM dendron concentration. Due to the potential biomedical applications of these systems, we were interested in systems with the lowest effective concentrations. In prior reports with carbosilane dendrons having palmitic groups at the focal point, 20 mM NaCl was found to be the optimal salt concentration to achieve self-assembly [33]. Because the Cl^- ion could exchange with I^- counterion from the dendrons and interfere with the micelle formation, NaI in the same proportions was also used and evaluated to study the possible influence of counterion exchange in the aggregation process. The results indicated a higher surface tension reduction in the presence of NaI than NaCl and slightly lower surface tension with 40 mM of salt than at 20 mM of salt (Table S1).

CMC measurements were performed at increasing dendron concentrations in aqueous NaI solution (40 mM) at 30 °C. Figure 3 displays the surface tension curves obtained for each dendron. The CMC values listed in Table 1 range from 4.4 to 9 μM for the cationic carbosilane dendrons.

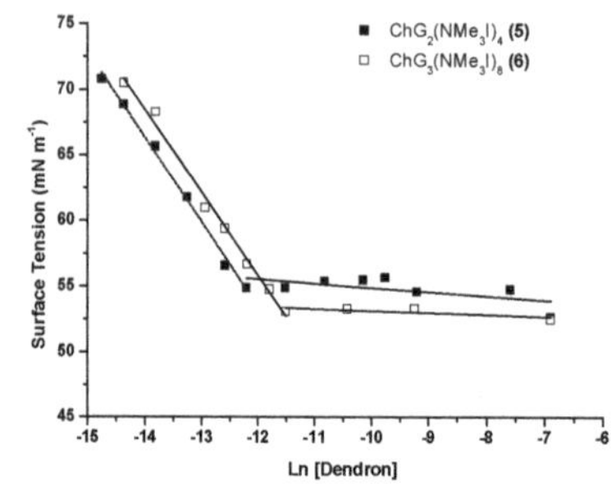

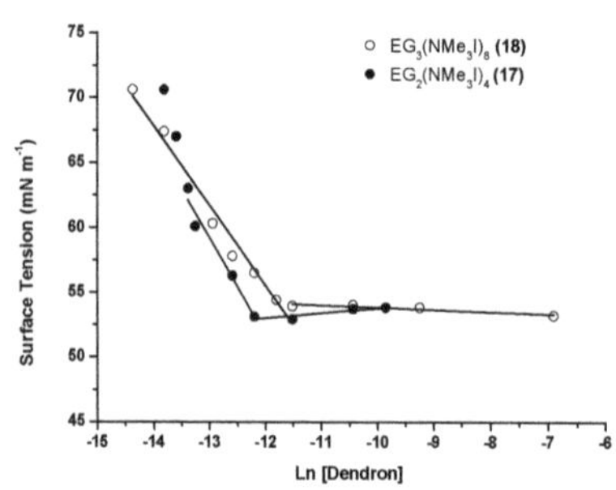

Figure 3. Surface tension measurements of amphiphilic dendrons with cholesterol (top; **5–6**) or vitamin E (bottom; **17–18**) at the focal point in 40 mM aqueous NaI.

Table 1. CMC and diameter values of amphiphilic dendrons with cholesterol (**5–6**) or vitamin E (**17–18**) at the focal point in 40 mM aqueous NaI and comparison with values of analogous previously published systems.

Dendron	CMC (μM)	Diameter (nm)	Γ (μmol/m²)	A (nm²/Molecule)	ΔG^0_{mic} (kJ/mol)
$ChG_2(NMe_3I)_4$ (**5**)	4.4 ± 0.7	9.2 ± 0.4	2.6	0.64	−40.5
$ChG_3(NMe_3I)_8$ (**6**)	9.0 ± 1.0	6.6 ± 0.1	2.5	0.65	−38.7
$EG_2(NMe_3I)_4$ (**17**)	5.1 ± 0.9	7.7 ± 0.2	3.1	0.54	−40.1
$EG_3(NMe_3I)_8$ (**18**)	8.0 ± 1.0	6.5 ± 0.3	2.5	0.67	−39.1
* $C_{16}G_2(NMe_3I)_4$	19 ± 1	5.6 ± 0.1	0.77	2.1	-
* $C_{16}G_3(NMe_3I)_8$	17 ± 1	5.6 ± 0.1	0.69	2.4	-
* $C_6G_3(NMe_3I)_8$	12 ± 1	3.8 ± 0.3	0,83	2.0	-

* Data obtained from Ref. [33].

CMC values slightly depend on the generation of the dendron but not on the focal point group. The second-generation dendrons had about two-fold-lower CMC values, implying that the second-generation dendron had a balance between lipophilicity (dendritic skeleton + tail) and hydrophilicity (number of ionic charges) that was more favorable for micelle formation. This behavior agrees with cationic bis-MPA dendrons modified with cholesterol (2.9–13 μM) [7,8] or cationic polylysine dendrons functionalized with tocopherol (1.3–15 μM) [25,26]. However, this observation is the opposite to that found for analogous cationic carbosilane dendrons with fatty acids (palmitic or hexanoic groups) at the focal point (see Table 1) [33]. The latter different profile can be attributed to the importance of a hydrophilic–lipophilic balance (HBL) in the micelle formation process of amphiphilic systems.

The Gibbs adsorption equation suitable for dilute ideal solutions can be considered for ionic micelles with an excess of salt. From the surface excess (Γ), approximate values for the area per molecule of dendrons at the air/water interface (A) can be obtained.

$$\Gamma_{CMC} = -\frac{1}{RT}\frac{\partial\gamma}{\partial \ln C} \tag{1}$$

$$A = \frac{1}{N\Gamma} \tag{2}$$

Results derived from Expressions 1 and 2 are listed in Table 1. As expected, all dendrons presented positive surface excess which reflects their preference to stay at the water/air interface instead of in the solution matrix, as expected for amphiphilic molecules. The area per molecule of dendron at the surface (A) ranged from 0.54 to 0.67 nm^2 and is significantly lower than those found for analogous carbosilane dendrons with palmitic groups at the focal point [33]. Similar values were determined for conventional surfactants such as dodecyl trimethylammonium bromide (0.56 nm^2 per molecule). In our case, the ionic head groups are larger in number and more charged, but we should keep in mind the presence of an excess of electrolytes. It is clear from the values in Table 1 that dendron molecules in this region of surface saturation are closely packed, with an orientation perpendicular to the surface. This fact could be explained by a more compact arrangement in the surface creating a highly dense particle compared to their palmitic analogous. Considering that the cationic head groups are the same, the cholesterol and vitamin E at the focal points favor the closest packing of head groups.

The spontaneity of the micellar aggregation process was confirmed through Gibbs free energy calculations (ΔG^0_{mic}) based on Expression 3, in which the correction factor i was set up as 1 due to the saturation of the stern layer derived from the high salt concentration employed in the experiment. Table 1 shows negative ΔG^0_{mic} values and more favorable processes in second-generation compounds, which agrees with their lower CMC data.

$$\Delta_{mic}G^0 = iRT\ln X_{CMC} \tag{3}$$

Hydrodynamic diameters were estimated using DLS for cationic micelles formed in saline. In the absence of drugs, the size distributions (see Figure S14) confirmed the aggregate formation. Hydrodynamic diameter values showed a decreasing tendency with their generation, contrary to the CMC trend (Table 1). These results can be explained through the dendron-tail model in which the amphiphilic balance between the dendron (polar head) and the non-polar tail, cholesterol or vitamin E in this work, controls the aggregation process. In this approach, larger polar head groups drive the formation of smaller micelles composed of fewer amphiphilic molecules. In any case, the diameters estimated using DLS are calculated considering spherical micelles. However, the values obtained are too high to be considered as spherical geometries and fit better with cylindrical micelles. The presence of NaI effectively screens the repulsive charges between the micelles, but potentially may also affect their aggregate structures. The reduction in effective head group area due to the screening of the electrostatic repulsion results in the increase in the packing geometry and the growth of cylindrical micelles. These shapes were described in our previous studies for cationic micelles prepared from carbosilane dendrons containing fatty acids at the focal point [34]. The polar head is made up of a hydrophobic carbosilane scaffold and hydrophilic terminal groups (-NMe_3I). Consequently, the growth from G2 to G3 dendrons not only increases the hydrophobicity (skeleton) but also the hydrophilicity (number of peripheral functional groups) explaining the smaller size obtained for the highest-generation compounds.

3.3. Drug Encapsulation

Drug encapsulations were performed for hydrophilic drugs including ibuprofen sodium salt, lidocaine, and procaine, as well as for the hydrophobic drug diclofenac. Only dendrons **5** and **17** were selected for these experiments based on their lowest CMC values. Both dendrons were able to load all of the drugs, although the protocols used depended on the nature of the drugs.

The encapsulation of aqueous-soluble drugs was determined through the modification of their absorbance in the presence of increasing concentrations of dendrons (0.5–50 μM). For all molecules, the absorption spectra showed an increase in the drug absorbance as the dendron concentration increased (see Figure S13). This behavior indicates the association of drug molecules with dendron micelles, although drugs can be incorporated in various ways in micelles: they may locate (i) inside the hydrophobic core of the micelles, (ii) be adsorbed on the surface of micelles, or (iii), in the case of drugs with polar and non-polar regions, they may be in the polar portion between the hydrophilic peripheral groups of dendrons and the non-polar region towards the micelle core. For hydrophilic drugs such as procaine hydrochloride or hydrochlorothiazide, it is well known that a bathochromic shift is observed when transferring from water to a less polar region such as in micelles [35,36]. The absorption maxima were found at wavelengths of 272, 270, and 290 nm for ibuprofen, lidocaine, and procaine, respectively. However, no bathochromic shifts were observed. Although these behaviors suggest that the drugs were adsorbed on the micellar surface, inclusion inside of the micelle cannot be ruled out because these dendritic micelles include rather large amounts of water, disrupting the hydrophobic core [34]. The representation of absorbances at these wavelengths versus dendron concentrations showed absorbance increases for dendron concentrations below the CMC values of the corresponding dendrons (Figure 4) and suggesting that drugs affect the CMC values.

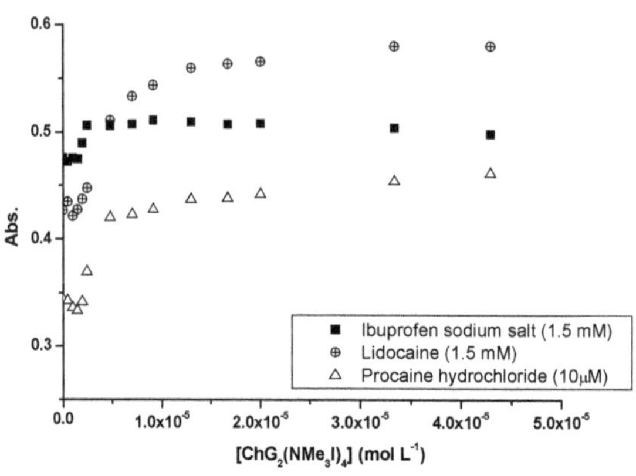

Figure 4. *Cont.*

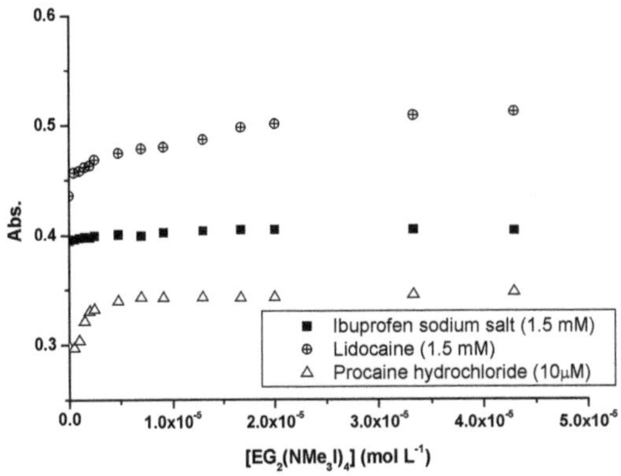

Figure 4. Variation of absorbance by increasing the dendron concentration at the maximum absorption wavelength for each drug.

The CMCs in the presence of drugs were measured, affording slightly lower values than those obtained in the absence of drugs (Figure 5), and confirming the influence of the drugs in the micelle formation process. The sizes of micelles were also affected by the drugs (Table 2). Particle size distributions in the presence of drugs can be seen in Figure S14. The drug incorporation increased the diameters of the micelles slightly, with the effect being least pronounced for ibuprofen and most pronounced for procaine.

Table 2. CMC and diameter values of dendrons with cholesterol (**5**) or vitamin E (**17**) at the focal point obtained in absence or presence of ibuprofen (1.5 mM), lidocaine (1.5 mM), or procaine (10 μM).

Dendron	CMC (μM)	Diameter (nm)	Dendron	CMC (μM)	Diameter (nm)
$ChG_2(NMe_3I)_4$ (**5**)	4.4 ± 0.7	9.2 ± 0.4	$EG_2(NMe_3I)_4$ (**17**)	4.8 ± 0.9	7.7 ± 0.2
5 + ibuprofen	2.4 ± 0.2	10.0 ± 0.6	**17** + ibuprofen	1.22 ± 0.02	10.7 ± 0.4
5 + lidocaine	2.4 ± 0.3	11.9 ± 0.8	**17** + lidocaine	3.0 ± 0.4	11.1 ± 0.2
5 + procaine	2.6 ± 0.2	12.9 ± 0.3	**17** + procaine	3.7 ± 0.5	11.0 ± 0.7
5 + diclofenac	-	9.1 ± 0.2	**17** + diclofenac	-	8.9 ± 0.2

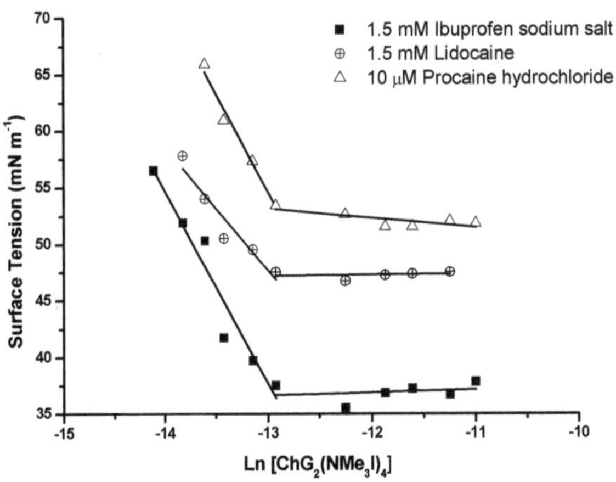

Figure 5. *Cont.*

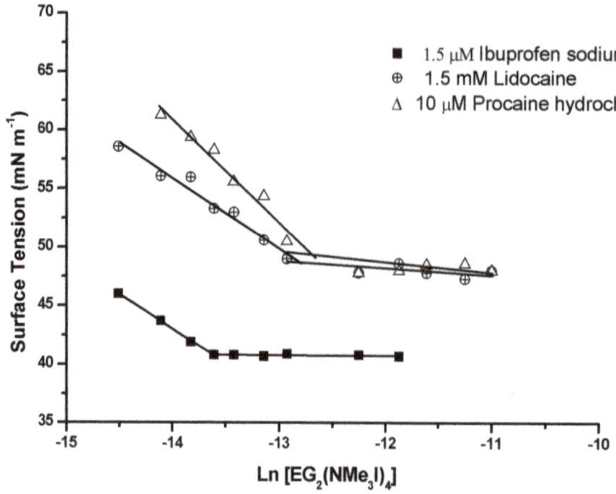

Figure 5. Surface tension measurements of amphiphilic dendrons with cholesterol (**top**) or vitamin E (**bottom**) at the focal point in 40 mM aqueous NaI and in the presence of drugs (■ ibuprofen ○ (1.5 mM), lidocaine (1.5 mM), or Δ procaine (10 μM).

From the data in Figure 4, we can observe that the difference between the absorbance of the drug completely bound to the micelle (plateau A_∞) and the absorbance of the drug in water (A_0) was the lowest for ibuprofen. All data considered, we can conclude that the binding affinity of ibuprofen to these dendrons is the lowest of all the drugs.

Partition constants (*K*) were calculated for procaine using a pseudo-phase model as described in the literature [36,37]. The relationships between $1/(A-A_0)$ and 1/([Drug] + [Dendron] −cmc) were not linear for lidocaine and ibuprofen. The drug concentrations for lidocaine and ibuprofen were much higher than the dendron concentration which prevents us from using this method. These high drug concentrations were necessary to obtain absorbance data. However, data obtained for procaine was the only one which could be adjusted to a linear fit (Figure 6). The log*K* values obtained were 6.7 and 7.4 for **5** and **17**, respectively. The results showed that **17** can more readily encapsulate procaine than **5**, probably due to the presence of additional hydrophobic interactions such as π-π stacking. These results suggest an improvement of more than one order of magnitude compared to other carbosilane dendritic systems previously described [31].

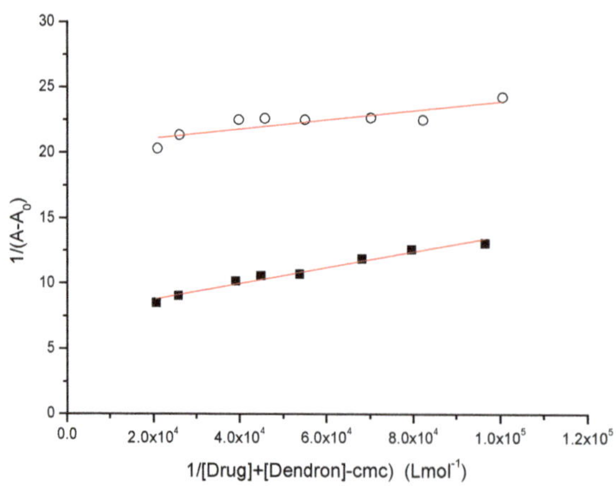

Figure 6. Relationship between $1/(A-A_0)$ and 1/([Drug] + [Dendron] −cmc) for procaine in dendron solutions (▪ $ChG_2(NMe_3I)_4$ (**5**); ○ $EG_2(NMe_3I)_4$ (**17**)).

For hydrophobic drugs, a solubility study of diclofenac with dendrons **5** and **17** was performed, confirming the capabilities of both dendrons to enhance the solubility of diclofenac through the formation of micelles (Supporting Figure S15). The encapsulation percentage was measured using HPLC (see encapsulation protocol). Micelles were prepared with different dendron/diclofenac molar ratios, showing their optimal encapsulation values at molar ratios of 3.3:1 and 5.5:1 for dendrons **5** and **17**, respectively (Supporting Figure S16).

These micelles presented a very good encapsulation efficiency of 92% for diclofenac (Figure S16), which was the best reported in the literature so far, compared to PLGA nanoparticles (55%), nanostructured lipids (67%), or span 60/cholesterol (82.1%) [38–40]. It is noteworthy that in all cases reported in the literature, diclofenac sodium salt was used. The neutral form used here is more hydrophobic, which may result in higher affinity for the internal micellar domain than its ionic analogue, resulting in higher efficiencies. Diclofenac loading did not modify the hydrodynamic diameters of the micelles for cholesterol-modified dendrons while it slightly increased the diameters observed for tocopherol-modified dendrons (Table 2). The stabilities in the solution of the micellar systems loaded with diclofenac were also evaluated. Both micellar solutions displayed good colloidal stability at 25 °C in both water and PBS (10 mM), maintaining their size and the encapsulated drug for at least 7 days (Supporting Figure S17).

We performed in vitro release studies of only dendron **5** micelles loaded with diclofenac, considering their exceptional encapsulation efficiency values achieved at lower dendron concentrations. The micelle system prepared with a **5**/diclofenac molar ratio of 3.3:1 was chosen for the study. As depicted in Figure 7, **5**+diclofenac micelles could slowly release diclofenac in a time-dependent manner, with 93% of total diclofenac released in 7 days.

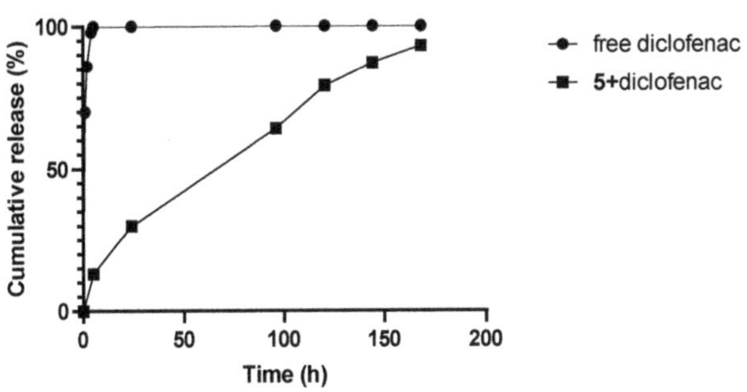

Figure 7. In vitro release profile of **5**+diclofenac micelles in PBS solution (pH = 7.4) at 37 °C.

3.4. Toxicicy Experiments

The toxicity of the dendritic systems in eukaryotic cells was also studied. Safe concentrations of the dendrons were determined using MTT assay in peripheral blood mononuclear cells (PBMCs). Acceptable cellular viability was established at 80%, while lower values were considered toxic. The results are shown in Figure 8 where the maximum tolerated concentrations were 20 µM for **5** and **17**, and 10 µM for **6** and **18**. Considering that the salt concentration in the cellular medium employed is higher than the 40 mM NaI used in the CMC determination, these data reflect different generation-dependent profiles in their toxicity. Toxicity of second-generation amphiphiles **5** and **17** were independent of micelle formation, given that some assayed concentrations higher than the CMC (4.4–4.8 µM) were non-toxic. However, the toxic limit of third-generation dendrons **6** and **18** was established around the CMC values (8.0–9.0 µM) showing toxicity under the micellar regime and suggesting that a possible effect of micelle formation on toxicity could not be ruled out. The cell viability obtained for these dendrons are in the range of those measured for PAMAM-based dendrons or carbosilane dendrons containing fatty acids at the focal points [28,33,41].

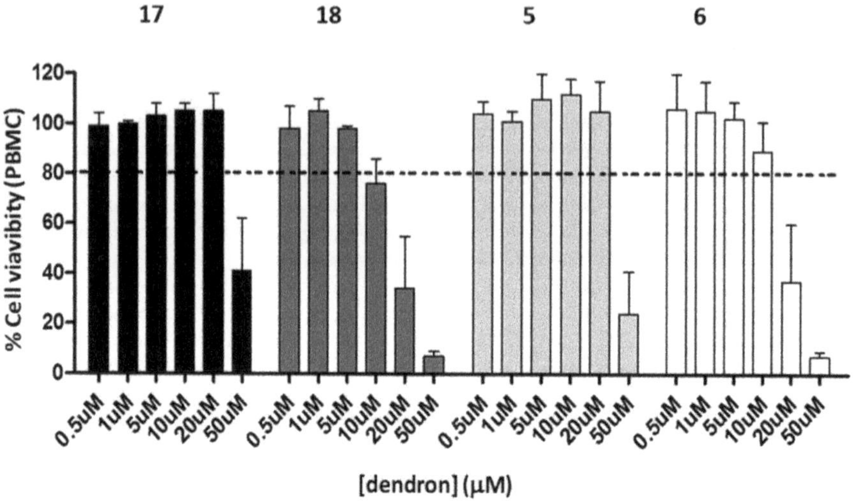

Figure 8. Cell viability in PBMCs of amphiphilic cationic compounds with cholesterol (**5–6**) or vitamin E (**17–18**) by MTT assay. The cells were treated with increasing concentrations of dendrons (ranged from 0.5 to 50 μM). The percent cell viability was calculated as optical density of treated/non-treated control (NT) × 100. In total 80% viability was set as the limit of toxicity. Data are represented as mean ± SD of three experiments achieved in triplicate.

4. Conclusions

Cationic families of dendritic amphiphiles were synthetized from cholesterol or vitamin E as hydrophobic molecules and carbosilane dendrons. Peripheral quaternary ammonium moieties were selected as the hydrophilic components of the structure and the effects of the different structures on the micellization process were examined. Second- and third-generation dendrons formed micelles, and this micellization process was favored by salt addition. Different concentrations (20 mM and 40 mM) and salt types (NaCl and NaI) were assayed, establishing the optimal conditions for aggregate formation in 40 mM NaI. The larger iodide anion (I^-) probably produces a favorable stabilization of repulsion forces between peripheral ammonium groups. CMC values reflected a generation dependence of self-assembly, with values of approximately 5 and 10 μM for the second and third generations, respectively, and with a negligible focal point effect. Thermodynamic parameter calculations confirmed the surfactant nature of the dendritic systems and the spontaneity of the micellar process through positive values of surface excess (Γ) and negative Gibbs free energy (ΔG^0_{mic}). According to the lowest CMC values found for second-generation amphiphiles, ΔG^0_{mic} corroborated that the micellization is energetically more favorable. Hydrophilic and hydrophobic drugs were satisfactorily loaded in micelles using different methods. The protocol employed for water-soluble drugs showed their encapsulation. This phenomenon was attributed to the reduction in CMC in the presence of the drug, which in turn resulted in a more favorable aggregation process. Partition constant (K) calculations were relevant only for procaine and showed a better encapsulation efficiency for the d-α-tocopherol modified dendron (**17**) than the cholesterol-based analogue (**5**). Regarding hydrophobic drugs, a very high diclofenac encapsulation was achieved with both cholesterol- and vitamin E-modified dendrons. The encapsulation efficiency of 92% found for diclofenac was the best described in the literature so far. In addition, DLS measurements revealed micelle size modification in the presence of hydrophilic drugs but none or very minimal change in the case of the hydrophobic ones. The toxicity of the amphiphilic systems was measured on PBMCs, showing that, unlike the third-generation system, the second-generation system was not toxic until 20 μM, which is above their CMC values, opening a window for their use in a micellar regimen where they can operate as drug delivery systems for different biomedical applications.

Supplementary Materials: The following supporting information can be downloaded at: https://www.mdpi.com/article/10.3390/pharmaceutics16040451/s1, Table S1. Surface tension values of 1 mM solution of dendrons **5** and **17** at different concentrations of NaCl and NaI. Figure S1. ^{1}H-NMR spectrum of dendron $ChG_1(SNMe_2)_2$ (**1**) in $CDCl_3$. Figure S2. ^{13}C-NMR spectrum of dendron $ChG_1(SNMe_2)_2$ (**1**) in $CDCl_3$. Figure S3. ^{1}H-NMR spectrum of dendron $ChG_1(SNMe_3I)_2$ (**4**) in CD_3OD. Figure S4. ^{13}C-NMR spectrum of dendron $ChG_1(SNMe_3I)_2$ (**4**) in CD_3OD. Figure S5. ^{1}H-NMR spectrum of dendron $EG_1(V)_2$ (**7**) in $CDCl_3$. Figure S6. ^{13}C-NMR spectrum of dendron $EG_1(V)_2$ (**7**) in $CDCl_3$. Figure S7. ^{1}H-NMR spectrum of dendron $EG_1(SNMe_2{\cdot}HCl)_2$ (**10**) in CD_3OD. Figure S8. ^{1}H-NMR spectrum of dendron $EG_1(SNMe_2)_2$ (**13**) in $CDCl_3$. Figure S9. ^{13}C-NMR spectrum of dendron $EG_1(SNMe_2)_2$ (**13**) in $CDCl_3$. Figure S10. ^{1}H-NMR spectrum of dendron $EG_1(SNMe_3I)_2$ (**16**) in CD_3OD. Figure S11. ^{13}C-NMR spectrum of dendron $EG1(SNMe_3I)_2$ (**16**) in CD_3OD. Figure S12. Surface tension measurements of dendrons $ChG_2(SNMe_3I)_4$ (**5**) and $EG_2(SNMe_3I)_4$ (**17**) at increasing concentrations without the presence of salt. Figure S13. UV-Vis absorption spectra of saline solution (40 mM of NaI) of increasing concentrations of dendrons **5** and **17** in presence of ibuprofen (1.5 mM), procaine (1.5 mM) or lidocaine (10 μM). Figure S14. Particle size distribution of amphiphilic dendrons **5** and **17** in absence or presence of ibuprofen (1.5 mM), lidocaine (1.5 mM) or procaine (10 μM) with 40 mM of NaI. Figure S15. Solubilization of diclofenac by dendron **5** or **17**. Figure S16. Relation between dendron **5** or **17** and encapsulation percentage. Optime dendron:diclofenac molar ratio 3.3:1 (**5**) and 5.5:1 (**17**). Figure S17. Time-dependent hydrodynamic size and % diclofenac encapsulated change **5**+diclofenac and **17**+diclofenac nanomicelles dispersed in water or PBS (10 mM).

Author Contributions: Study conception and discussed and planned the experiments: E.R.G., J.C., M.V., R.G. and S.A. Synthesis: G.M. and T.L.-C. Physical–chemical studies: G.M., M.V., S.A. and J.C. Cytotoxicity studies: G.M. and M.Á.M.-F. Discussion on the results: E.R.G., M.V., J.C. and R.G. Manuscript writing: T.L.-C., M.V. and R.G. Comments on the manuscript: M.Á.M.-F., E.R.G. and J.C. Supervision: E.R.G., M.V., J.C. and R.G. Funding: J.C. and R.G. All authors have read and agreed to the published version of the manuscript.

Funding: This research was funded by grants from PID2020-112924RB-I00 (Ministerio de Ciencia, Educación y Universidades), consortium Radioprotect-CM (P2022/BMD-7406) from Comunidad de Madrid and CCG19/CC-063 from University of Alcalá. CIBER-BBN is an initiative funded by the VI National R&D&I Plan 2008–2011, Iniciativa Ingenio 2010, Consolider Program, and CIBER Actions and financed by the Instituto de Salud Carlos III with assistance from the European Regional Development Fund.

Data Availability Statement: The data presented in this study are available in this article (and Supplementary Materials).

Conflicts of Interest: The authors declare no conflicts of interest. The funders had no role in the design of the study; in the collection, analyses, or interpretation of data; in the writing of the manuscript; or in the decision to publish the results.

References

1. Haberland, M.E.; Reynolds, J.A. Self-association of cholesterol in aqueous solution. *Proc. Natl. Acad. Sci. USA* **1973**, *70*, 2313. [CrossRef]
2. Mandal, D.; Das, S. Glucose-triggered dissolution of phenylboronic acid-functionalized cholesterol-based niosomal self-assembly for tuneable drug release. *New J. Chem.* **2019**, *43*, 7855. [CrossRef]
3. Xu, M.; Zhang, C.Y.; Wu, J.; Zhou, H.; Bai, R.; Shen, Z.; Deng, F.; Liu, Y.; Liu, J. PEG-Detachable Polymeric Micelles Self-Assembled from Amphiphilic Copolymers for Tumor-Acidity-Triggered Drug Delivery and Controlled Release. *ACS Appl. Mater. Interfaces* **2019**, *11*, 5701. [CrossRef]
4. Liu, M.; Luo, X.; Qiu, Q.; Kang, L.; Li, T.; Ding, J.; Xiong, Y.; Zhao, Z.; Zan, J.; Chang, C.; et al. Redox- and pH-Sensitive Glycan (Polysialic Acid) Derivatives and F127 Mixed Micelles for Tumor-Targeted Drug Delivery. *Mol. Pharm.* **2018**, *15*, 5534. [CrossRef]

5. Ferrer-Tasies, L.; Moreno-Calvo, E.; Cano-Sarabia, M.; Aguilella-Arzo, M.; Angelova, A.; Lesieur, S.; Ricart, S.; Faraudo, J.; Ventosa, N.; Veciana, J. Quatsomes: Vesicles Formed by Self-Assembly of Sterols and Quaternary Ammonium Surfactants. *Langmuir* **2013**, *29*, 6519. [CrossRef] [PubMed]
6. Barnard, A.; Posocco, P.; Pricl, S.; Calderon, M.; Haag, R.; Hwang, M.E.; Shum, V.W.T.; Pack, D.W.; Smith, D.K. Degradable Self-Assembling Dendrons for Gene Delivery: Experimental and Theoretical Insights into the Barriers to Cellular Uptake. *J. Am. Chem. Soc.* **2011**, *133*, 20288. [CrossRef] [PubMed]
7. Barnard, A.; Calderon, M.; Tschiche, A.; Haag, R.; Smith, D.K. Effects of a PEG additive on the biomolecular interactions of self-assembled dendron nanostructures. *Org. Biomol. Chem.* **2012**, *10*, 8403. [CrossRef]
8. Barnard, A.; Posocco, P.; Fermeglia, M.; Tschiche, A.; Calderon, M.; Pricl, S.; Smith, D.K. Double-degradable responsive self-assembled multivalent arrays—Temporary nanoscale recognition between dendrons and DNA. *Org. Biomol. Chem.* **2014**, *12*, 446. [CrossRef] [PubMed]
9. Lai, Y.-S.; Kao, C.-L.; Chen, Y.-P.; Fang, C.-C.; Hu, C.-C.; Chu, C.-C. Photodegradable self-assembling PAMAM dendrons for gene delivery involving dendriplex formation and phototriggered circular DNA release. *New J. Chem.* **2016**, *40*, 2601. [CrossRef]
10. Ou, J.-Y.; Shih, Y.-C.; Wang, B.-Y.; Chu, C.-C. Photodegradable coumarin-derived amphiphilic dendrons for DNA binding: Self-assembly and phototriggered disassembly in water and air-water interface. *Colloids Surf. B* **2019**, *175*, 428. [CrossRef]
11. Preedy, V.R.; Watson, R.R. (Eds.) *The Encyclopedia of Vitamin E*; CABI Publishing: Wallingford, UK, 2007; p. 962.
12. Sen, C.K.; Khanna, S.; Roy, S. Tocotrienols: Vitamin E beyond tocopherols. *Life Sci.* **2006**, *78*, 2088. [CrossRef] [PubMed]
13. Liu, Y.; Fu, S.; Lin, L.; Cao, Y.; Xie, X.; Yu, H.; Chen, M.; Li, H. Redox-sensitive Pluronic F127-tocopherol micelles: Synthesis, characterization, and cytotoxicity evaluation. *Int. J. Nanomed.* **2017**, *12*, 2635. [CrossRef]
14. Zhang, H.; Li, W.; Guo, X.; Kong, F.; Wang, Z.; Zhu, C.; Luo, L.; Li, Q.; Yang, J.; Du, Y.; et al. Specifically Increased Paclitaxel Release in Tumor and Synergetic Therapy by a Hyaluronic Acid–Tocopherol Nanomicelle. *ACS Appl. Mater. Interfaces* **2017**, *9*, 20385. [CrossRef]
15. Zhang, X.; Liang, N.; Gong, X.; Kawashima, Y.; Cui, F.; Sun, S. Tumor-targeting micelles based on folic acid and α-tocopherol succinate conjugated hyaluronic acid for paclitaxel delivery. *Colloids Surf. B Biointerfaces* **2019**, *177*, 11. [CrossRef]
16. Figueira, T.N.; Mendonça, D.A.; Gaspar, D.; Melo, M.N.; Moscona, A.; Porotto, M.; Castanho, M.A.R.B.; Veiga, A.S. Structure–Stability–Function Mechanistic Links in the Anti-Measles Virus Action of Tocopherol-Derivatized Peptide Nanoparticles. *ACS Nano* **2018**, *12*, 9855. [CrossRef] [PubMed]
17. Liu, X.; Chen, Y.; Chen, X.; Su, J.; Huang, C. Enhanced efficacy of baicalin-loaded TPGS polymeric micelles against periodontitis. *Mater. Sci. Eng. C* **2019**, *101*, 387. [CrossRef] [PubMed]
18. Banala, V.T.; Urandur, S.; Sharma, S.; Sharma, M.; Shukla, R.P.; Marwaha, D.; Gautam, S.; Dwivedi, M.; Mishra, P.R. Targeted co-delivery of the aldose reductase inhibitor epalrestat and chemotherapeutic doxorubicin via a redox-sensitive prodrug approach promotes synergistic tumor suppression. *Biomater. Sci.* **2019**, *7*, 2889. [CrossRef]
19. Dong, K.; Lei, Q.; Qi, H.; Zhang, Y.; Cui, N.; Wu, X.; Xie, L.; Yan, X.; Lu, T. Amplification of Oxidative Stress in MCF-7 Cells by a Novel pH-Responsive Amphiphilic Micellar System Enhances Anticancer Therapy. *Mol. Pharm.* **2019**, *16*, 689. [CrossRef]
20. Yang, C.; Wu, T.; Qi, Y.; Zhang, Z. Recent advances in the application of vitamin E TPGS for drug delivery. *Theranostics* **2018**, *8*, 464. [CrossRef]
21. Mandracchia, D.; Tripodo, G.; Trapani, A.; Ruggieri, S.; Annese, T.; Chlapanidas, T.; Trapani, G.; Ribatti, D. Inulin based micelles loaded with curcumin or celecoxib with effective anti-angiogenic activity. *Eur. J. Pharm. Sci.* **2016**, *93*, 141. [CrossRef]
22. Wang, Y.; Shen, W.; Shi, X.; Fu, F.; Fan, Y.; Shen, W.; Cao, Y.; Zhang, Q.; Qi, R. Alpha-Tocopheryl Succinate-Conjugated G5 PAMAM Dendrimer Enables Effective Inhibition of Ulcerative Colitis. *Adv. Healthc. Mater.* **2017**, *6*, 1700276. [CrossRef]
23. Zhu, J.; Zheng, L.; Wen, S.; Tang, Y.; Shen, M.; Zhang, G.; Shi, X. Targeted cancer theranostics using alpha-tocopheryl succinate-conjugated multifunctional dendrimer-entrapped gold nanoparticles. *Biomaterials* **2014**, *35*, 7635. [CrossRef]
24. Bhatt, H.; Kiran Rompicharla, S.V.; Ghosh, B.; Biswas, S. α-Tocopherol Succinate-Anchored PEGylated Poly(amidoamine) Dendrimer for the Delivery of Paclitaxel: Assessment of in Vitro and in Vivo Therapeutic Efficacy. *Mol. Pharm.* **2019**, *16*, 1541. [CrossRef]
25. Wang, X.; Shi, C.; Zhang, L.; Bodman, A.; Guo, D.; Wang, L.; Hall, W.A.; Wilkens, S.; Luo, J. Affinity-controlled protein encapsulation into sub-30 nm telodendrimer nanocarriers by multivalent and synergistic interactions. *Biomaterials* **2016**, *101*, 258. [CrossRef]
26. Wang, X.; Shi, C.; Zhang, L.; Lin, M.Y.; Guo, D.; Wang, L.; Yang, Y.; Duncan, T.M.; Luo, J. Structure-Based Nanocarrier Design for Protein Delivery. *ACS Macro Lett.* **2017**, *6*, 267. [CrossRef]
27. Percec, V.; Wilson, D.A.; Leowanawat, P.; Wilson, C.J.; Hughes, A.D.; Kaucher, M.S.; Hammer, D.A.; Levine, D.H.; Kim, A.J.; Bates, F.S.; et al. Self-assembly of Janus dendrimers into uniform dendrimersomes and other complex architectures. *Science* **2010**, *328*, 1009–1014. [CrossRef] [PubMed]
28. Chen, C.; Posocco, P.; Liu, X.; Cheng, Q.; Laurini, E.; Zhou, J.; Liu, C.; Wang, Y.; Tang, J.; Col, V.D.; et al. Mastering Dendrimer Self-Assembly for Efficient siRNA Delivery: From Conceptual Design to In Vivo Efficient Gene Silencing. *Small* **2016**, *12*, 3667–3676. [CrossRef]
29. Kostiainen, M.A.; Kasyutich, O.; Cornelissen, J.J.L.M.; Nolte, R.J.M. Self-assembly and optically triggered disassembly of hierarchical dendron-virus complexes. *Nat. Chem.* **2010**, *2*, 394–399. [CrossRef] [PubMed]

30. Martin, A.L.; Li, B.; Gillies, E.R. Surface Functionalization of Nanomaterials with Dendritic Groups: Toward Enhanced Binding to Biological Targets. *J. Am. Chem. Soc.* **2009**, *131*, 734–741. [CrossRef] [PubMed]
31. Mencia, G.; Lozano-Cruz, T.; Valiente, M.; Jimenez, J.L.; de la Mata, F.J.; Muñoz-Fernández, M.A.; Cano, J.; Gillies, E.; Gómez, R. Evaluation of pH-dependent amphiphilic carbosilane dendrons in micelle formation, drug loading and HIV-1 infection. *Org. Biomol. Chem.* **2020**, *18*, 9639–9652. [CrossRef] [PubMed]
32. Fuentes-Paniagua, E.; Peña-González, C.E.; Galán, M.; Gómez, R.; de la Mata, F.J.; Sánchez-Nieves, J. Thiol-Ene Synthesis of Cationic Carbosilane Dendrons: A New Family of Synthons. *Organometallics* **2013**, *32*, 1789. [CrossRef]
33. Gutiérrez-Ulloa, C.E.; Buyanova, M.Y.; Apartsin, E.K.; Venyaminova, A.G.; de la Mata, F.J.; Valiente, M.; Gómez, R. Amphiphilic carbosilane dendrons as a novel synthetic platform toward micelle formation. *Org. Biomol. Chem.* **2017**, *15*, 7352. [CrossRef] [PubMed]
34. Chiappisi, L.; Keiderling, U.; Gutierrez-Ulloa, C.E.; Gómez, R.; Valiente, M.; Gradzielski, M. Aggregation behavior of surfactants with cationic and anionic dendronic head groups. *J. Colloid Interf. Sci.* **2019**, *534*, 430–439. [CrossRef] [PubMed]
35. Enache, M.; Volanschi, E. Spectral studies on the molecular interaction of anticancer drug mitoxantrone with CTBA micelles. *J. Pharm. Sci.* **2011**, *100*, 558. [CrossRef] [PubMed]
36. Hosseinzadeh, R.; Gheshlagi, M.; Tahmasebi, R.; Hojjati, F. Spectrophotometric study of interaction and solubilization of procaine hydrochloride in micellar systems. *Cent. Eur. J. Chem.* **2009**, *7*, 90–95. [CrossRef]
37. Ćudina, O.; Karljiković-Rajić, K.; Ruvarac-Burgarčić, I.; Janković, I. Interaction of hydrochlorothiazide with cationic surfactant micelles of cetyltrimethylammonium bromide. *Colloids Surf. A Physicochem. Eng. Asp.* **2005**, *256*, 225. [CrossRef]
38. Dalpiaz, A.; Sacchetti, F.; Baldisserotto, A.; Pavan, B.; Maretti, E.; Iannuccelli, V.; Leo, E. Application of the "in-oil nanoprecipitation" method in the encapsulation of hydrophilic drugs in PLGA nanoparticles. *J. Drug Deliv. Sci. Technol.* **2016**, *32*, 283. [CrossRef]
39. Sapkota, M.; Karmakar, G.; Nahak, P.; Guha, P.; Roy, B.; Koirala, S.; Chettri, P.; Das, K.; Misono, T.; Torigoe, K.; et al. Effect of polymer charge on the formation and stability of anti-inflammatory drug loaded nanostructured lipid carriers: Physicochemical approach. *RSC Adv.* **2015**, *5*, 65697. [CrossRef]
40. Bhavya, R.; Upendra, N.; Jain, D.A. Development and characterization of non-ionic surfactant vesicles for ophthalmic drug delivery of diclofenac potassium. *J. Drug Delivery Ther.* **2014**, 1–6. [CrossRef]
41. Mirsharghi, S.; Knudsen, K.D.; Bagherifam, S.; Nyström, B.; Boas, U. Preparation and self-assembly of amphiphilic polylysine dendrons. *New J. Chem.* **2016**, *40*, 3597. [CrossRef]

pharmaceutics

MDPI

Review

In Vivo Applications of Dendrimers: A Step toward the Future of Nanoparticle-Mediated Therapeutics

Krzysztof Sztandera [1,2], José Luis Rodríguez-García [3] and Valentín Ceña [1,2,*]

1 Unidad Asociada Neurodeath, Instituto de Nanociencia Molecular, Universidad de Castilla-La Mancha, 02006 Albacete, Spain; krzysztof.sztandera@uclm.es
2 Centro de Investigación Biomédica en Red en Enfermedades Neurodegenerativas, Instituto de Salud Carlos III, 28029 Madrid, Spain
3 Department of Internal Medicine, General University Hospital of Albacete, 02006 Albacete, Spain; jlrg61@gmail.com
* Correspondence: valentin.cena@gmail.com

Abstract: Over the last few years, the development of nanotechnology has allowed for the synthesis of many different nanostructures with controlled sizes, shapes, and chemical properties, with dendrimers being the best-characterized of them. In this review, we present a succinct view of the structure and the synthetic procedures used for dendrimer synthesis, as well as the cellular uptake mechanisms used by these nanoparticles to gain access to the cell. In addition, the manuscript reviews the reported in vivo applications of dendrimers as drug carriers for drugs used in the treatment of cancer, neurodegenerative diseases, infections, and ocular diseases. The dendrimer-based formulations that have reached different phases of clinical trials, including safety and pharmacokinetic studies, or as delivery agents for therapeutic compounds are also presented. The continuous development of nanotechnology which makes it possible to produce increasingly sophisticated and complex dendrimers indicates that this fascinating family of nanoparticles has a wide potential in the pharmaceutical industry, especially for applications in drug delivery systems, and that the number of dendrimer-based compounds entering clinical trials will markedly increase during the coming years.

Keywords: dendrimers; cellular uptake; in vivo; drug delivery; gene delivery; theragnostic

1. Introduction

Over the last few years, the development of nanotechnology has significantly increased. Nanotechnology allows researchers to synthesize many different nanostructures with controlled sizes, shapes, and properties. Such nanostructures include, among others, metal nanoparticles [1], polymeric micelles [2], polymersomes [3], dendrimers [4,5], and liposomes [6], with dendrimers being the best-characterized of these to date [7]. The name "dendrimer" comes from the combination of the Greek words "dendros" meaning "tree or branching", and "meros" meaning "part of". The high number of chemically modifiable terminal groups in their surface, as well as the void spaces present in their interior makes dendrimers excellent delivery agents for different therapeutic agents, including genetic material and drugs. Initial attempts to synthesize these branched polymers were first made in the 1940s. However, it was not until 1985 that the team of Donald Tomalia first described and synthesized poly(amidoamine) or PAMAM dendrimers [8]. To date, more than 100 families of dendrimers differing in their initiator cores, branching units and terminal moieties have been synthesized and evaluated [9]. Some of them, such as PAMAM [10], poly-L-lysine (PLL), bis-methyl propionic acid [11], and poly(propyleneimine) (PPI) dendrimers [12], have been commercialized while others like phosphorus dendrimers [13], Janus dendrimers [14], peptide dendrimers [15], rotaxane dendrimers [16], and carbosilane dendrimers [17] among others [18–22] have not. Amphiphillic Janus dendrimers and glycodendrimers are water-soluble mimics of biological membranes, including cell membrane glycans that self-assemble into unilamellar or onion-like dendrimersomes with predictable dimensions [23]. This dendrimer family has shown efficacy for the in vivo targeted delivery of mRNA to different organs based on changes in their chemical structure [24].

2. Dendrimer Structure

These interesting nanoparticles are three-dimensional sphere-shaped and monodispersed polymers with symmetrical branches [25]. They consist of three components: the central core, branches, and terminal groups (Figure 1). Branches are attached to the central core and end in terminal moieties that play a role as a dendrimer scaffold. As the number of branches increases, the dendrimer generation grows, and after generation 4 (G4), these nanoparticles adopt a globular structure [10] resembling the natural vesicles found in cells.

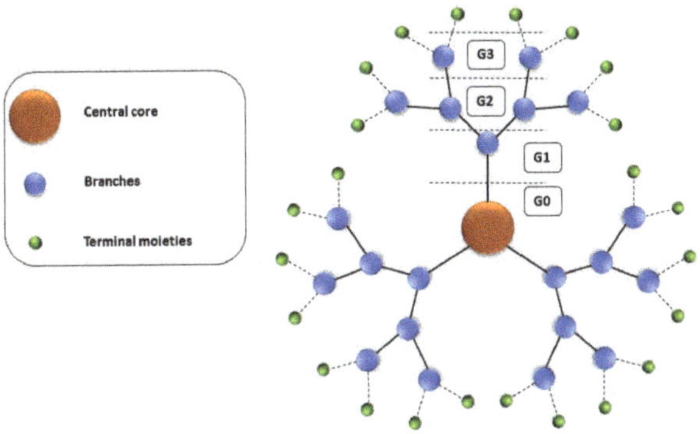

Figure 1. Scheme of the dendrimer structure. For a detailed explanation, see the text.

The synthesis of dendrimers can be strictly controlled, which provides high-purity homogeneous, monodispersed products with a well-defined structure, size, density, and uniform molecular weight [8,26,27]. This distinguishes them from classical linear polymers, that usually generate polydisperse products with different molecular weights.

There are two main ways to synthesize dendrimers: a divergent and a convergent approach (Figure 2). In the first method, monomers are added to the central core to engender the desired dendrimer generation. In contrast, during convergent synthesis, large segments (whole branches) are synthesized and then joined together to generate the dendrimer [26]. The use of click chemistry in the synthesis of dendrimers is also becoming increasingly popular. This system allows for the quick modification of substances without interfering with their structure [28]. Indeed, several reports about click chemistry in dendrimer synthesis with the use of thiol–yne, azide–alkyne, and Diels–Alder reactions have already been published [29–31].

Dendrimer synthesis requires a repeated series of reactions that increase dendrimer size and generation. Of note, there is a threshold generation level whereafter the attachment of further elements is impossible because the terminal groups form a closed membrane, with this phenomenon being referred to as the starburst effect [31]. Therefore, the synthesis of G10 is considered the highest possible level [32]. Furthermore, appropriate monomer selection is crucial in the development of dendrimers because the size, solubility, biocompatibility, multivalency, and ability to interact with biological systems depend on these initial units [33–35]. Moreover, manipulation of the dendrimer surface can prolong their blood circulation time or change their biodistribution in vivo.

The terminal groups of dendrimers can also be functionalized with biologically active molecules to provide them with wider application possibilities [36,37], thereby allowing them to encapsulate compounds (Figure 3). These cavities are usually hydrophobic and can generate hydrogen bonds to the transported compounds [38–40], which protects drugs from biodegradation before reaching the desired site of action [38]. However, because this premise is based on hydrophobic interactions, only hydrophobic compounds are used in this way. In addition to the use of internal cavities for storage, a wide range of terminal groups can also be conjugated covalently on the surface of dendrimers through specific linkers, including those sensitive to changes in pH or temperature, enzymatic or redox reactions, light irradiation, or hypoxia [41]. Non-covalent interactions between the terminal groups of dendrimers and different compounds do not interfere with the structure of these compounds but could be unstable in vivo. Thus, covalent bonding is the most stable connection between dendrimers and drugs but requires chemical modification of the compound by attaching linkers which could, in turn, change their properties [42] (Figure 3). The perspectives for the use of dendrimer-based systems as nanomedicines [43], biological adhesives [44], imaging agents [45], and in gene therapy [46] are all very promising. Dendrimers can be also used as vectors for the delivery of genes [47], nucleic acids [48], and drugs [49]. Moreover, research is currently underway to use dendrimers as adjuvants in vaccines [50] based on evidence that nanoparticles protect drugs from biodegradation, prolong their half-life in blood, improve their solubility, and provide targeted delivery [51].

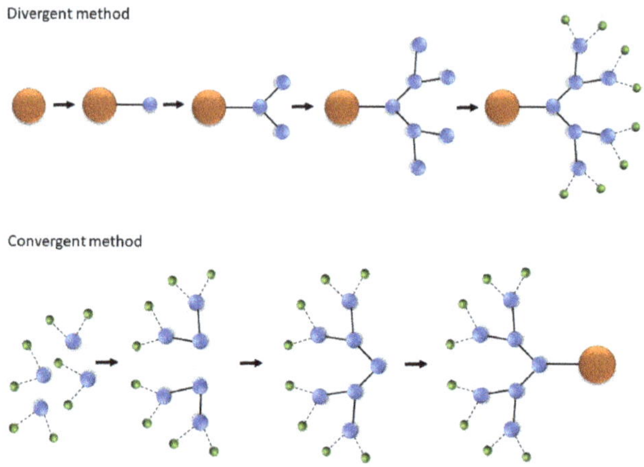

Figure 2. Scheme of the divergent and convergent methods for dendrimer synthesis. Symbols are the same as in Figure 1. For a detailed explanation, see the text.

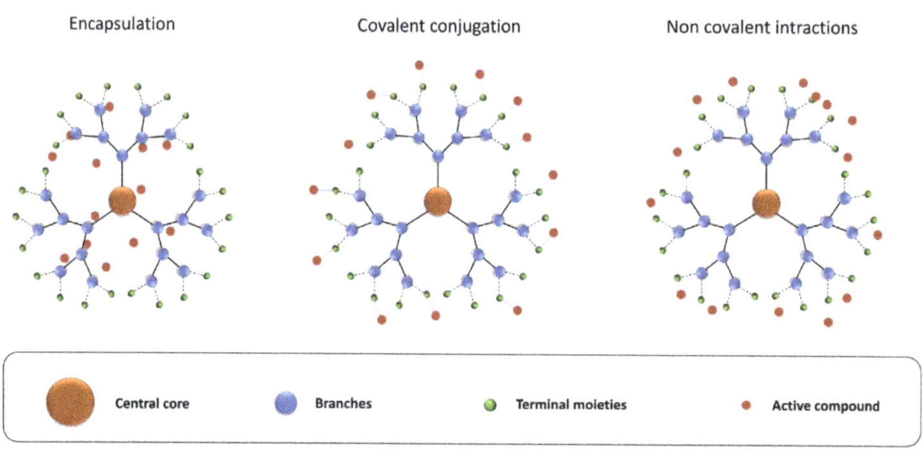

Figure 3. Main strategies for transporting active compounds by dendrimers. For a detailed explanation, see the text.

3. Cellular Dendrimer Uptake

The main use of dendrimers to date is in the transport and delivery of different compounds to cell interiors. Thus, intracellular uptake is one of their most studied properties. Two main mechanisms are responsible for the intracellular transport of dendrimers: clathrin-mediated endocytosis (CME) and caveolin-mediated endocytosis (CVME). However, under some specific conditions, macropinocytosis can also be engaged in this process (Figure 4). During CME, clathrin is recruited to specialized regions of the cell membrane where it coats endocytic vesicles measuring 70–150 nm [52]. After internalization by the cell, the vesicles lose the clathrin coat and form early endosomes which later evolve into late endosomes and fuse with lysosomes [53]. This internalization pathway is common for receptor–ligand complexes such as low-density lipoprotein (LDL) particles [54] or epithelial growth factor [55], virus entry [56], and the uptake of neurotransmitters [57]. In turn, CMVE starts by generating 60–80 nm invaginations of the cell membrane in which proteins participating in endocytosis (e.g., caveolin-1) bind to lipid rafts. These vesicles either fuse with other caveolin vesicles to form caveosomes or with early endosomes, which can be transported to the Golgi apparatus or the smooth endoplasmic reticulum [58]. This pathway is used for, among other substances, the internalization of cholesterol [59], TGF-β receptor signaling [60] or toxins [61]. Macropinocytosis starts by creating vacuoles, termed macropinosomes, of variable sizes. After these enter cells, their pH decreases and they fuse with late endosomes or lysosomes [58]. This pathway is mainly used for the uptake of proteins [62], viruses [63], and antigens [64].

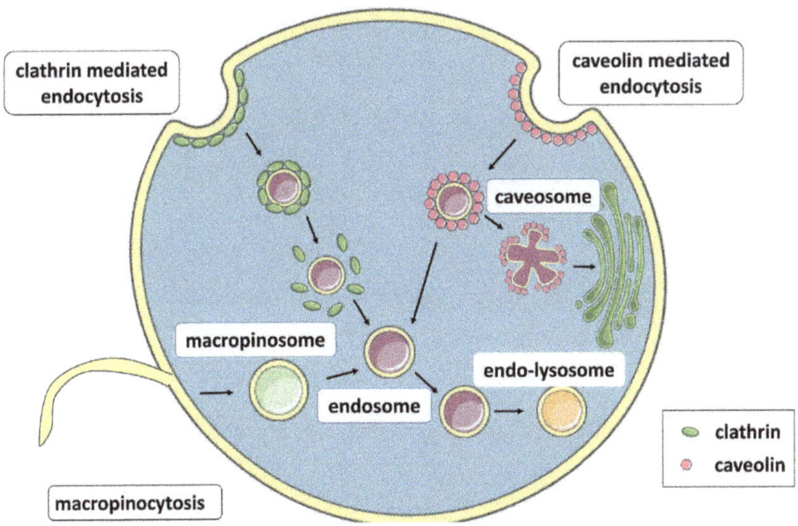

Figure 4. Main pathways for the intracellular uptake of dendrimers. For a detailed explanation, see the text.

The type and efficacy of the cellular uptake of dendrimers is strongly dependent on the cell type, generation route, and surface charge of the nanoparticles in question. For instance, G4 PAMAM dendrimers are better internalized than lower generations [58]. Moreover, epithelial cells have a negative charge on their surface because of the presence of phosphate groups. Combined with a positive charge on the surface of cationic dendrimers, this creates electrostatic interactions that increase the efficiency of endocytosis [65]. Thus, it is extremely important to choose a dendrimer with an appropriate surface charge for every cell type. For example, PAMAM dendrimers with -NH_2 moieties in MCF-7 cells are internalized by CME and micropinocytosis. However, in the case of A549 cells, they are internalized by both the CME and CVME pathways [66]. Furthermore, the chemical modification of dendrimers is also relevant: for instance, naked G4.5 PAMAM dendrimers are usually internalized through the CME, whereas after PEGylation (the modification of biological molecules by covalent conjugation with polyethylene glycol [PEG]), the main endocytic pathway changes to CVME [67].

The ideal nanocarriers should protect cargo compounds from biodegradation and release them into the targeted area. Moreover, they must also be biocompatible and not cause side effects [67]. Because of their shape, structure, and nanometric size, dendrimers can also penetrate into tumoral environments and be retained in the interstitium of tumors, a property termed the enhanced permeability and retention effect [51]. In addition, the possibility of almost unlimited dendrimer modifications by, for example, conjugation with antibodies, carbohydrates, folic acid (FA), or PEG, or by attaching active components through encapsulation, conjugation, or noncovalent interactions, makes these nanoparticles a promising alternative to regular cancer treatments [51]. In fact, nanosystems comprising dendrimers and drugs that result in improved cellular uptake and increased retention time compared to free drug delivery systems have been widely described in the academic literature [68–70].

4. In Vivo Use of Dendrimers

The cytotoxic activity, hemolytic properties, cellular uptake, or ability to transport and release different cargo compounds of many dendrimers have already been studied in vitro [9,71]. However, studies in isolated groups of cells do not accurately model the difficulties nanoparticles must overcome to reach their targets in vivo. These include biological barriers such as the blood–brain barrier (BBB), short plasma circulation times, hepatic or renal clearance, and limited distribution to sites of drug action [72]. Hence, more complex in vivo models of disease are now shedding new light on the usability of dendrimers in living systems. Studies performed at this stage aim to evaluate acute toxicity, dose dependence, and long-term toxicity in animal models, with parameters including pharmacodynamics and pharmacokinetics also being important.

4.1. Dendrimers as Carriers for Active Compounds

There is intense interest in dendrimers as delivery vehicles, especially for anti-cancer, anti-neurodegenerative, and anti-inflammation drugs [73–76], with the most important role of dendrimers in these systems being the efficient transport of drugs to the site of action. The almost infinite possibilities for dendrimer functionalization mean that compounds such as antibodies [77,78], folic acid [79], amino acids [80,81], sugar groups [82,83], or other specific ligands can be attached to their surface so that these nanosystems can target specific cells and tissues (Figure 5) [84]. For instance, these dendrimers could be designed to target cells with specific receptors or other substances secreted specifically by a given tumor type. Indeed, such modifications might also enable these molecules to cross the BBB [85]. Moreover, the use of pH-sensitive linkers can be used to release the drugs they carry only in a specific environment [86]. Thus, all the above-mentioned strategies could be combined to help improve drug efficiency and decrease side effects.

To date, most in vivo studies have focused on PAMAM dendrimers, although a few other dendrimer types have also been evaluated. For example, Chen et al. used phosphorus dendrimers to prepare micelles in order to encapsulate doxorubicin (DOX). They showed that this nanosystem can decrease the size of breast cancer tumor xenografts in mice by upregulating Bax, PTEN, and p53 [87]. Another group also used DOX combined with peptide dendrimers to target pancreatic ductal adenocarcinoma xenografts in mice, resulting in increased accumulation and internalization of the drug into these tumors. Additionally, these authors found that the efficacy of DOX was greater when it was co-administered with the dendrimer [88]. Furthermore, they reported that in a zebrafish model, the release of DOX in response to γ-radiation was increased when delivered by PAMAM dendrimers modified with L-cysteine because the latter acts as a radiosensitizer that allows for the release of the drug and inhibits cancer growth [89].

The use of PAMAM dendrimers to deliver other anti-cancer agents has also been extensively studied. For example, Bhadra et al. exploited naked and PEGylated PAMAM dendrimers to transport 5-fluorouracil and verified that this nanosystem was stable and biocompatible in albino rats by measuring the serum levels of the drug. Thus, this nanosystem proved to be safe for animals; and moreover, PEGylation reduced drug leakage and hemolysis, thereby indicating that PAMAM dendrimers are suitable for the prolonged delivery of 5-fluorouracil [90]. Additionally, Gupta et al. employed PAMAM dendrimers to transport berberine, a drug with potential anti-cancer activity. They prepared two formulations: in the first, berberine was conjugated with the dendrimers, while in the second, the drug was encapsulated inside the PAMAM structure. They then went on to evaluate the biocompatibility and safety of these formulations in albino rats, observing that the conjugated form was safer than the encapsulated one in this animal model. Moreover, the half-life of berberine when delivered in the conjugated form was also significantly increased when compared to free delivery of the drug [91].

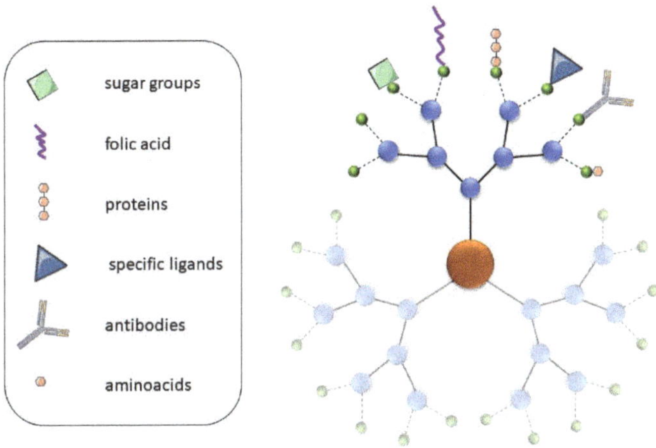

Figure 5. The targeting methods of dendrimers. For a detailed explanation, see the text.

In another study, PPI dendrimers anchored with polysorbate 80 were used to deliver docetaxel in a brain tumor mouse model. These authors found that this nanosystem reduced the tumor volume and moreover, the median survival rate was almost twice as high as in the case of mice treated with PPI-DOX (without polysorbate 80), and more than double when compared to the free delivery of DOX [92]. Finally, when G5 L-lysine dendrimers were used as a vehicle for SN-38 (an active irinotecan metabolite) in a murine colorectal cancer xenograft model, sustained blood levels of SN-38 were detected, which led to significant tumor regression. Moreover, this conjugate exhibited reduced gastrointestinal toxicity compared to free delivery of the drug. They also observed that a regimen of 4 mg/kg SN-38 in 4 doses at weekly intervals extended the survival of the mice to 70 days after delivery of the final dose [93]. More in vivo studies on the use of dendrimers as carriers of anticancer drugs are described in Table 1.

Table 1. In vivo studies of dendrimers as carriers for anti-cancer drugs. Transported active drugs are indicated in an italic font.

Dendrimer	Modification/ *Active Drug*	Outcome	Ref.
PAMAM	*cisplatin*	• selective accumulation in the tumor • decreased toxicity in comparison with free cisplatin	[94]
	PEG and *5 fluorouracil*	• lack of significant hematological disturbances	[90]
	β-cyclodextrin and oligoarginine peptide entrapped gold nanoparticles and *dexamethasone*	• improved hearing in C57/BL6 mice • more effective tympanic injection than posterior ear injection, muscle injection, and tail vein injection	[95]
	L-cysteine and *doxorubicin*	• L-cysteine acts as a radiosensitizer • inhibition of cancer growth	[89]
	berberine	• longer half-life and AUC	[91]
	folic acid and borneol	• tumor growth inhibition • median survival time prolonged compared to free doxorubicin	[96]
	cholesteryl chloroformate and alkyl-PEG	• significantly decreased tumor growth rate	[97]
	dendrimer–gold hybrid structure	• effective anti-tumor agent • accurate CT imaging • usability in combined detection of therapy of different adenocarcinomas via an active, MUC-1-mediated targeting pathway	[98]
PPI	Polysorbate 80	• anti-cancer activity in brain tumor • longer survival time of the case of DTX–P80-PPI than DTX–PPI • higher targeting efficiency and biodistribution of ligand-conjugated dendrimer into the brain	[92]
phosphorus dendrimers	*doxorubicin (DOX)*	• good intrinsic anticancer activity • collective action with DOX to take down breast cancer via the upregulation of Bax, PTEN, and p53 proteins for enhanced cell apoptosis	[87]
Janus dendrimers	*doxorubicin (DOX)*	• minimal systemic toxicity • half-life approx. 16 h • 9 times higher tumor uptake in comparison with free DOX • complete tumor regression • 100% survival of the mice • antitumor effect of dendrimer–DOX similar to liposomal DOX	[99]
	cytarabine and daunorubicin	• superior therapeutic activity compared to free drug cocktails • prolonged maintenance of synergistic drug ratios in the bone marrow	[100]
peptide dendrimers	*doxorubicin*	• increased doxorubicin concentration in the tumor • enhanced anticancer efficacy of doxorubicin and gemcitabine	[88]

Table 1. *Cont.*

Dendrimer	Modification/ *Active Drug*	Outcome	Ref.
polylysine dendrimers	*polyoxazoline*	• prolonged circulation of the dendrimer • survival period of the mice extended beyond 70 days following the final dose	[93]
rotaxane dendrimer	*chlorambucil*	• accumulation in the reticuloendothelial system • enriching spleen and liver	[16]

The effect of dendrimer-based preparation has been also studied on animal models of ocular, metabolic, or inflammation diseases. Simvastatin was entrapped into amino-terminated, hydroxyl-terminated, and pegylated PAMAM dendrimers to compare its cholesterol-reducing effects with the free drug in male albino rats. Since entrapment increased simvastatin solubility, it was described that the drug residence time when used in this dendrimer formulation was 3–5 times longer than when the free drug was used. Additionally, drug absorption and elimination rates also decreased significantly, indicating the controlled release of simvastatin from these dendrimer formulations [101]. In a similar vein, phosphorus dendrimers were used to transport azabisphosphonate to target monocytes where they produced anti-inflammatory effects in a model of rheumatoid arthritis in both IL-1ra(−/−) mice (genetically modified mice with silenced gene encoding interleukin-1 receptor antagonist) and mice undergoing K/BxN serum transfer, an animal model of arthritis where the serum from arthritic transgenic K/BxN mice is transferred to naive mice and manifestations of arthritis occur a few days later. This nanosystem suppressed disease by reducing the levels of inflammatory cytokines. Moreover, inhibition of the colony-stimulating factor receptor promoted the maintenance of normal synovial membranes and cartilage, and prevented bone erosion and anti-osteoclastic activity, both in mouse and human cells [102]. In another study, PAMAM dendrimers were used as carriers for pilocarpine nitrate and tropicamide, resulting in prolonged drug residence time for the ophthalmic route when compared to free delivery of the drug [103]. Neutral high-generation phosphorus dendrimers bearing 48 (G3) or 96 (G4) bisphosphonate groups on their surface showed no toxicity and good solubility, as well as chemical stability in aqueous solutions. Furthermore, the anti-inflammatory activity of these neutral phosphorus dendrimers was high in a mouse model of sub-chronic inflammation [76]. Finally, in other works, amino-bis(methylene phosphonate)-capped phosphorus dendrimers prevented the development of experimental autoimmune encephalomyelitis and inhibited the progression of the established disease [104] (Table 2).

Table 2. In vivo studies of dendrimers as carriers for drugs in non-cancer diseases. Transported active drugs are indicated in an italic font.

Dendrimer	Modification/ *Active Drug*	Outcome	Ref.
Phosphorus dendrimer	azabisphosphonate (ABP)	• efficient anti-inflammatory activity	[76]
	azabisphosphonate (ABP)	• anti-inflammatory activity • selective targeting to monocytes • anti-osteoclastic activity	[102]
	amino-bis(methylene phosphonate)	• preventing of autoimmune encephalomyelitis development • inhibition of established disease progression • redirection of pathogenic myelin-specific CD4+ T cell response toward IL-10 production	[104]

Table 2. *Cont.*

Dendrimer	Modification/ *Active Drug*	Outcome	Ref.
Phosphorus dendrimer	amino-bis(methylene phosphonate)	• inhibition of the onset and development of experimental arthritis • lack of adverse response • lack of lesion or non-physiological occurrence	[105]
	carteolol	• no eye irritation • 2.5 times larger quantity of mix of carteolol and dendrimer in comparison with free carteolol	[106]
Janus dendrimers	carboxybetain and α-lactalbumin	• prolonged pharmacokinetic profiles of payloads in comparison with the PEGylated nanocarriers	[107]
PAMAM	amino-terminated	• improved diabetes-induced vascular remodeling and dysfunction • inhibited EGFR-ERK1/2-ROCK signaling	[108]
	amino-terminated	• intraperitoneal and subcutaneous administration are the most effective in suppressing the long-term markers of hyperglycemia • the lowest incidence of side effects was observed after subcutaneous administration • subcutaneous injection is the best way to compromise moderate PAMAM toxicity and effective reduction in the markers of long-term severe hyperglycemia	[109]
		• reduced levels of blood glucose glycated hemoglobin or protein oxidation, cholesterol, and triglycerides • higher terminal blood glucose in PAMAM-treated animals	
	amino-terminated	• reduction of blood glucose concentration and hallmarks of late diabetic complications • reduced diabetes-induced permeabilization of BBB • enrichment of the biochemical hallmarks of severe hyperglycemia.	[110]
	simvastatin	• reduction in the increase in cholesterol level approx. 2 times and in triglyceride and low-density lipoprotein levels • better pharmacokinetic performance in comparison with free drug • three-to-five times higher residence time in comparison with free drug • controlled release of simvastatin decreasing absorption and elimination rates	[101]
Lysine dendrimers	mannose	• accelerated diabetes wound repair after topical administration • increased closure rate, collagen deposition, and angiogenesis, production of TGF-β1	[111]

4.2. Dendrimers in Infectious Diseases

The antiviral activity of dendrimers is based on mimicking the anionic cell surface, and so dendrimers developed taking this approach also have a negative surface charge.

Consequently, viruses bind to dendrimers not to cells, leading to a decrease in the viral infection rate. For example, PLL dendrimers with naphthyl residues were able to inhibit herpes simplex virus infection [112]; and moreover, PAMAM dendrimers modified with naphthyl sulfonate exhibited anti-HIV activity. In both cases, dendrimers inhibited virus entry into cells and replication. Furthermore, other PAMAM dendrimers combined with sialic acid have been studied as inhibitors of influenza A virus infection [113].

Excessive use of antibiotics has been one of the most important factors leading to the emergence of new antibiotic-resistant pathogen variants, meaning that research into new types of anti-bacterial agents remains of vital importance. In this context, dendrimers with a positive surface charge have shown antibacterial activity by binding to the anionic surface of bacterial membranes and damaging it, thereby causing lysis. For instance, PPI dendrimers with alkyl ammonium moieties have been studied to counteract anti-Gram-positive and anti-Gram-negative bacteria [114]. Furthermore, PLL dendrimers with mannosyl surface groups inhibited the adhesion of Escherichia coli to blood cells, making them good candidates as antibacterial drugs [115].

To date, only a few in vivo studies have been carried out to examine the activity of dendrimers against viruses and bacteria. In this sense, lysine dendrimers formulated with SPL7013 were used in mouse and guinea pig models to evaluate anti-herpes simplex virus activity, where they provided protection against infection at 10 mg/mL doses. However, further studies on guinea pigs showed that the optimal dose ranges from 30 to 50 mg/mL [116]. In another study, Landers et al. exploited a G4 PAMAM dendrimer carrying sialic acid to treat infection with three influenza variants in a mouse model. They showed that this nanosystem prevented infection by the H3N2 subtype but was unable to prevent pneumonitis caused by the other two virus types [113]. Elsewhere, researchers synthesized poly(phosphorhydrazone) dendrimers carrying mannose units with oligommanoside caps differing in size, number, and length. They showed that G3 dendrimers with 48 trimannoside caps reduced the neutrophil influx by targeting the DC-SIGN murine homolog, SIGN-related 1. Thus, this nanosystem showed great promise for the treatment of lung inflammation caused by Mycobacterium tuberculosis infection [117]. Even more interestingly, a G2 polyanionic carbosilane dendrimer, G2-S16, with a silica core and 16 sulfonate end-groups exerted anti-HIV-1 activity at an early stage of viral replication, blocking the viral protein gp120/CD4 interaction. Furthermore, topical vaginal administration of a 3% G2-S16 gel prevented HIV-1JR-CSF transmission by 84% in humanized (h)-BLT mice with no presence of HIV-1 RNA in vaginal lesions, thereby taking us one step forward the development of G2-S16-based vaginal microbicides to prevent vaginal HIV-1 transmission in humans [118].

4.3. Dendrimers in Gene Delivery

Gene therapy involves two basic actions: enhancing the expression of or silencing a specific gene, and depending on the application in question, different nucleic acids acting upon the cytosol and/or nucleus are used [119]. For silencing a specific gene, antisense oligonucleotides, or small-interfering RNA (siRNA) are generally used, reaching some of the later the clinical setting [120]. Viral vectors were initially employed for the delivery of genetic material [121,122]. However, because of their immunogenicity, carcinogenicity, and difficulties in large-scale production, their biocompatibility and efficacy has been challenged. Considering all the above, a limited number of approved and commercially used gene therapies are currently available [123]. Thus, the search for the ideal synthetic carrier for genetic material delivery is still underway. The main goals for any novel synthetic nanocarrier would be to efficiently deliver genetic material to patient cells without causing toxicity [124]. Of note, current in vitro studies indicate that dendrimers could be more efficient carriers for genetic materials than biological vectors [125]. Several in vivo studies have been conducted in the central nervous system (Table 3). For instance, PEGylated PAMAM dendrimers carrying angiopep-2, a ligand for lipoprotein receptor-related protein 1 that would facilitate BBB crossing, were used to target glioma cells and deliver tumor necrosis factor-related apoptosis-inducing ligand (TRAIL) as the therapeutic agent. This nanosystem exhibited good BBB penetration, and a favorable biodistribution and pharmacodynamic profile [126].

Elsewhere, cationic phosphorus dendrimers were used to deliver plasmid DNA encoding enhanced green fluorescent protein (GFP). Of note, this nanosystem did not show systemic toxicity after intratumoral injection of the formulation, suggesting that dendriplexes such as these could be good candidates for gene therapy [127]. Another study showed that compared to PAMAM dendrimers, polyethyleneimine (PEI) dendrimers transferred DNA to the airways in BALB/c mouse models more efficiently [128]. Similarly, Mekuria et al. used PAMAM dendrimers to create nanoclusters able to transfer DNA encoding GFP and p53. These authors proved that these dendriplexes were non-toxic to animals and also showed a high gene transfer rate [129]. In other work, poly(ether imine) (PETIM) dendrimers were also used to transport genetic material to enhance the immunogenicity and efficacy of a plasmid-based rabies vaccine in Swiss albino mice. The nanoformulations evaluated produced an earlier onset of a high-titer protective antibody response to rabies virus, thereby suggesting that PETIM dendriplexes were effective carriers for gene-based vaccines [130]. Moreover, Sheikh et al. utilized a polylysine-modified PEI (PEI-PLL) dendrimer to transport the vascular endothelial growth factor (VEGF) gene in a rat model of Parkinson disease where it prevented apoptosis and microglial activation [131].

Table 3. In vivo studies of dendrimers as carriers of genetic material. Transported active drugs are indicated in an italic font.

Dendrimer	Modification/ *Active Drug*	Outcome	Ref.
Phosphorus dendrimer	pyrrolidine ammonium	• lack of systemic toxicity	[127]
Janus dendrimers	*mRNA*	• higher transfection efficiency than the positive control • organ specificity	[132]
	siRNA	• ability to deliver Hsp27 siRNA to a castration-resistant prostate cancer mode • gene silencing and potent anticancer activity	[133]
	mRNA	• protonated ionizable amines play role in c hanging delivery from the lung to the spleen and/or liver • replacing the interconnecting ester with the amide changed the delivery back to the lung	[134]
	mRNA	• targeting the spleen, liver, and lymph nodes • simplest synthetic vectors and the first system delivering equally to multiple organs	[135]
PAMAM	polyamidoamine	• increased transfection in the lung • more flexible structure after complexes activation	[136]
	fractured polyamidoamine	• lower gene delivery efficiency in comparison with PEI dendrimers	[128]
	lipids	• increased GFP expression • improved serum biochemistry and hematological profile • no tissue necrosis	[137]

Table 3. *Cont.*

Dendrimer	Modification/ *Active Drug*	Outcome	Ref.
PAMAM	alkyl-carboxylate chain, PEG, and cholesteryl chloroformate	• non-toxic, safe vector • inhibition of tumor growth • efficient gene delivery in TRAIL therapy	[138]
	4,4′-dithiodibutryic acid (DA)	• lack of systemic toxicity • efficient delivery of pDNA-p53 • efficient cell cycle arrest at the G1 phase with upregulated p53 and p21 mRNA and protein expressions	[130]
	triethanolamine core	• efficient delivery of siRNA • gene silencing of Hsp27 • significant anticancer activity in the prostate cancer	[139]
	hydroxyl-terminated	• protecting of payload from degradation • effective delivery of siRNA to the cells • knockdown of GFP expression	[140]
	plasmid DNA	• increased immunogenicity in comparison with the plasmid vector	[141]
Carbosilane dendrimer	*siRNA* *FITC*	• detection of dendriplexes inside the brain • efficient transport of siRNA into the brain	[142]
Phospholipid peptide dendrimers	-	• more efficient intracellular uptake and endosome release • better siRNA releasing ability • more potent gene silencing and anticancer effects	[143]
Poly(ether imine)	*plasmid vaccine*	• providing 100% protection against virus infection	[130]
PPI	*plasmid DNA*	• induction of specific immunoglobulins and Th1 response	[144]
Modified dendrimer nanoparticle	*RNA*	• efficient immunization	[145]
PEI-PLL	*VEGF gene*	• prevented apoptosis and microglial activation in Parkinson's disease • beneficial effects of PEI-PLL-mediated VEGF gene delivery in the dopaminergic system	[131]

4.4. Dendrimers as Diagnostic Agents

The number of patient cases requiring diagnostic imaging is steadily increasing. Therefore, it will also be essential to develop specific and efficient methods to speed up diagnosis and enable timelier treatments to begin. The imaging agents currently used in magnetic resonance imaging, (MRI), computed tomography (CT), and scintigraphy are of low specificity, have a short half-life, and some toxicity [146], and so their combination with dendrimers is being explored to help overcome these limitations (Table 4). Indeed, dendrimers can increase the efficacy of imaging by, for example, increasing accumulation of the imaging agent in tumor lesions [51]. Moreover, by functionalizing the surface of nanoparticles, these nanosystems can be leveraged to target the specific proteins expressed in certain cell types [78]. Finally, in addition to improving the properties of imaging agents, dendrimers can act as drugs per se to support treatment [147]. Thus, all these approaches can be used to deliver imaging agents to target cells with more specificity, while also limiting the dose needed and, consequently, the side effects of the currently used imaging agents. For example, in one study, PAMAM dendrimers that target epidermal growth factor receptor-2 were used as a contrast agent for CT and MRI of HER-2-positive breast cancer. These authors showed that the use of this nanosystem significantly enhanced MRI signal intensity by about 20% and doubled the CT resolution and contrast in a mouse model, thereby suggesting that it can efficiently target and image HER-2-positive tumors [78].

PAMAM dendrimer-based gold nanoparticles have also been evaluated as a dual-modality contrast agent for MRI and CT imaging of breast cancer to efficiently provide imaging of a xenograft tumor model [148]. Moreover, a more complex nanosystem comprising PAMAM dendrimer-entrapped gold nanoparticles loaded with gadolinium chelator/Gd(III) complexes for targeted dual-mode MRI and CT imaging of small tumors and carrying a RGD peptide produced good imaging results in tumors overexpressing $\alpha v\beta 3$ integrin [149]. Similarly, the use of amphiphilic Janus dendrimer-based dendrimersomes to transport an MRI contrast agent and prednisolone resulted in anti-tumor activity in an animal model of melanoma [150]. Finally, a multifunctional dendrimer entrapping gold nanoparticles and gadolinium, and also carrying FA to target xenografts was generated using the keratin-forming HeLa tumor cell line. When tested, this nanosystem showed good potential as an imaging agent, suggesting that such systems could be used to design imaging agents for the diagnosis of different cancer types [151].

Table 4. In vivo studies of dendrimers in diagnostics. Transported active drugs are indicated in an italic font.

Dendrimer	Modification/ *Active Drug*	Outcome	Ref.
PAMAM	encapsulated gold nanoparticles, chelated gadolinium, and *anti-human HER-2 antibody*	• enhancing of MRI signal intensity by approx. 20% • improving CT resolution two times	[78]
	thiolated cyclopeptide-based gold nanoparticle *entrapped gold nanoparticles loaded with gadolinium chelator/Gd(III) complexes*	• usability as a dual-mode nanoprobe for targeted CT/MR imaging of different types of $\alpha v\beta 3$ integrin-overexpressing cancer	[149]
	poly(amidoamine)/gold nanoparticles *gadolinium chelate*	• biocompatibility • efficient cellular uptake • usability in dual-mode MR/CT imaging of the xenograft tumor model after intravenous injection of the particles	[148]
	FA-modified *entrapped gold nanoparticles loaded with gadolinium*	• high intensity of radiation suppression • improved MRI contrast • usability in dual mode nanoprobes for targeted CT/MR imaging xenograft tumor model in vivo via the FA receptor-mediated active targeting pathway	[149]
	gadolinium-loaded dendrimer-entrapped gold nanoparticles	• extended blood circulation time • total clearance within 24 h • usability in dual-mode CT/MR imaging of the heart, liver, kidney, and bladder	[152]
	surface-PEGylated Gd-PAMAM dendrimers	• higher relaxivities • stability in the blood • decreased plasma clearance • usability as a carrier for diagnostic or theranostic agents	[153]

Table 4. *Cont.*

Dendrimer	Modification/ *Active Drug*	Outcome	Ref.
PAMAM	N-succinimidyl (S)-acetyl(thiotetraethylene glycol with *Gadolinium*	• possessed a circulation half-life of >1.6 h • significant contrast enhancement in the abdominal aorta and kidneys for as long as 4 h • reduced circulation time as a result of thiol–disulfide exchange, and the degradation products were rapidly excreted via renal filtration	[154]
	Arg-Gly-Asp (RGD)-modified conjugated with *Fe_3O_4 NPs*	• high affinity for C6 cells that overexpress $\alpha_v\beta_3$ receptors in mice • excellent potential for use as contrast agents for targeted T_2 MR imaging of specific tumors.	[155]
Janus dendrimers	*$GdDOTAGA(C18)_2$ and prednisolone phosphate*	• contrast enhancement in the tumor area • good efficiency and displayed anti-tumor activity • usability in theranostic applications	[150]
	$GdDOTAGA(C18)_2$	• improved relaxivity • long-term in vivo retention of the nanoprobe	[156]
poly(propylene imine) dendrimers	densely organized maltose shell (MAL DS) *tetraazacyclododecane tetraacetic acid (DOTA) ligands*	• fast metabolization and total clearance in 48 h • efficient contrast agent for MR imaging aorta, renal artery, kidney, and bladder	[157]
peptide dendrimers	*gadolinium*	• higher signal intensity enhancement • much higher Gd(III) concentration in blood • usability as an MRI probe	[158]
triazine dendrimer	*gadolinium*	• high in vivo r1 relaxivity, desirable pharmacokinetics, and well-defined structure	[159]
folic acid- and gadolinium-labeled dendrimer	FA/graphene oxide *gadolinium*	• long blood circulation time • excellent magnetic resonance angiography (MRA) images with high-resolution vascular structures	[160]
polyester dendrimer	zwitterionized	• minimal long-term Gd^{3+} retention in all organs and tissues • degraded into small fragments • significant capability of enhancing the MRI of metastases in the liver	[161]

5. Future Perspectives

The continuous development of nanotechnology makes it possible to produce increasingly sophisticated and complex dendrimers that have a wide spectrum of applications in medicine. Moreover, chemical modifications of their surfaces can further expand their capabilities as nanocarriers. Additionally, some dendrimers can act as drugs in and of themselves, as indicated in Section 4.1, thereby also contributing to treatment effectivity. Of note, further work will be essential to thoroughly understand the biological properties and actions of dendrimers on living organisms. To date, several in vitro studies in which dendrimers have proven to be excellent carriers have already been published. Unfortunately, not all the results from this initial research could be confirmed in in vivo preclinical phase drug development trials focusing on selecting optimal drugs and dosages, or in pharmacokinetic and pharmacodynamic studies. Thus, to date, there is scarce information about the chemical stability and long-term toxicity of these nanosystems, and standardized methods to evaluate nanoparticles are also scarce.

Therefore, so far, only a few dendrimer-based formulations have reached clinical trials, including safety and pharmacokinetic studies for hydroxyl-polyamidoamine dendrimer-N-actylcysteine conjugates (NCT03500627), hydroxyl-terminated PAMAM (NCT05105607), or as delivery agents for therapeutic compounds to treat COVID disease (NCT05208996), OP-101, a hydroxyl-polyamidoamine dendrimer-N-acetylcysteine conjugate [162], Phase I/II poly-L-lysine dendrimers for advanced non-Hodgkin lymphoma alone (NCT04214093) or in combination with voriconazole (NCT05205161), and poly-L-Lysine conjugated to a complex of 188Rhenium–ligand (nitro-imidazole-methyl-1,2,3-triazol-methyl-di-[2-pycolyl] amine) for inoperable liver tumor resistant to other therapies (NCT03255343). Although some compounds have successfully moved from in vivo studies to clinical trials, to date, only one dendrimer-based formulation has passed clinical trials to reach the market: VivaGel® (SPL7013), a G4 polylysine dendrimer that was approved for the treatment of bacterial vaginosis and protection against HIV [10]. However, the large amount of research data already published on dendrimers indicates that this fascinating family of nanoparticles has wide-ranging potential in the pharmaceutical industry, especially for applications in drug delivery systems. Indeed, the use of cutting-edge technologies has made it possible to develop advanced systems for delivering active agents into living systems. However, further research on dendrimers will still be needed to allow for medicine to reach previously unknown levels of sophistication through nanosystems, thereby making it possible to manage diseases that currently lack effective treatments.

Author Contributions: Conceptualization, K.S. and V.C.; Methodology, K.S. and J.L.R.-G.; Validation, J.L.R.-G. and V.C.; Formal Analysis, V.C.; Resources, V.C.; Writing—Original Draft Preparation, K.S.; Writing—Review and Editing, V.C.; Supervision, V.C.; Project Administration, V.C.; Funding Acquisition, V.C. All authors have read and agreed to the published version of the manuscript.

Funding: This research was funded by MCINN and JCCM, with funding from the European Union NextGenerationEU (PRTR-C17.I1); project PID2020-120134RB-I00 from MINECO/AEI/FEDER/UE (MCIN/AEI/10.13039/501100011033), and University of Castilla-La Mancha project 2022-GRIN-34370 to V.C. K.S. is thankful for the support from the Foundation for Polish Science (FNP).

Institutional Review Board Statement: Not applicable.

Informed Consent Statement: Not applicable.

Data Availability Statement: No new data were generated for this manuscript.

Conflicts of Interest: The authors declare no conflicts of interest.

References

1. Sztandera, K.; Gorzkiewicz, M.; Klajnert-Maculewicz, B. Gold Nanoparticles in Cancer Treatment. *Mol. Pharm.* **2019**, *16*, 1–23. [CrossRef]
2. Aliabadi, H.M.; Lavasanifar, A. Polymeric micelles for drug delivery. *Expert Opin. Drug Deliv.* **2006**, *3*, 139–162. [CrossRef]
3. Sztandera, K.; Gorzkiewicz, M.; Wang, X.; Boye, S.; Appelhans, D.; Klajnert-Maculewicz, B. pH-stable polymersome as nanocarrier for post-loaded rose bengal in photodynamic therapy. *Colloids Surf. B Biointerfaces* **2022**, *217*, 112662. [CrossRef]
4. Mignani, S.; Shi, X.; Ceña, V.; Rodrigues, J.; Tomas, H.; Majoral, J.P. Engineered non-invasive functionalized dendrimer/dendron-entrapped/complexed gold nanoparticles as a novel class of theranostic (radio)pharmaceuticals in cancer therapy. *J. Control. Release.* **2024**, *332*, 346–366. [CrossRef]
5. Percec, V.; Sahoo, D. From Frank-Kasper, Quasicrystals, and Biological Membrane Mimics to Reprogramming In Vivo the Living Factory to Target the Delivery of mRNA with One-Component Amphiphilic Janus Dendrimers. *Biomacromolecules* **2024**, *25*, 1353–1370. [CrossRef]
6. Bozzuto, G.; Molinari, A. Liposomes as nanomedical devices. *Int. J. Nanomed.* **2015**, *10*, 975–999. [CrossRef]
7. Svenson, S.; Tomalia, D.A. Dendrimers in biomedical applications--reflections on the field. *Adv. Drug Deliv. Rev.* **2005**, *57*, 2106–2129. [CrossRef]
8. Tomalia, D.A.; Baker, H.; Dewald, J.; Hall, M.; Kallos, G.; Martin, S.; Roeck, J.; Ryder, J.; Smith, P. A new class of polymers: Starburst-dendritic macromolecules. *Polym. J.* **1985**, *17*, 117–132. [CrossRef]

9. Wang, J.; Li, B.; Qiu, L.; Qiao, X.; Yang, H. Dendrimer-based drug delivery systems: History, challenges, and latest developments. *J. Biol. Eng.* **2022**, *16*, 18. [CrossRef]
10. Fox, L.J.; Richardson, R.M.; Briscoe, W.H. PAMAM dendrimer—Cell membrane interactions. *Adv. Colloid. Interface Sci.* **2018**, *257*, 1–18. [CrossRef]
11. Stenstrom, P.; Manzanares, D.; Zhang, Y.; Cena, V.; Malkoch, M. Evaluation of Amino-Functional Polyester Dendrimers Based on Bis-MPA as Nonviral Vectors for siRNA Delivery. *Molecules* **2018**, *23*, 2028. [CrossRef]
12. Singh, V.; Sahebkar, A.; Kesharwani, P. Poly (propylene imine) dendrimer as an emerging polymeric nanocarrier for anticancer drug and gene delivery. *Eur. Polym. J.* **2021**, *158*, 110683. [CrossRef]
13. Mignani, S.; Shi, X.; Cena, V.; Shcharbin, D.; Bryszewska, M.; Majoral, J.P. In vivo therapeutic applications of phosphorus dendrimers: State of the art. *Drug Discov. Today* **2021**, *26*, 677–689. [CrossRef]
14. Lu, J.; Atochina-Vasserman, E.N.; Maurya, D.S.; Shalihin, M.I.; Zhang, D.; Chenna, S.S.; Adamson, J.; Liu, M.; Ur, H.; Shah, R.; et al. Screening Libraries to Discover Molecular Design Principles for the Targeted Delivery of mRNA with One-Component Ionizable Amphiphilic Janus Dendrimers Derived from Plant Phenolic Acids. *Pharmaceutics* **2023**, *15*, 1572. [CrossRef]
15. Sadler, K.; Tam, J.P. Peptide dendrimers: Applications and synthesis. *Rev. Mol. Biotechnol.* **2002**, *90*, 195–229. [CrossRef]
16. Kwan, C.S.; Leung, K.C.F. Development and advancement of rotaxane dendrimers as switchable macromolecular machines. *Mater. Chem. Front.* **2020**, *4*, 2825–2844. [CrossRef]
17. Sánchez-Nieves, J.; Ortega, P.; Muñoz-Fernández, M.Á.; Gómez, R.; De La Mata, F.J. Synthesis of carbosilane dendrons and dendrimers derived from 1,3,5-trihydroxybenzene. *Tetrahedron* **2010**, *66*, 9203–9213. [CrossRef]
18. Xu, X.; Yuan, H.; Chang, J.; He, B.; Gu, Z. Cooperative Hierarchical Self-Assembly of Peptide Dendrimers and Linear Polypeptides into Nanoarchitectures Mimicking Viral Capsids. *Angew. Chem.* **2012**, *124*, 3184–3187. [CrossRef]
19. Türp, D.; Nguyen, T.T.T.; Baumgarten, M.; Müllen, K. Uniquely versatile: Nano-site defined materials based on polyphenylene dendrimers. *New J. Chem.* **2012**, *36*, 282–298. [CrossRef]
20. Feliu, N.; Walter, M.V.; Montañez, M.I.; Kunzmann, A.; Hult, A.; Nyström, A.; Malkoch, M.; Fadeel, B. Stability and biocompatibility of a library of polyester dendrimers in comparison to polyamidoamine dendrimers. *Biomaterials* **2012**, *33*, 1970–1981. [CrossRef]
21. Simanek, E.E. Two Decades of Triazine Dendrimers. *Molecules* **2021**, *26*, 4774. [CrossRef]
22. Turnbull, W.B.; Stoddart, J.F. Design and synthesis of glycodendrimers. *J. Biotechnol.* **2002**, *90*, 231–255. [CrossRef]
23. Zhang, S.; Sun, H.J.; Hughes, A.D.; Moussodia, R.O.; Bertin, A.; Chen, Y.; Pochan, D.J.; Heiney, P.A.; Klein, M.L.; Percec, V. Self-assembly of amphiphilic Janus dendrimers into uniform onion-like dendrimersomes with predictable size and number of bilayers. *Proc. Natl. Acad. Sci. USA* **2014**, *111*, 9058–9063. [CrossRef]
24. Sahoo, D.; Atochina-Vasserman, E.N.; Maurya, D.S.; Arshad, M.; Chenna, S.S.; Ona, N.; Vasserman, J.A.; Ni, H.; Weissman, D.; Percec, V. The Constitutional Isomerism of One-Component Ionizable Amphiphilic Janus Dendrimers Orchestrates the Total and Targeted Activities of mRNA Delivery. *J. Am. Chem. Soc.* **2024**, *146*, 3627–3634. [CrossRef]
25. Pérez-Ferreiro, M.; Abelairas, A.M.; Criado, A.; Gómez, I.J.; Mosquera, J. Dendrimers: Exploring Their Wide Structural Variety and Applications. *Polymers* **2023**, *15*, 4369. [CrossRef]
26. Tomalia, D.A. Birth of a new macromolecular architecture: Dendrimers as quantized building blocks for nanoscale synthetic polymer chemistry. *Prog. Polym. Sci.* **2005**, *30*, 294–324. [CrossRef]
27. Bosman, A.W.; Janssen, H.M.; Meijer, E.W. About Dendrimers: Structure, Physical Properties, and Applications. *Chem. Rev.* **1999**, *99*, 1665–1688. [CrossRef]
28. Franc, G.; Kakkar, A.K. Diels-alder "click" chemistry in designing dendritic macromolecules. *Chem.—A Eur. J.* **2009**, *15*, 5630–5639. [CrossRef]
29. Shen, Y.; Ma, Y.; Li, Z. Facile synthesis of dendrimers combining aza-Michael addition with thiol-yne click chemistry. *J. Polym. Sci. Part A Polym. Chem.* **2013**, *51*, 708–715. [CrossRef]
30. Ghirardello, M.; Öberg, K.; Staderini, S.; Renaudet, O.; Berthet, N.; Dumy, P.; Hed, Y.; Marra, A.; Malkoch, M.; Dondoni, A. Thiol-ene and thiol-yne-based synthesis of glycodendrimers as nanomolar inhibitors of wheat germ agglutinin. *J. Polym. Sci. Part A Polym. Chem.* **2014**, *52*, 2422–2433. [CrossRef]
31. Hizal, G.; Tunca, U.; Sanyal, A. Discrete macromolecular constructs via the Diels-Alder "click" reaction. *J. Polym. Sci. Part A Polym. Chem.* **2011**, *49*, 4103–4120. [CrossRef]
32. Bober, Z.; Bartusik-Aebisher, D.; Aebisher, D. Application of Dendrimers in Anticancer Diagnostics and Therapy. *Molecules* **2022**, *27*, 3237. [CrossRef]
33. Mintzer, M.A.; Grinstaff, M.W. Biomedical applications of dendrimers: A tutorial. *Chem. Soc. Rev.* **2011**, *40*, 173–190. [CrossRef]
34. Biricova, V.; Laznickova, A. Dendrimers: Analytical characterization and applications. *Bioorganic Chem.* **2009**, *37*, 185–192. [CrossRef] [PubMed]
35. Fréchet, J.M.J. Functional polymers and dendrimers: Reactivity, molecular architecture, and interfacial energy. *Science* **1994**, *263*, 1710–1715. [CrossRef] [PubMed]
36. Trinchi, A.; Muster, T.H. A review of surface functionalized amine terminated dendrimers for application in biological and molecular sensing. *Supramol. Chem.* **2007**, *19*, 431–445. [CrossRef]
37. Fischer, M.; Vogtle, F. Dendrimers: From design to application—A progress report. *Angew. Chem.—Int. Ed.* **1999**, *38*, 884–905. [CrossRef]

38. Gillies, E.R.; Fréchet, J.M.J. Dendrimers and dendritic polymers in drug delivery. *Drug Discov. Today* **2005**, *10*, 35–43. [CrossRef] [PubMed]
39. D'Emanuele, A.; Attwood, D. Dendrimer-drug interactions. *Adv. Drug Deliv. Rev.* **2005**, *57*, 2147–2162. [CrossRef] [PubMed]
40. Kojima, C.; Kono, K.; Maruyama, K.; Takagishi, T. Synthesis of polyamidoamine dendrimers having poly(ethylene glycol) grafts and their ability to encapsulate anticancer drugs. *Bioconjugate Chem.* **2000**, *11*, 910–917. [CrossRef] [PubMed]
41. Leriche, G.; Chisholm, L.; Wagner, A. Cleavable linkers in chemical biology. *Bioorganic Med. Chem.* **2012**, *20*, 571–582. [CrossRef]
42. Sztandera, K.; Marcinkowska, M.; Gorzkiewicz, M.; Janaszewska, A.; Laurent, R.; Zabłocka, M.; Mignani, S.; Majoral, J.P.; Klajnert-Maculewicz, B. In search of a phosphorus dendrimer-based carrier of rose bengal: Tyramine linker limits fluorescent and phototoxic properties of a photosensitizer. *Int. J. Mol. Sci.* **2020**, *21*, 4456. [CrossRef]
43. Moreira, D.A.; Santos, S.D.; Leiro, V.; Pego, A.P. Dendrimers and Derivatives as Multifunctional Nanotherapeutics for Alzheimer's Disease. *Pharmaceutics* **2023**, *15*, 1054. [CrossRef] [PubMed]
44. Kongcharoen, H.; Coester, B.; Yu, F.; Aziz, I.; Poh, W.C.; Tan, M.W.M.; Tonanon, P.; Ciou, J.H.; Chan, B.; Webster, R.D.; et al. Magnetically Directed Co-nanoinitiators for Cross-Linking Adhesives and Enhancing Mechanical Properties. *ACS Appl. Mater. Interfaces* **2021**, *13*, 57851–57863. [CrossRef]
45. Zhou, X.; Xu, X.; Hu, Q.; Wu, Y.; Yu, F.; He, C.; Qian, Y.; Han, Y.; Tang, J.; Hu, H. Novel manganese and polyester dendrimer-based theranostic nanoparticles for MRI and breast cancer therapy. *J. Mater. Chem. B* **2022**, *11*, 648–656. [CrossRef] [PubMed]
46. Pedziwiatr-Werbicka, E.; Serchenya, T.; Shcharbin, D.; Terekhova, M.; Prokhira, E.; Dzmitruk, V.; Shyrochyna, I.; Sviridov, O.; Peña-González, C.E.; Gómez, R.; et al. Dendronization of gold nanoparticles decreases their effect on human alpha-1-microglobulin. *Int. J. Biol. Macromol.* **2018**, *108*, 936–941. [CrossRef] [PubMed]
47. Garoff, H.; Simons, K. Location of the spike glycoproteins in the Semliki Forest virus membrane. *Proc. Natl. Acad. Sci. USA* **1974**, *71*, 3988–3992. [CrossRef]
48. Zhang, P.; Li, Z.; Cao, W.; Tang, J.; Xia, Y.; Peng, L.; Ma, J. A PD-L1 Antibody-Conjugated PAMAM Dendrimer Nanosystem for Simultaneously Inhibiting Glycolysis and Promoting Immune Response in Fighting Breast Cancer. *Adv. Mater.* **2023**, *35*, e2305215. [CrossRef]
49. Gorzkiewicz, M.; Marcinkowska, M.; Studzian, M.; Karwaciak, I.; Pulaski, L.; Klajnert-Maculewicz, B. Mesalazine–PAMAM Nanoparticles for Transporter-Independent Intracellular Drug Delivery: Cellular Uptake and Anti-Inflammatory Activity. *Int. J. Nanomed.* **2023**, *18*, 2109–2126. [CrossRef]
50. Chowdhury, S.; Toth, I.; Stephenson, R.J. Dendrimers in vaccine delivery: Recent progress and advances. *Biomaterials* **2022**, *280*, 121303. [CrossRef]
51. Bertrand, N.; Wu, J.; Xu, X.; Kamaly, N.; Farokhzad, O.C. Cancer nanotechnology: The impact of passive and active targeting in the era of modern cancer biology. *Adv. Drug Deliv. Rev.* **2014**, *66*, 2–25. [CrossRef] [PubMed]
52. McMahon, H.T.; Boucrot, E. Molecular mechanism and physiological functions of clathrin-mediated endocytosis. *Nat. Rev. Mol. Cell Biol.* **2011**, *12*, 517–533. [CrossRef] [PubMed]
53. Manzanares, D.; Cena, V. Endocytosis: The Nanoparticle and Submicron Nanocompounds Gateway into the Cell. *Pharmaceutics* **2020**, *12*, 371. [CrossRef] [PubMed]
54. Goldstein, J.L.; Brown, M.S. The LDL receptor. *Arter. Thromb. Vasc. Biol.* **2009**, *29*, 431–438. [CrossRef]
55. Sigismund, S.; Confalonieri, S.; Ciliberto, A.; Polo, S.; Scita, G.; Di Fiore, P.P. Endocytosis and signaling: Cell logistics shape the eukaryotic cell plan. *Physiol. Rev.* **2012**, *92*, 273–366. [CrossRef] [PubMed]
56. Lakadamyali, M.; Rust, M.J.; Zhuang, X. Ligands for clathrin-mediated endocytosis are differentially sorted into distinct populations of early endosomes. *Cell* **2006**, *124*, 997–1009. [CrossRef] [PubMed]
57. Saheki, Y.; De Camilli, P. Synaptic vesicle endocytosis. *Cold Spring Harb. Perspect. Biol.* **2012**, *4*, a005645. [CrossRef] [PubMed]
58. Pelkmans, L.; Bürli, T.; Zerial, M.; Helenius, A. Caveolin-stabilized membrane domains as multifunctional transport and sorting devices in endocytic membrane traffic. *Cell* **2004**, *118*, 767–780. [CrossRef]
59. Mayor, S.; Parton, R.G.; Donaldson, J.G. Clathrin-independent pathways of endocytosis. *Cold Spring Harb. Perspect. Biol.* **2014**, *6*, a016758. [CrossRef]
60. Di Guglielmo, G.M.; Le Roy, C.; Goodfellow, A.F.; Wrana, J.L. Distinct endocytic pathways regulate TGF-beta receptor signalling and turnover. *Nat. Cell Biol.* **2003**, *5*, 410–421. [CrossRef]
61. Rossetto, O.; Pirazzini, M.; Montecucco, C. Botulinum neurotoxins: Genetic, structural and mechanistic insights. *Nat. Rev. Microbiol.* **2014**, *12*, 535–549. [CrossRef]
62. Commisso, C.; Davidson, S.M.; Soydaner-Azeloglu, R.G.; Parker, S.J.; Kamphorst, J.J.; Hackett, S.; Grabocka, E.; Nofal, M.; Drebin, J.A.; Thompson, C.B.; et al. Macropinocytosis of protein is an amino acid supply route in Ras-transformed cells. *Nature* **2013**, *497*, 633–637. [CrossRef]
63. Mercer, J.; Helenius, A. Gulping rather than sipping: Macropinocytosis as a way of virus entry. *Curr. Opin. Microbiol.* **2012**, *15*, 490–499. [CrossRef] [PubMed]
64. Norbury, C.C.; Chambers, B.J.; Prescott, A.R.; Ljunggren, H.G.; Watts, C. Constitutive macropinocytosis allows TAP-dependent major histocompatibility complex class I presentation of exogenous soluble antigen by bone marrow-derived dendritic cells. *Eur. J. Immunol.* **1997**, *27*, 280–288. [CrossRef]
65. Albertazzi, L.; Serresi, M.; Albanese, A.; Beltram, F. Dendrimer internalization and intracellular trafficking in living cells. *Mol. Pharm.* **2010**, *7*, 680–688. [CrossRef]

66. Perumal, O.P.; Inapagolla, R.; Kannan, S.; Kannan, R.M. The effect of surface functionality on cellular trafficking of dendrimers. *Biomaterials* **2008**, *29*, 3469–3476. [CrossRef] [PubMed]
67. Bastien, E.; Schneider, R.; Hackbarth, S.; Dumas, D.; Jasniewski, J.; Röder, B.; Bezdetnaya, L.; Lassalle, H.P. PAMAM G4.5-chlorin e6 dendrimeric nanoparticles for enhanced photodynamic effects. *Photochem. Photobiol. Sci.* **2015**, *14*, 2203–2212. [CrossRef]
68. Tabasi, H.; Babaei, M.; Abnous, K.; Taghdisi, S.M.; Saljooghi, A.S.; Ramezani, M.; Alibolandi, M. Metal–polymer-coordinated complexes as potential nanovehicles for drug delivery. *J. Nanostruct. Chem.* **2021**, *11*, 501–526. [CrossRef]
69. Oddone, N.; Lecot, N.; Fernández, M.; Rodriguez-Haralambides, A.; Cabral, P.; Cerecetto, H.; Benech, J.C. In vitro and in vivo uptake studies of PAMAM G4.5 dendrimers in breast cancer. *J. Nanobiotechnol.* **2016**, *14*, 45. [CrossRef]
70. Konda, S.D.; Aref, M.; Wang, S.; Brechbiel, M.; Wiener, E.C. Specific targeting of folate-dendrimer MRI contrast agents to the high affinity folate receptor expressed in ovarian tumor xenografts. *Magn. Reson. Mater. Phys. Biol. Med.* **2001**, *12*, 104–113. [CrossRef]
71. Kharwade, R.; Badole, P.; Mahajan, N.; More, S. Toxicity and Surface Modification of Dendrimers: A Critical Review. *Curr. Drug Deliv.* **2022**, *19*, 451–465. [CrossRef] [PubMed]
72. Shcharbin, D.; Janaszewska, A.; Klajnert-Maculewicz, B.; Ziemba, B.; Dzmitruk, V.; Halets, I.; Loznikova, S.; Shcharbina, N.; Milowska, K.; Ionov, M.; et al. How to study dendrimers and dendriplexes III. Biodistribution, pharmacokinetics and toxicity in vivo. *J. Control. Release* **2014**, *181*, 40–52. [CrossRef] [PubMed]
73. Mahdavijalal, M.; Ahmad Panahi, H.; Moniri, E. Synthesis of PAMAM dendrimers anchored to WS2 nano-sheets for controlled delivery of docetaxel: Design, characterization and in vitro drug release. *J. Drug Deliv. Sci. Technol.* **2023**, *79*, 104066. [CrossRef]
74. Sastri, K.T.; Gupta, N.V.; Sharadha, M.; Chakraborty, S.; Kumar, H.; Chand, P.; Balamuralidhara, V.; Gowda, D.V. Nanocarrier facilitated drug delivery to the brain through intranasal route: A promising approach to transcend bio-obstacles and alleviate neurodegenerative conditions. *J. Drug Deliv. Sci. Technol.* **2022**, *75*, 103656. [CrossRef]
75. Benseny-Cases, N.; Álvarez-Marimon, E.; Aso, E.; Carmona, M.; Klementieva, O.; Appelhans, D.; Ferrer, I.; Cladera, J. In situ identification and G4-PPI-His-Mal-dendrimer-induced reduction of early-stage amyloid aggregates in Alzheimer's disease transgenic mice using synchrotron-based infrared imaging. *Sci. Rep.* **2021**, *11*, 18368. [CrossRef]
76. Posadas, I.; Romero-Castillo, L.; El, B.N.; Manzanares, D.; Mignani, S.; Majoral, J.P.; Cena, V. Neutral high-generation phosphorus dendrimers inhibit macrophage-mediated inflammatory response in vitro and in vivo. *Proc. Natl. Acad. Sci. USA* **2017**, *114*, E7660–E7669. [CrossRef]
77. Oliveira, I.M.; Goncalves, C.; Oliveira, E.P.; Simon-Vazquez, R.; da Silva Morais, A.; Gonzalez-Fernandez, A.; Reis, R.L.; Oliveira, J.M. PAMAM dendrimers functionalised with an anti-TNF alpha antibody and chondroitin sulphate for treatment of rheumatoid arthritis. *Mater. Sci. Eng. C Mater. Biol. Appl.* **2021**, *121*, 111845. [CrossRef]
78. Chen, J.S.; Chen, J.; Bhattacharjee, S.; Cao, Z.; Wang, H.; Swanson, S.D.; Zong, H.; Baker, J.R.; Wang, S.H. Functionalized nanoparticles with targeted antibody to enhance imaging of breast cancer in vivo. *J. Nanobiotechnol.* **2020**, *18*, 135. [CrossRef]
79. Soltany, P.; Miralinaghi, M.; Pajoum Shariati, F. Folic acid conjugated poly (Amidoamine) dendrimer grafted magnetic chitosan as a smart drug delivery platform for doxorubicin: In-vitro drug release and cytotoxicity studies. *Int. J. Biol. Macromol.* **2024**, *257*, 127564. [CrossRef]
80. Tan, G.; Li, J.; Liu, D.; Pan, H.; Zhu, R.; Yang, Y.; Pan, W. Amino acids functionalized dendrimers with nucleus accumulation for efficient gene delivery. *Int. J. Pharm.* **2021**, *602*, 120641. [CrossRef]
81. Schito, A.M.; Schito, G.C.; Alfei, S. Synthesis and Antibacterial Activity of Cationic Amino Acid-Conjugated Dendrimers Loaded with a Mixture of Two Triterpenoid Acids. *Polymers* **2021**, *13*, 521. [CrossRef] [PubMed]
82. Jatczak-Pawlik, I.; Gorzkiewicz, M.; Studzian, M.; Zinke, R.; Appelhans, D.; Klajnert-Maculewicz, B.; Pulaski, L. Nanoparticles for Directed Immunomodulation: Mannose-Functionalized Glycodendrimers Induce Interleukin-8 in Myeloid Cell Lines. *Biomacromolecules* **2021**, *22*, 3396–3407. [CrossRef] [PubMed]
83. Sharma, R.; Liaw, K.; Sharma, A.; Jimenez, A.; Chang, M.; Salazar, S.; Amlani, I.; Kannan, S.; Kannan, R.M. Glycosylation of PAMAM dendrimers significantly improves tumor macrophage targeting and specificity in glioblastoma. *J. Control. Release* **2021**, *337*, 179–192. [CrossRef] [PubMed]
84. Wang, X.; Zhang, M.; Li, Y.; Cong, H.; Yu, B.; Shen, Y. Research Status of Dendrimer Micelles in Tumor Therapy for Drug Delivery. *Small* **2023**, *19*, e2304006. [CrossRef] [PubMed]
85. de la Torre, C.; Jativa, P.; Posadas, I.; Manzanares, D.; Blanco, J.L.J.; Mellet, C.O.; Fernandez, J.M.G.; Cena, V. A beta-Cyclodextrin-Based Nanoparticle with Very High Transfection Efficiency Unveils siRNA-Activated TLR3 Responses in Human Prostate Cancer Cells. *Pharmaceutics* **2022**, *14*, 2424. [CrossRef]
86. Caminade, A.M.; Turrin, C.O. Dendrimers for drug delivery. *J. Mater. Chem. B* **2014**, *2*, 4055–4066. [CrossRef]
87. Chen, L.; Cao, L.; Zhan, M.; Li, J.; Wang, D.; Laurent, R.; Mignani, S.; Caminade, A.M.; Majoral, J.P.; Shi, X. Engineered Stable Bioactive per Se Amphiphilic Phosphorus Dendron Nanomicelles as a Highly Efficient Drug Delivery System to Take Down Breast Cancer in Vivo. *Biomacromolecules* **2022**, *23*, 2827–2837. [CrossRef]
88. Huang, S.; Huang, X.; Yan, H. Peptide dendrimers as potentiators of conventional chemotherapy in the treatment of pancreatic cancer in a mouse model. *Eur. J. Pharm. Biopharm.* **2022**, *170*, 121–132. [CrossRef]
89. Wu, S.Y.; Chou, H.Y.; Yuh, C.H.; Mekuria, S.L.; Kao, Y.C.; Tsai, H.C. Radiation-Sensitive Dendrimer-Based Drug Delivery System. *Adv. Sci.* **2018**, *5*, 1700339. [CrossRef]
90. Bhadra, D.; Bhadra, S.; Jain, S.; Jain, N.K. A PEGylated dendritic nanoparticulate carrier of fluorouracil. *Int. J. Pharm.* **2003**, *257*, 111–124. [CrossRef]

91. Gupta, L.; Sharma, A.K.; Gothwal, A.; Khan, M.S.; Khinchi, M.P.; Qayum, A.; Singh, S.K.; Gupta, U. Dendrimer encapsulated and conjugated delivery of berberine: A novel approach mitigating toxicity and improving in vivo pharmacokinetics. *Int. J. Pharm.* **2017**, *528*, 88–99. [CrossRef]
92. Gajbhiye, V.; Jain, N.K. The treatment of Glioblastoma Xenografts by surfactant conjugated dendritic nanoconjugates. *Biomaterials* **2011**, *32*, 6213–6225. [CrossRef]
93. England, R.M.; Hare, J.I.; Barnes, J.; Wilson, J.; Smith, A.; Strittmatter, N.; Kemmitt, P.D.; Waring, M.J.; Barry, S.T.; Alexander, C.; et al. Tumour regression and improved gastrointestinal tolerability from controlled release of SN-38 from novel polyoxazoline-modified dendrimers. *J. Control. Release* **2017**, *247*, 73–85. [CrossRef] [PubMed]
94. Kirkpatrick, G.J.; Plumb, J.A.; Sutcliffe, O.B.; Flint, D.J.; Wheate, N.J. Evaluation of anionic half generation 3.5-6.5 poly(amidoamine) dendrimers as delivery vehicles for the active component of the anticancer drug cisplatin. *J. Inorg. Biochem.* **2011**, *105*, 1115–1122. [CrossRef]
95. Luo, J.; Lin, X.X.; Li, L.L.; Tan, J.Q.; Li, P. β-Cyclodextrin and Oligoarginine Peptide-Based Dendrimer-Entrapped Gold Nanoparticles for Improving Drug Delivery to the Inner Ear. *Front. Bioeng. Biotechnol.* **2022**, *10*, 844177. [CrossRef]
96. Xu, X.; Li, J.; Han, S.; Tao, C.; Fang, L.; Sun, Y.; Zhu, J.; Liang, Z.; Li, F. A novel doxorubicin loaded folic acid conjugated PAMAM modified with borneol, a nature dual-functional product of reducing PAMAM toxicity and boosting BBB penetration. *Eur. J. Pharm. Sci.* **2016**, *88*, 178–190. [CrossRef] [PubMed]
97. Pishavar, E.; Ramezani, M.; Hashemi, M. Co-delivery of doxorubicin and TRAIL plasmid by modified PAMAM dendrimer in colon cancer cells, in vitro and in vivo evaluation. *Drug Dev. Ind. Pharm.* **2019**, *45*, 1931–1939. [CrossRef]
98. Alibolandi, M.; Hoseini, F.; Mohammadi, M.; Ramezani, P.; Einafshar, E.; Taghdisi, S.M.; Ramezani, M.; Abnous, K. Curcumin-entrapped MUC-1 aptamer targeted dendrimer-gold hybrid nanostructure as a theranostic system for colon adenocarcinoma. *Int. J. Pharm.* **2018**, *549*, 67–75. [CrossRef]
99. Li, N.; Guo, C.; Duan, Z.; Yu, L.; Luo, K.; Lu, J.; Gu, Z. A stimuli-responsive Janus peptide dendron-drug conjugate as a safe and nanoscale drug delivery vehicle for breast cancer therapy. *J. Mater. Chem. B* **2016**, *4*, 3760–3769. [CrossRef]
100. Tardi, P.; Johnstone, S.; Harasym, N.; Xie, S.; Harasym, T.; Zisman, N.; Harvie, P.; Bermudes, D.; Mayer, L. In vivo maintenance of synergistic cytarabine:daunorubicin ratios greatly enhances therapeutic efficacy. *Leuk. Res.* **2009**, *33*, 129–139. [CrossRef]
101. Kulhari, H.; Kulhari, D.P.; Prajapati, S.K.; Chauhan, A.S. Pharmacokinetic and pharmacodynamic studies of poly(amidoamine) dendrimer based simvastatin oral formulations for the treatment of hypercholesterolemia. *Mol. Pharm.* **2013**, *10*, 2528–2533. [CrossRef]
102. Hayder, M.; Poupot, M.; Baron, M.; Nigon, D.; Turrin, C.O.; Caminade, A.M.; Majoral, J.P.; Eisenberg, R.A.; Fournié, J.J.; Cantagrel, A.; et al. A phosphorus-based dendrimer targets inflammation and osteoclastogenesis in experimental arthritis. *Sci. Transl. Med.* **2011**, *3*, 81ra35. [CrossRef]
103. Vandamme, T.F.; Brobeck, L. Poly(amidoamine) dendrimers as ophthalmic vehicles for ocular delivery of pilocarpine nitrate and tropicamide. *J. Control. Release* **2005**, *102*, 23–38. [CrossRef]
104. Hayder, M.; Varilh, M.; Turrin, C.O.; Saoudi, A.; Caminade, A.M.; Poupot, R.; Liblau, R.S. Phosphorus-Based Dendrimer ABP Treats Neuroinflammation by Promoting IL-10-Producing CD4+ T Cells. *Biomacromolecules* **2015**, *16*, 3425–3433. [CrossRef]
105. Fruchon, S.; Mouriot, S.; Thiollier, T.; Grandin, C.; Caminade, A.M.; Turrin, C.O.; Contamin, H.; Poupot, R. Repeated intravenous injections in non-human primates demonstrate preclinical safety of an anti-inflammatory phosphorus-based dendrimer. *Nanotoxicology* **2015**, *9*, 433–441. [CrossRef]
106. Spataro, G.; Malecaze, F.; Turrin, C.O.; Soler, V.; Duhayon, C.; Elena, P.P.; Majoral, J.P.; Caminade, A.M. Designing dendrimers for ocular drug delivery. *Eur. J. Med. Chem.* **2010**, *45*, 326–334. [CrossRef] [PubMed]
107. Wang, L.; Shi, C.; Wang, X.; Guo, D.; Duncan, T.M.; Luo, J. Zwitterionic Janus Dendrimer with distinct functional disparity for enhanced protein delivery. *Biomaterials* **2019**, *215*, 119233. [CrossRef]
108. Akhtar, S.; Chandrasekhar, B.; Yousif, M.H.M.; Renno, W.; Benter, I.F.; El-Hashim, A.Z. Chronic administration of nano-sized PAMAM dendrimers in vivo inhibits EGFR-ERK1/2-ROCK signaling pathway and attenuates diabetes-induced vascular remodeling and dysfunction. *Nanomedicine: Nanotechnol. Biol. Med.* **2019**, *18*, 78–89. [CrossRef]
109. Labieniec-Watala, M.; Przygodzki, T.; Sebekova, K.; Watala, C. Can metabolic impairments in experimental diabetes be cured with poly(amido)amine (PAMAM) G4 dendrimers?—In the search for minimizing of the adverse effects of PAMAM administration. *Int. J. Pharm.* **2014**, *464*, 152–167. [CrossRef] [PubMed]
110. Karolczak, K.; Rozalska, S.; Wieczorek, M.; Labieniec-Watala, M.; Watala, C. Poly(amido)amine dendrimers generation 4.0 (PAMAM G4) reduce blood hyperglycaemia and restore impaired blood-brain barrier permeability in streptozotocin diabetes in rats. *Int. J. Pharm.* **2012**, *436*, 508–518. [CrossRef] [PubMed]
111. Jiang, Y.; Zhao, W.; Xu, S.; Wei, J.; Lasaosa, F.L.; He, Y.; Mao, H.; Bolea Bailo, R.M.; Kong, D.; Gu, Z. Bioinspired design of mannose-decorated globular lysine dendrimers promotes diabetic wound healing by orchestrating appropriate macrophage polarization. *Biomaterials* **2022**, *280*, 121323. [CrossRef]
112. Bourne, N.; Stanberry, L.R.; Kern, E.R.; Holan, G.; Matthews, B.; Bernstein, D.I. Dendrimers, a new class of candidate topical microbicides with activity against herpes simplex virus infection. *Antimicrob. Agents Chemother.* **2000**, *44*, 2471–2474. [CrossRef]
113. Landers, J.J.; Cao, Z.; Lee, I.; Piehler, L.T.; Myc, P.P.; Myc, A.; Hamouda, T.; Galecki, A.T.; Baker, J.R. Prevention of influenza pneumonitis by sialic acid-conjugated dendritic polymers. *J. Infect. Dis.* **2002**, *186*, 1222–1230. [CrossRef]

114. Chen, C.Z.; Cooper, S.L. Interactions between dendrimer biocides and bacterial membranes. *Biomaterials* **2002**, *23*, 3359–3368. [CrossRef] [PubMed]
115. Nagahori, N.; Lee, R.T.; Nishimura, S.I.; Pagé, D.; Roy, R.; Lee, Y.C. Inhibition of adhesion of type 1 fimbriated Escherichia coli to highly mannosylated ligands. *ChemBioChem* **2002**, *3*, 836–844. [CrossRef] [PubMed]
116. Bernstein, D.I.; Stanberry, L.R.; Sacks, S.; Ayisi, N.K.; Gong, Y.H.; Ireland, J.; Mumper, R.J.; Holan, G.; Matthews, B.; McCarthy, T.; et al. Evaluations of Unformulated and Formulated Dendrimer-Based Microbicide Candidates in Mouse and Guinea Pig Models of Genital Herpes. *Antimicrob. Agents Chemother.* **2003**, *47*, 3784–3788. [CrossRef] [PubMed]
117. Blattes, E.; Vercellone, A.; Eutamène, H.; Turrin, C.O.; Théodorou, V.; Majoral, J.P.; Caminade, A.M.; Prandi, J.; Nigou, J.; Puzo, G. Mannodendrimers prevent acute lung inflammation by inhibiting neutrophil recruitment. *Proc. Natl. Acad. Sci. USA* **2013**, *110*, 8795–8800. [CrossRef] [PubMed]
118. Sepulveda-Crespo, D.; Serramia, M.J.; Tager, A.M.; Vrbanac, V.; Gomez, R.; De La Mata, F.J.; Jimenez, J.L.; Munoz-Fernandez, M.A. Prevention vaginally of HIV-1 transmission in humanized BLT mice and mode of antiviral action of polyanionic carbosilane dendrimer G2-S16. *Nanomedicine* **2015**, *11*, 1299–1308. [CrossRef]
119. Crooke, S.T.; Witztum, J.L.; Bennett, C.F.; Baker, B.F. RNA-Targeted Therapeutics. *Cell Metab.* **2018**, *27*, 714–739. [CrossRef]
120. Perez-Carrion, M.D.; Posadas, I.; Cena, V. Nanoparticles and siRNA: A new era in therapeutics? *Pharmacol. Res.* **2024**, *201*, 107102. [CrossRef]
121. Ribeil, J.-A.; Hacein-Bey-Abina, S.; Payen, E.; Magnani, A.; Semeraro, M.; Magrin, E.; Caccavelli, L.; Neven, B.; Bourget, P.; El Nemer, W.; et al. Gene Therapy in a Patient with Sickle Cell Disease. *N. Engl. J. Med.* **2017**, *376*, 848–855. [CrossRef]
122. Rosenberg, J.B.; Kaminsky, S.M.; Aubourg, P.; Crystal, R.G.; Sondhi, D. Gene therapy for metachromatic leukodystrophy. *J. Neurosci. Res.* **2016**, *94*, 1169–1179. [CrossRef]
123. Shahryari, A.; Saghaeian Jazi, M.; Mohammadi, S.; Razavi Nikoo, H.; Nazari, Z.; Hosseini, E.S.; Burtscher, I.; Mowla, S.J.; Lickert, H. Development and Clinical Translation of Approved Gene Therapy Products for Genetic Disorders. *Front. Genet.* **2019**, *10*, 868. [CrossRef]
124. Sung, Y.K.; Kim, S.W. Recent advances in the development of gene delivery systems. *Biomater. Res.* **2019**, *23*, 8. [CrossRef]
125. Xu, Q.; Wang, C.H.; Pack, D.W. Polymeric carriers for gene delivery: Chitosan and poly(amidoamine) dendrimers. *Curr. Pharm. Des.* **2010**, *16*, 2350–2368. [CrossRef]
126. Huang, S.; Li, J.; Han, L.; Liu, S.; Ma, H.; Huang, R.; Jiang, C. Dual targeting effect of Angiopep-2-modified, DNA-loaded nanoparticles for glioma. *Biomaterials* **2011**, *32*, 6832–6838. [CrossRef]
127. Chen, L.; Li, J.; Fan, Y.; Qiu, J.; Cao, L.; Laurent, R.; Mignani, S.; Caminade, A.M.; Majoral, J.P.; Shi, X. Revisiting Cationic Phosphorus Dendrimers as a Nonviral Vector for Optimized Gene Delivery Toward Cancer Therapy Applications. *Biomacromolecules* **2020**, *21*, 2502–2511. [CrossRef]
128. Rudolph, C.; Lausier, J.; Naundorf, S.; Müller, R.H.; Rosenecker, J. In vivo gene delivery to the lung using polyethylenimine and fractured polyamidoamine dendrimers. *J. Gene Med.* **2000**, *2*, 269–278. [CrossRef]
129. Mekuria, S.L.; Li, J.; Song, C.; Gao, Y.; Ouyang, Z.; Shen, M.; Shi, X. Facile Formation of PAMAM Dendrimer Nanoclusters for Enhanced Gene Delivery and Cancer Gene Therapy. *ACS Appl. Bio Mater.* **2021**, *4*, 7168–7175. [CrossRef]
130. Ullas, P.T.; Madhusudana, S.N.; Desai, A.; Sagar, B.K.C.; Jayamurugan, G.; Rajesh, Y.B.R.D.; Jayaraman, N. Enhancement of immunogenicity and efficacy of a plasmid DNA rabies vaccine by nanoformulation with a fourth-generation amine-terminated poly(ether imine) dendrimer. *Int. J. Nanomed.* **2014**, *9*, 627–634. [CrossRef]
131. Sheikh, M.A.; Malik, Y.S.; Xing, Z.; Guo, Z.; Tian, H.; Zhu, X.; Chen, X. Polylysine-modified polyethylenimine (PEI-PLL) mediated VEGF gene delivery protects dopaminergic neurons in cell culture and in rat models of Parkinson's Disease (PD). *Acta Biomater.* **2017**, *54*, 58–68. [CrossRef]
132. Zhang, D.; Atochina-Vasserman, E.N.; Maurya, D.S.; Huang, N.; Xiao, Q.; Ona, N.; Liu, M.; Shahnawaz, H.; Ni, H.; Kim, K.; et al. One-Component Multifunctional Sequence-Defined Ionizable Amphiphilic Janus Dendrimer Delivery Systems for mRNA. *J. Am. Chem. Soc.* **2021**, *143*, 12315–12327. [CrossRef]
133. Yu, T.; Liu, X.; Bolcato-Bellemin, A.L.; Wang, Y.; Liu, C.; Erbacher, P.; Qu, F.; Rocchi, P.; Behr, J.P.; Peng, L. An Amphiphilic Dendrimer for Effective Delivery of Small Interfering RNA and Gene Silencing In Vitro and In Vivo. *Angew. Chem.* **2012**, *124*, 8606–8612. [CrossRef]
134. Zhang, D.; Atochina-Vasserman, E.N.; Maurya, D.S.; Liu, M.; Xiao, Q.; Lu, J.; Lauri, G.; Ona, N.; Reagan, E.K.; Ni, H.; et al. Targeted Delivery of mRNA with One-Component Ionizable Amphiphilic Janus Dendrimers. *J. Am. Chem. Soc.* **2021**, *143*, 17975–17982. [CrossRef] [PubMed]
135. Lu, J.; Atochina-Vasserman, E.N.; Maurya, D.S.; Sahoo, D.; Ona, N.; Reagan, E.K.; Ni, H.; Weissman, D.; Percec, V. Targeted and Equally Distributed Delivery of mRNA to Organs with Pentaerythritol-Based One-Component Ionizable Amphiphilic Janus Dendrimers. *J. Am. Chem. Soc.* **2023**, *145*, 18760–18766. [CrossRef] [PubMed]
136. Navarro, G.; Tros de Ilarduya, C. Activated and non-activated PAMAM dendrimers for gene delivery in vitro and in vivo. *Nanomed. Nanotechnol. Biol. Med.* **2009**, *5*, 287–297. [CrossRef]
137. Tariq, I.; Ali, M.Y.; Sohail, M.F.; Amin, M.U.; Ali, S.; Bukhari, N.I.; Raza, A.; Pinnapireddy, S.R.; Schäfer, J.; Bakowsky, U. Lipodendriplexes mediated enhanced gene delivery: A cellular to pre-clinical investigation. *Sci. Rep.* **2020**, *10*, 21446. [CrossRef] [PubMed]

138. Pishavar, E.; Attaranzadeh, A.; Alibolandi, M.; Ramezani, M.; Hashemi, M. Modified PAMAM vehicles for effective TRAIL gene delivery to colon adenocarcinoma: In vitro and in vivo evaluation. *Artif. Cells Nanomed. Biotechnol.* **2018**, *46*, S503–S513. [CrossRef]
139. Liu, X.; Liu, C.; Laurini, E.; Posocco, P.; Pricl, S.; Qu, F.; Rocchi, P.; Peng, L. Efficient delivery of sticky siRNA and potent gene silencing in a prostate cancer model using a generation 5 triethanolamine-core PAMAM dendrimer. *Mol. Pharm.* **2012**, *9*, 470–481. [CrossRef]
140. Liyanage, W.; Wu, T.; Kannan, S.; Kannan, R.M. Dendrimer-siRNA Conjugates for Targeted Intracellular Delivery in Glioblastoma Animal Models. *ACS Appl. Mater. Interfaces* **2022**, *14*, 46290–46303. [CrossRef]
141. Karpenko, L.I.; Apartsin, E.K.; Dudko, S.G.; Starostina, E.V.; Kaplina, O.N.; Antonets, D.V.; Volosnikova, E.A.; Zaitsev, B.N.; Bakulina, A.Y.; Venyaminova, A.G.; et al. Cationic polymers for the delivery of the ebola dna vaccine encoding artificial t-cell immunogen. *Vaccines* **2020**, *8*, 718. [CrossRef] [PubMed]
142. Serramía, M.J.; Álvarez, S.; Fuentes-Paniagua, E.; Clemente, M.I.; Sánchez-Nieves, J.; Gómez, R.; De La Mata, J.; Muñoz-Fernández, M.Á. In vivo delivery of siRNA to the brain by carbosilane dendrimer. *J. Control. Release* **2015**, *200*, 60–70. [CrossRef]
143. Dong, Y.; Chen, Y.; Zhu, D.; Shi, K.; Ma, C.; Zhang, W.; Rocchi, P.; Jiang, L.; Liu, X. Self-assembly of amphiphilic phospholipid peptide dendrimer-based nanovectors for effective delivery of siRNA therapeutics in prostate cancer therapy. *J. Control. Release* **2020**, *322*, 416–425. [CrossRef] [PubMed]
144. Dutta, T.; Garg, M.; Jain, N.K. Poly(propyleneimine) dendrimer and dendrosome mediated genetic immunization against hepatitis B. *Vaccine* **2008**, *26*, 3389–3394. [CrossRef] [PubMed]
145. Chahal, J.S.; Fang, T.; Woodham, A.W.; Khan, O.F.; Ling, J.; Anderson, D.G.; Ploegh, H.L. An RNA nanoparticle Vaccine against Zika virus elicits antibody and CD8+ T cell responses in a mouse model. *Sci. Rep.* **2017**, *7*, 252. [CrossRef]
146. Longmire, M.; Choyke, P.; Kobayashi, H. Dendrimer-Based Contrast Agents for Molecular Imaging. *Curr. Top. Med. Chem.* **2008**, *8*, 1180–1186. [CrossRef] [PubMed]
147. Posadas, I.; Romero-Castillo, L.; Ronca, R.A.; Karpus, A.; Mignani, S.; Majoral, J.P.; Munoz-Fernandez, M.; Cena, V. Engineered Neutral Phosphorous Dendrimers Protect Mouse Cortical Neurons and Brain Organoids from Excitotoxic Death. *Int. J. Mol. Sci.* **2022**, *23*, 4391. [CrossRef] [PubMed]
148. Li, K.; Wen, S.; Larson, A.C.; Shen, M.; Zhang, Z.; Chen, Q.; Shi, X.; Zhang, G. Multifunctional dendrimer-based nanoparticles for in vivo MR/CT dual-modal molecular imaging of breast cancer. *Int. J. Nanomed.* **2013**, *8*, 2589–2600. [CrossRef]
149. Chen, Q.; Wang, H.; Liu, H.; Wen, S.; Peng, C.; Shen, M.; Zhang, G.; Shi, X. Multifunctional Dendrimer-Entrapped Gold Nanoparticles Modified with RGD Peptide for Targeted Computed Tomography/Magnetic Resonance Dual-Modal Imaging of Tumors. *Anal. Chem.* **2015**, *87*, 3949–3956. [CrossRef]
150. Filippi, M.; Catanzaro, V.; Patrucco, D.; Botta, M.; Tei, L.; Terreno, E. First in vivo MRI study on theranostic dendrimersomes. *J. Control. Release* **2017**, *248*, 45–52. [CrossRef]
151. Chen, Q.; Li, K.; Wen, S.; Liu, H.; Peng, C.; Cai, H.; Shen, M.; Zhang, G.; Shi, X. Targeted CT/MR dual mode imaging of tumors using multifunctional dendrimer-entrapped gold nanoparticles. *Biomaterials* **2013**, *34*, 5200–5209. [CrossRef]
152. Wen, S.; Li, K.; Cai, H.; Chen, Q.; Shen, M.; Huang, Y.; Peng, C.; Hou, W.; Zhu, M.; Zhang, G.; et al. Multifunctional dendrimer-entrapped gold nanoparticles for dual mode CT/MR imaging applications. *Biomaterials* **2013**, *34*, 1570–1580. [CrossRef]
153. Kojima, C.; Turkbey, B.; Ogawa, M.; Bernardo, M.; Regino, C.A.S.; Bryant, L.H.; Choyke, P.L.; Kono, K.; Kobayashi, H. Dendrimer-based MRI contrast agents: The effects of PEGylation on relaxivity and pharmacokinetics. *Nanomed. Nanotechnol. Biol. Med.* **2011**, *7*, 1001–1008. [CrossRef]
154. Huang, C.H.; Nwe, K.; Al Zaki, A.; Brechbiel, M.W.; Tsourkas, A. Biodegradable polydisulfide dendrimer nanoclusters as MRI contrast agents. *ACS Nano* **2012**, *6*, 9416–9424. [CrossRef]
155. Yang, J.; Luo, Y.; Xu, Y.; Li, J.; Zhang, Z.; Wang, H.; Shen, M.; Shi, X.; Zhang, G. Conjugation of iron oxide nanoparticles with RGD-modified dendrimers for targeted tumor MR imaging. *ACS Appl. Mater. Interfaces* **2015**, *7*, 5420–5428. [CrossRef]
156. Filippi, M.; Remotti, D.; Botta, M.; Terreno, E.; Tei, L. GdDOTAGA(C18)2: An efficient amphiphilic Gd(III) chelate for the preparation of self-assembled high relaxivity MRI nanoprobes. *Chem. Commun.* **2015**, *51*, 17455–17458. [CrossRef]
157. Xiong, Z.; Wang, Y.; Zhu, J.; He, Y.; Qu, J.; Effenberg, C.; Xia, J.; Appelhans, D.; Shi, X. Gd-Chelated poly(propylene imine) dendrimers with densely organized maltose shells for enhanced MR imaging applications. *Biomater. Sci.* **2016**, *4*, 1622–1629. [CrossRef]
158. Luo, K.; Liu, G.; She, W.; Wang, Q.; Wang, G.; He, B.; Ai, H.; Gong, Q.; Song, B.; Gu, Z. Gadolinium-labeled peptide dendrimers with controlled structures as potential magnetic resonance imaging contrast agents. *Biomaterials* **2011**, *32*, 7951–7960. [CrossRef]
159. Lim, J.; Turkbey, B.; Bernardo, M.; Bryant, L.H.; Garzoni, M.; Pavan, G.M.; Nakajima, T.; Choyke, P.L.; Simanek, E.E.; Kobayashi, H. Gadolinium MRI contrast agents based on triazine dendrimers: Relaxivity and in vivo pharmacokinetics. *Bioconjug. Chem.* **2012**, *23*, 2291–2299. [CrossRef]
160. Zhang, G.; Du, R.; Qian, J.; Zheng, X.; Tian, X.; Cai, D.; He, J.; Wu, Y.; Huang, W.; Wang, Y.; et al. A tailored nanosheet decorated with a metallized dendrimer for angiography and magnetic resonance imaging-guided combined chemotherapy. *Nanoscale* **2018**, *10*, 488–498. [CrossRef]

161. Zhou, X.; Ye, M.; Han, Y.; Tang, J.; Qian, Y.; Hu, H.; Shen, Y. Enhancing MRI of liver metastases with a zwitterionized biodegradable dendritic contrast agent. *Biomater. Sci.* **2017**, *5*, 1588–1595. [CrossRef] [PubMed]
162. Gusdon, A.M.; Faraday, N.; Aita, J.S.; Kumar, S.; Mehta, I.; Choi, H.A.; Cleland, J.L.; Robinson, K.; McCullough, L.D.; Ng, D.K.; et al. Dendrimer nanotherapy for severe COVID-19 attenuates inflammation and neurological injury markers and improves outcomes in a phase2a clinical trial. *Sci. Transl. Med.* **2022**, *14*, eabo2652. [CrossRef] [PubMed]

pharmaceutics

MDPI

Article

Dendritic Glycerol-Cholesterol Amphiphiles as Drug Delivery Systems: A Comparison between Monomeric and Polymeric Structures

Jocelyn Fernanda Romero, Svenja Herziger, Mariam Cherri, Mathias Dimde, Katharina Achazi, Ehsan Mohammadifar * and Rainer Haag *

Institute of Chemistry and Biochemistry, Freie Universität Berlin, Takustr. 3, 14195 Berlin, Germany; fernandarh@zedat.fu-berlin.de (J.F.R.); svenja.herziger@fu-berlin.de (S.H.); mcherri6@zedat.fu-berlin.de (M.C.); matze111@zedat.fu-berlin.de (M.D.); katharina.achazi@fu-berlin.de (K.A.)

* Correspondence: ehsan@zedat.fu-berlin.de (E.M.); haag@chemie.fu-berlin.de (R.H.)

Abstract: The application of micelles as drug delivery systems has gained a great deal of attention as a means to overcome the current several drawbacks present in conventional cancer treatments. In this work, we highlight the comparison of polymeric and monomeric amphiphilic systems with a similar hydrophilic–lipophilic balance (HLB) in terms of their biocompatibility, aggregation behavior in aqueous solution, and potential in solubilizing hydrophobic compounds. The polymeric system consists of non-ionic polymeric amphiphiles synthesized via sequential RAFT polymerization of polyglycerol first-generation [G1] dendron methacrylate and cholesterol methacrylate to obtain poly(G1-polyglycerol dendron methacrylate)-block-poly(cholesterol methacrylate) (pG1MA-b-pCMA). The monomeric system is a polyglycerol second-generation [G2] dendron end-capped to a cholesterol unit. Both amphiphiles form spherical micellar aggregations in aqueous solution, with differences in size and the morphology in which hydrophobic molecules can be encapsulated. The polymeric and monomeric micelles showed a low critical micelle concentration (CMC) of 0.2 and 17 μg/mL, respectively. The results of our cytotoxicity assays showed that the polymeric system has significantly higher cell viability compared to that of the monomeric amphiphiles. The polymeric micelles were implemented as drug delivery systems by encapsulation of the hydrophobic small molecule doxorubicin, achieving a loading capacity of 4%. In summary, the results of this study reveal that using cholesterol as a building block for polymer synthesis is a promising method of preparation for efficient drug delivery systems while improving the cell viability of monomeric cholesterol.

Keywords: polyglycerol dendron; cholesterol; RAFT polymerization; polymeric amphiphiles; drug delivery

1. Introduction

Diverse shapes and architectures have been designed as drug delivery systems (DDSs) as an alternative method for anti-cancer drug delivery, aiming to enhance the biocompatibility and tumor targeting that conventional treatments cannot offer [1–3]. The ability to transport highly hydrophobic drugs has been another challenge, as delivery systems often show critical issues when interacting with cell membranes [4].

The design of polymeric transport systems from versatile synthetic routes has gained a great deal of attention [5,6], leading to varied architectures such as amphiphilic polymers that are able to self-assemble into polymeric micelles, bilayers, or polymersomes [7,8]. The spontaneous formation of those self-assembled structures relies on the hydrophilic–lipophilic balance (HLB) of the chemical structure, and is observed when the concentration in an aqueous solution is above the critical micelle concentration (CMC) [9].

Recently, a synthetic amphiphilic random copolymer bearing cholesterol moieties (12 wt. %) capable of self-assembly into polymersomes was investigated by Martin et al. [10].

The polymersomes resulted in a ten-fold increase in cellular uptake of dextran into HeLa cells compared to free dextran, improving cellular membrane crossing via endocytosis [10]. The hydroxyl group on the cholesterol structure allows for straightforward synthesis of cholesterol derivatives, with different functional groups usually incorporated into the molecules in two different fashions: either as cholesterol end-capped molecules [11,12] or as chain modified polymers bearing cholesteryl moieties [13,14]. These cholesteryl moieties can be implemented as pendant groups thanks to their high compatibility with anticancer drugs and ability to ameliorate the interaction with the cell membrane as hydrophobic domains of a DDS [4,11,13,15].However, a high concentration of cholesterol-bearing structures shows high cell toxicity; therefore, incorporating the cholesterol with an adjusted HLB ratio can improve the cell viability while enabling the cellular uptake [10]. In this context, a well-defined cholesterol-based "monodisperse" amphiphilic system with precise knowledge about the composition and behavior of biological entities is relevant [16, 17]. A great synthetic-route candidate for accomplishing well defined amphiphilic block copolymers is reversible addition–fragmentation chain transfer (RAFT) polymerization [18–21]. The absence of metal catalysts is an attractive feature of this type of polymerization for biomedical purposes [22–24]. In a recent study, a cholesterol end-capped macro-RAFT agent was added to a PNIPAAm backbone to obtain polymeric micelles. The final system did not disrupt red blood cell membranes at concentrations up to 0.25 mg/mL [25].

The prolonged circulation in the blood of micellar systems is mainly a consequence of the physiological behavior of the micelles' hydrophilic outer shell, which plays a principal role in terms of stability, cellular uptake, and in certain cases reticuloendothelial system (RES) uptake [26,27]. Our group has reported several amphiphilic systems containing polyglycerol (PG) dendrons as hydrophilic parts, which is due to the hydrophilicity and biocompatibility provided to the system by their tree-like structure along with the several terminal hydroxyl groups on the periphery [28,29]. Moreover, their simple chemical structure makes them excellent candidates for incorporation as pendant groups [30]. Recently, Trappmann et al. [31] reported the synthesis of nonionic amphiphilic molecules containing different generations of PG dendrons as hydrophilic parts. These molecules are capable of self-assembly into ring-like, fiber-like, and spherical aggregations for possible application as transport carriers. In another study, nonionic amphiphiles composed of polyglycerol [G2] dendron and single alkyl chains were investigated [32]. The noncytotoxic amphiphilic structures showed superior solubilization properties of hydrophobic molecules than standard excipients used in commercially available surfactant formulations [32].

The aim of this study is to investigate two analogous tailored micellar structures containing PG dendrons as the hydrophilic part and cholesterol moieties as the hydrophobic part (Figure 1). The first structure (left) is an AB-type block copolymer amphiphile synthesized via RAFT polymerization containing poly(G1-polyglycerol dendron methacrylate) and poly(cholesterol methacrylate) blocks. The second structure (right) is a monomeric amphiphile containing a G2-polyglycerol dendron end-capped with one cholesterol unit. In this study, we compare these two structures based on their solubility, size, shape, and cytotoxicity properties. As a proof of concept, the capability of the polymeric structure as a drug carrier is presented as well.

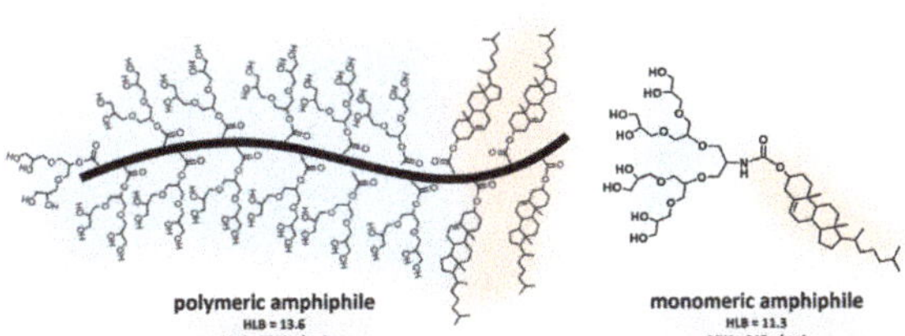

Figure 1. Chemical structure of pG1MAOH-b-pCMA polymeric amphiphiles (**left**) and G2OH-CHOL monomeric amphiphiles (**right**).

2. Materials and Methods

Chemicals, materials, and methods are described in detail in Appendix A.

2.1. Synthesis of Polymeric Amphiphiles

2.1.1. Synthesis of Acetal-Protected G1-Methacrylate Monomer

In a Schlenk flask, G1-OH (5 g, 15.6 mmol) was dissolved in 50 mL DCM. Triethylamine (Et_3N, 10 equiv., 21.8 mL) was added to the mixture and cooled down to 0 °C with an ice bath. Methacryloyl chloride (2 equiv., 3 mL) was added dropwise over 30 min with a syringe pump for 1 h. The reaction occurred overnight, letting it reach room temperature. The crude was extracted with DI water three times, dried over $MgSO_4$, and purified by column chromatography (silica, cyclohexane/EtOAc 65/35 v/v). ^{1}H NMR is shown in Figure S1. Yield: 76%, slightly yellow viscous liquid.

2.1.2. Synthesis of Cholesterol Methacrylate (CMA) Monomer

Cholesterol methacrylate (CMA) was synthesized as reported by Zhou et al. [33]. In a Schlenk flask, cholesterol (5 g) was dissolved in 50 mL THF. In reflux, Et_3N (10 equiv., 17.2 mL) was added to the reaction flask at 80 °C. Methacryloyl chloride (2 equiv., 2.5 mL) was added dropwise over 30 min. The mixture was reacted overnight for 20 h and then cooled to room temperature. The crude was concentrated and dissolved in 100 mL of DCM. Liquid–liquid extraction was performed with 200 mL of DI water, HCl (0.5 M), DI water, saturated $NaHCO_3/H_2O$ (90/10 v/v), DI water, and brine. The organic phase was dried over $MgSO_4$ and purified by flash column chromatography (silica, cyclohexane/DCM 70/30 v/v). ^{1}H NMR is shown in Figure S2. Yield: 90%, white powder.

2.1.3. First Step: Synthesis of pG1MA Homopolymer

In a Schlenk flask, the G1MA monomer (1 g, 2.6 mmol) was dissolved in 8 mL of toluene. The solution was deoxygenated by bubbling nitrogen into the solution over 30 min. DDMAT (78.2 mg, 0.21 mmol) and AIBN (0.167 equiv., 6 mg) were quickly added to the reaction flask while bubbling with argon for at least 30 min. The reaction mixture was placed into an oil bath stirring at 70 °C, stirred for 24 h under an argon atmosphere, and quenched with liquid nitrogen, then 2 mL of acetone was added to the flask and the product was purified by dialysis in acetone (2 days, RC membrane, MWCO 3.5 kDa). The final product was characterized by ^{1}H NMR (Figure S3) and GPC ($M_n \triangleq$ 5.0 kDa, Đ≙ 1.5). Yield: 61%, yellow viscous liquid.

2.1.4. Second Step: Synthesis of pG1MA-b-pCMA Block Copolymer

In this step, pG1MA (600 mg) was used as a macro-RAFT agent after previously drying overnight in a Schlenk flask. Toluene (0.6 mL) was added to the reaction flask, followed by the addition of CMA monomer (6 equiv., 380 mg) and AIBN (0.167 equiv., 0.35 mg). The mixture was stirred and purged for at least 30 min. The reaction flask was placed in an oil bath at 70 °C and degassed for over 30 min more. After 20 h of reaction, the reaction mixture was quenched with liquid nitrogen and purified by dialysis in acetone (2 days, RC membrane, MWCO 3.5 kDa). The final product was characterized by ^{1}H NMR (Figure S4) and GPC ($M_n \triangleq$ 6.9 kDa, Đ≙ 1.4). Yield: 41%, yellowish paste.

2.1.5. Synthesis of pG1MAOH-b-pCMA Polymeric Amphiphiles by Deprotection of Dendritic Polyglycerol Units

pG1MA-b-pCHOL polymer (400 mg) was first dissolved in methanol (4 mL). HCl (37%) was added carefully to make up a final acid concentration of 3.7%. The solution was stirred overnight at room temperature and the mixture was purified by dialysis in water (2 days, RC membrane, MWCO 3.5 kDa). The product was lyophilized. Successful deprotection was confirmed by the absence of acetal-group proton signals in the ^{1}H NMR spectrum in D_2O (Figure S5). Yield: 81%, white powder.

2.2. Synthesis of Monomeric Amphiphiles

2.2.1. Synthesis of Acetal-Protected G2-CHOL

First, cholesterol chloroformate (1.3 g, 2.9 mmol) was dissolved in dry DCM (15 mL). Et_3N (0.46 mL, 3.6 mmol) and acetal-protected G2-NH_2 (500 mg, 0.7 mmol) were subsequently added to the reaction flask (synthesis described in Appendix B). The mixture was stirred for 18 h at room temperature. After concentration, the crude product was purified by column chromatography (NP, DCM/MeOH 90/10 *v*/*v*). The final product was characterized by ^{1}H NMR (Figure S6). Yield: 61%, colorless oily solid.

2.2.2. Synthesis of G2OH-CHOL Monomeric Amphiphiles by Deprotection of Dendritic Polyglycerol Units

Acetal-protected G2-CHOL (500 mg, 0.5 mmol) was dissolved in methanol (15 mL). After Dowex-H (2 eq/wt.) was added, the reaction mixture was stirred for 3 h at 50 °C. The residue was filtered off and the filtrate was concentrated in vacuo. The crude product was purified by HPLC (RP, MeOH/H_2O 15/85 *v*/*v*). Successful deprotection was confirmed by the absence of acetal-group proton signals in the ^{1}H NMR spectrum in D_2O (Figure S7). Yield: 86%, light yellow viscous oil.

2.3. Preparation of Doxorubicin (Free Base)

DOX·HCl (100 mg, 0.172 mmol) was dissolved in 200 mL of water, then Et_3N (1 mL; 7.2 mmol; 42.0 equiv.) was added. The DOX-free base was extracted three times using chloroform (200 mL). The organic phase was dried over Na_2SO_4, the solvent was removed under reduced pressure, and the product was dried overnight under vacuum. The product was obtained in quantitative yield and stored in the freezer. ESI-MS: *m/z*; calculated: 544.2 g/mol.; found: 544.1 g/mol ($[M+H]^+$).

2.4. Micelle Formation and Characterization

A suspension of 5 mg of the respective amphiphiles was prepared in a solution mixture of 0.5 mL of acetone (HPLC grade) and 50 µL of Milli-Q water. The solution was ultrasonicated until no further precipitation was observed. This solution was added dropwise to a vial containing 4.95 mL of Milli-Q water, then acetone was removed under rotary evaporation to obtain micelles with a final concentration of 1 mg/mL. The size and polydispersity index of the micelle solution were recorded by Dynamic Light Scattering (DLS) in low-volume cuvettes at a constant temperature of 37 °C. The ζ-potential was recorded in folded capillary zeta cells at 25 °C. The samples were calibrated for 2 min before each measurement. The critical micelle concentration (CMC) was determined by DLS for pG1MAOH-b-pCMA polymeric micelles and by surface tension for G2OH-CHOL monomeric micelles. DLS studies were performed by observing the derived count rate (in kpcs) at 37 °C for two-folded serial dilutions starting with a concentration of 1 mg/mL of the amphiphiles. The samples were calibrated for 2 min before measurement. Surface tension experiments were recorded in a Dataphysics OCA 20 tensiometer at 25 °C using the pendant drop method. The surface tension of amphiphilic solutions in Milli-Q water was recorded and calculated using the Young–Laplace equation. Samples were vortexed (10 min) and equilibrated 24 h prior to measurement. The surface tension was measured in intervals of 20 s. The experiments were stopped when the surface tension value reached a plateau and did not change for several minutes (in general, after 30–90 min).

2.5. Cryo-Tem Imaging

Perforated carbon film-covered microscopical 200 mesh grids (R1/4 batch of Quantifoil, MicroTools GmbH, Jena, Germany) were cleaned with chloroform and hydrophilized by 60 s glow discharging at 10 mA in a Safematic CCU-010 device (Safematic GmbH, Zizers, Switzerland). Subsequently, 4 µL aliquots of the sample solution were applied to the grids. The samples were vitrified by automatic blotting and plunge freezing with an FEI Vitrobot Mark IV (Thermo Fisher Scientific Inc., Waltham, MA, USA) using liquid ethane as a cryogen. The vitrified specimens were transferred to the autoloader of an FEI TALOS ARCTICA electron microscope (Thermo Fisher Scientific Inc., Waltham, MA, USA). This microscope is equipped with a high-brightness field-emission gun (XFEG) operated at an acceleration voltage of 200 kV. Micrographs were acquired on an FEI Falcon 3 direct electron detector (Thermo Fisher Scientific Inc., Waltham, MA, USA) using a 100 μm objective aperture. Graphical analysis of the images was performed using Image J v1.53k.

2.6. Encapsulation Studies

Doxorubicin (free base) (DOX) drug was encapsulated in the polymeric micelles by the film method, as described by Prasad et al. [34]. First, a stock solution of DOX was prepared in methanol (C = 1 mg/mL) and 3 mL of drug solution was evaporated under a reduced vacuum forming a film at the bottom of the vial. Then, 20 mL of polymeric micelle solution (C = 1 mg/mL) was added to the vial containing the drug film. The mixture was stirred overnight and filtered through Sephadex G-25 to remove the non-encapsulated drug. The polymeric micelles loaded with DOX were measured by UV-vis at 488 nm. The drug-loading content was calculated from the Lambert–Beer law using a calibration curve of free DOX (Figure S8).

2.7. Cytotoxicity Studies

All cell experiments were conducted according to German genetic engineering laws and German biosafety guidelines in the laboratory (safety level 2).

Cell viability was determined using a Cell Counting Kit-8 (CCK-8 Kit, Sigma; Art. 96992) kit according to the manufacturer's instructions. A549 cells were obtained from Leibniz-Institut DSMZ—Deutsche Sammlung von Mikroorganismen und Zellkulturen GmbH and cultured in Dulbecco's Modified Eagle Medium (DMEM high glucose GlutaMAX, Gibco; Art. 10566016) supplemented with 10% (*v*/*v*) Fetal Bovine Serum (FBS), 100 U/mL penicillin, and 100 μg/mL streptomycin. A549 cells were routinely cultivated in a 96-well plate at a density of 5×10^4 cells/mL in 90 μL DMEM medium per well overnight at 37 °C and 5% CO_2 until 70% confluency was reached, then subcultured twice a week.

Serial dilutions of the sample in deionized water were prepared; 10 μL of each sample dilution in serial dilutions, including positive (1% SDS) and negative (DMEM) and solvent (H_2O) controls, were added and incubated for another 24 h at 37 °C and 5% CO_2. For background subtraction, wells containing no cells and only samples were used. After 48 h of incubation, the CCK-8 solution was added (10 μL/well) and the absorbance (450 nm/650 nm) was measured after approximately 3 h incubation of the dye using a Tecan plate reader (SPARK, Tecan Group Ltd., Männedorf, Switzerland). Measurements were performed in technical and biological triplicates. The cell viability was calculated by setting the non-treated control to 100% and the negative control to 0% after subtracting the background signal using Microsoft Excel software v2309. The mean values of all three measurements were plotted and the results were used to determine the half-maximal inhibitory concentration (IC_{50}) using the "log[inhibitor] vs. normalized response (three parameters)" model in GraphPad Prism.

2.8. Cellular Uptake Studies

The cells were propagated as described above. For confocal laser scanning microscopy (CLSM), A549 cells (5×10^4 cells/mL) were seeded in eight-well ibidi slides (ibidi treat) in 270 μL DMEM. After cell attachment for 4–24 h, a post-seeding 30 μL of the compound-containing solution was added for 20 h. Before imaging, the cells were stained with Hoechst 33342 (1 μg/mL), washed with PBS, and covered with fresh cell culture medium (DMEM). Confocal images were taken with a Leica DMI6000CSB SP8 inverted confocal laser scanning microscope (Leica, Wetzlar, Germany) with a 63×/1.4 HC PL APO CS2 oil immersion objective using the manufacturer's provided LAS X software in sequential mode with the following channel settings: Transmission Ch (grey intensity values), excitation laser line 405 nm, detection of transmitted light (photomultiplier); Ch1 (Hoechst 33342): excitation laser line 405 nm, detection range 408–558 nm (hybrid detector); Ch2 (Doxorubicin free base): excitation laser line 561 nm, detection range 564–670 nm (hybrid detector).

3. Results

3.1. Synthesis of Polymeric Amphiphiles

A block copolymer of two methacrylate-based monomers was synthesized by sequential RAFT polymerization, with the expectation of AB-type polymerization of the hydrophobic and hydrophilic blocks. As a building block of the hydrophilic part, the acetal-protected polyglycerol [G1] dendron methacrylate (abbreviated as G1MA monomer) was synthesized via the esterification reaction of the acetal-protected polyglycerol [G1] dendron (G1-OH) and methacryloyl chloride. This dendritic precursor was used in its acetal-protected version to avoid any side reactions or intramolecular transfer of the hydroxyl protons. Deprotection of the acetal groups was performed at the end to achieve the hydrophilic block. As a hydrophobic monomer, cholesterol methacrylate (abbreviated CMA monomer) was synthesized as reported by Zhou et al. [33].

The synthetic route overview of the polymeric structure is depicted in Figure 2A. To synthesize the copolymer, the G1MA monomer was polymerized at the first step using 2-(dodecylthiocarbonothioylthio)-2-methylpropionic acid (abbreviated as DDMAT) as a RAFT agent to obtain the pG1MA homopolymer. The pG1MA was purified by dialysis against acetone and used further as a macro-RAFT agent for the polymerization of the CMA monomer in the presence of a small amount of AIBN, which acted as a co-initiator to obtain the pG1MA-b-pCMAdiblock copolymer. In the end, the acid-catalyzed deprotection of the G1MA block was performed afterward in order to obtain the pG1MAOH-b-pCMA polymeric amphiphiles.

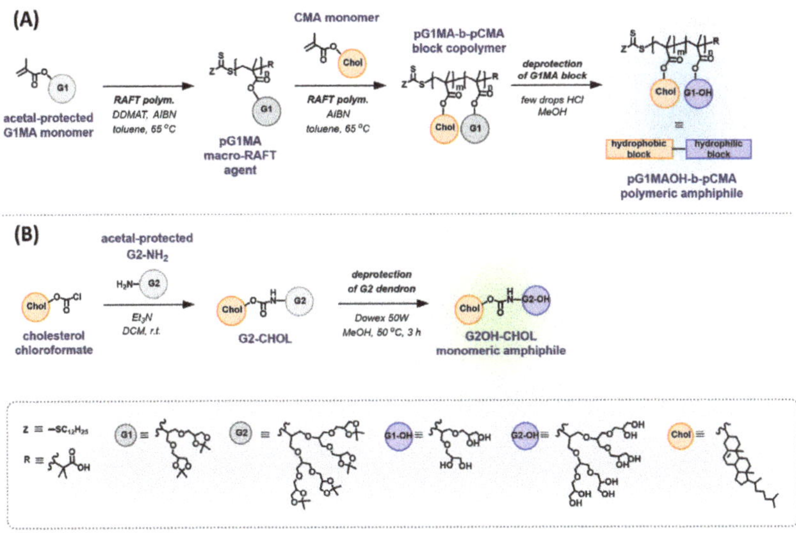

Figure 2. (**A**) Synthetic route of the pG1MA-b-pCMA block copolymer followed by deprotection of the G1MA block to form pG1MAOH-b-pCMA polymeric amphiphiles. (**B**) Synthetic route of the G2-CHOL structure followed by deprotection of the G2 dendron to form G2OH-CHOL monomeric amphiphiles.

The homopolymerization of G1MA was monitored by the signal's shift of the proton adjacent to the ester group from 5.2 ppm to 4.9 ppm in the ^{1}H NMR spectra of the crude product (Figure A2). A high monomer conversion of 94% was observed from the ^{1}H NMR of the crude product, as described in Appendix C. After purification by dialysis, pG1MA homopolymer was characterized by ^{1}H NMR (Figure 3A) and GPC, the latter showing the targeted molecular weight (M_n≅ 5.0 kDa) and the narrow polydispersity index (Đ≅ 1.5) of the produced homopolymer (Figure 3B, yellow line).

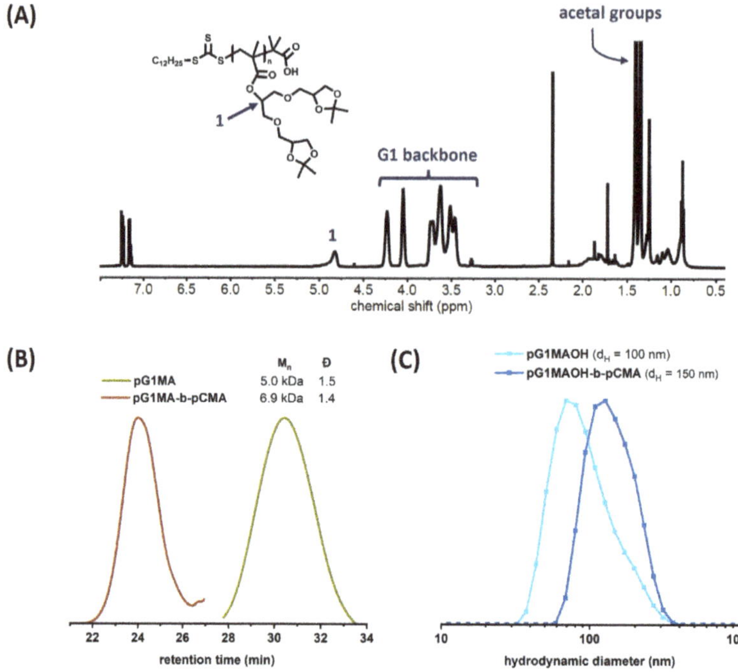

Figure 3. (**A**) ^{1}H NMR of the pG1MA homopolymer. (**B**) GPC chromatograms of pG1MA homopolymer (yellow) and pG1MA-b-pCMA block copolymer (orange), showing an increase in the M_n value from 5.0 to 6.9 kDa. (**C**) Size distributions (% by volume) from DLS for the pG1MAOH-b-pCMA polymeric micelles (dark blue) and pG1MAOH deprotected homopolymer (light blue) in solution.

pG1MA was used as a macro-RAFT agent in the second step for polymerization of the CMA monomer. Polymerization was carried out with a [macro-RAFT]:[CMA]:[AIBN] molar ratio of 1:6:0.167 in toluene at 65 °C for 20 h and quenched by immersing the reaction flask in liquid nitrogen. The copolymer formation was followed by GPC, observing an increase in the molecular weight from 5 kDa to 6.9 kDa (Figure 3B), resulting in an extent of four cholesterol repeating units to the homopolymer backbone.

The protecting acetal groups from the G1MA block present in the copolymer were hydrolyzed to form the hydrophilic block (Figure 2A). The reaction was acid-catalyzed by dissolving the polymer in methanol, followed by slow dropwise addition of the corresponding amount of hydrochloric acid (37%) to the solution. As a control, deprotection of the pG1MA homopolymer was carried out following the same procedure to obtain hydrophilic pG1MAOH homopolymer.

Figure 4 depicts the ^{1}H NMR for the polymeric amphiphiles (above) compared to the ^{1}H NMR spectra of pG1MAOH control (below) in deuterated water. Deprotection was confirmed in both cases based on the disappearance of the acetal-group proton signal at δ = 1.4 ppm. Regarding the polyglycerol [G1] dendron backbone (3.4–4.2 ppm) and the polymer backbone (1–1.5 ppm), both spectra show a similar shape, with a small shift to higher values in the case of the polymeric amphiphiles (see Figure 4 above). Further, in the chemical structure of the polymeric amphiphile (Figure 4 above) it can be noted that the thiocarbonothioyl thio group (marked in the yellow square) is chemically connected to the polycholesterol block. On the contrary, in the pG1MAOH homopolymer structure (Figure 4 below), the sulfur-containing functional group is directly attached to the hydrophilic polyglycerol [G1] dendron block, leading to the small peak observed at 3.3 ppm (the red star). The absence of this peak in the NMR spectra of the polymeric amphiphile suggests successful copolymer formation, in which the peak at 3.3 ppm should not be present.

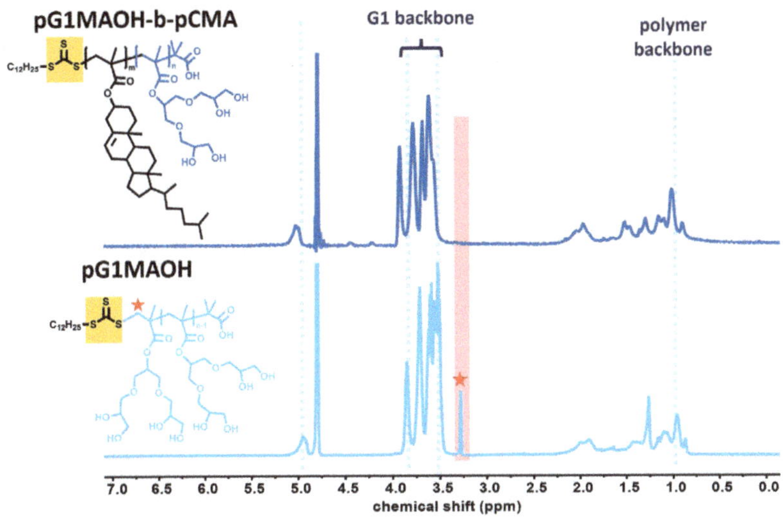

Figure 4. ^{1}H NMR in D_2O of pG1MAOH-b-pcMA polymeric amphiphiles (**above**) and pG1MAOH control (**below**). The yellow square highlights the thiocarbonothioyl thio group connected to the hydrophobic polycholesterol block (**above**) and to the hydrophilic polyglycerol [G1] dendron block (**below**), leading to the small peak (red star) observed at 3.3 ppm for the latter case.

3.2. Synthesis of Monomeric Amphiphiles

The monomeric amphiphiles consist of the hydrophobic steroidal part of one cholesterol unit in combination with one polyglycerol [G2] dendron unit. For synthesis, the precursor acetal-protected polyglycerol G2-NH_2 dendron (abbreviated G2-NH_2) was synthesized as the hydrophilic unit following the previously reported synthetic route [35] in five steps (see Appendix B). After purification, the acetal-protected G2-NH_2 dendron was reacted in a single step with the commercially available cholesteryl chloroformate in a base-mediated substitution reaction. The acetal-protected structure was deprotected following the procedure reported by Wyzogrodska et al. [35] to obtain the G2OH-CHOL monomeric amphiphiles. An overview of the synthetic route is shown in Figure 2B.

3.3. Formation and Characterization of Micelles

The polymeric amphiphiles were subjected to nanoprecipitation in aqueous media to investigate their self-assembly behavior. This behavior occurs when the concentration of the amphiphilic block copolymer exceeds the critical micelle concentration (CMC). Above this concentration, the polymeric structure shows an association due to the desired minimal contact with water forming a stable assembly with low free energy, indicating micellar stability [36]. After nanoprecipitation, it is expected that micelle formation will result from the hydrophobic interactions of the cholesterol blocks forming an inner core, minimizing contact with water molecules, with the outer shell composed of the hydrophilic block of the copolymer. DLS was used to investigate the formation of polymeric micelles at a concentration of 1 mg/mL in water. A monomodal size distribution presented a hydrodynamic diameter of around 150 nm by volume. The ζ-potential (Figure S9) was measured to be −5 mV, corroborating the formation of a non-ionic polymeric micellar system. The CMC of the polymeric micelles was determined by DLS, observing a value of 0.2 μg/mL (Figure S10).

As a control, the pG1MA homopolymer was deprotected following the same procedure to obtain the hydrophilic homopolymer (abbreviated pG1MAOH). The size distribution of the pG1MAOH control aggregates in water was investigated to compare the impact of adding cholesterol units to the polymer structure. DLS results demonstrated a hydrodynamic diameter of around 100 nm for the pG1MAOH control solution in water at 1 mg/mL (Figure 3C). As expected, a small increase in the hydrodynamic diameter was observed in the case of the copolymer amphiphiles when the cholesterol block was included.

On the other hand, monomeric micelles revealed a CMC of 17.0 μg/mL as determined by a surface tension experiment (Figure S11), and presented a monomodal size distribution with a hydrodynamic diameter of around 10 nm (Figure S12). Regarding the hydrophilic–lipophilic balance (HLB) of the systems, monomeric and polymeric amphiphiles showed comparable values of 11.3 and 13.6, respectively, calculated as described in Appendix D. Table 1 summarizes the characterization results of the pG1MAOH-b-pCMA polymeric micelles and the G2OH-CHOL monomeric micelles.

Table 1. Characterization of polymeric and monomeric micelles.

Micelles System	MW (g/mol)	CMC (μg/mL)	$d_H \pm$ SD (nm)	HLB [1]
polymeric	5940	0.2 [2]	145 ± 7	13.6
monomeric	948	17.0 [3]	10 ± 1	11.3

MW: molecular weight. CMC: critical micelle concentration. d_H: hydrodynamic size. SD: standard deviation. HLB: hydrophilic-lipophilic balance. [1] Calculated with Equation (A5). [2] Determined by DLS. [3] Determined by surface tension.

The morphology of the micellar solutions was observed by cryogenic Transmission Electronic Microscopy (cryo-TEM). The images showed the self-assembly of the polymeric micelles into spherical aggregations, as shown in Figure 5A1,A2. The diameters of 100 particles were determined and found to be approximately 80 nm (Figure 5A3), corresponding to the typical values of non-ionic polymeric micelles [7]. In the case of the monomeric micelles, small and well-distributed spherical micelles were identified, as shown in Figure 5B1,B2. Similarly, the diameters of 100 particles were determined and found to be around 6 nm (Figure 5B3), showing similar values to other non-ionic dendritic polyglycerol amphiphilic structures [37]. This indicates that the spherical particles are likely composed of a small number of self-assembled amphiphiles [38].

In both cases, the diameters of the particles observed by cryo-TEM were smaller compared to the DLS measurements. This decrease in size can be explained by the differences between the two methods. DLS measures the hydrodynamic diameter is measured, which means that the particles' hydration shell is considered. On the other hand, the hydration shell is not visualized in cryo-TEM experiments; therefore, smaller diameters were obtained for the micelles.

3.4. Cell Viability

A preliminary assessment of cytotoxicity (Figure 6) was carried out via CCK-8 Kit assays on A549 cells treated with empty polymeric micelles (blue) and monomeric micelles (green). Ten-fold serial dilutions of the samples were prepared in both cases, starting with 1000 μg/mL micellar solution. As revealed by Figure 6, the monomeric micelles show a severe cytotoxic effect, with less than 10% viable cells at 1000 μg/mL and up to 75% viable cells for a concentration of 10 μg/mL, which is considered very low for employment in biological systems and is below the CMC value (17 μg/mL). According to the literature, the toxic effect of excess cellular free cholesterol results mainly from two protective mechanisms against its accumulation, namely, cholesterol esterification and cellular efflux of cholesterol, and may be due to certain cholesterol-derived oxysterols as well [39]. Thus, the toxic effect of the monomeric micelles can be attributed to the fact that the polyglycerol [G2] dendron end-capped with cholesterol molecules can be inserted into cell membranes following a similar mechanism as free cholesterol [40], resulting in low viability of the treated cells. On the other hand, the polymeric micelles reveal 80% cell viability after 48 h even at high concentrations (1000 µg/mL).

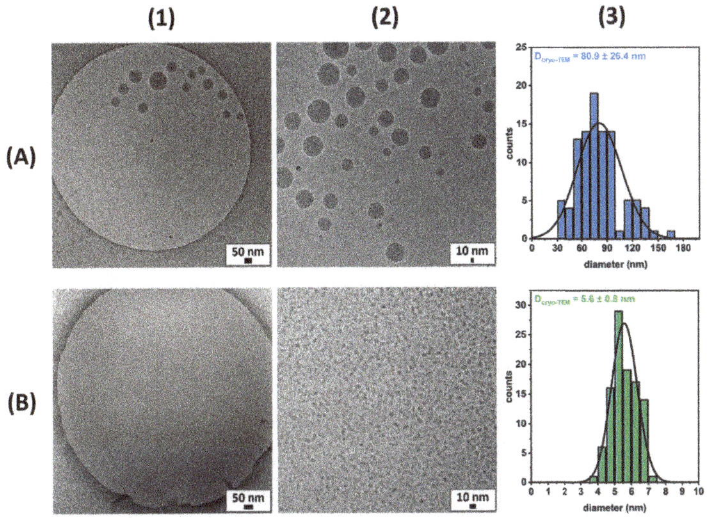

Figure 5. Cryo-TEM micrographs of pG1MAOH-b-pCMA polymeric micelles at (**A1**) 28,000× and (**A2**) 45,000× magnification and G2OH-CHOL monomeric micelles at (**B1**) 58,300× magnification and (**B2**) digital zoom; histograms of 100-micelle size from the analysis of cryo-TEM images of (**A3**) polymeric micelles and (**B3**) monomeric micelles.

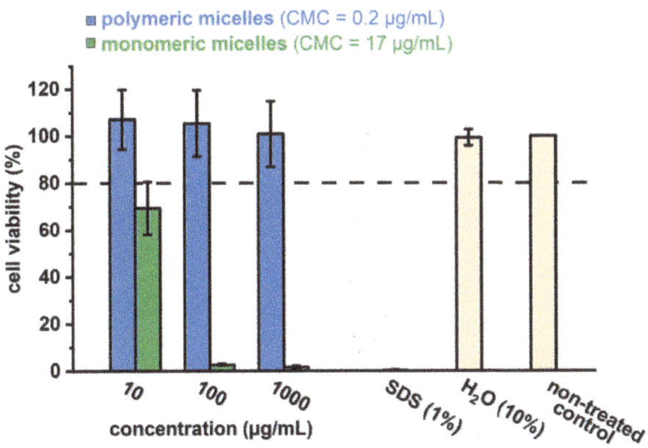

Figure 6. Cell viability of A549 cells treated with polymeric micelles (blue), monomeric micelles (green), and control (light orange). Each bar represents the mean of three independent experiments with the standard deviation.

3.5. Characterization and In Vitro Studies of DOX-Loaded Polymeric Micelles

The good biocompatibility of the polymeric micelles led us to investigate their efficacy as drug carriers by encapsulating DOX (free base) as a drug model. Here, a hydrophobic interaction between the cholesterol block and the drug was expected to be the driving force of drug loading. The micelles were loaded with 20 wt% of the drug and purified before characterization. The loading capacity (LC) and encapsulation efficiency (EE) of the micelles were calculated as stated in Appendix E. The polymeric micellar system showed a loading capacity of 4% and an encapsulation efficiency of 14%. DLS characterization of the DOX-loaded micellar solution revealed a monomodal particle distribution (Figure S13) with a slightly smaller hydrodynamic diameter of loaded micelles (140 nm) compared to empty micelles (around 150 nm). The shrinking behavior of the encapsulated system could be due to the hydrophobic host–drug interaction. Further, cryo-TEM micrographs of the DOX-loaded polymeric micelles were investigated, where a spherical micellar shape was again observed (Figure S14). These results show that there is no significant impact on size and morphology after the encapsulation of doxorubicin in the polymeric micelles. The viability of A549 cells treated with DOX-loaded polymeric micelles was compared to non-loaded polymeric micelles and free DOX (Figure S15) to inspect the possibility of DOX being released from the micelles and promoting cell death. Therefore, the IC_{50} values were determined through plot fitting using a nonlinear regression model (inhibitor) vs. the normalized response, first for the non-loaded and DOX-loaded micelles based on the polymeric micelles concentration (Figure 7A), and then for the DOX-loaded micelles and free DOX based on DOX concentration (Figure 7B). Based on the micelles concentration, the IC_{50} of the empty micelles was 1555.0 µg/mL, in comparison to 264.5 µg/mL for the loaded ones, indicating that the DOX-containing micelles are indeed more toxic than the empty micelles. Based on the free DOX concentration, the DOX-loaded in the micelles had an IC_{50} of 5.3 µg/mL, while the IC_{50} of free DOX was 9.8 µg/mL. This implies that DOX might be effectively encapsulated, solubilized, and sustainably released from the micelles and that the encapsulation does not affect the activity of the drug or its effect on the cells. The IC_{50} values are summarized in Table 2.

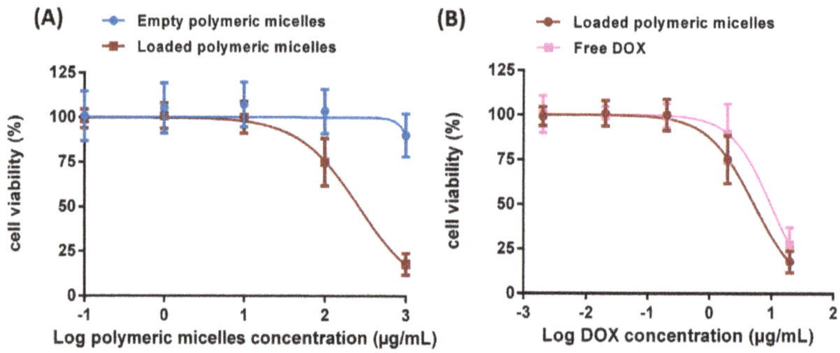

Figure 7. Cell viability of A549 cells after 48 h treatment with (**A**) empty polymeric micelles (blue) and DOX-loaded polymeric micelles (red) based on polymeric micelle concentration, and (**B**) DOX-loaded polymeric micelles (red) and free DOX (pink) based on DOX concentration. Each point represents the mean of three independent experiments with the standard deviation.

Table 2. IC_{50} values based on the polymeric micelles concentration and DOX concentration for A549 cells.

	IC_{50} (µg/mL Polymeric Micelles)	**IC_{50} (µg/mL DOX)**
empty micelles	1555.0	–
DOX-loaded micelles	264.5	5.3
free DOX	–	9.8

Confocal laser scanning microscopy (CLSM) was used to monitor the cellular uptake of living A549 cells after 20 h treatment with the DOX-loaded and empty polymeric micelles as well as the uptake of free DOX after incubation. The red fluorescence observed in the cell nucleus treated with DOX-loaded polymeric micelles (Figure 8A) suggests that free doxorubicin was released from the polymeric micelles, taken up inside the cells, and mainly distributed in the cytoplasm and within the nuclei, as the polymeric micelles are too large (d_H = 145 nm) to enter the nucleus. Additionally, the red fluorescence of cells treated with DOX-loaded polymeric micelles (Figure 8A) is qualitatively more intense than free DOX (Figure 8C) at the same tested concentration of DOX (2%), suggesting enhanced uptake by A459 cells and an improvement in the bioavailability of doxorubicin (free base).

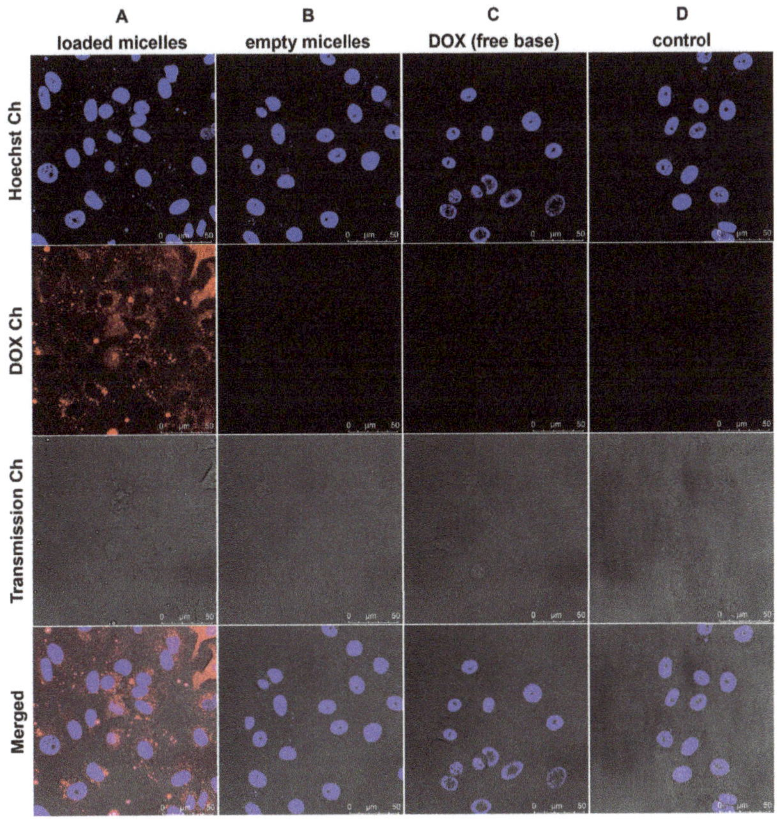

Figure 8. Confocal Laser Scanning Microscopy (CLSM) images of A549 cells treated for 20 h with (**A**) DOX-loaded polymeric micelles (100 µg/mL polymeric micelles + 2% DOX formulation), (**B**) empty polymeric micelles (100 µg/mL), and (**C**) free DOX (2 µg/mL). (**D**) Non-treated cells served as a control. Blue shows Hoechst staining in the nuclei, while red shows DOX. For all images, the scale bar represents 5 µm.

4. Discussion

Herein, we have employed RAFT polymerization to synthesize well-defined non-ionic polymeric amphiphiles composed of polyglycerol dendrons as the hydrophilic block and polycholesterol as the hydrophobic block. The amphiphiles are capable of self-assembly behavior, as confirmed by cryo-TEM images. The micelle diameter was around 80 nm as measured by cryo-TEM, and the hydrodynamic diameter was 150 nm as measured by DLS. In addition, a polyglycerol–cholesterol monomeric structure was synthesized with a similar hydrophilic–lipophilic balance on the part of the polymeric amphiphiles. Their morphology was observed by cryo-TEM, revealing smaller spherical micelles of 6 nm in diameter, while the hydrodynamic size was shown to be 10 nm by DLS measurement. The CMC of both systems was detected in a typical micellar range of 0.1–10 mg/L. As a proof of concept, the polymeric micelles were tested as possible drug carriers, using doxorubicin as a hydrophobic drug model. The obtained loading capacity was 4%, while the morphology and the hydrodynamic size remained similar to those of empty carriers.

The cytotoxicity studies of the polymeric micelles using the A549 cell line suggest good biocompatibility up to relatively high concentrations (1000 μg/mL). In comparison, the monomeric micelles revealed a severe cytotoxic effect at the same concentration, suggesting that monomeric micelles may penetrate the cell membrane by following a mechanism similar to free cholesterol. On the other hand, the presented polymeric micelles combine a low CMC (0.2 μg/mL) and a highly tested biocompatible concentration (1000 μg/mL), suggesting a broad safe window of micellar concentrations for application as a biocompatible drug delivery system. The cellular uptake of the DOX-loaded polymeric micelles was examined via confocal laser scanning microscopy. Our observations indicated that the carriers are taken up efficiently by A549 cells, showing a possible sustained release of doxorubicin, as indicated by the accumulation of DOX in the cell nucleus.

All of these properties, together with the incorporation of cholesterol as pendant groups in the design of a polymeric structure, suggest a promising method of preparation for efficient drug delivery systems while improving the cell toxicity of the monomeric cholesterol structure.

Supplementary Materials: The following supporting information can be downloaded at: https://www.mdpi.com/article/10.3390/pharmaceutics15102452/s1. Figure S1: ^{1}H NMR spectrum of the acetal-protected G1 methacrylate (G1MA) monomer. Figure S2: ^{1}H NMR spectrum of the cholesterol methacrylate (CMA) monomer. Figure S3: ^{1}H NMR spectrum of the pG1MA homopolymer. Figure S4: ^{1}H NMR spectrum of the pG1MA-b-pCMA block copolymer. Figure S5: ^{1}H NMR spectrum of the pG1MAOH-b-pCMA polymeric amphiphiles. Figure S6: ^{1}H NMR spectrum of the acetal-protected G2-CHOL. Figure S7: ^{1}H NMR spectrum of the G2OH-CHOL monomeric amphiphiles. Figure S8: (A) *Uv/vis* measurements at different concentrations of DOX free base and (B) calibration curve obtained at 488 nm. Figure S9: Zeta potential of pG1MAOH-b-pCMA polymeric micelles. Figure S10: CMC determination of pG1MAOH-b-pCMA polymeric micelles. Figure S11: CMC determination of G2OH-CHOL monomeric micelles. Figure S12: Size distributions (% by volume) from DLS for the G2OH-CHOL monomeric micelles. Figure S13: Size distributions (% by volume) from DLS for the DOX@pG1MAOH-b-pCMA. Figure S14: Cryo-TEM micrographs of DOX-loaded polymeric micelles at 28,000× magnification (left) and 45,000× magnification (right). Figure S15: Cell viability of A549 cells treated with polymeric micelles (blue), DOX-loaded polymeric micelles (red), and free DOX (pink). Each bar represents the mean of three independent experiments with standard deviation.

Author Contributions: Conceptualization, methodology, synthesis of polymeric amphiphiles, data interpretation, writing—original draft preparation, visualization: J.F.R. Methodology, synthesis of monomeric amphiphiles, data interpretation: S.H. Conceptualization, methodology, data interpretation, supervision, writing—original draft preparation: M.C. TEM images and data interpretation: M.D. In vitro studies, data interpretation, writing—review and editing: K.A. Conceptualization, data interpretation, supervision, writing—review and editing, project administration: E.M. Conceptualization, guidance, resources, funding acquisition: R.H. All authors have read and agreed to the published version of the manuscript.

Funding: This study was funded by the Deutsche Forschungsgemeinschaft (DFG, German Research Foundation)—Project ID 431232613—SFB 1449.

Institutional Review Board Statement: Not applicable.

Informed Consent Statement: Not applicable.

Data Availability Statement: All data are contained within the article or Supplementary Materials.

Acknowledgments: We would like to acknowledge BCP Core Facility BioSupraMolfor assistance in NMR, IR, ESI-MS, and CLSM characterization; Cathleen Hudziak for GPC measurements; Marleen Selent for HPLC purification of G1-OH; Fabian Nusshardt for ESI-MS of DOX (free base); Christoph Tschucke and Kai Ludwig for cryo-TEM micrographs of monomeric micelles; Elisa Quaas for cell viability and cellular uptake studies; and Taylor Page for English review of the manuscript.

Conflicts of Interest: The authors declare no conflict of interest.

Abbreviations

The following abbreviations are used in this manuscript:

CMC	Critical Micelle Concentration
DDS	Drug Delivery System
DOX	Doxorubicin
EE	Encapsulation Efficiency
LC	Loading Capacity
MW	Molecular Weight
RAFT	Reversible Addition–Fragmentation Chain Transfer

Appendix A. Chemicals, Materials, and Methods

Appendix A.1. Chemicals and Materials

Acetal-protected polyglycerol [G1] dendron (G1-OH) was synthesized as reported by Alpugan et al. [41] and purified by High-Pressure Liquid Chromatography (HPLC). Acetal-protected second-generation polyglycerol dendron-NH_2 (G2-NH_2) was synthesized and purified as described in Appendix B. All commercially available compounds were used as received without further purification. All reactions were carried out with extra-dry over molecular sieve conditions solvents. Solvents for work-up procedures and column chromatography (i.e., DCM, acetone, chloroform, hexane, EtOAc) were of analytical grade. Millipore water (Milli-Q) was obtained from a Merck Millipore Milli-Q Integral System. All polymers were purified by dialysis using pretreated regenerated cellulose (RC) tubing (MWCO 3.5 kDa) Spectra/Por 7® dialysis membranes.

Appendix A.2. Methods

Nuclear Magnetic Resonance (NMR) spectra were recorded on either a Bruker AVANCE III 500 (Bruker Corporation, Billerica, MA, USA), a Jeol ECP 500 (JEOL GmbH, Freising, Germany), or a Bruker AVANCE III 700 (Bruker Corporation). Chemical shifts are reported in δ (ppm) and referenced to the respective deuterated solvents.

The Gel Permeation Chromatography (GPC) system was equipped with a Shimadzu Prominenze-i LC-2030 model, a model Shimadzu RID-20A refractive index detector (Nakagyo-ku, Kyōto, Japan), and a three-column set of PPS PolarSil analytical columns (5 µm particle size, 1000 Å, 300 Å, and 100 Å 8×300 mm columns). Calibration of the column system was carried out using monodispersed linear polystyrene standards. The system was equilibrated at 40 °C using a mixture of DMF, LiBr (0.3 wt%), and AcOH (0.6 wt%) as both polymer solvent and eluent. The flow rate was set to 1 mL/min. The polymer solutions were prepared at a known concentration (5–8 mg/mL) and an injection volume of 100 µL was used. The solutions were allowed to swell for at least 30 min before filtration with 0.2 µm RC syringe filters.

Dynamic Light Scattering (DLS) characterization was performed using a Malvern Zetasizer Ultra (Malvern Instruments Limited, Malvern, UK) equipped with a 10 mW He-Ne laser operating at a wavelength of 632.8 nm. The scattered light was detected using the backscattering setting at an angle of 173° (NIBS, noninvasive backscatter). The measurements were carried out in disposable plastic cuvettes at a constant temperature of 37 °C in triplicates. All samples were calibrated for 2 min before the experiment was performed.

UV-Vis Spectroscopy was recorded with a LAMBDA 365 *Uv*/*vis* Spectrophotometer using disposable plastic cells in a wavelength range of 400–1100 nm.

Appendix B. Synthesis of Acetal-Protected G2-NH$_2$ Precursor

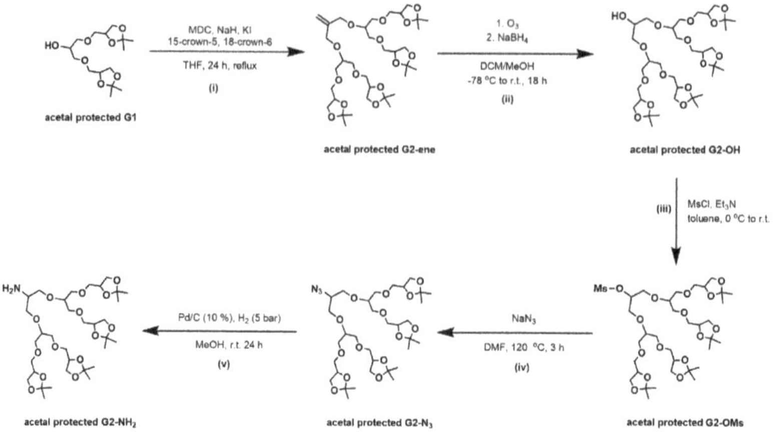

Figure A1. Synthesis of acetal-protected G2-NH$_2$ precursor in five steps: (i) synthesis of acetal-protected G2-ene, (ii) synthesis of acetal-protected G2-OH, (iii) synthesis of acetal-protected G2-OMs, (iv) synthesis of acetal-protected G2-N$_3$, and (v) synthesis of acetal-protected G2-NH$_2$.

(i) Synthesis of acetal-protected G2-ene. Acetal-protected G1-OH (2.0 g, 6.2 mmol) was dissolved in 20 mL dry THF under an argon atmosphere. After the addition of NaH (60% in mineral oil, 620 mg, 15.5 mmol) and catalytic amounts of 15-crown-5, the reaction solution was stirred for 1.5 h at 40 °C. Afterwards, methallyl dichloride (MDC, 310 mg, 2.5 mmol) and catalytic amounts of potassium iodide (KI) and 18-crown-6 were added and the reaction solution was refluxed for 16 h. The reaction was monitored by TLC. After all starting material had been consumed, the reaction solution was cooled to room temperature and quenched with water. The aqueous layer was extracted with DCM and the combined organic layers were washed with brine and dried over Na_2SO_4. The crude product was concentrated and purified by column chromatography (silica, hexane/i-propanol 92/8 v/v). Yield: 74%, light yellow oil. ^{1}H NMR: (CD_3OD, 400 MHz) δ = 5.21–5.17 (m, 2H), 4.28–4.20 (m, 4H) , 4.16 (d, J = 9.2 Hz, 3H), 4.05 (dd, J = 8.1, 6.6 Hz, 5H), 3.78–3.46 (m, 22H), 1.38 (s, 12H), 1.33 (s, 12H) ppm. ^{13}C NMR: (CD_3OD, 101 MHz) δ = 144.77, 114.64, 110.50, 79.90, 78.55, 76.25, 76.15, 73.40, 72.90, 72.56, 72.43, 72.35, 71.66, 71.16, 67.76, 67.59, 49.00, 27.11, 25.69 ppm. IR (ATR) ν: 2985, 2932, 2870, 1654, 1456, 1370, 1253, 1212, 1075, 1050, 974, 974, 916, 841 cm $^{-1}$. MS (ESI): m/z = calculated 715.4 ([M+Na]$^+$) 731.4 ([M+K]$^+$); measured 715.4 ([M+Na]$^+$) 731.4 ([M+K]$^+$).

(ii) Synthesis of acetal-protected G2-OH. Acetal-protected G2-ene (830 mg, 1.1 mmol) was dissolved in dry DCM (8 mL) and dry methanol (8 mL). Ozone was bubbled through the reaction solution at −78 °C. After the reaction mixture turned blue, excess ozone was removed by flushing the solution with oxygen and stirring vigorously. Next, $NaBH_4$ (416 mg, 11 mmol) was added and the reaction solution was stirred for 16 h while warming to room temperature. The reaction solution was quenched with saturated NH_4Cl solution at 0 °C followed by stirring for 1 h. The aqueous layer was extracted with DCM. The combined organic layers were washed with water and dried over Na_2SO_4 before being concentrated in vacuo. Yield: 90%, colorless oil. ^{1}H NMR: (CD_3OD, 400 MHz) δ = 4.29–4.20 (m, 4H) , 4.02–4.08 (m, 4H), 3.87–3.79 (m, 1H), 3.77–3.46 (m, 24H), 1.39 (s, 12H), 1.33 (s, 12H) ppm. ^{13}C NMR: (CD_3OD, 101 MHz) δ = 110.51, 110.45, 79.87, 76.12, 73.42, 72.44, 71.15, 70.88, 67.72, 67.58, 27.11, 25.68 ppm. IR (ATR) ν: 3487, 2985, 2872, 1456, 1370, 1254, 1212, 1050, 974, 841, 734 cm^{-1}. MS (ESI): m/z = calculated 719.4 ([M+Na]$^+$) 735.4 ([M+K]$^+$); measured 719.4 ([M+Na]$^+$) 735.3 ([M+K]$^+$).

(iii) Synthesis of acetal-protected G2-OMs. Acetal-protected G2-OH (600 mg, 0.86 mmol) was dissolved in dry toluene (8 mL) at 0 °C. After the subsequent addition of

Et_3N (0.14 mL, 1.03 mmol) and MsCl (0.073 mL, 0.95 mmol), the reaction was stirred for 18 h while warming to room temperature. The reaction was monitored by TLC. After all starting material had been consumed, the reaction mixture was filtered and the filtrate was concentrated in vacuo. The crude product was used without further purification. Yield: 84%, colorless oil.

(iv) Synthesis of acetal-protected G2-N$_3$. Acetal-protected G2-OMs (491 mg, 0.63 mmol) was dissolved in dry DMF (3 mL) under an argon atmosphere. After NaN_3 (206 mg, 3.1 mmol) was added, the reaction mixture was stirred for 4 h at 120 °C. The reaction mixture was filtered and concentrated in vacuo. The crude product was purified by column chromatography (silica, hexane/EtOAc 1/6 v/v). Yield: 81%, colorless oil. ^{1}H NMR: (CD_3OD, 400 MHz) δ = 4.29–4.21 (m, 4H) , 4.02–4.08 (m, 4H), 3.79–3.50 (m, 27H), 1.39 (s, 12H), 1.33 (s, 12H) ppm. ^{13}C NMR: (CD_3OD, 101 MHz) δ = 110.46, 80.02, 79.83, 76.23, 76.12, 73.42, 72.48, 72.17, 71.18, 67.74, 67.57, 62.25, 27.12, 25.71 ppm. IR (ATR) ν: 2985, 2933, 2872, 2096, 1738, 1456, 1370, 1252, 1212, 1057, 1049, 974, 840 cm^{-1}. MS (ESI): m/z = calculated 744.4 ([M+Na]$^+$) 760.4 ([M+K]$^+$); measured 744.4 ([M+Na]$^+$) 760.4 ([M+K]$^+$).

(v) Synthesis of acetal-protected G2-NH$_2$. Acetal-protected G2-N$_3$ (1.7 g, 2.2 mmol) was dissolved in methanol (50 mL) in a reactor vessel. After cautious addition of 10 wt% Pd/C (400 mg, 0.4 mmol of Pd), the reactor was closed and 5 bar of hydrogen was added. The reaction solution was stirred overnight and monitored by TLC. After all starting material had been consumed, the reaction solution was filtered through a celite pad and a syringe filter (0.45 nM) before being concentrated in vacuo. Yield: 99%, colorless oil. ^{1}H NMR: (DMSO, 400 MHz) δ = 4.19–4.11 (m, 4H) , 4.00-3.94 (m, 4H), 3.64–3.56 (m, 6H), 3.53–3.32 (m, 20H), 1.31 (s, 12H), 1.26 (s, 12H) ppm. ^{13}C NMR: (DMSO, 101 MHz) δ = 108.45, 77.84, 74.40, 74.27, 71.79, 70.73, 66.13, 65.96, 50.66, 48.61, 26.62, 25.40 ppm. IR (ATR) ν: 3384, 2984, 2870, 1680, 1456, 1370, 1253, 1211, 1074, 1050, 974, 841 cm^{-1}. MS (ESI): m/z = calculated 696.4 ([M+Na]$^+$) 718.3 ([M+Na]$^+$) 734.3 ([M+K]$^+$); measured 696.4 ([M+K]$^+$) 718.4 ([M+Na]$^+$) 734.4 ([M+K]$^+$).

Appendix C. Calculation of Monomer Conversion

The monomer conversion of pG1MA homopolymerization was calculated by

$$\mathrm{p} = \frac{\int H_{\mathrm{polymer}}}{\int H_{\mathrm{monomer}} + \int H_{\mathrm{polymer}}}, \tag{A1}$$

where $\int H$ is the integral of the proton adjacent to the ester functional group. In Figure A2, the proton corresponding to the monomer is marked in purple at 5.2 ppm and the proton corresponding to the polymer is marked in yellow at 4.9 ppm.

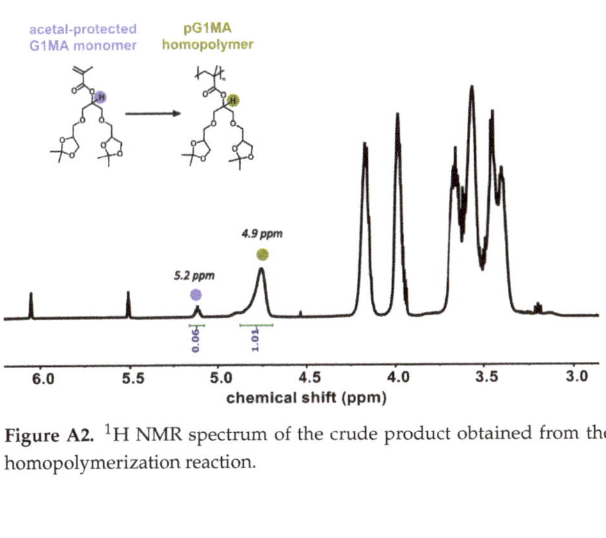

Figure A2. ^{1}H NMR spectrum of the crude product obtained from the acetal-protected pG1MA homopolymerization reaction.

Appendix D. Calculation of the Degree of Polymerization, Molecular Weights, and HLB Values

The molecular weights of the pG1MA homopolymer and pG1MA-b-pCMA copolymer were determined via GPC (Figure 3C).

The degree of polymerization of the hydrophilic part ($X_{n,H}$) was calculated from the GPC results of the pG1MA homopolymer ($M_{n,\,pG1MA}$) as follows:

$$X_{n,H} = \frac{M_{n,\,pG1MA}}{MW_{G1MA}}, \quad \text{(A2)}$$

where MW_{G1MA} is the molecular weight of the G1MA monomer.

The degree of polymerization of the lipophilic part ($X_{n,L}$) was calculated from the difference in the number-average molecular weights of the copolymer and the homopolymer (ΔM_n):

$$X_{n,L} = \frac{\Delta M_n}{MW_{CMA}} = \frac{M_{n,\,pG1MA\text{-}b\text{-}pCMA} - M_{n,\,pG1MA}}{MW_{CMA}}, \quad \text{(A3)}$$

where MW_{CMA} is the molecular weight of the CMA monomer.

The theoretical molecular weight of the pG1MAOH deprotected homopolymer and the pG1MAOH-b-pCMA polymeric amphiphiles were calculated assuming the complete removal of acetal groups in the G1MA backbone using the following equation:

$$M_n = M_{n,\,protected} - 2 \cdot p_H \cdot m_{acetal}, \quad \text{(A4)}$$

where $M_{n,\,protected}$ is the molecular weight before deprotection, p_H is the degree of polymerization of the hydrophilic part, and m_{acetal} is the acetal mass loss when deprotection occurs. The second term refers to the presence of two acetal groups per G1MA repeating unit.

The Hydrophilic–Lipophilic Balance (HLB) of non-ionic amphiphiles can be calculated with Griffin's method [42] using Equation (A5):

$$HLB = 20 \cdot \frac{MW_H}{M_n}, \quad \text{(A5)}$$

where MW_H is the molecular weight of the hydrophilic part in the amphiphilic structure and M_n is the molecular weight of the complete structure.

Table A1. Summary of molecular weights and HLB values.

Compound	M_n (g/mol)	p_H	p_L	MW_H (g/mol)	HLB [1]
pG1MA	5000	12	–	–	–
pG1MA-b-pCMA	6900	12	4	–	–
pG1MAOH-b-pCMA	5940 [2]	12	4	4040	13.6
pG1MAOH	4040 [2]	12	–	4040	–
G2OH-CHOL	948	–	–	536	11.3

MW: molecular weight. p_H: degree of polymerization of the hydrophilic part. p_L: degree of polymerization of the lipophilic part. HLB: hydrophilic–lipophilic balance. [1] Calculated with Equation (A5). [2] Theoretical M_n values calculated with Equation (A4).

Appendix E. Loading Capacity (LC) and Encapsulation Efficiency (EE) Calculation

The loading capacity (LC) and encapsulation efficiency (EE) were respectively calculated using

$$LC(\%) = \frac{m_{\text{encapsulated DOX}}}{m_{\text{amphiphile}}} \cdot 100, \quad \text{(A6)}$$

$$EE(\%) = \frac{m_{\text{encapsulated DOX}}}{m_{\text{initial DOX added}}} \cdot 100. \quad \text{(A7)}$$

References

1. Pucci, C.; Martinelli, C.; Ciofani, G. Innovative approaches for cancer treatment: Current perspectives and new challenges. *Ecancer* **2019**, *13*, 1–26. [CrossRef] [PubMed]
2. Shi, J.; Votruba, A.R.; Farokhzad, O.C.; Langer, R. Nanotechnology in drug delivery and tissue engineering: From discovery to applications. *Nano Lett.* **2010**, *10*, 3223–3230. [CrossRef] [PubMed]
3. Dagogo-Jack, I.; Shaw, A.T. Tumour heterogeneity and resistance to cancer therapies. *Nat. Rev. Clin. Oncol.* **2018**, *15*, 81–94. [CrossRef] [PubMed]
4. Zhang, R.; Qin, X.; Kong, F.; Chen, P.; Pan, G. Improving cellular uptake of therapeutic entities through interaction with components of cell membrane. *Drug Deliv.* **2019**, *26*, 328–342. [CrossRef] [PubMed]
5. Liechty, W.B.; Kryscio, D.R.; Slaughter, B.V.; Peppas, N.A. Polymers for drug delivery systems. *Annu. Rev. Chem. Biomol. Eng.* **2010**, *1*, 149–173. [CrossRef] [PubMed]
6. Kumari, P.; Ghosh, B.; Biswas, S. Nanocarriers for cancer-targeted drug delivery. *J. Drug Target.* **2016**, *24*, 179–191. [CrossRef] [PubMed]
7. Xu, W.; Ling, P.; Zhang, T. Polymeric Micelles, a Promising Drug Delivery System to Enhance Bioavailability of Poorly Water-Soluble Drugs. *J. Drug Deliv.* **2013**, *2013*, 340315 . [CrossRef] [PubMed]
8. Zhang, X.y.; Zhang, P.y. Polymersomes in Nanomedicine—A Review. *Curr. Nanosci.* **2016**, *13*, 124–129. [CrossRef]
9. Nagarajan, R.; Ganesh, K. Block copolymer self-assembly in selective solvents: Spherical micelles with segregated cores. *J. Chem. Phys.* **1989**, *90*, 5843–5856. [CrossRef]
10. Martin, C.; Marino, N.; Curran, C.; McHale, A.P.; Callan, J.F.; Callan, B. Cholesteryl to improve the cellular uptake of polymersomes within HeLa cells. *Int. J. Pharm.* **2016**, *511*, 570–578. [CrossRef]
11. Kumari, P.; Muddineti, O.S.; Rompicharla, S.V.K.; Ghanta, P.; Adithya, K.B.; Ghosh, B.; Biswas, S. Cholesterol-conjugated poly(D, L-lactide)-based micelles as a nanocarrier system for effective delivery of curcumin in cancer therapy. *Drug Deliv.* **2017**, *24*, 209–223. [CrossRef] [PubMed]
12. Song, Y.; Tian, Q.; Huang, Z.; Fan, D.; She, Z.; Liu, X.; Cheng, X.; Yu, B.; Deng, Y. Self-assembled micelles of novel amphiphilic copolymer cholesterol-coupled F68 containing cabazitaxel as a drug delivery system. *Int. J. Nanomed.* **2014**, *9*, 2307–2317. [CrossRef]
13. Lee, A.L.; Venkataraman, S.; Sirat, S.B.; Gao, S.; Hedrick, J.L.; Yang, Y.Y. The use of cholesterol-containing biodegradable block copolymers to exploit hydrophobic interactions for the delivery of anticancer drugs. *Biomaterials* **2012**, *33*, 1921–1928. [CrossRef]
14. Misiak, P.; Markiewicz, K.H.; Szymczuk, D.; Wilczewska, A.Z. Polymeric drug delivery systems bearing cholesterol moieties: A review. *Polymers* **2020**, *12*, 2620. [CrossRef] [PubMed]
15. Tran, T.H.; Nguyen, C.T.; Gonzalez-Fajardo, L.; Hargrove, D.; Song, D.; Deshmukh, P.; Mahajan, L.; Ndaya, D.; Lai, L.; Kasi, R.M.; et al. Long Circulating Self-Assembled Nanoparticles from Cholesterol-Containing Brush-Like Block Copolymers for Improved Drug Delivery to Tumors. *Biomacromolecules* **2014**, *15*, 4363–4375. [CrossRef] [PubMed]
16. Thunemann, A.F.; Gruber, A.; Klinger, D. Amphiphilic Nanogels: Fuzzy Spheres with a Pseudo-Periodic Internal Structure. *Langmuir* **2020**, *36*, 10979–10988. [CrossRef] [PubMed]
17. Wan, Q.; Huang, B.; Li, T.; Xiao, Y.; He, Y.; Du, W.; Wang, B.Z.; Dakin, G.F.; Rosenbaum, M.; Goncalves, M.D.; et al. Selective targeting of visceral adiposity by polycation nanomedicine. *Nat. Nanotechnol.* **2022**, *17*, 1311–1321. [CrossRef] [PubMed]
18. Perrier, S. 50th Anniversary Perspective: RAFT Polymerization—A User Guide. *Macromolecules* **2017**, *50*, 7433–7447. [CrossRef]
19. He, S.J.; Zhang, Y.; Cui, Z.H.; Tao, Y.Z.; Zhang, B.L. Controlled radical polymerization of cholesteryl acrylate and its block copolymer with styrene via the RAFT process. *Eur. Polym. J.* **2009**, *45*, 2395–2401. [CrossRef]
20. Keddie, D.J. A guide to the synthesis of block copolymers using reversible-addition fragmentation chain transfer (RAFT) polymerization. *Chem. Soc. Rev.* **2014**, *43*, 496–505. [CrossRef] [PubMed]
21. Magami, S.M.; Abdulganiyyu, U. Raft approach to the copolymerisation of methyl methacrylate based polymeric micelles. *Bayero J. Pure Appl. Sci.* **2017**, *10*, 197. [CrossRef]
22. Semsarilar, M.; Perrier, S. 'Green' reversible addition-fragmentation chain-transfer (RAFT) polymerization. *Nat. Chem.* **2010**, *2*, 811–820. [CrossRef] [PubMed]
23. Boyer, C.; Bulmus, V.; Davis, T.P.; Ladmiral, V.; Liu, J.; Perrier, S. Bioapplications of RAFT polymerization. *Chem. Rev.* **2009**, *109*, 5402–5436. [CrossRef] [PubMed]
24. Moad, G.; Rizzardo, E.; Thang, S.H. Living radical polymerization by the RAFT process—A second update. *Aust. J. Chem.* **2009**, *62*, 1402–1472. [CrossRef]
25. Misiak, P.; Niemirowicz- Laskowska, K.; Markiewicz, K.H.; Misztalewska-Turkowicz, I.; Wielgat, P.; Kurowska, I.; Siemiaszko, G.; Destarac, M.; Car, H.; Wilczewska, A.Z. Evaluation of cytotoxic effect of cholesterol end-capped poly(N-isopropylacrylamide)s on selected normal and neoplastic cells. *Int. J. Nanomed.* **2020**, *15*, 7263–7278. [CrossRef] [PubMed]
26. Adams, M.L.; Lavasanifar, A.; Kwon, G.S. Amphiphilic block copolymers for drug delivery. *J. Pharm. Sci.* **2003**, *92*, 1343–1355. [CrossRef]
27. Yoncheva, K.; Calleja, P.; Agüeros, M.; Petrov, P.; Miladinova, I.; Tsvetanov, C.; Irache, J.M. Stabilized micelles as delivery vehicles for paclitaxel. *Int. J. Pharm.* **2012**, *436*, 258–264. [CrossRef] [PubMed]
28. Prasad, S.; Achazi, K.; Böttcher, C.; Haag, R.; Sharma, S.K. Fabrication of nanostructures through self-assembly of non-ionic amphiphiles for biomedical applications. *RSC Adv.* **2017**, *7*, 22121–22132. [CrossRef]

29. Rodrigo, A.C.; Malhotra, S.; Böttcher, C.; Adeli, M.; Haag, R. Dendritic polyglycerol cyclodextrin amphiphiles and their self-assembled architectures to transport hydrophobic guest molecules. *RSC Adv.* **2014**, *4*, 61656–61659. [CrossRef]
30. Haag, R.; Kratz, F. Polymer therapeutics: Concepts and applications. *Angew. Chem.-Int. Ed.* **2006**, *45*, 1198–1215. [CrossRef]
31. Trappmann, B.; Ludwig, K.; Radowski, M.R.; Shukla, A.; Mohr, A.; Rehage, H.; Böttcher, C.; Haag, R. A new family of nonionic dendritic amphiphiles displaying unexpected packing parameters in micellar assemblies. *J. Am. Chem. Soc.* **2010**, *132*, 11119–11124. [CrossRef]
32. Richter, A.; Wiedekind, A.; Krause, M.; Kissel, T.; Haag, R.; Olbrich, C. Non-ionic dendritic glycerol-based amphiphiles: Novel excipients for the solubilization of poorly water-soluble anticancer drug Sagopilone. *Eur. J. Pharm. Sci.* **2010**, *40*, 48–55. [CrossRef] [PubMed]
33. Zhou, Y.; Kasi, R.M. Synthesis and Characterization of Polycholesteryl Methacrylate–Polyhydroxyethyl Methyacrylate Block Copolymers. *J. Polym. Sci. Part A Polym. Chem.* **2008**, *46*, 6801–6809. [CrossRef]
34. Prasad, S.; Achazi, K.; Schade, B.; Haag, R.; Sharma, S.K. Nonionic Dendritic and Carbohydrate Based Amphiphiles: Self-Assembly and Transport Behavior. *Macromol. Biosci.* **2018**, *18*, 1800019. [CrossRef] [PubMed]
35. Wyszogrodzka, M.; Haag, R. A convergent approach to biocompatible polyglycerol "click" dendrons for the synthesis of modular core-shell architectures and their transport behavior. *Chem.-Eur. J.* **2008**, *14*, 9202–9214. [CrossRef]
36. Patravale, V.B.; Upadhaya, P.G.; Jain, R.D. *Preparation and Characterization of Micelles*; Humana Press Inc.: Totowa, NJ, USA, 2019; Volume 2000, pp. 19–29. [CrossRef]
37. Rashmi.; Singh, A.K.; Achazi, K.; Schade, B.; Böttcher, C.; Haag, R.; Sharma, S.K. Synthesis of non-ionic bolaamphiphiles and study of their self-assembly and transport behaviour for drug delivery applications. *RSC Adv.* **2018**, *8*, 31777–31782. [CrossRef] [PubMed]
38. Tschiche, A.; Staedtler, A.M.; Malhotra, S.; Bauer, H.; Böttcher, C.; Sharbati, S.; Calderón, M.; Koch, M.; Zollner, T.M.; Barnard, A.; et al. Polyglycerol-based amphiphilic dendrons as potential siRNA carriers for in vivo applications. *J. Mater. Chem. B* **2014**, *2*, 2153–2167. [CrossRef]
39. Tabas, I. Consequences of cellular cholesterol accumulation: Basic concepts and physiological implications. *J. Clin. Investig.* **2002**, *110*, 905–911. [CrossRef]
40. Krause, M.R.; Regen, S.L. The Structural Role of Cholesterol in Cell Membranes: From Condensed Bilayers to Lipid Rafts. *Accounts Chem. Res.* **2014**, *47*, 3512–3521. [CrossRef] [PubMed]
41. Alpugan, S.; Garcia, G.; Poyer, F.; Durmuş, M.; Maillard, P.; Ahsen, V.; Dumoulin, F. Dendrimeric-like hexadecahydroxylated zinc phthalocyanine. *J. Porphyrins Phthalocyanines* **2013**, *17*, 596–603. [CrossRef]
42. Griffin, W.C. Calculation of HLB values of non-ionic surfactants. *J. Soc. Cosmet. Chem.* **1954**, *5*, 249–256.

pharmaceutics

MDPI

Article

Systemic Dendrimer-Peptide Therapies for Wet Age-Related Macular Degeneration

Tony Wu, Chang Liu and Rangaramanujam M. Kannan *

Center for Nanomedicine, Wilmer Eye Institute, Johns Hopkins University School of Medicine, Baltimore, MD 21287, USA; twu29@jhu.edu (T.W.); cliu188@jhu.edu (C.L.)

* Correspondence: krangar1@jhmi.edu

Abstract: Wet age-related macular degeneration (AMD) is an end-stage event in a complex pathogenesis of macular degeneration, involving the abnormal growth of blood vessels at the retinal pigment epithelium driven by vascular endothelial growth factor (VEGF). Current therapies seek to interrupt VEGF signaling to halt the progress of neovascularization, but a significant patient population is not responsive. New treatment modalities such as integrin-binding peptides (risuteganib/Luminate/ALG-1001) are being explored to address this clinical need but these treatments necessitate the use of intravitreal injections (IVT), which carries risks of complications and restricts its availability in less-developed countries. Successful systemic delivery of peptide-based therapeutics must overcome obstacles such as degradation by proteinases in circulation and off-target binding. In this work, we present a novel dendrimer-integrin-binding peptide (D-ALG) synthesized with a noncleavable, "clickable" linker. In vitro, D-ALG protected the peptide payload from enzymatic degradation for up to 1.5 h (~90% of the compound remained intact) in a high concentration of proteinase (2 mg/mL) whereas ~90% of free ALG-1001 was degraded in the same period. Further, dendrimer conjugation preserved the antiangiogenic activity of ALG-1001 in vitro with significant reductions in endothelial vessel network formation compared to untreated controls. In vivo, direct intravitreal injections of ALG-1001 and D-ALG produced reductions in the CNV lesion area but in systemically dosed animals, only D-ALG produced significant reductions of CNV lesion area at 14 days. Imaging data suggested that the difference in efficacy may be due to more D-ALG remaining in the target area than ALG-1001 after administration. The results presented here offer a clinically relevant route for peptide therapeutics by addressing the major obstacles that these therapies face in delivery.

Keywords: integrin; peptide conjugates; AMD; hydroxyl PAMAM dendrimer; targeted delivery; neovascularization

1. Introduction

Millions of elderly patients face the risk of vision loss due to age-related macular degeneration (AMD) and approximately 10% of these patients will develop wet AMD [1–4]. Wet AMD is a late-stage event in the complex pathological evolution of AMD, in which choroidal neovascularization pushes blood vessels from the choroid through the Bruch's membrane to displace or destroy the retinal pigment epithelium (RPE) [5–7]. A prominent factor in the pathogenesis of wet AMD is the elevated expression of vascular endothelial growth factor (VEGF) in the eye, which encourages the growth of new blood vessels [8–11]. As a result, most current standards of care for wet AMD target extracellular VEGF directly through intravitreal injections of anti-VEGF antibodies such as aflibercept [12–16]. However, a significant portion of patients (~1/3) do not respond to these therapies [17–19] and vision can still decline despite optimal patient adherence to the treatment regimen [20].

Other therapeutic modalities such as integrin-binding peptides are being developed to halt the progression of wet AMD in patients [21–23]. These peptide antagonists bind strongly to cell surface integrins such as αVβ3, α5β1, and α5β3 and inhibit the downstream signaling of these integrins [24–26]. Specifically, these integrin antagonists reduce the activation of the ERK and PI3K/Akt pathways, which in turn attenuate the expression of a variety of proinflammatory and proangiogenic cytokines such as VEGF-A, TNF-α, and IL1β [27–30]. Luminate (or ALG-1001) is one such integrin-binding peptide that has proven successful in halting neovascularization and is currently undergoing clinical trials for applications in AMD and in diabetic macular edema (DME) [28,31,32]. However, peptide-based antagonists suffer from a wide range of delivery challenges including rapid enzymatic degradation and renal clearance, and lack of cell-targeting [33,34]. Thus, these therapies are currently restricted to intravitreal injections, which not only limits their availability to patients in less developed countries [35] but also carry risks of endophthalmitis, elevated intraocular pressures (IOP), and irritation [36–39].

Systemic treatments for AMD may enable treatments during the early stages of the disease [40] while bypassing the challenges associated with intravitreal injections. In recent years, hydroxyl-terminated, neutrally charged dendrimers have emerged as a promising biocompatible platform for drug delivery, with multiple products in clinical trials. In numerous animal model and human studies, dendrimer conjugation of small molecule drugs improved their safety profile and increased their efficacy in the target area [40–45]. The inherent ability of the dendrimer to be taken up by reactive macrophages and microglia allows for a higher local concentration to be achieved while the rapid clearance of dendrimer conjugates from the blood reduces unnecessary exposure in nontargeted cells and tissues [46–48]. Recent phase 2a clinical trials of hydroxyl PAMAM dendrimer-NAC conjugates in hospitalized severe COVID-19 patients showed that a single intravenous dose of this conjugates led to an 82% survival, the attenuation of hyperinflammation, and a significant reduction in blood biomarkers of brain injury associated with COVID, compared to the standard of care. This suggests that the safety and inflammatory cell-targeting viability of this approach can be leveraged clinically to improve patient outcome [49]. Further, dendrimer conjugation of peptides have also been employed to enable superior cell surface binding because multivalency prevents the binding of the SARS-CoV-2 spike protein with the ACE2 receptor at 1–3 magnitudes lower concentration compared to the free peptide [50]. In this work, we demonstrate that the advantages conferred to small molecule drugs by dendrimer conjugation can be extended to small-molecule biologics [51–53]. Dendrimer conjugation to ALG-1001 peptide preserves the activity of the peptide, increases its stability, prolongs its residence time in the target tissue, and offers systemic administration as an alternative route to intravitreal injections, thereby expanding the availability of the therapy worldwide.

2. Materials and Methods

2.1. Chemicals and Reagents

Hydroxyl-terminated, ethylenediamine-core PAMAM dendrimer (generation 6, pharmaceutical grade) in methanol solution was purchased from Dendritech (Midland, MI, USA). Prior to use, the dendrimer solution was evaporated on a rotary evaporator. The dialysis membrane (MWCO 1 kDa) was purchased from Spectrum Chemicals (New Brunswick, NJ, USA). ALG-1001 and ALG-1001 modified with azide linker were purchased from Bio-Synthesis (Lewisville, TX, USA). Deuterated solvents (DMSO-d_6), methanol (CD_3OD), and water (D_2O) were purchased from Sigma-Aldrich. Proteinase K stock solution and Dulbecco's modified Eagle medium (DMEM, low glucose with L-glutamine) were purchased from ThermoFisher (Waltham, MA, USA). Human umbilical vein endothelial cells and the required media kit were purchased from Lonza (Basel, Switzerland). Phenol Red-free Matrigel was purchased from Corning (Tewksberry, MA, USA).

2.2. *Instrumentation*

2.2.1. Nuclear Magnetic Resonance

A Bruker 500 MHz spectrometer was used to obtain ^{1}H NMR spectra at ambient temperatures. Chemical shifts are reported in parts per million relative to tetramethylsilane, which was used as an internal standard, and the residual protic solvent peaks were used for chemical shifts' calibration. DMSO-d_6 (δ = 2.50 ppm). The resonance multiplicity in the spectra is indicated as "s" (singlet), "d" (doublet), "t" (triplet), and "m" (multiplet). Broad resonances are expressed by "b".

2.2.2. High-Performance Liquid Chromatography

Waters HPLC (Milford, MA, USA) equipped with a 1525 binary pump, and in-line degasser AF, a 717 plus autosampler, and a 2998 photodiode array detector interfaced with Waters Empower 2 software was used to determine the purities of compounds. The column was a Waters Symmetry C18 reversed-phase column with a particle size of 5 μm, a length of 25 cm, and an internal diameter of 4.6. mm. The chromatograms were monitored at 210, 650, and 530 nm using the photodiode array (PDA) detector. The analysis was performed with a gradient flow starting at 95:5 (H_2O/ACN) increasing to 50:50 (H_2O/ACN) in 30 min and returning to 95:5 (H_2O/ACN) in 10 min at a flow rate of 1 mL/min.

2.3. *Synthesis of Dendrimer Conjugates*

2.3.1. Synthesis of Dendrimer-Hexyne

5-Hexynoic acid and DMAP were added to a solution of D-OH in anhydrous DMF and stirred at RT for 15 min. EDC·HCl was added to the resulting clear solutions in 3 equal portions and the solution was stirred overnight at room temperature. The reaction mixture was purified by dialysis through a 2 kDa MW cut-off cellulose dialysis membrane against DMF with solvent change at 8 h intervals. After 24 h, the mixture was dialyzed against water for 24 h with solvent change at 12 h intervals. The final aqueous solution was lyophilized to get the product as a white solid.

^{1}H NMR (500 MHz, DMSO) δ 8.06–7.79 (m, internal amide 510H), 4.73 (s, surface OH, 232H), 4.01 (s, ester linked, 22H), 3.40 (d, dendrimer-CH_2), 3.33 (d, dendrimer-CH_2), 3.18–3.11 (m, dendrimer-CH_2), 2.64 (s, dendrimer-CH_2), 2.43 (s, dendrimer-CH_2), 2.20 (s, dendrimer-CH_2), 1.68 (t, acetylene, 30H). Retention time: 19.58 min

2.3.2. Synthesis of BOC-GABA-D-Hexyne

D-hexyne was dissolved in anhydrous DMF, and BOC-GABA-OH and DMAP were added. The solution was stirred for 15 min before the addition of EDC·HCl in 3 equal, separate portions. The solution was stirred overnight, purified by dialysis, and lyophilized to get the product as a white solid.

^{1}H NMR (500 MHz, DMSO-d_6) δ 8.06–7.79 (m, internal amide 510H), 4.73 (s, surface OH, 199H), 4.06 (s, ester linked, 40H), 3.40 (d, dendrimer-CH_2), 3.33 (d, dendrimer-CH_2), 3.18–3.11 (m, dendrimer-CH_2), 2.64 (s, dendrimer-CH_2), 2.43 (s, dendrimer-CH_2), 2.20 (s, dendrimer-CH_2), 1.68 (t, acetylene, 27H), 1.36 (s, BOC, 68H).

2.3.3. Synthesis of GABA-D-Hexyne

The deprotection of BOC-GABA-D-hexyne was performed under anhydrous conditions. The compound was placed in a round bottom flask, and anhydrous DCM was added under a nitrogen atmosphere. The solution was constantly stirred and sonicated to form a cloudy, sticky suspension. TFA was then added to the suspension in a 4:1 ratio (DCM:TFA), and the solution was stirred overnight. DCM was then evaporated using a rotary evaporator. TFA was removed by repeatedly diluting the reaction mixture with methanol and evaporating the resultant solution. The product was then placed under high vacuum for 3 h and used without further purification.

2.3.4. Synthesis of Cy5-D-Hexyne

GABA-D-hexyne was dissolved in anhydrous DMF, followed by DIPEA, and finally the addition of Cy5 NHS ester. The reaction was stirred overnight, and the reaction mixture was dialyzed through a 2 kDa membrane against DMF for 24 h. The mixture was then dialyzed against water for an additional 24 h and lyophilized to obtain a solid, blue product.

^{1}H NMR (500 MHz, DMSO-d$_6$) δ 8.06–7.79 (m, internal amide 510H), 7.35 (m, Cy5 H), 7.25 (m, Cy5 H), 7.05 (m, Cy5 H), 6.6 (m, Cy5 H), 6.3 (m, Cy5 H), 4.73 (s, surface OH, 199H), 4.06 (s, ester linked, 40H), 3.40 (d, dendrimer-CH$_2$), 3.33 (d, dendrimer-CH$_2$), 3.18–3.11 (m, dendrimer-CH$_2$), 2.64 (s, dendrimer-CH$_2$), 2.43 (s, dendrimer-CH$_2$), 2.20 (s, dendrimer-CH$_2$), 1.68 (t, acetylene, 27H). Retention time: 18.01 min

2.3.5. Synthesis of D-ALG1001 and Cy5-D-ALG1001

ALG-1001 was dissolved in ultrapure water and added to an aqueous solution of D-hexyne for unlabeled conjugates. ALG-1001-Cy3 was dissolved in ultrapure water and added to an aqueous solution of Cy5-D-hexyne for dual-labeled conjugates. We then added a solution of copper sulfate and stirred the solution for 10 min at RT before adding sodium ascorbate. For purification, both reactions were left at room temperature overnight then dialyzed against water for 24 h. Each solution was lyophilized to obtain a powder product.

^{1}H NMR (500 MHz, DMSO-d$_6$) of D-ALG: 8.12–7.78 (m, internal amide H), 4.45–4.06 (m, peptide α carbon), 4.00 (s, ester linked, 37H), 3.78 (m, polyethylene glycol H), 3.40 (d, dendrimer-CH$_2$), 3.33 (d, dendrimer-CH$_2$), 3.18–3.11 (m, dendrimer-CH$_2$), 2.64 (s, dendrimer-CH$_2$), 1.64–1.59 (m, GABA linker-CH$_2$ and peptide side chain). Retention time: 16.60 min

^{1}H NMR (500 MHz, DMSO-d$_6$) of Cy5-D-ALG-Cy3: 8.12–7.78 (m, internal amide H), 7.01 (m, aromatic 5H), 6.59 (s, GABA amide H, 10H), 4.73 (s, surface OH, 233H), 4.06 (s, ester linked, 16H), 3.40 (d, dendrimer-CH$_2$), 3.33 (d, dendrimer-CH$_2$), 3.18–3.11 (m, dendrimer-CH$_2$), 2.64 (s, dendrimer-CH$_2$), 1.64–1.59 (m, GABA linker-CH2, 6H), 1.36 (s, Boc group, 20H). Retention time: 17.99 min

2.4. In Vitro Stability under Enzymatic Degradation

Proteinase K stock solution was purchased from ThermoFisher and used as is. ALG-1001 and D-ALG solutions were prepared at a concentration of 2 mg/mL, and proteinase K was added to each solution such that the final concentration of proteinase K was 2 mg/mL. The mixture was incubated at 37 °C and at set time points, 100 μL of the mixture was removed and analyzed through HPLC. To determine compound degradation, the integrations of peaks at elution times associated with ALG-1001 and D-ALG were used and normalized to the injected analyte peak at the 0 h time point.

2.5. Cell Culture

HUVEC cells were obtained from Lonza and cultured in EGM-2 endothelial cell growth medium (Lonza). Murine macrophages (RAW264.7) between passages 5–9 were cultured in Dulbecco's modified Eagle's medium (DMEM, Life technologies, Grand Island, NY, USA) supplemented with 10% fetal bovine serum (Invitrogen Corp., Carlsbad, CA, USA) and 1% penicillin/streptomycin (Invitrogen Corp., Carlsbad, CA, USA). All cells were maintained at 37 °C and 5% CO$_2$ with a humidified incubator.

2.6. In Vitro Evaluation of D-ALG Efficacy

2.6.1. Vessel Formation Assay

First, 96-well plates were coated with 75 μL of Matrigel and left at room temperature for 15 min before being placed into 37 °C incubators for an additional 30 min. Then, D-ALG1001 was dissolved at twice the desired concentration and 50 μL of the drug solution was added to the wells. HUVEC cells were then added to each well at a density of 70,000 cells/cm^2. Live-cell images were taken at 12 h for analysis.

2.6.2. Wound-Healing Assay

HUVEC cells were seeded at a density of 5×10^4 cells per well in 24-well plates and set aside for at least 72 h for a uniform monolayer of cells to form. Cells were treated with D-ALG1001 and ALG-1001 for 24 h. A centimeter-long scratch was introduced to the cell monolayer with the tip of a 200 µL pipette tip. Images were taken on a Nikon.

2.6.3. VEGF Activation for Western Blotting and PCR

HUVEC cells were seeded at a density of 5×10^4 cells per well in 24-well plates 24 h before treatment. Cells were treated with D-ALG1001 and ALG-1001 for 24 h before activation with VEGF for 5 min. Cells were collected and lysed for Western blotting using T-Per buffer (ThermoFisher) supplemented with PhosStop and proteinase inhibitor cocktail. Cells were lysed with Trizol and processed as previously described for qPCR analysis.

2.6.4. In Vitro Inflammation Model

RAW264.7 cells were seeded at a density of 1×10^5 cells per well in 12-well plates 48 h before treatment. Cells were incubated with D-ALG1001 and ALG-1001 for 24 h, the treatment media was aspirated, then LPS at a concentration of 10,000 endotoxin units/mL was added to stimulate inflammatory response. Samples were collected 3 h after LPS stimulation for qPCR analysis.

2.7. In Vivo Evaluation of D-ALG at Attenuating Choroidal Neovascularization

2.7.1. In Vivo Laser CNV Rat Models

All animal procedures were approved by the Johns Hopkins Animal Care and Use Committee. Brown Norway rats between 8 and 12 weeks old were obtained and housed at constant temperature and humidity (20 ± 1 °C, 50 ± 5% humidity). Animals were anesthetized through intraperitoneal injections of a ketamine/xylazine cocktail (ketamine 50 mg/kg and xylazine 10 mg/kg). Pupils were dilated with topical 2.5% phenylephrine hydrochloride solution followed by 0.5% tetracaine hydrochloride solution. To induce CNV formation, four equally spaced lesions were created in the Bruch's membrane with a built-in laser system on the Micron III SLO. Laser power was set to 240–250 W with a duration of 70 ms. A gonio ophthalmic solution was applied postoperatively to prevent the eyes from drying and forming cataracts.

On the day of CNV induction (Day 0), D-ALG1001 and ALG1001 was administered intraperitoneally at a dose of 150 µg on a peptide basis. Subsequent doses were administered every 4 days. At days 7 and 14, mice were sacrificed and enucleated. Eyes used for CNV image were fixed in 10% formalin for 1 h. Eyes used for qPCR, ELISA, and Western blotting were immediately stored at −80 °C until use.

2.7.2. Tissue Preparation for Western Blotting and qPCR

In brief, 500 µL of T-Per supplemented with PhosStop and proteinase inhibitor cocktail was added to tubes containing dissected choroid. A scoop of 1.6 mm steel homogenization beads was added to each sample and then placed in TissueLyserLT (Qiagen, Germantown, MD, USA) at an oscillation frequency of 50 cycles/s for 15 min.

For qPCR, 200 µL of Trizol was added to tubes containing choroid and a scoop of 1.6 mm steel homogenization beads was added. The samples were placed in TissueLyserLT at an oscillation frequency of 50 cycles/s for 15 min.

2.7.3. Pathway Activation Analysis with Western Blot and ELISA

In brief, the concentration of protein was determined with the BCA protein assay kit (Thermo Scientific, Rockford, IL, USA). Equal amounts of protein were denatured and resolved on 4–15% TGX gels (Bio-Rad, Hercules, CA, USA). Gels were transferred to nitrocellulose membranes, blocked with 3% BSA at RT for 1 h and probed for GAPDH, FAK, pFAK, MAPK, and pMAPK at 4 °C overnight. Membranes were washed thrice before incubation with HRP-conjugated secondary antibodies followed by incubation with chemiluminescent substrate for visualization.

For protein extracted from tissues, total FAK and FAK (Phospho) [pY397] ELISA kits (Invitrogen) were used to quantify the level of protein expression, and the measured protein expression was normalized to the total protein amount of each sample as determined from BCA assays.

2.7.4. qPCR Analysis

In brief, 100 μL of chloroform was added to the Trizol suspension, and the aqueous phase was separated with a centrifuge at 10K RPM at 4 °C for 15 min. Then, 400 μL of 2-propanol was added to the aqueous solution and spun again to pellet the RNA. The RNA was washed with 70% ethanol solution, pelleted again, and resuspended in DEPC water.

To convert RNA to complementary DNA, 2 μg of RNA was converted using a High-Capacity cDNA Reverse Transcription Kit (Applied Biosystems, Foster City, CA, USA). Samples were analyzed using StepOne Plus real-time PCR system (Applied Biosystems) with SYBR Green reagent (ThermoFisher Scientific). Relative expression was quantified with ΔΔCt calculations normalized to controls. Primers for GAPDH was obtained from Bio-Rad Laboratories (Hercules, CA, USA). Primers for TNFα (forward: CCA GTG TGG GAA GCT GTC TT; reverse: AAG CAA AAG AGG AGG CAA CA), IL1β (forward: AGC TTC AAA TCT CGA AGC AG; reverse: TGT CCT CAT CCT GGA AGG TC) were purchased from Integrated DNA Technologies (Coralville, IA, USA).

2.7.5. Biodistribution

For biodistribution studies, a dose of Cy5-D-ALG1001-Cy3 and ALG-1001-Cy3 at 150 μg/100 μL was administered to each animal intraperitoneally on the day of CNV induction (day 0). Animals were sacrificed at 1-, 2-, 3-, and 4-day time points and enucleated.

2.7.6. Imaging

After fixation, the posterior segment of the eye was dissected out and the retina separated from the choroid. Tissues stained with FITC-labeled isolectin (GS IB_4) (Life Technologies, Eugene, OR, USA) for blood vessels and monocytes. Eyes were mounted by introducing four radial relaxation cuts. Samples for biodistribution were imaged under a confocal 710 microscope (Carl Zeiss, Oberkochen, Germany). Samples for CNV quantification were imaged with an Axiovert phase contrast microscope. All images were processed with ImageJ.

2.7.7. Statistical Analysis

Data were presented as means ± SEM and analyses were performed in GraphPad Prism (version 9; La Jolla, CA, USA). Treatment groups across time point or doses were analyzed through an analysis of variance (ANOVA) tests. Significant differences among single groups were determined with Student's t tests: * $p < 0.05$, ** $p < 0.01$ and *** $p < 0.001$.

3. Results

3.1. Synthesis and Characterization of D-ALG1001 Intermediates and Conjugates

We utilized a high-yield click reaction to efficiently attach the ALG-1001 peptide to the dendrimer platform under mild conditions, which is amenable to preserving the structural stability and activity of the peptide (Figure 1A) [54–60]. First, we modified the dendrimer surface functional groups with a hexynoic acid linker and confirmed the modification by ^{1}HNMR with the presence of 20 protons at 4.0 ppm and 1.7 ppm (Figure 1B). The dendrimer surface was minimally modified to preserve its near-neutral charge and its inherent ability to penetrate tissues.

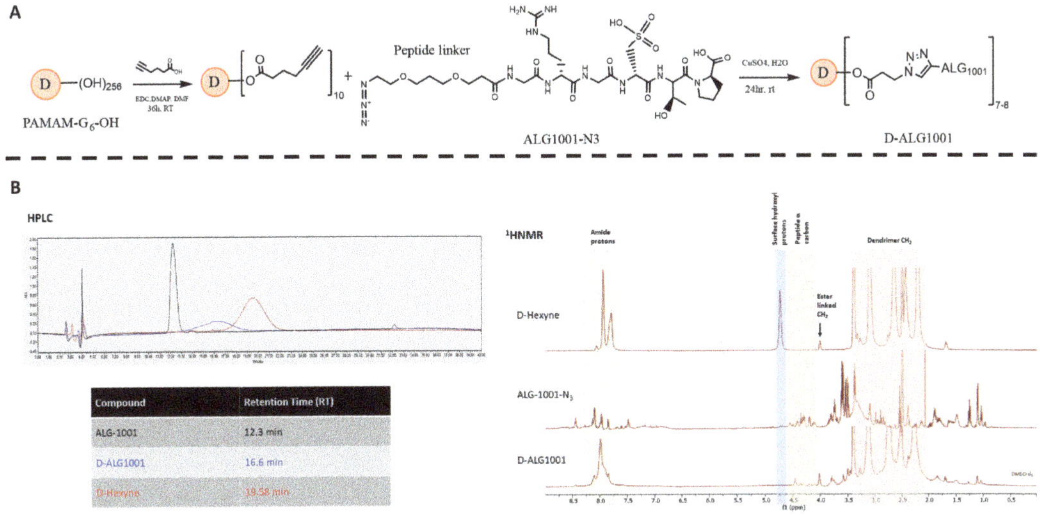

Figure 1. Synthesis and characterization of D-ALG1001. (**A**) Synthesis scheme of D-ALG1001: surface of generation-6 hydroxyl-terminated dendrimer was functionalized with alkyne-terminated linkers. ALG-1001 peptide was then attached using a copper-catalyzed click reaction to yield D-ALG conjugates. (**B**) The D-ALG conjugate was characterized by HPLC (**left**) with a retention time of 16.6 min compared to precursor materials ALG-1001 (12.3 min) and D-hexyne (19.58 min) with the chromatogram trace color corresponding to the text color. ^{1}H NMR characterization of the precursor and final conjugate (**right**) shows the appearance of characteristic signals.

For biodistribution studies using Cy5 fluorophore, the dendrimer surface was further modified with GABA-Boc linkers. The presence of additional protons at 4.0 ppm, 1.7 ppm, and 1.2 ppm confirmed the modification. The resulting intermediate was deprotected and the free amine was used to couple with Cy5 ester to obtain a fluorescently labeled dendrimer (Figures S1–S7).

ALG-1001 peptide was purchased with a short polyethylene glycol (PEG) azide linker attached to the C terminus and used without further preparation. For biodistribution studies, the N terminus of the peptide was also modified with Cy3 fluorophore for tracking. A copper (I)-catalyzed alkyne-azide click (CuAAC) reaction was used to attach ALG-1001 to dendrimers, and ^{1}HNMR spectra confirmed the attachment of ALG-1001 by showing the presence of the peptide protons.

3.2. *In Vitro Stability under Enzymatic Degradation*

Coincubation of ALG-1001 and proteinase K, a broad acting protease, resulted in a rapid degradation of free ALG-1001 with about 50% degraded at 30 min and 90% at 90 min. On the other hand, the dendrimer conjugation of the ALG-1001 peptide coincubated with proteinase K did not result in HPLC peak shifts in retention time or produce additional peaks indicating the degradation of the compound at incubation times shorter than 90 min. The conjugation conferred resistance to enzymatic degradation possibly due to steric hinderance from the dendrimer carrier. Only around 10% of D-ALG was degraded at 90 min (Figure 2). This resistance toward enzymatic degradation, even at a high enzyme concentration (2 mg/mL) suggests that dendrimer conjugation increases the stability and may increase the circulation time of intact peptides in vivo by helping it escape degradation pathways. The concentration used (2 mg/mL) was about 20–40× higher than the concentration used for routine protease digestion protocols (50–100 µg/mL). The 2 mg/mL concentration was also 5× higher concentration than the 400 µg/mL used in assessing the stability of NF55/pDNA nanoparticles in which the compound resisted degradation for 3 h at most [61].

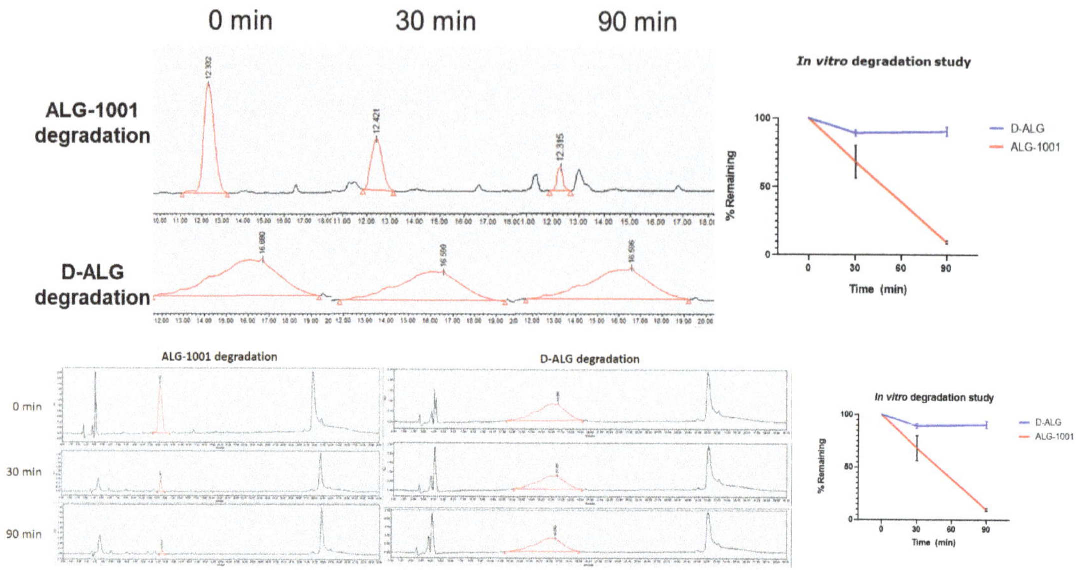

Figure 2. In vitro enzymatic degradation in the presence of proteinase K. HPLC chromatographs of D-ALG and ALG-1001 after coincubation with proteinase K show a decrease in the AUC of the peak associated with the free ALG-1001 peptide (**top**). The trace of D-ALG shows a negligible decrease in AUC (**middle**). The peaks corresponding to ALG-1001 and D-ALG are outlined in red. The curve plotting the amount degraded is shown by normalizing peaks of analyte taken at set time points to the starting peak obtained at 0 min (**bottom**). About 90% of ALG-1001 was degraded by 90 min whereas only 10% of D-ALG was degraded.

The generation-6 PAMAM dendrimers conjugates had a blood circulation time of ~4–8 h, reaching target cells over this time duration [46,62]. Therefore, the dendrimer conjugation may enable peptides to be largely delivered intact into target cells, at levels above what could be expected for free peptides, enabling us to address a major roadblock in the clinical translation of peptide-based therapeutics [63–65].

3.3. In Vitro Vessel Formation Assay

To compare the dose–response efficacy of free and D-ALG in a physiologically relevant model, we utilized an in vitro model of blood vessel formation [66]. HUVEC cells were treated with a gradient concentration of D-ALG and ALG-1001 for 24 h at three different magnitudes of doses. The cells were then seeded on Matrigel after which cells naturally migrate to form blood vessel-like tubule structures. The images were analyzed with the Angiogenesis Analyzer plug-in on ImageJ to extract relevant metrics that measure the connectivity and integrity of tube networks (Figure 3A and Figure S8).

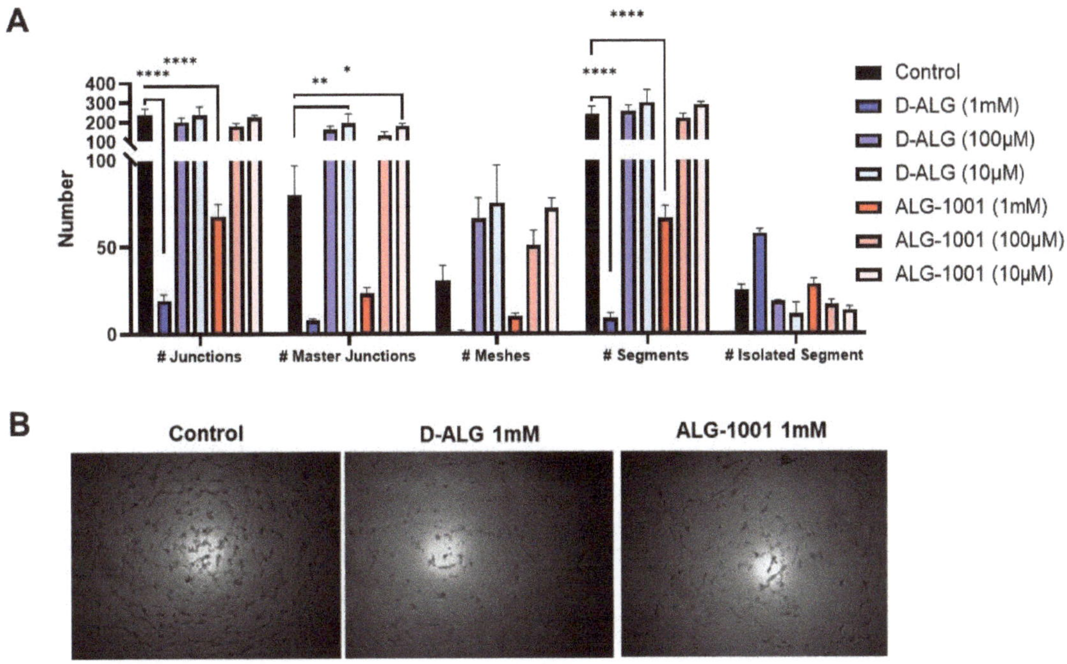

Figure 3. In vitro inhibition of vessel formation. (**A**) Image analysis of HUVECs seeded onto a Matrigel matrix using the Angiogenesis Analyzer plug-in for ImageJ. The relevant metrics extracted for the integrity and expanse of vessel formation were the number (#) of times vessels intersected one another (junctions), the number (#) of spaces enclosed by vessels (meshes), the number (#) of connected vessels (segments), and the number (#) of isolated vessels (isolated segments). Significant disruptions in vessel formation resulted in reduced junctions, segments, and meshes while the number of isolated segments increased. Cells treated with 1 mM ALG-1001 and D-ALG significantly reduced vessel formation compared to untreated cells. * $p < 0.05$, ** $p < 0.01$, and **** $p < 0.0001$ (**B**) Representative images of vessel formation from untreated cells (control), and cells treated with D-ALG and ALG-1001 at a 1 mM concentration.

While lower doses were not effective, cells treated with 1 mM of D-ALG and ALG-1001 exhibited an increased disruption in tube formation with more isolated segments and a smaller area or meshes enclosed by tubes. Interestingly, the trend suggested dendrimer conjugation may increase the efficacy of ALG-1001 at disrupting network formation. HUVECs treated with 1 mM of D-ALG had fewer points of intersection between vessels (junctions), fewer connected segments, and more isolated segments compared to those treated with 1 mM of ALG-1001.

3.4. Wound-Healing Assay

In addition to cell morphological and motility changes measured by tube formation assays, we investigated the activity of D-ALG and ALG-1001 in a wound-healing assay. Previous studies have utilized this method to assess cell migration and proliferation [67–71]. Monolayers of HUVECs were pretreated with D-ALG or ALG-1001 followed by scratching the monolayer with a pipette tip. Images were taken at the time of the wound and at 24 h after injury. The proliferative activity of endothelial cells can be measured by the area that was healed postinjury to the monolayer. Untreated cells managed to heal up to 80% of the initial damage after 24 h, while cells treated with D-ALG and ALG-1001 healed up to 50% of the initial wound area. Further, cells treated with a high dose of D-ALG at 1 mM only recovered 20% of the initial damage, suggesting a reduced ability of HUVECs to regenerate (Figure S9). Because neovascularization is driven in part by the proliferation and migration of endothelial cells in the disease area, reductions in these activities as observed in cells treated with D-ALG can modulate endothelial cell contributions to the neovascularization process. Further, comparing the efficacy between D-ALG and free ALG-1001 suggests that treatment with D-ALG is more efficacious than the free peptide at reducing neovascularization-related cellular processes.

3.5. Western Blot on Endothelial Cell Activation

To elucidate the mechanism through which D-ALG and free ALG-1001 influence angiogenic function, we pretreated the cells with D-ALG and free ALG-1001 for 24 h. The cells were then stimulated with a high dose of exogenous VEGF for 5 min after which the samples were collected for Western blotting. We probed for the expression of total FAK, phospho-FAK (Y397), ERK1/2, phospho-ERK1/2, and cyclophilin B (CycB) with CycB acting as the internal control.

Compared to untreated, VEGF stimulated controls, the trend suggested that cells treated with D-ALG and ALG-1001 expressed lower levels of phospho-ERK1/2 and phospho-FAK at doses of 100 μM on a peptide basis. Both ERK1/2 and FAK pathways are important players in angiogenesis and their activation promotes endothelial cell proliferation and migration (Figure 4). The trend in the reduction in phosphorylated proteins suggests an attenuation in the activation of these networks in response to VEGF.

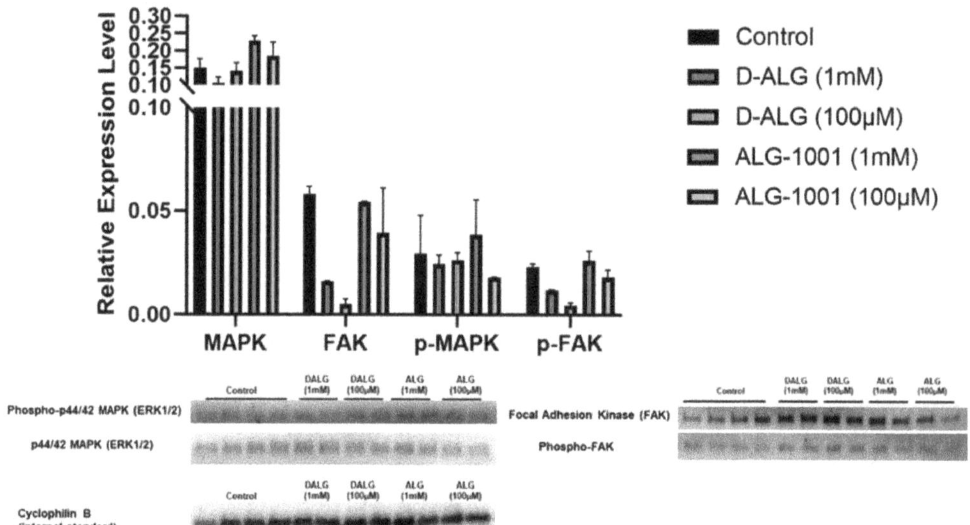

Figure 4. Activation of ERK and FAK pathway in response to VEGF stimulation. Relative protein expression was calculated by analyzing protein bands associated with ERK (42 and 44 kDa) and FAK (110 kDa) and normalizing the content to an internal control (cyclophilin B) (**top**). Representative images of blots are shown (**bottom**).

In addition to examining pathway activation, we also studied the effects of D-ALG and ALG-1001 on VEGF-A expression by endothelial cells (Figure S10). Cells treated with VEGF-A significantly increased the production of VEGF-A compared to unstimulated controls. Cells coincubated with VEGF-A and either free ALG-1001 or D-ALG did not have statistically significant increases in VEGF production compared to the control, suggesting a minor attenuation in endothelial activation in response to VEGF.

3.6. Attenuation of Inflammatory Response in Murine Microglia

Other important players in angiogenesis are macrophages and microglia which produce proinflammatory and proangiogenic cytokines during the angiogenic process. To elucidate the effect of D-ALG and ALG-1001 on macrophage activation, we pretreated RAW264.7 macrophage cells with a high and low dose of D-ALG and free ALG-1001 24 h prior to LPS stimulation. The treatment media was first aspirated to simulate the transient nature of in vivo delivery, and cells were activated with LPS for 3 h.

Cells activated with LPS displayed a robust increase in the expression of proinflammatory cytokines IL1β and TNFα as detected through qPCR when compared to unstimulated controls (Figure 5). With D-ALG treatment, the expression of IL1β was reduced by ~90% and TNFα by 80% in both the low (100 μM) and high dose (1 mM). In comparison, ALG-1001 reduced the expression of TNFα only by a relatively moderate 20%, only at the highest dose as well. We observed no impact on IL1β production with free ALG-1001 treatment alone. This major difference in the efficacy between free ALG-1001 and the dendrimer conjugate may be due to two potential differences: (1) the dendrimer platform is demonstrated to be much more efficient at delivering therapeutics to activated macrophages compared to free drugs; (2) attaching multiple ligands on the dendrimer surface may allow for multivalency effects, increasing the interaction of the peptide and surface integrin.

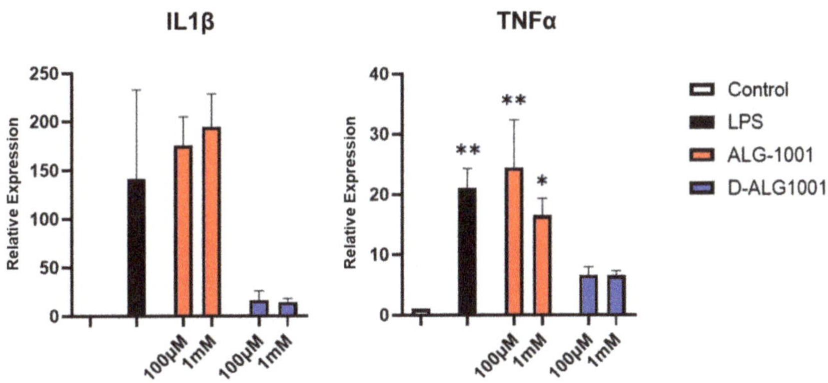

Figure 5. Expression of proinflammatory cytokine of RAW264.7 cells in response to LPS stimulation. Compared to untreated controls, RAW cells stimulated with LPS produced robust expressions of IL1β and TNFα. Pretreatment with ALG-1001 produced a slight effect at attenuating TNFα expression at 1 mM concentration; on the other hand, treating with D-ALG brought the level of TNFα to a level not statistically different than untreated controls. *p*-values denoted here compare the level of IL1β and TNFα expression to untreated controls. * $p < 0.05$, ** $p < 0.01$.

3.7. Biodistribution of Systemically Administered ALG-1001 and D-ALG in Laser CNV Model

Fluorescently labeled Cy3-ALG-1001 peptide and dual-labeled Cy5-dendrimer-ALG-Cy3 were systemically injected on day 0 (same day as CNV induction in the laser CNV model) and choroidal tissues were collected at set time points. Confocal microscopy was used to monitor the presence of ALG-1001 peptide (Cy3), dendrimer carrier (Cy5), and CNV formation (isolectin).

Within the first 24 h of systemic administration, free ALG-1001 peptide reached the CNV area and remained there for up to 2 days as seen from detected Cy3 signals (Figure 6). In comparison, D-ALG was able to not only reach the CNV area within 24 h after systemic injection but also remain in the target area up to at least 4 days postadministration from the colocalized presence of both Cy5 and Cy3 signals. The prolonged residence time may suggest that dendrimer conjugation allowed the target area itself to serve as a drug depot, prolonging the efficacy of the peptide therapeutic. This prolonged residence time may be due to a better resistance to enzymatic degradation, and/or due to cellular uptake into the resident macrophages in the target area that is an intrinsic property of dendrimers.

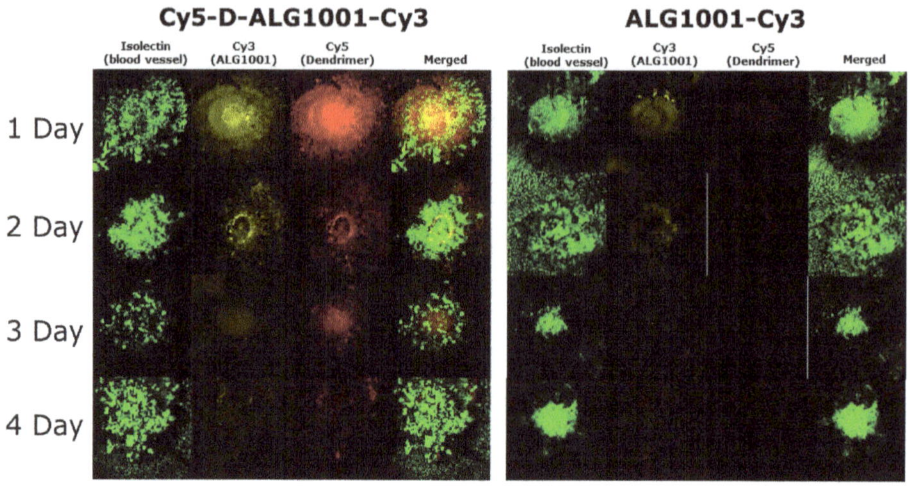

Figure 6. Biodistribution of intraperitoneally injected Cy5-D-ALG-Cy3 and ALG-1001-Cy3 at areas of choroidal neovascularization. CNVs were stained with isolectin (green), ALG-1001 was labeled with Cy3 (yellow), and the dendrimer was labeled with Cy5 (red). Cy5-D-ALG-Cy3 conjugates stayed in the target area over a period of 4 days with the signal staying around the CNV area. A majority of ALG-1001-Cy3 stayed in the target area over 2 days, and most were cleared by day 3.

3.8. Systemically Administered D-ALG Attenuates FAK and ERK Activation

To evaluate the activation of FAK and ERK pathways, eyes were enucleated at set time points, and the choroidal tissue dissected out. Tissues were submerged in a mixture of T-per, proteinase inhibitor, and PhosStop with stainless-steel homogenization beads and homogenized to produce protein extracts. Total FAK, total ERK, p-FAK (Y397), and p-44/42 ERK ELISA kits were used to quantify the amount of total and phosphorylated proteins in FAK and ERK pathways. In animals treated with D-ALG, a trend in the reduction in total FAK and p-FAK proteins was observed over both 7 and 14 days compared to untreated controls, suggesting a prolonged attenuation of the FAK pathway (Figure 7A). The treatment of ALG-1001 also resulted in a trend in the reduction in p-FAK across both time points. However, the level of total FAK protein in ALG-1001-treated animals was elevated at day 14. Both D-ALG- and ALG-1001-treated animals resulted in a similar trend in the decrease in p44/42 ERK production, while total ERK remained relatively constant at day 7 across treatment groups. On day 14, there was a slight trend in the reduction in total ERK in D-ALG- and ALG-1001-treated animals compared to untreated animals.

To compare the expression of proinflammatory and proangiogenic cytokines, RNA was extracted, and qPCR was performed to determine the relative expression of VEGF-A, TNFα, and IL1β (Figure 7B). In D-ALG treated animals, we observed a trend that VEGF-A production was reduced over both 7 and 14 days, whereas free ALG-1001 treated animals expressed lower VEGF-A production at 14 days only. Comparing trends in inflammatory cytokines, D-ALG produced lower TNFα level at 7 days only, while ALG-1001-treated animals had lower TNFα levels across both time points. The trend of IL1β expression was only reduced at day 14 for ALG-1001- and D-ALG-treated animals.

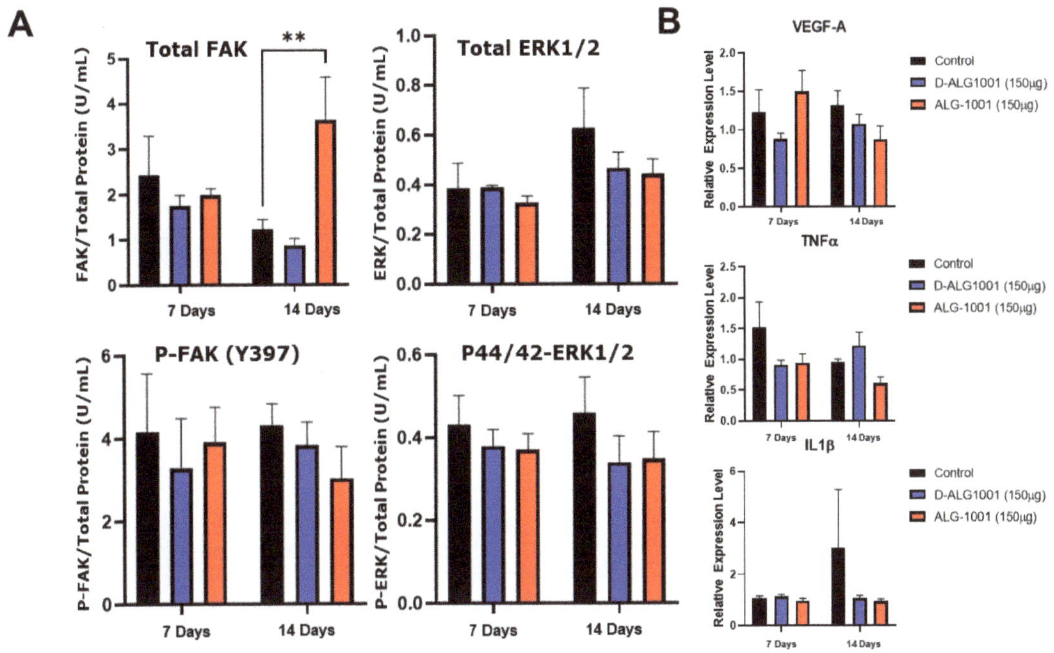

Figure 7. Quantification of ERK and FAK pathway activation and expression of proinflammatory/angiogenic cytokines. (**A**) Quantification of FAK, phosphor-FAK (Y397), p44/42 ERK, phospho-p44/42 ERK proteins using ELISA kits. Trends indicate a reduced phosphorylation of p44/42 ERK over both 7 and 14 days compared to controls in both treatment groups. In D-ALG-treated animals, there is also a trend in reduced phosphor-FAK protein expression across both time points. ** $p < 0.01$ (**B**) Quantification of VEGF-A, TNFα, and IL1β through qPCR. The trend shows a reduction in VEGF-A and TNFα at day 7 for animals treated with D-ALG and a reduction in IL1β production on day 14. ALG-1001-treated animals had a trend of lower TNFα at both time points and lower VEGF-A and IL1β on day 14.

3.9. In Vivo Attenuation of CNV Formation

A Micron III SLO scope and a laser attachment were used to induce CNV formation in mice. The laser CNV model was chosen due to its consistency in creating CNV and the progression of the CNV process [72,73]. We first evaluated whether dendrimer conjugation impeded the peptide from attenuating CNV by first injecting free ALG-1001 and D-ALG intravitreally after CNV induction. The eyes were then collected on day 7 and the CNV area quantified. Both D-ALG and ALG-1001 significantly inhibited the formation of CNV when administered intravitreally (Figure S11).

We then evaluated whether the improved protection and targeting of D-ALG allowed for less invasive administration routes. A laser was used to induce CNV at day 0, and the first dose (150 μg peptide basis) of ALG-1001 and D-ALG was administered intraperitoneally. The animals were dosed once every 4 days at 150 μg of peptide basis (7.5 mg/kg). Choroidal flatmounts of eyes at day 7 and 14 were imaged, and the CNV area was calculated using ImageJ.

In untreated control animals, the CNV area reached a size of 13,000 μm^2 by day 7 and 14,000 μm^2 by day 14 after CNV induction (Figure 8). The systemic injection of ALG-1001 produced a robust attenuation of the CNV formation (~60% reduction) on day 7, but the CNV area recovered at day 14. In comparison, the systemic administration of D-ALG suppressed the formation of CNV by ~50% both on day 7 and day 14, with day 14 reaching statistical significance. This improvement in CNV reduction and its sustained effect up to

14 days, following a single intraperitonial administration of D-ALG-1001, is a significant advance and may be attributed to the ability of D-ALG to protect the peptide payload and lengthen the residence time at the target CNV area [74].

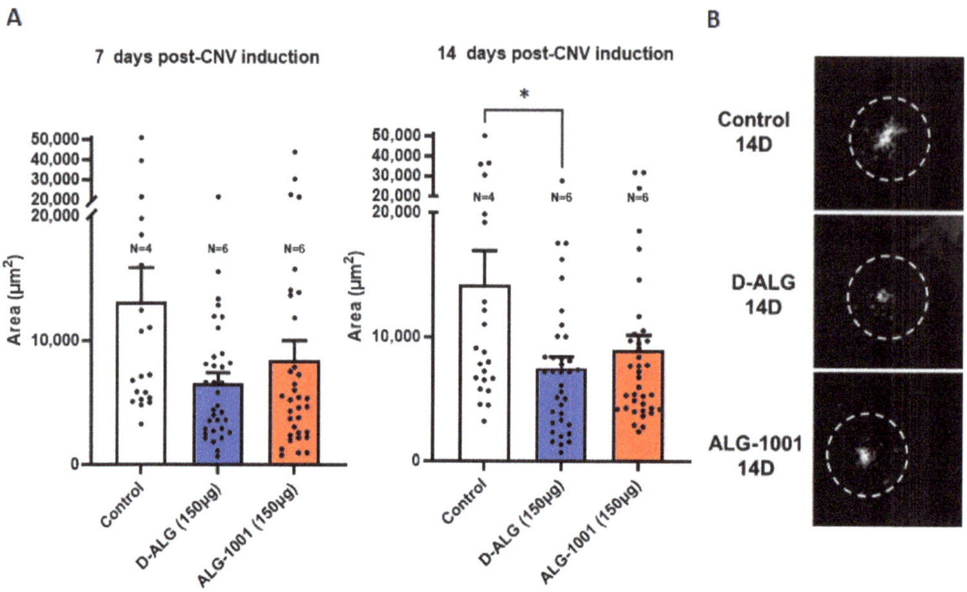

Figure 8. In vivo inhibition of CNV formation in a laser CNV mouse model, following intraperitonial administration of free ALG-1001 and D-ALG-1001. (**A**) Area of CNV as quantified using ImageJ. The trend suggests D-ALG- and ALG-1001-treated animals had smaller CNV areas compared to untreated animals at day 7. The degree of CNV reduction is retained in D-ALG-treated animals on day 14 and the difference reaches statistical significance. (**B**) Representative images of CNV on day 14. * $p < 0.05$.

4. Discussion and Conclusions

Peptide drugs face many challenges relating to plasma stability and intracellular delivery to target cells, which has hampered their clinical translation. We used hydroxyl PAMAM dendrimers, which have shown potential in phase 2 trials, to deliver peptides to areas of neovascularization from systemic administration. Dendrimer conjugation of ALG-1001 peptide was accomplished through a highly efficient copper-assisted click reaction under mild conditions and characterized through HPLC and NMR. Through the integration of NMR peaks, we calculated that 6–7 peptides were attached per dendrimer carrier (~6 wt% payload). We observed an increased resistance to enzymatic degradation with dendrimer conjugation in vitro after incubation with a broad-acting proteinase, where the conjugated peptide was stable up to at least 90 min in plasma.

At high, equivalent doses, D-ALG conjugates inhibited vessel formation an order of magnitude better than the free peptide. In addition, D-ALG1001 attenuated not only the activation of the FAK pathway in endothelial cells but also the expression of proinflammatory cytokines in LPS-stimulated murine macrophages. We hypothesize that attaching multiple peptide moieties on a single dendrimer allowed the integrin clusters to be engaged more effectively, enhancing the antiangiogenic and anti-inflammatory activity of ALG-1001 through this multivalency effect.

When systemically administered in vivo, differences in the distribution and bioavailability of D-ALG and free ALG-1001 peptide could be better elucidated. Fluorescently labeled D-ALG was detectable in the CNV area up to 4 days after intraperitoneal injection; on the other hand, free ALG-1001 signal was undetectable after day 2. The increased residence time at the target area allowed for less frequent injections for D-ALG. An intraperitoneal injection of 150 µg of D-ALG (on a peptide basis) every four days resulted in a 50% reduction in the CNV area, whereas free ALG-1001 peptide reduced CNV formation by 40% on day 7 and lost potency at later time points (20% CNV reduction on day 14 for free ALG-1001 vs. 50% CNV reduction on day 14 for D-ALG). In comparison, the continuous systemic delivery of JSM6427, a small molecule α5β1 antagonist, using an implanted pump resulted in a 40% CNV area reduction [75]. Similarly, in separate studies by Das et al. and Toriyama et al., exploring Å6 peptide and CGRP peptides, respectively, daily injections were necessary to reduce CNV area by 30% [76,77].

The work presented here demonstrates that dendrimer conjugation can not only deliver biologics intact to the target area after systemic administration but also increase its residence time and efficacy. As a result, a less stringent dosing schedule is needed to effectively control CNV formation. The work presented here suggests that dendrimer conjugation is a valid strategy to significantly improve the stability of biologics and as a vehicle for the systemic, targeted delivery of these powerful therapeutics.

Supplementary Materials: The following supporting information can be downloaded at: https://www.mdpi.com/article/10.3390/pharmaceutics15102428/s1, Figure S1: ^{1}H NMR spectrum of compound 1 in DMSO-d_6; Figure S2: ^{1}H NMR spectrum of ALG-1001 in DMSO-d_6; Figure S3: ^{1}H NMR spectrum of compound 3 in DMSO-d_6; Figure S4: ^{1}H NMR spectrum of compound 4 in DMSO-d_6; Figure S5: ^{1}H NMR spectrum of compound 5 in DMSO-d_6; Figure S6: ^{1}H NMR spectrum of compound 6 in DMSO-d_6; Figure S7: HPLC chromatograph of dendrimer intermediates, dendrimer-ALG conjugates, ALG-1001 peptide, and proteinase K (serine protease). Conjugation of ALG-1001 peptide to the dendrimer result in a ~3 minute-shift in retention time whereas the Cy5-labeled dendrimer-ALG1001 conjugate did not result in a minimal shift of 0.1 minutes compared to the precursor Cy5-labeled dendrimer. To confirm peptide attachment, UV spectrum of fluorescently labeled compounds were extracted with photodiode array detector. The Cy5-labeled precursor had peaks at 200 and 650 nm which correspond to dendrimer and Cy5 peaks respectively. The Cy5-labeled dendrimer-ALG-1001 conjugate had peaks at 200, 550, and 650 nm which correspond to dendrimer, Cy3, and Cy5 respectively and indicated successful conjugation of the Cy3-labeled peptide to the Cy5-labeled dendrimer; Figure S8: Quantification of vessel formation through image network analysis. Treatment with D-ALG and ALG-1001 at high doses result in statistically significant disruptions in vessel formation as measured through number of nodes, total length, and total isolated length; Figure S9: Quantification of in vitro wound healing assay. Growth of cell monolayer was analyzed 0 and 24 h after a scratch was introduced. Resultant change in monolayer area was normalized to the starting scratch area. Treatment with ALG-1001 and D-ALG result in statistically significant decrease in healing/proliferation rate of cells compared to the control; Figure S10: Expression of VEGF-A by human umbilical vein endothelial cells (HUVEC) was measured through qPCR. Statistical significance denote difference to the unstimulated and untreated cells (control). Stimulation with LPS induced a statistically significant increase in VEGF-A expression and treatment with ALG-1001 or D-ALG1001 attenuated the increase; Figure S11: In vivo inhibition of CNV formation via intravitreal injection. CNV area quantified using ImageJ. Dendrimer conjugation preserves the in vivo activity of ALG-1001 peptide when administered locally (intravitreally).

Author Contributions: Conceptualization, T.W. and R.M.K.; methodology, T.W., C.L., R.M.K.; software, T.W. and C.L.; validation, all authors; formal analysis, T.W. and C.L.; data curation, T.W. and C.L.; writing—review and editing, all authors; supervision, R.M.K.; project administration, R.M.K.; funding acquisition, R.M.K. All authors have read and agreed to the published version of the manuscript.

Funding: This research received no external funding.

Institutional Review Board Statement: The animal study protocol was approved by the Institutional Review Board of Johns Hopkins Institutional Animal Care and Use Committee (MO20M75, Date of Approval: 29 October 2020).

Informed Consent Statement: Not applicable.

Data Availability Statement: The data presented in this study are available on request from the corresponding author.

Conflicts of Interest: T.W and R.M.K. are co-inventors are patents relating to the compositions described in this manuscript.

References

1. Hobbs, S.D.; Pierce, K. Wet Age-related Macular Degeneration (Wet AMD). In *StatPearls*; StatPearls Publishing: Treasure Island, FL, USA, 2022.
2. Pugazhendhi, A.; Hubbell, M.; Jairam, P.; Ambati, B. Neovascular macular degeneration: A review of etiology, risk factors, and recent advances in research and therapy. *Int. J. Mol. Sci.* **2021**, *22*, 1170. [CrossRef]
3. Deng, Y.; Qiao, L.; Du, M.; Qu, C.; Wan, L.; Li, J.; Huang, L. Age-related macular degeneration: Epidemiology, genetics, pathophysiology, diagnosis, and targeted therapy. *Genes Dis.* **2022**, *9*, 62–79. [CrossRef] [PubMed]
4. Nowak, J.Z. Age-related macular degeneration (AMD): Pathogenesis and therapy. *Pharmacol. Rep.* **2006**, *58*, 353–363.
5. Chang, L.K.; Sarraf, D. Tears of the retinal pigment epithelium: An old problem in a new era. *Retina* **2007**, *27*, 523–534. [CrossRef]
6. Grossniklaus, H.E.; Green, W.R. Choroidal neovascularization. *Am. J. Ophthalmol.* **2004**, *137*, 496–503. [CrossRef]
7. Campochiaro, P.A. Ocular neovascularization. *J. Mol. Med.* **2013**, *91*, 311–321. [CrossRef]
8. Witmer, A.N.; Vrensen, G.F.J.M.; Van Noorden, C.J.F.; Schlingemann, R.O. Vascular endothelial growth factors and angiogenesis in eye disease. *Prog. Retin. Eye Res.* **2003**, *22*, 1–29. [CrossRef]
9. Miller, J.W.; Le Couter, J.; Strauss, E.C.; Ferrara, N. Vascular endothelial growth factor a in intraocular vascular disease. *Ophthalmology* **2013**, *120*, 106–114. [CrossRef] [PubMed]
10. Tobe, T.; Okamoto, N.; Vinores, M.A.; Derevjanik, N.L.; Vinores, S.A.; Zack, D.J.; Campochiaro, P.A. Evolution of neovascularization in mice with overexpression of vascular endothelial growth factor in photoreceptors. *Investig. Ophthalmol. Vis. Sci.* **1998**, *39*, 180–188.
11. Schlingemann, R.O. Role of growth factors and the wound healing response in age-related macular degeneration. *Graefes Arch. Clin. Exp. Ophthalmol.* **2004**, *242*, 91–101. [CrossRef] [PubMed]
12. Kovach, J.L.; Schwartz, S.G.; Flynn, H.W.; Scott, I.U. Anti-VEGF Treatment Strategies for Wet AMD. *J. Ophthalmol.* **2012**, *2012*, 786870. [CrossRef] [PubMed]
13. Avery, R.L.; Gordon, G.M. Systemic Safety of Prolonged Monthly Anti-Vascular Endothelial Growth Factor Therapy for Diabetic Macular Edema: A Systematic Review and Meta-analysis. *JAMA Ophthalmol.* **2016**, *134*, 21–29. [CrossRef] [PubMed]
14. Ohno-Matsui, K.; Ikuno, Y.; Lai, T.Y.Y.; Gemmy Cheung, C.M. Diagnosis and treatment guideline for myopic choroidal neovascularization due to pathologic myopia. *Prog. Retin. Eye Res.* **2018**, *63*, 92–106. [CrossRef]
15. Treatments for Wet AMD (Advanced Neovascular AMD) | National Eye Institute. Available online: https://www.nei.nih.gov/learn-about-eye-health/eye-conditions-and-diseases/age-related-macular-degeneration/wet-amd-type-late-age-related-macular-degeneration-read-about-treatments-wet-amd-anti-vegf (accessed on 6 May 2022).
16. Age-Related Macular Degeneration (AMD) | Johns Hopkins Medicine. Available online: https://www.hopkinsmedicine.org/health/conditions-and-diseases/agerelated-macular-degeneration-amd (accessed on 6 May 2022).
17. Mettu, P.S.; Allingham, M.J.; Cousins, S.W. Incomplete response to Anti-VEGF therapy in neovascular AMD: Exploring disease mechanisms and therapeutic opportunities. *Prog. Retin. Eye Res.* **2021**, *82*, 100906. [CrossRef]
18. Nagai, N.; Suzuki, M.; Uchida, A.; Kurihara, T.; Kamoshita, M.; Minami, S.; Shinoda, H.; Tsubota, K.; Ozawa, Y. Non-responsiveness to intravitreal aflibercept treatment in neovascular age-related macular degeneration: Implications of serous pigment epithelial detachment. *Sci. Rep.* **2016**, *6*, 29619. [CrossRef] [PubMed]
19. Gau, D.; Vignaud, L.; Francoeur, P.; Koes, D.; Guillonneau, X.; Roy, P. Inhibition of ocular neovascularization by novel anti-angiogenic compound. *Exp. Eye Res.* **2021**, *213*, 108861. [CrossRef]
20. Vogt, D.; Deiters, V.; Herold, T.R.; Guenther, S.R.; Kortuem, K.U.; Priglinger, S.G.; Wolf, A.; Schumann, R.G. Optimal Patient Adherence and Long-Term Treatment Outcomes of Neovascular Age-Related Macular Degeneration in Real-Life. *Curr. Eye Res.* **2022**, *47*, 889–896. [CrossRef]
21. Van Hove, I.; Hu, T.-T.; Beets, K.; Van Bergen, T.; Etienne, I.; Stitt, A.W.; Vermassen, E.; Feyen, J.H.M. Targeting RGD-binding integrins as an integrative therapy for diabetic retinopathy and neovascular age-related macular degeneration. *Prog. Retin. Eye Res.* **2021**, *85*, 100966. [CrossRef]
22. Bhatwadekar, A.D.; Kansara, V.; Luo, Q.; Ciulla, T. Anti-integrin therapy for retinovascular diseases. *Expert Opin. Investig. Drugs* **2020**, *29*, 935–945. [CrossRef]
23. Wolf, A.T.; Harris, A.; Oddone, F.; Siesky, B.; Verticchio Vercellin, A.; Ciulla, T.A. Disease progression pathways of wet AMD: Opportunities for new target discovery. *Expert Opin. Ther. Targets* **2022**, *26*, 5–12. [CrossRef]
24. Hu, T.-T.; Vanhove, M.; Porcu, M.; Van Hove, I.; Van Bergen, T.; Jonckx, B.; Barbeaux, P.; Vermassen, E.; Feyen, J.H.M. The potent small molecule integrin antagonist THR-687 is a promising next-generation therapy for retinal vascular disorders. *Exp. Eye Res.* **2019**, *180*, 43–52. [CrossRef] [PubMed]
25. Wang, Y.; Xiao, W.; Zhang, Y.; Meza, L.; Tseng, H.; Takada, Y.; Ames, J.B.; Lam, K.S. Optimization of RGD-Containing Cyclic Peptides against $\alpha v\beta 3$ Integrin. *Mol. Cancer Ther.* **2016**, *15*, 232–240. [CrossRef]

26. Wang, W.; Wang, F.; Lu, F.; Xu, S.; Hu, W.; Huang, J.; Gu, Q.; Sun, X. The antiangiogenic effects of integrin alpha5beta1 inhibitor (ATN-161) in vitro and in vivo. *Investig. Ophthalmol. Vis. Sci.* **2011**, *52*, 7213–7220. [CrossRef]
27. Chappelow, A.V.; Kaiser, P.K. Neovascular age-related macular degeneration: Potential therapies. *Drugs* **2008**, *68*, 1029–1036. [CrossRef]
28. Shaw, L.T.; Mackin, A.; Shah, R.; Jain, S.; Jain, P.; Nayak, R.; Hariprasad, S.M. Risuteganib-a novel integrin inhibitor for the treatment of non-exudative (dry) age-related macular degeneration and diabetic macular edema. *Expert Opin. Investig. Drugs* **2020**, *29*, 547–554. [CrossRef]
29. Joshi, P.; Chung, C.Y.; Aukhil, I.; Erickson, H.P. Endothelial cells adhere to the RGD domain and the fibrinogen-like terminal knob of tenascin. *J. Cell Sci.* **1993**, *106 Pt 1*, 389–400. [CrossRef]
30. Fibronectin and Integrin. Available online: https://www.ks.uiuc.edu/Research/fibronectin/ (accessed on 2 April 2021).
31. Maturi, R.; Jaffe, G.J.; Ehlers, J.P.; Kaiser, P.K.; Boyer, D.S.; Heier, J.S.; Kornfield, J.A.; Kuppermann, B.D.; Quiroz-Mercado, H.; Aubel, J.; et al. Safety and Efficacy of Risuteganib in Intermediate Non-exudative Age-Related Macular Degeneration. *Investig. Ophthalmol. Vis. Sci.* **2020**, *61*, 1944.
32. Zhou, D.; Chwa, M.; Shao, Z.; Koo, J.M.; Park, J.Y.; Karageozian, H.L.; Karageozian, V.H.; Kenney, C.M.; Kornfield, J.A. Mechanism of Action of Risuteganib for Retinal Diseases through Protection of Retinal Pigment Epithelium (RPE) and Enhancement of Mitochondrial Functions. *Investig. Ophthalmol. Vis. Sci.* **2020**, *61*, 4949.
33. Mandal, A.; Pal, D.; Agrahari, V.; Trinh, H.M.; Joseph, M.; Mitra, A.K. Ocular delivery of proteins and peptides: Challenges and novel formulation approaches. *Adv. Drug Deliv. Rev.* **2018**, *126*, 67–95. [CrossRef] [PubMed]
34. Varela-Fernández, R.; Díaz-Tomé, V.; Luaces-Rodríguez, A.; Conde-Penedo, A.; García-Otero, X.; Luzardo-Álvarez, A.; Fernández-Ferreiro, A.; Otero-Espinar, F.J. Drug delivery to the posterior segment of the eye: Biopharmaceutic and pharmacokinetic considerations. *Pharmaceutics* **2020**, *12*, 269. [CrossRef]
35. Zarei, M.; Roohipoor, R.; Mahmoudzadeh, R.; Yaseri, M.; Riazi-Esfahani, H. Epidemiology of intravitreal injections in iran: Indications and referral patterns in a tertiary hospital. *Clin. Ophthalmol.* **2020**, *14*, 1201–1206. [CrossRef]
36. Falavarjani, K.G.; Nguyen, Q.D. Adverse events and complications associated with intravitreal injection of anti-VEGF agents: A review of literature. *Eye* **2013**, *27*, 787–794. [CrossRef]
37. Nagai, H.; Hirano, Y.; Yoshida, M.; Ogura, Y. Incidence of the Complications After Intravitreal Injections. *Investig. Ophthalmol. Vis. Sci.* **2010**, *51*, 5120.
38. Miller, A.; Wilneff, M.A.; Yazji, A.; Petrinec, E.; Carbone, M.; Miller, C.; McCrossin, C.; Donkor, R.; Miller, D.G. Analysis of urgent follow up visits and complications after intravitreal injections: A retrospective cohort study. *Int. J. Retina Vitreous* **2022**, *8*, 8. [CrossRef]
39. Jonas, J.B.; Spandau, U.H.; Schlichtenbrede, F. Short-term complications of intravitreal injections of triamcinolone and bevacizumab. *Eye* **2008**, *22*, 590–591. [CrossRef] [PubMed]
40. Kambhampati, S.P.; Bhutto, I.A.; Wu, T.; Ho, K.; McLeod, D.S.; Lutty, G.A.; Kannan, R.M. Systemic dendrimer nanotherapies for targeted suppression of choroidal inflammation and neovascularization in age-related macular degeneration. *J. Control. Release* **2021**, *335*, 527–540. [CrossRef] [PubMed]
41. Arteaga Cabeza, O.; Zhang, Z.; Smith Khoury, E.; Sheldon, R.A.; Sharma, A.; Zhang, F.; Slusher, B.S.; Kannan, R.M.; Kannan, S.; Ferriero, D.M. Neuroprotective effects of a dendrimer-based glutamate carboxypeptidase inhibitor on superoxide dismutase transgenic mice after neonatal hypoxic-ischemic brain injury. *Neurobiol. Dis.* **2021**, *148*, 105201. [CrossRef] [PubMed]
42. Emmerich, K.B.; White, D.T.; Kambhamptati, S.P.; Lee, G.Y.; Fu, T.-M.; Sahoo, A.; Saxena, M.T.; Betzig, E.; Kannan, R.M.; Mumm, J.S. Dendrimer-targeted immunosuppression of microglia reactivity super-accelerates photoreceptor regeneration in the zebrafish retina. *bioRxiv* **2020**. [CrossRef]
43. DeRidder, L.; Sharma, A.; Liaw, K.; Sharma, R.; John, J.; Kannan, S.; Kannan, R.M. Dendrimer-tesaglitazar conjugate induces a phenotype shift of microglia and enhances β-amyloid phagocytosis. *Nanoscale* **2021**, *13*, 939–952. [CrossRef] [PubMed]
44. Liaw, K.; Reddy, R.; Sharma, A.; Li, J.; Chang, M.; Sharma, R.; Salazar, S.; Kannan, S.; Kannan, R.M. Targeted systemic dendrimer delivery of CSF-1R inhibitor to tumor-associated macrophages improves outcomes in orthotopic glioblastoma. *Bioeng. Transl. Med.* **2021**, *6*, e10205. [CrossRef] [PubMed]
45. Kannan, R.M.; Pitha, I.; Parikh, K.S. A new era in posterior segment ocular drug delivery: Translation of systemic, cell-targeted, dendrimer-based therapies. *Adv. Drug Deliv. Rev.* **2023**, *200*, 115005. [CrossRef]
46. Zhang, F.; Trent Magruder, J.; Lin, Y.-A.; Crawford, T.C.; Grimm, J.C.; Sciortino, C.M.; Wilson, M.A.; Blue, M.E.; Kannan, S.; Johnston, M.V.; et al. Generation-6 hydroxyl PAMAM dendrimers improve CNS penetration from intravenous administration in a large animal brain injury model. *J. Control. Release* **2017**, *249*, 173–182. [CrossRef]
47. Zhang, F.; Nance, E.; Alnasser, Y.; Kannan, R.; Kannan, S. Microglial migration and interactions with dendrimer nanoparticles are altered in the presence of neuroinflammation. *J. Neuroinflamm.* **2016**, *13*, 65. [CrossRef]
48. Nance, E.; Zhang, F.; Mishra, M.K.; Zhang, Z.; Kambhampati, S.P.; Kannan, R.M.; Kannan, S. Nanoscale effects in dendrimer-mediated targeting of neuroinflammation. *Biomaterials* **2016**, *101*, 96–107. [CrossRef]
49. Gusdon, A.M.; Faraday, N.; Aita, J.S.; Kumar, S.; Mehta, I.; Choi, H.A.; Cleland, J.L.; Robinson, K.; McCullough, L.D.; Ng, D.K.; et al. Dendrimer nanotherapy for severe COVID-19 attenuates inflammation and neurological injury markers and improves outcomes in a phase2a clinical trial. *Sci. Transl. Med.* **2022**, *14*, eabo2652. [CrossRef] [PubMed]

50. Jeong, W.-J.; Bu, J.; Mickel, P.; Han, Y.; Rawding, P.A.; Wang, J.; Kang, H.; Hong, H.; Král, P.; Hong, S. Dendrimer-Peptide Conjugates for Effective Blockade of the Interactions between SARS-CoV-2 Spike Protein and Human ACE2 Receptor. *Biomacromolecules* **2023**, *24*, 141–149. [CrossRef] [PubMed]
51. Yang, B.S.; Mallick, S.; Kwon, Y.-E.; Kim, Y.-J.; Kim, G.H.; Choi, J.S. PAMAM Dendrimer Conjugated with Cell-penetrating Peptide-derived Oligopeptides for Enhanced Cell Uptake and Gene Delivery. *Bull. Korean Chem. Soc.* **2015**, *36*, 2477–2483. [CrossRef]
52. Chi, L.A.; Asgharpour, S.; Correa-Basurto, J.; Bandala, C.R.; Martínez-Archundia, M. Unveiling the G4-PAMAM capacity to bind and protect Ang-(1-7) bioactive peptide by molecular dynamics simulations. *J. Comput. Aided Mol. Des.* **2022**, *36*, 653–675. [CrossRef] [PubMed]
53. Liyanage, W.; Wu, T.; Kannan, S.; Kannan, R.M. Dendrimer-siRNA Conjugates for Targeted Intracellular Delivery in Glioblastoma Animal Models. *ACS Appl. Mater. Interfaces* **2022**, *14*, 46290–46303. [CrossRef]
54. Lee, J.W.; Han, S.C.; Ji, W.H.; Jin, S.-H.; Kim, J.H. Synthesis of diblock codendrimer by double click chemistry. *Bull. Korean Chem. Soc.* **2012**, *33*, 4103–4108. [CrossRef]
55. Arseneault, M.; Wafer, C.; Morin, J.-F. Recent advances in click chemistry applied to dendrimer synthesis. *Molecules* **2015**, *20*, 9263–9294. [CrossRef] [PubMed]
56. Samarasimhareddy, M.; Shamir, M.; Shalev, D.E.; Hurevich, M.; Friedler, A. A rapid and efficient building block approach for click cyclization of peptoids. *Front. Chem.* **2020**, *8*, 405. [CrossRef] [PubMed]
57. Ahmad Fuaad, A.A.H.; Azmi, F.; Skwarczynski, M.; Toth, I. Peptide conjugation via CuAAC "click" chemistry. *Molecules* **2013**, *18*, 13148–13174. [CrossRef]
58. Li, H.; Aneja, R.; Chaiken, I. Click chemistry in peptide-based drug design. *Molecules* **2013**, *18*, 9797–9817. [CrossRef] [PubMed]
59. Hollinger, K.R.; Sharma, A.; Tallon, C.; Lovell, L.; Thomas, A.G.; Zhu, X.; Wiseman, R.; Wu, Y.; Kambhampati, S.P.; Liaw, K.; et al. Dendrimer-2PMPA selectively blocks upregulated microglial GCPII activity and improves cognition in a mouse model of multiple sclerosis. *Nanotheranostics* **2022**, *6*, 126–142. [CrossRef]
60. Tang, W.; Becker, M.L. "Click" reactions: A versatile toolbox for the synthesis of peptide-conjugates. *Chem. Soc. Rev.* **2014**, *43*, 7013–7039. [CrossRef]
61. Freimann, K.; Arukuusk, P.; Kurrikoff, K.; Pärnaste, L.; Raid, R.; Piirsoo, A.; Pooga, M.; Langel, Ü. Formulation of Stable and Homogeneous Cell-Penetrating Peptide NF55 Nanoparticles for Efficient Gene Delivery In Vivo. *Mol. Ther. Nucleic Acids* **2018**, *10*, 28–35. [CrossRef]
62. Liaw, K.; Zhang, F.; Mangraviti, A.; Kannan, S.; Tyler, B.; Kannan, R.M. Dendrimer size effects on the selective brain tumor targeting in orthotopic tumor models upon systemic administration. *Bioeng. Transl. Med.* **2020**, *5*, e10160. [CrossRef]
63. McGregor, D.P. Discovering and improving novel peptide therapeutics. *Curr. Opin. Pharmacol.* **2008**, *8*, 616–619. [CrossRef]
64. Weinstock, M.T.; Francis, J.N.; Redman, J.S.; Kay, M.S. Protease-resistant peptide design-empowering nature's fragile warriors against HIV. *Biopolymers* **2012**, *98*, 431–442. [CrossRef]
65. Lei, R.; Hou, J.; Chen, Q.; Yuan, W.; Cheng, B.; Sun, Y.; Jin, Y.; Ge, L.; Ben-Sasson, S.A.; Chen, J.; et al. Self-Assembling Myristoylated Human α-Defensin 5 as a Next-Generation Nanobiotics Potentiates Therapeutic Efficacy in Bacterial Infection. *ACS Nano* **2018**, *12*, 5284–5296. [CrossRef]
66. DeCicco-Skinner, K.L.; Henry, G.H.; Cataisson, C.; Tabib, T.; Gwilliam, J.C.; Watson, N.J.; Bullwinkle, E.M.; Falkenburg, L.; O'Neill, R.C.; Morin, A.; et al. Endothelial cell tube formation assay for the in vitro study of angiogenesis. *J. Vis. Exp.* **2014**, *91*, e51312. [CrossRef]
67. Liang, C.-C.; Park, A.Y.; Guan, J.-L. In vitro scratch assay: A convenient and inexpensive method for analysis of cell migration in vitro. *Nat. Protoc.* **2007**, *2*, 329–333. [CrossRef]
68. Yarrow, J.C.; Perlman, Z.E.; Westwood, N.J.; Mitchison, T.J. A high-throughput cell migration assay using scratch wound healing, a comparison of image-based readout methods. *BMC Biotechnol.* **2004**, *4*, 21. [CrossRef] [PubMed]
69. Abbi, S.; Ueda, H.; Zheng, C.; Cooper, L.A.; Zhao, J.; Christopher, R.; Guan, J.-L. Regulation of focal adhesion kinase by a novel protein inhibitor FIP200. *Mol. Biol. Cell* **2002**, *13*, 3178–3191. [CrossRef]
70. Underwood, P.A.; Bean, P.A.; Gamble, J.R. Rate of endothelial expansion is controlled by cell:cell adhesion. *Int. J. Biochem. Cell Biol.* **2002**, *34*, 55–69. [CrossRef] [PubMed]
71. Jonkman, J.E.N.; Cathcart, J.A.; Xu, F.; Bartolini, M.E.; Amon, J.E.; Stevens, K.M.; Colarusso, P. An introduction to the wound healing assay using live-cell microscopy. *Cell Adh. Migr.* **2014**, *8*, 440–451. [CrossRef] [PubMed]
72. Lambert, V.; Lecomte, J.; Hansen, S.; Blacher, S.; Gonzalez, M.-L.A.; Struman, I.; Sounni, N.E.; Rozet, E.; de Tullio, P.; Foidart, J.M.; et al. Laser-induced choroidal neovascularization model to study age-related macular degeneration in mice. *Nat. Protoc.* **2013**, *8*, 2197–2211. [CrossRef]
73. Fabian-Jessing, B.K.; Jakobsen, T.S.; Jensen, E.G.; Alsing, S.; Hansen, S.; Aagaard, L.; Askou, A.L.; Bek, T.; Corydon, T.J. Animal models of choroidal neovascularization: A systematic review. *Investig. Ophthalmol. Vis. Sci.* **2022**, *63*, 11. [CrossRef]
74. Shah, R.S.; Soetikno, B.T.; Lajko, M.; Fawzi, A.A. A Mouse Model for Laser-induced Choroidal Neovascularization. *J. Vis. Exp.* **2015**, *106*, e53502. [CrossRef]
75. Umeda, N.; Kachi, S.; Akiyama, H.; Zahn, G.; Vossmeyer, D.; Stragies, R.; Campochiaro, P.A. Suppression and regression of choroidal neovascularization by systemic administration of an alpha5beta1 integrin antagonist. *Mol. Pharmacol.* **2006**, *69*, 1820–1828. [CrossRef] [PubMed]

76. Koh, H.J.; Bessho, K.; Cheng, L.; Bartsch, D.-U.; Jones, T.R.; Bergeron-Lynn, G.; Freeman, W.R. Inhibition of choroidal neovascularization in rats by the urokinase-derived peptide A6. *Investig. Ophthalmol. Vis. Sci.* **2004**, *45*, 635–640. [CrossRef] [PubMed]
77. Toriyama, Y.; Iesato, Y.; Imai, A.; Sakurai, T.; Kamiyoshi, A.; Ichikawa-Shindo, Y.; Kawate, H.; Yamauchi, A.; Igarashi, K.; Tanaka, M.; et al. Pathophysiological function of endogenous calcitonin gene-related peptide in ocular vascular diseases. *Am. J. Pathol.* **2015**, *185*, 1783–1794. [CrossRef] [PubMed]

pharmaceutics

MDPI

Review

Dendritic Structures Functionalized with Boron Clusters, in Particular Carboranes, and Their Biological Properties †

Anne-Marie Caminade [1,2,*], Max Milewski [1,2,3] and Evamarie Hey-Hawkins [3]

1 Laboratoire de Chimie de Coordination (LCC-CNRS) 205 Route de Narbonne, CEDEX 4, 31077 Toulouse, France; max.milewski@lcc-toulouse.fr
2 LCC-CNRS, Université de Toulouse, CNRS, 31077 Toulouse, France
3 Faculty of Chemistry and Mineralogy, Institute of Inorganic Chemistry, Leipzig University, Johannisallee 29, 04103 Leipzig, Germany; mm41cety@studserv.uni-leipzig.de or hey@rz.uni-leipzig.de
* Correspondence: anne-marie.caminade@lcc-toulouse.fr

† Dedicated to the 85th Anniversary of Donald A. Tomalia.

Abstract: The presence of a large number of boron atoms in boron clusters make them attractive tools for the treatment of cancer using boron neutron capture therapy (BNCT). Since the quantity of boron atoms present in the target cell directly affects the effectiveness of BNCT, the idea of gathering a high number of boron atoms in a single entity has emerged many years ago. In this perspective, using hyper-branched macromolecules such as dendrimers appears as an interesting solution. In this review, we will first present the synthesis of diverse dendritic entities (dendrimers, dendrons, and Janus dendrimers) that incorporate boron clusters, in particular carboranes, anywhere in their structure. Four parts of this review present the synthesis of dendrimers having boron clusters on the surface, or inside their structure, of dendrons and of Janus dendrimers, bearing boron clusters. Practically all these boronated dendritic structures were synthesized with the objective to study their biological properties, but in fact only a few of them have been tested against cancerous cells, and even a smaller number was tested in BNCT experiments. The biological experiments are discussed in the fifth part of this review. A good efficiency is generally observed with the boronated dendrimers, even in animal models, with an increase in their mean survival time (MST).

Keywords: boron clusters; carborane; dendrimer; boron neutron capture therapy (BNCT); cancer

1. Introduction

Boron clusters display a wide range of structures and intriguing properties. They have been used as materials, but also as antiseptic, antiviral, antitumor, and antifungal agents [1]. Carboranes (*closo*-dicarbadodecaboranes, also named carbaboranes) are a special class of boron clusters composed of two CR groups (R = mainly H) included in a $B_{10}H_{10}$ cluster [2]. The very first papers in the field of carboranes were published in 1963 [3,4]. They displayed the synthesis of *ortho*-carborane, by reaction of $B_{10}H_{14}$ with acetylene, in the presence of a Lewis base. Other isomers of $B_{10}C_2H_{12}$ can be obtained by thermal rearrangement of the *ortho* isomer in an autoclave under inert conditions. The *meta* isomer is irreversibly obtained upon heating to 465–500 °C [5], whereas the *para* isomer is obtained at temperatures above 615 °C, but this latter reaction is reversible [6] (Scheme 1).

Carboranes display a rich chemistry, at the level of the C−H groups, but also in some cases at the level of B−H groups. The chemistry of carboranes has been reviewed [7,8], in particular with emphasis on their biological properties [9]. Indeed, the large number of boron atoms present in these boron clusters made them desirable instruments for cancer treatment using boron neutron capture therapy (BNCT). The starting materials for BNCT are based on ^{10}B, which is a nonradioactive constituent of the natural elemental boron. Irradiation of ^{10}B with low energy thermal neutrons yields high linear energy transfer (LET) α particles (^{4}He) and recoiling ^{7}Li nuclei [10] (Scheme 2).

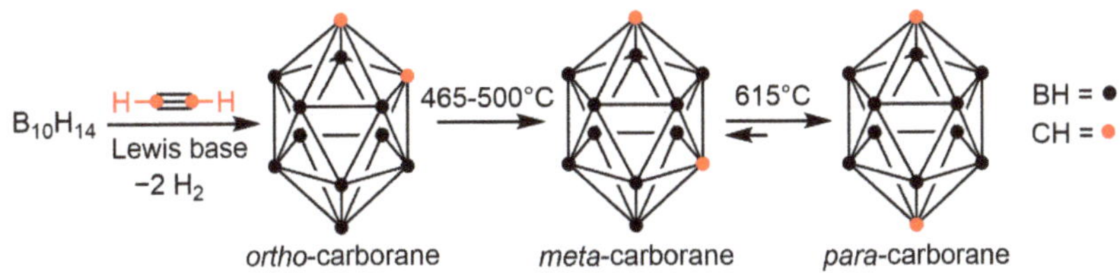

Scheme 1. Synthesis of *ortho-*, *meta-*, and *para*-carborane (1,2-, 1,7-, and 1,12-*closo*-dicarbadodecaborane, respectively).

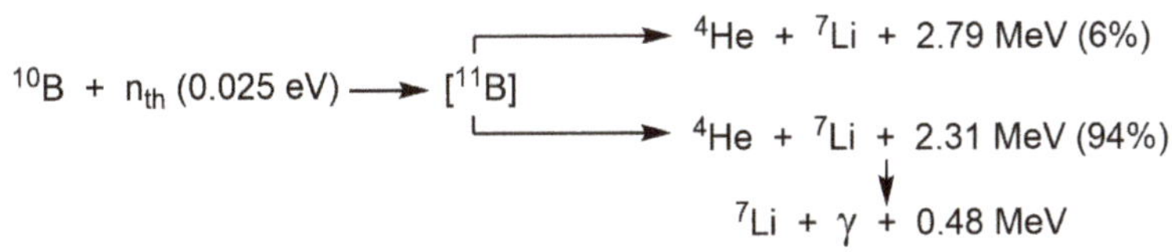

Scheme 2. Reaction of ^{10}B with low energy thermal neutrons used in BNCT.

In order to sustain a deadly $^{10}B(n,\alpha)^{7}Li$ capture reaction, enough thermal neutrons must be captured by ^{10}B (neutron capture cross-section is 3840 barn) to produce the high LET particles due to their constrained path lengths in tissues (5–9 μm). For this reason, a sufficient amount of ^{10}B must be delivered to the tumor ($\approx$20 μg/g or $\approx 10^9$ atoms/cell), making boron clusters appealing delivery systems for this purpose. In particular, sodium borocaptate ($Na_2B_{12}H_{11}SH$) and *p*-boronophenylalanine (BPA), have been used in BNCT clinical studies [11].

Having more boron atoms in close proximity should increase the efficiency of BNCT. Dendrimers appear as a perfect solution. Indeed, dendrimers are hyper-branched macromolecules synthesized step-by-step, generally by a divergent process from a multifunctional core [12], having a large number of functions on their surface, which can be modified at will. The name "dendrimer" was coined by Donald A. Tomalia [13], to whom this review is dedicated, in gratitude for his inspiring work. He created the PAMAM dendrimers (PolyAMidoAMine), which are the most popular type of dendrimers [14].

Several reviews have already gathered some aspects of boron clusters linked to dendrimers, especially carboranes, but either the review is limited to the work produced by the authors of the review, and contains small molecules or cobalt derivatives (cobalt bis(dicarbollide) (or COSAN) derivatives) together with dendrimers [15–17], or dendrimers are only a part of the review [18–20], or only a small part of the review about dendrimers concerns boron clusters [21].

In this original review, we will present boron clusters, especially carboranes, anywhere in the structure of dendritic compounds, i.e., dendrimers and dendrons (dendritic wedges). We will consider only compounds in which the number of terminal functions is superior to the number of branches emanating from the core, as illustrated in Figure 1. This review is organized depending on the location of the boron clusters: on the surface of dendrimers (case A), at one or several layers inside the structure of dendrimers (case B), at the core or the surface of dendrons (case C), and on part of the surface of Janus dendrimers (case D). A last part will concern the biological properties (mainly but not exclusively for BNCT) of the dendritic compounds displayed in the previous parts.

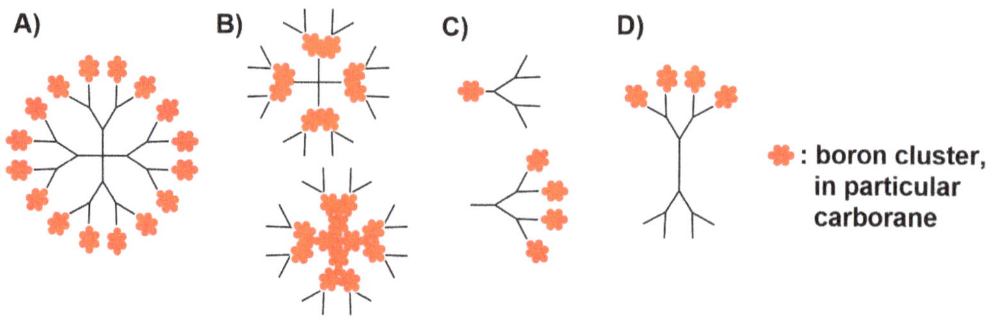

Figure 1. Different locations of boron clusters in dendritic compounds: surface of dendrimers (**A**), branches of dendrimers (**B**), core or surface of dendrons (**C**), and part of the surface of Janus dendrimers (**D**).

2. Boron Clusters on the Surface of Dendrimers

Different types of dendrimers have been functionalized with boron clusters on their surface. This part will be organized depending on the type of the internal structure. The first, most widely used, and oldest examples concern PAMAM dendrimers. Other examples concern carbosilane dendrimers, dendrimers having a porphyrin or a phenylene core, and miscellaneous types of dendrimers.

2.1. Boronated PAMAM Dendrimers

Second and fourth generation PAMAM dendrimers, bearing 12 (generation 2) or 48 (generation 4) NH_2 surface functions have been functionalized with the isocyanato polyhedral borane shown in Scheme 3, affording the dendrimer **1a-G4** for the fourth generation. Analyses indicated that only some NH_2 groups reacted, thus some of the remaining NH_2 groups were used for the stochastic grafting of *m*-maleimidobenzoyl *N*-hydroxysulfosuccinimide ester, suitable for further reactions. For instance, the grafting to a monoclonal antibody (MoAb IB 16-6, which is directed against the murine B16 melanoma), afforded dendrimer **1b-G4**. A total of 8150 atoms of boron per molecule of antibody were measured, showing that in fact several dendrimers were grafted per MoAb unit [22].

Analogous types of reactions were carried out for the grafting of epidermal growth factor [23], folic acid and PEG (polyethylene glycol of variable length) [24], or vascular endothelial growth factor [25] to boronated PAMAM dendrimers. These dendrimers and related boronated PAMAM dendrimers bearing different types of MoAb were essentially synthesized for studying their biological properties, as will be discussed in Part 5 of this review.

2.2. Boronated Carbosilane Dendrimers

Contrarily to PAMAM dendrimers, which have been functionalized stochastically with boron clusters, carbosilane dendrimers have been functionalized on all their terminal functions with only *ortho*-carboranes. Different types of reactions have been used. In a first example, the carborane was first functionalized with a methyl or phenyl group on one carbon atom, and then with an alkyl-SiH function, which adds to the vinyl groups of carbosilane dendrimers, using the Karstedt catalyst (platinum derivative of divinyl disiloxane). The first generation **2-G1** was isolated in about 60% yield (Scheme 4) [26].

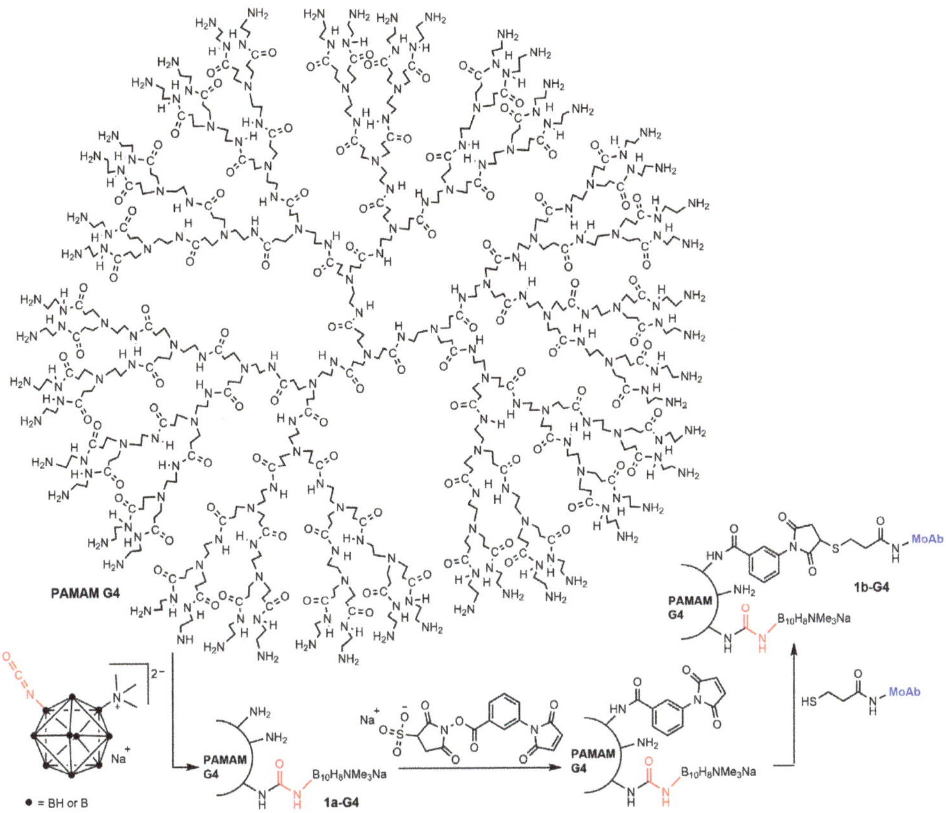

Scheme 3. Full chemical structure of a generation 4 PAMAM dendrimer, and the stochastic grafting of B_{10} boron clusters and of a monoclonal antibody (MoAb) on its surface.

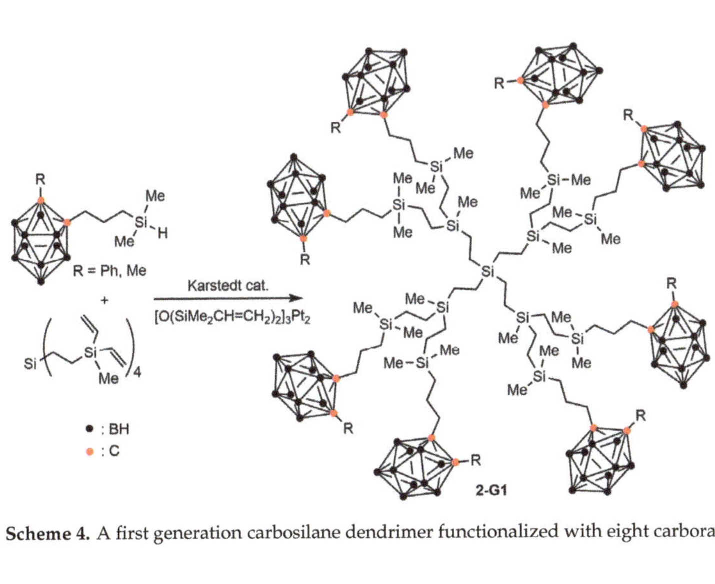

Scheme 4. A first generation carbosilane dendrimer functionalized with eight carboranes.

Larger boronated carbosilane dendrimers were synthesized by Copper(I)-catalyzed Huisgen-type azide-alkyne click cycloaddition reactions (CuAAC). The carborane was functionalized with a methyl group and an ethynyl group. The carbosilane dendrimers, from generation 0 to generation 3, were functionalized with azides as terminal functions. The CuAAC reaction afforded the expected dendrimers **3-G1** (nine carboranes) to **3-G3** (eighty-one carboranes) in about 80% yield. Scheme 5 displays the full structure of the first generation, and the linear structure with parentheses after each branching point for the third generation. Attempts to synthesize higher-generation dendrimers yielded insoluble materials. These dendrimers are particularly thermally stable, with only 10% mass loss at temperatures up to 392 °C for dendrimer **3-G3**. Low intensity emissions were observed between 280 and 480 nm with these carborane dendrimers [27].

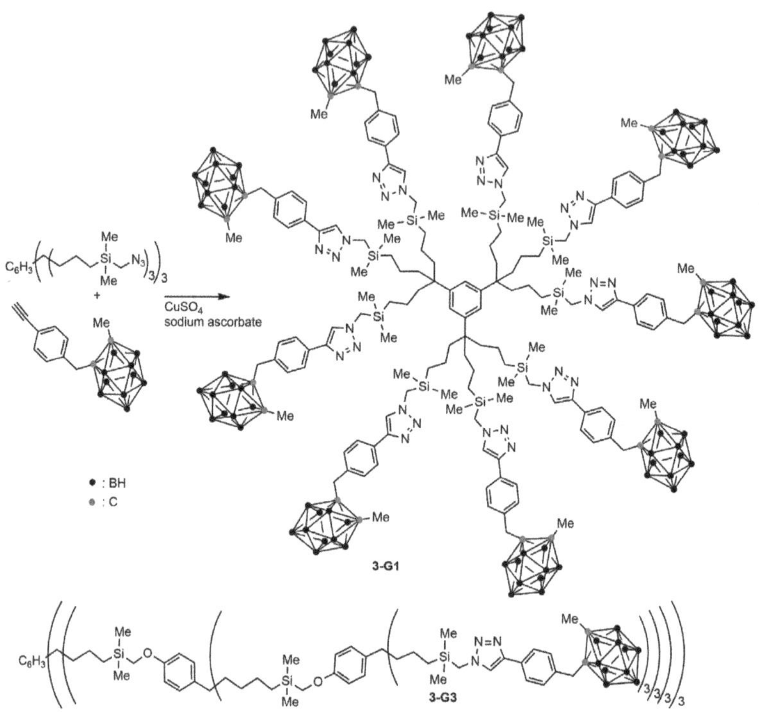

Scheme 5. Carbosilane dendrimers functionalized with carboranes by CuAAC click reactions.

A larger family of boronated carbosilane dendrimers was obtained from a carborane in which the carbon atoms were not used for the grafting to the dendrimers, contrarily to the previous cases. Hydrothiolation of carbosilane dendrimers capped with allyl groups and with 9-mercapto-*meta*-carborane initiated by UV irradiation in the presence of 2,2-dimethoxy-2-phenylacetophenone (DMPA) afforded carborane−carbosilane dendrimers of the zero, first, third, and fifth generations in about 60% yield. The full structure of the first generation **4-G1** and the linear structure with parentheses of the fifth generation **4-G5** are displayed in Scheme 6 [28]. The thermal properties and the rheological behavior of these dendrimers in relation with analogous polymers were recently compared [29].

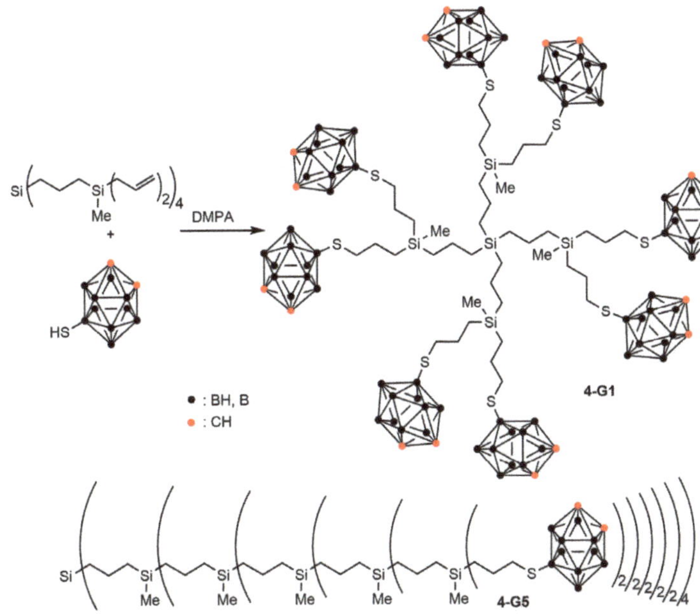

Scheme 6. Carborane–carbosilane dendrimers functionalized by hydrothiolation.

2.3. Boronated Dendrimers Having a Porphyrin Core

A series of different carborane dendrimers bearing a porphyrin as core were synthesized as shown in Scheme 7. In these cases, a kind of divergent synthetic process was used as two carboranes were first linked to a benzaldehyde derivative. This was then used in condensation reactions with dipyrromethene in the presence of trifluoroacetic acid (TFA), to afford the porphyrin **5a-G1** functionalized with four carboranes, in 34% yield. Addition of $ZnCl_2$ afforded the corresponding zinc complex **5b-G1** (Scheme 7, way A). Both the free porphyrin and the complex are insoluble in water, but they can be easily converted into the corresponding water-soluble *nido*-carboranylporphyrins by base degradation with pyridine/piperidine, followed by cation exchange with a Dowex resin [30]. An analogous process was applied to pyrrole instead of dipyrromethene, affording the porphyrin **6a-G1** functionalized with eight carboranes, isolated in 15% yield (Scheme 7, way B). The complexation of zinc (compound **6b-G1**) and the degradation to obtain water-soluble *nido*-carborane derivatives was carried out with compounds **6a,b-G1**, as was carried out for compound **5-G1** [31].

Another series of porphyrin-cored carborane dendrimers was synthesized in a different way, by grafting the carboranes to the surface of porphyrin dendrimers. Generations 0 (four carboranes), 1 (eight carboranes), 2 (sixteen carboranes), and 3 (thirty-two carboranes) were synthesized by a regioselective hydrosilylation reaction on the allyl functions of the dendrimers, with carboranylsilanes in the presence of the Karstedt catalyst, as illustrated for generation 2 (**7-G2**) in Scheme 8. All the carboranyl–carbosilane dendrimers were isolated in good to excellent yields in the range of 60–88%. Studying the photoluminescence properties revealed that the photoluminescence characteristics of the porphyrin core are unaffected by the presence of carboranes [32].

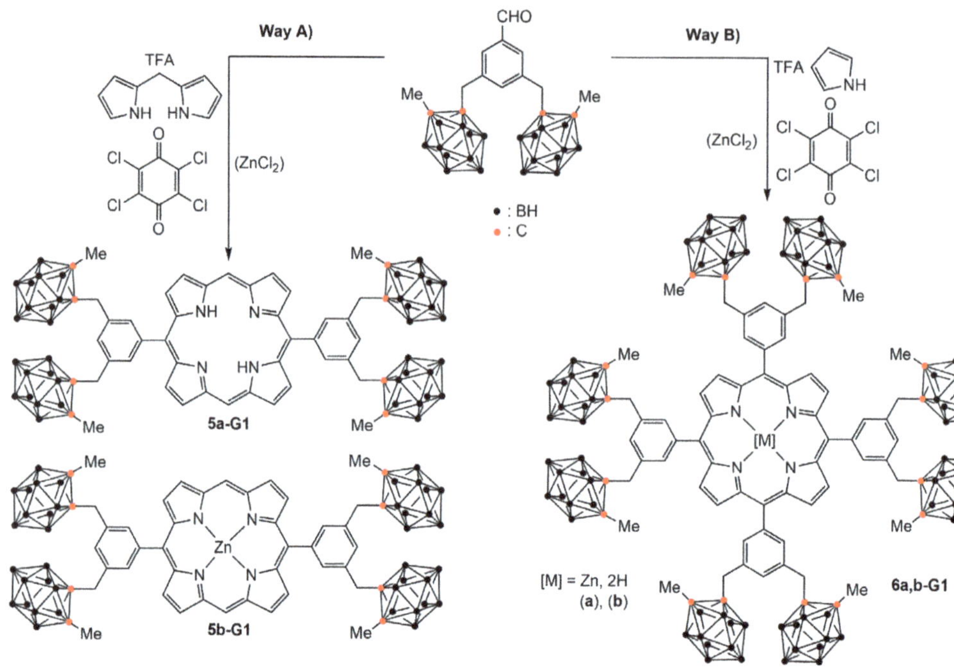

Scheme 7. Porphyrin-cored first generation carborane dendrimers, either free (b) or complexing Zn (a).

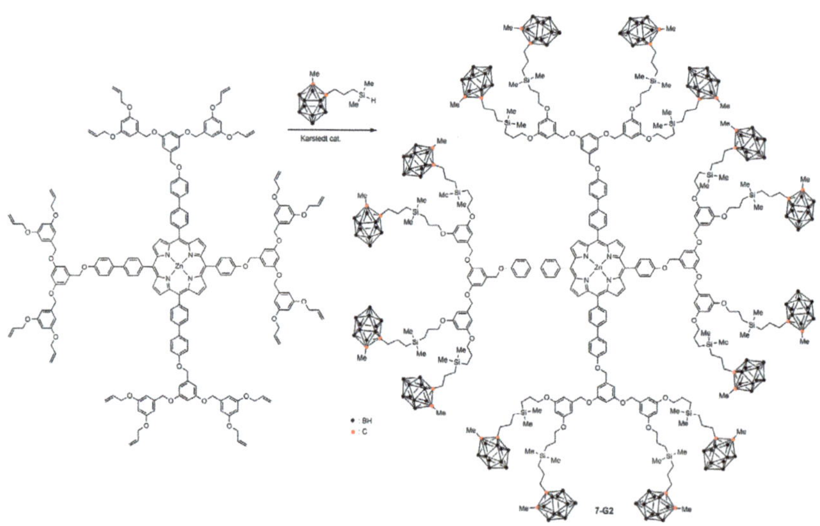

Scheme 8. Synthesis of a generation 2 carborane dendrimer built from a porphyrin core. Generations 0, 1, and 3 were also synthesized.

2.4. Boronated Dendrimers Having a Phenylene Core

As in the case of the porphyrin core, boronated dendrimers having a phenylene core were synthesized by a convergent method or by a divergent process. In the first method, a trimerization reaction of arylketones bearing two carborane units mediated by silicon tetrachloride afforded the first generation dendrimers **8a,b-G1** in 55% (**a**) and 40% (**b**) yield, respectively (Scheme 9). In order to have water-soluble compounds, alcoholic NaOH was used to induce the removal of one of the vertex boron atoms to yield a monoanionic *nido*-carborane [33].

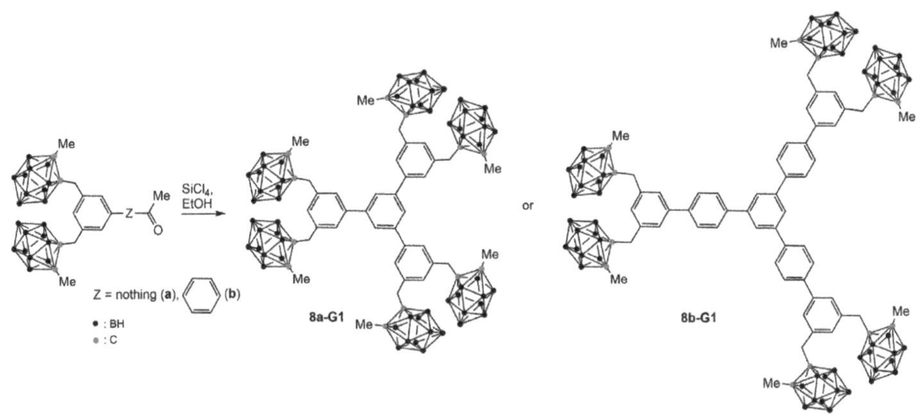

Scheme 9. Trimerization of a ketone for the synthesis of first generation carborane dendrimers.

Another family of boronated dendrimers was obtained by CuAAC reactions between a dendrimer having six or nine alkyne functions and a carborane functionalized with an azide. Dendrimer **9a-G1** bearing six carborane units was isolated in 78% yield, whereas dendrimer **9b-G1** bearing nine carborane units was isolated in 76% yield (Scheme 10) [34].

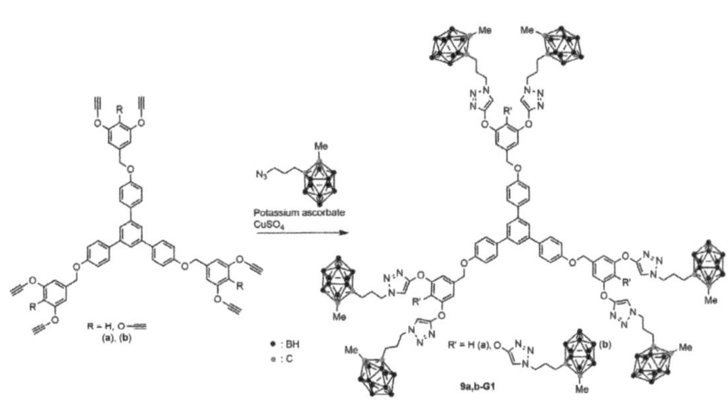

Scheme 10. Synthesis of first generation carborane dendrimers obtained by CuAAC reactions, bearing either six (**9a-G1**) or nine (**9b-G1**) carboranes.

Four different carborane dendrimers (**10a-d-G1**) were obtained by hydrosilylation reactions between carboranes functionalized with a silane, and a dendrimer bearing nine allyl groups. They were isolated with yields in the range of 60–85% (Scheme 11). The removal of one boron vertex from each cluster leads to water-soluble macromolecules. Photoluminescent properties with high quantum yields, but depending on the nature of the clusters, were observed [35].

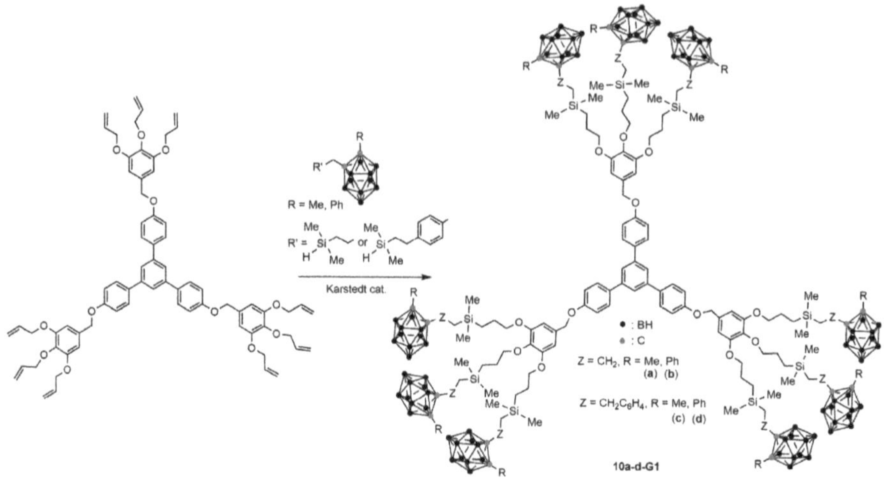

Scheme 11. Hydrosilylation reactions for the synthesis of first generation carborane dendrimers **10a-G1** (Z = CH_2, R = Me), **10b-G1** (Z = CH_2, R = Ph), **10c-G1** (Z = $CH_2C_6H_4$, R = Me), and **10d-G1** (Z = CH_2 C_6H_4, R = Ph).

2.5. Miscellaneous Boronated Dendrimers

Different other types of carborane dendrimers were built from aliphatic polyester dendrimers, grown from 1,1,1-tris(hydroxyphenyl) ethane (Scheme 12A) or pentaerythritol (Scheme 12B) as core in the presence of EDC (1-[3-(dimethylamino)propyl]-3-ethylcarbodiimide) and DPTS (4-(dimethylamino)pyridinium-*p*-toluene sulfonate) as coupling agents. The dendrimers were isolated with yields ranging from 79 to 93%. Contrarily to all the previous cases which used *ortho*-carboranes, *para*-carboranes were used in these cases. The presence of TBDPS (*tert*-butyldiphenylsilyl) (**11-G2**) or benzyl ether (**12-G2**) as terminal functions enables the growth of new polyester branches as will be shown in Part 3.2. [36].

A small carborane dendrimer (**13-G1**) was obtained from an arylether dendrimer and isolated in 82% yield (Scheme 13). As already indicated for other types of carborane dendrimers, water-soluble compounds were obtained by degrading the *closo*-cluster to the *nido*-cluster under basic conditions using KOH in EtOH. All these *closo*- and *nido*-carborane dendrimers show strong fluorescence emission in different solvents [37].

A series of triazine-cored small dendritic molecules containing three (not shown), six (**14a-G1**), or nine (**14b-G1**) peripheral carborane clusters were synthesized through CuAAC reactions and isolated in 75%, 71%, and 66% yield, respectively (Scheme 14). Thermal analyses demonstrated that dendrimers **14a-G1** and **14b-G1** maintained 53 and 54 wt% of residue at 700 °C, respectively [38].

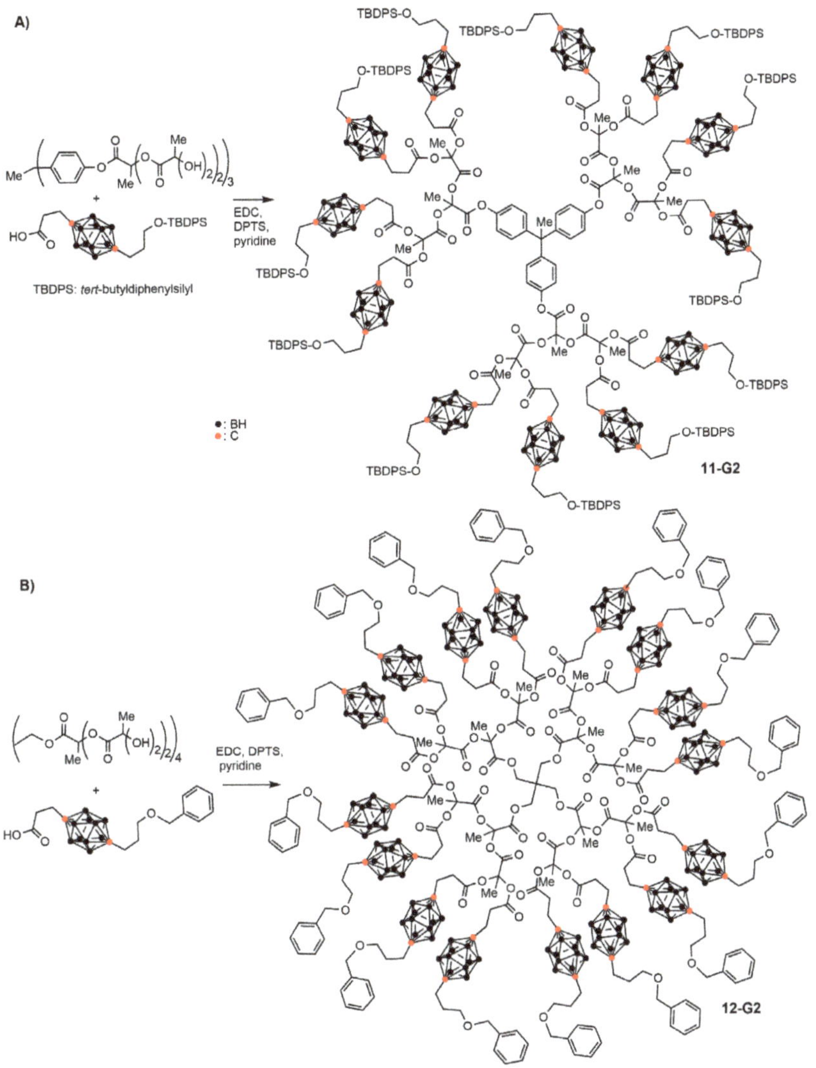

Scheme 12. Synthesis of two types of *para*-carborane polyester dendrimers, functionalized on their surface with either TBDPS (**A**) or benzyl ether (**B**).

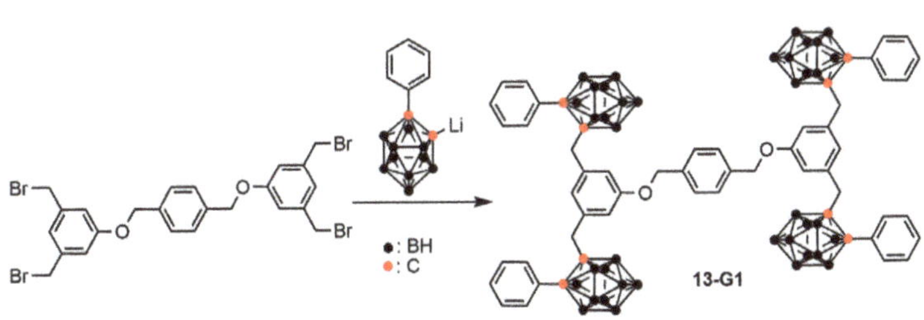

Scheme 13. A small arylether dendrimer functionalized with carboranes.

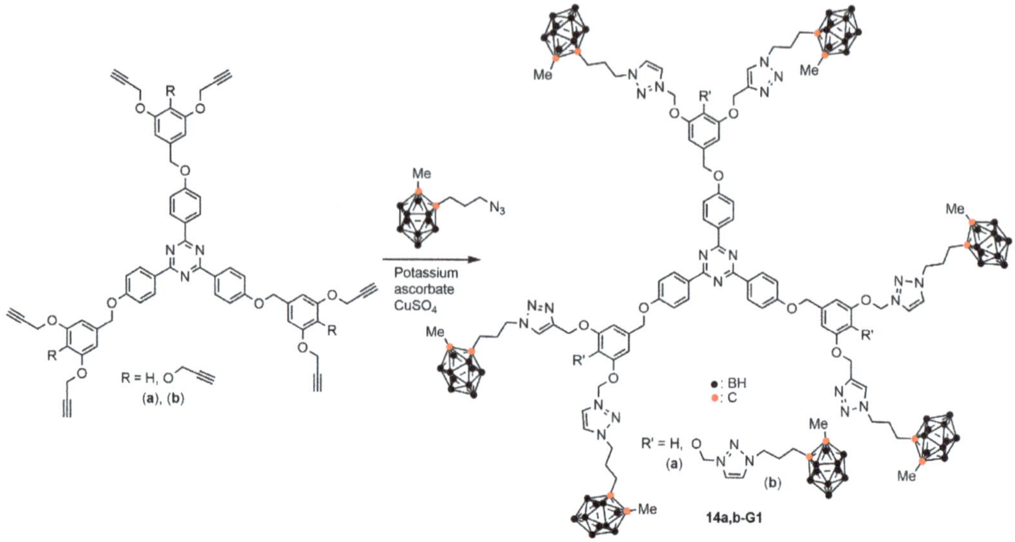

Scheme 14. Triazine-cored arylether dendrimers functionalized with six (**14a-G1**) or nine (**14b-G1**) carborane units.

3. Boron Clusters inside Dendrimers

As shown in the previous paragraphs, there are numerous examples of dendrimers functionalized on their surface by boron clusters, essentially *ortho*-carborane derivatives. Less research has been carried out on dendrimers functionalized in the internal structure by boron clusters. The very first example concerned the post-synthetic modification of the internal structure of hydrocarbon dendrimers, but in all the other cases, the borane clusters are introduced during the synthetic process.

3.1. Carboranes inside Hydrocarbon-Based Dendrimers

Hydrocarbon dendrimers equipped with an internal layer of alkyne moieties were reacted with decaborane to afford different 1,2-dicarba-*closo*-dodecaboranes (Scheme 15), using the method shown in Scheme 1. This process was carried out with both, the first (four carboranes) and the second generation **15a-G2**, having twelve carboranes inside its structure, and being isolated in 77% yield. The terminal benzyl ether moieties were converted to peripheral alcohols, which were subsequently transformed to sulfate groups, to afford the water-soluble carborane dendrimer **15b-G2** [39]. The alcohol terminal groups were also converted to carboxylic acids [40].

The post-synthetic modification shown in Scheme 15 is an exception to obtain carboranes inside the structure of dendrimers. In all the other cases, dendritic branches are grown from functionalized carboranes on the surface of dendrimers.

3.2. Carboranes inside Polyester-Based Dendrimers

Dendrimer **12-G2** (Scheme 12) possesses benzyl ether terminal functions, which were cleaved with Pd/C in the presence of H_2, to obtain alcohol terminal functions, suitable for further divergent growth. Reaction with 2,2-bis(hydroxymethyl)propanoic acid (bis-MPA) was followed by deprotection with Pd/C in the presence of H_2, to yield alcohol terminal functions. Repetition of both steps resulted in the growth of the dendritic branches, up to the fifth generation **16-G5** (Scheme 16) [36]. Analogous smaller dendrimers bearing four carboranes (**G2**) and eight carboranes (**G4**) were studied together with **16-G5** to determine their thermally-induced phase transition in aqueous media [41].

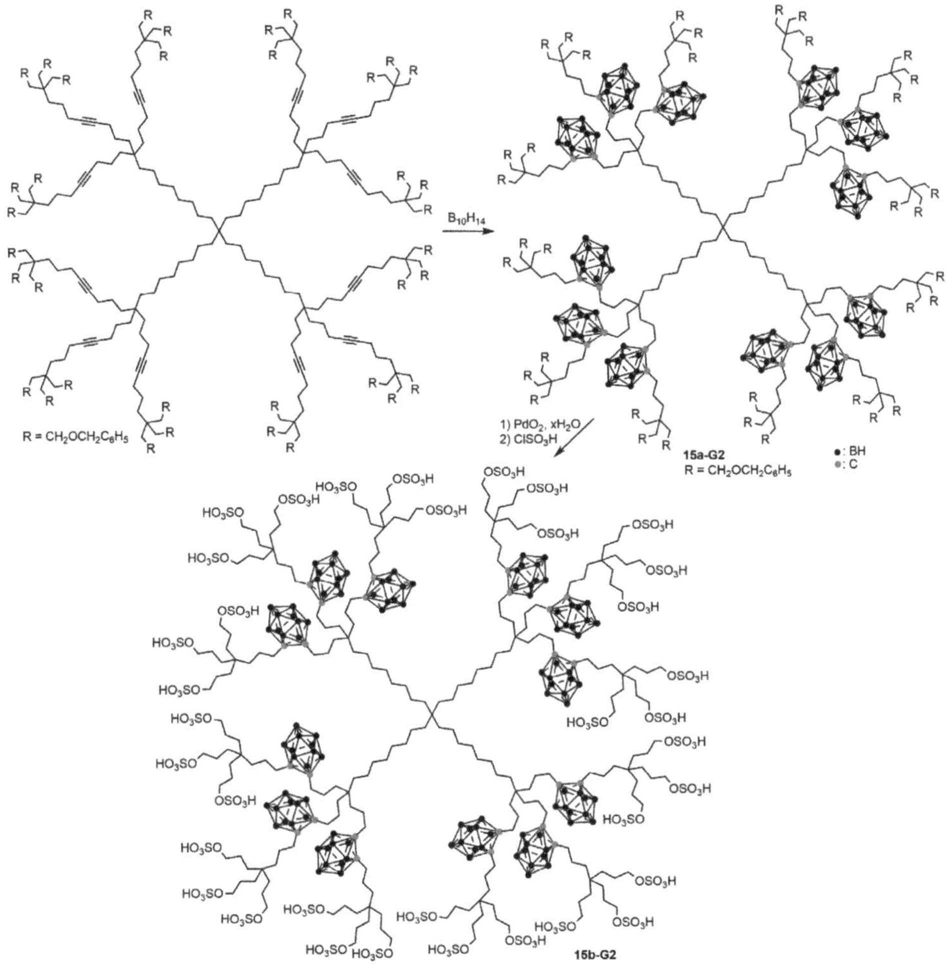

Scheme 15. Addition of decaborane to internal alkynes of hydrocarbon dendrimers, and subsequent transformation of the terminal functions to obtain a water-soluble dendrimer.

3.3. Carboranes inside Various Small Dendrimers

A small carborane dendrimer was first obtained by a cyclotrimerization reaction, analogous to the one shown in Scheme 9, and was then functionalized with trivinylsilane, to afford the phenylene-cored dendrimer **17-G1**, as shown in Scheme 17. This compound was isolated in 61% yield, and could be a precursor for the synthesis of larger carbosilane dendrimers [42].

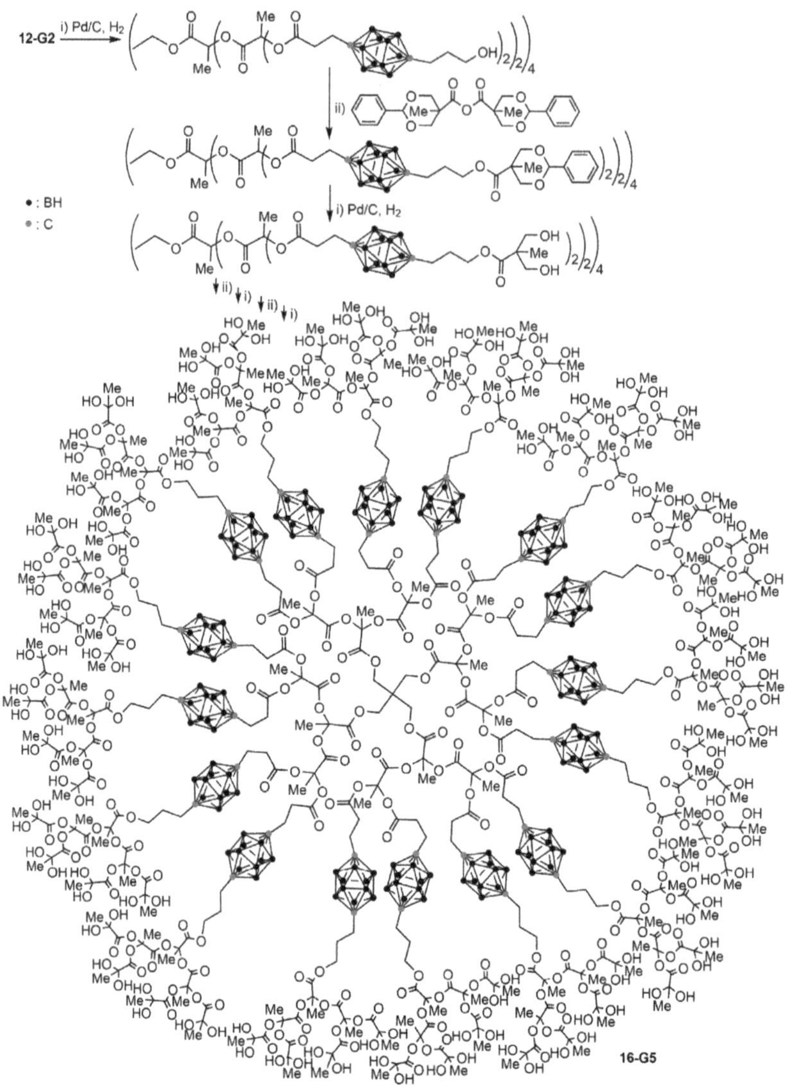

Scheme 16. Step-by-step synthesis of dendrimer **16-G5** from dendrimer **12-G2** by repetition of step i) Pd/C, H_2, and step ii) 2,2-bis(hydroxymethyl)propanoic acid.

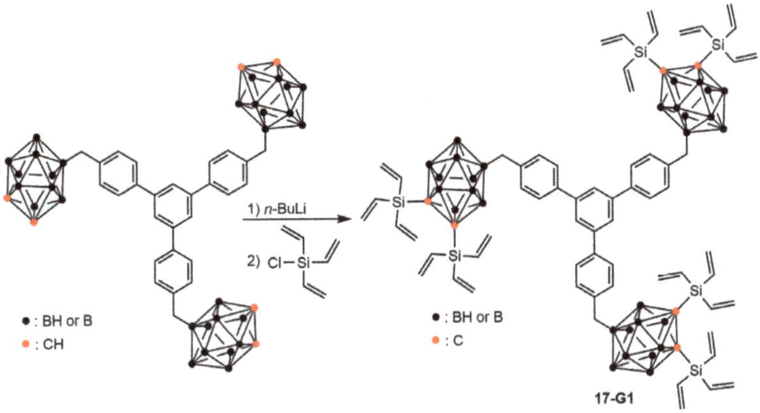

Scheme 17. A small carbosilane dendrimer having carboranes inside its structure.

Another carbosilane dendrimer bearing four *meta*-carboranes linked through a B–S bond was functionalized with chloro(dimethyl) vinylsilane to afford the first generation dendrimer **18-G1**, isolated in 90% yield (Scheme 18) [43].

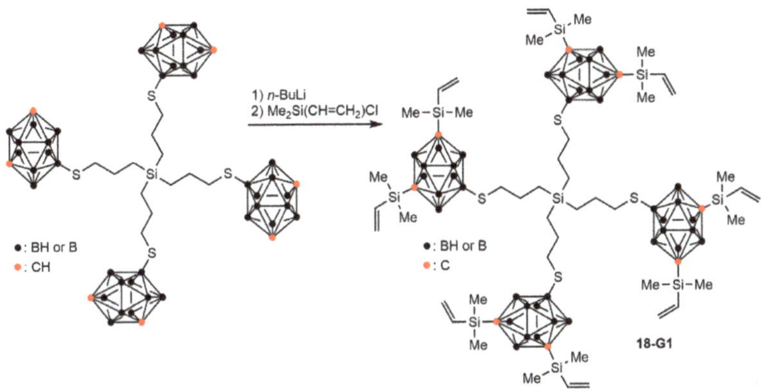

Scheme 18. Another example of a small carbosilane–carborane dendrimer.

A recent paper displays the grafting of two or three alkynes per carborane on a phenylene-cored dendrimer to obtain dendrimers **19a-G1** and **19b-G1**, respectively. Dendrimers **19a,b-G1** were subsequently used in CuAAC reactions with a protected glucosyl azide, isolated in 55–60% yield. Deprotection in the last step afforded the glycodendrimers functionalized with three internal carboranes and six (**19c-G1**) or nine (**19d-G1**) glucose derivatives on the surface, isolated in 73–80% yield (Scheme 19) [44].

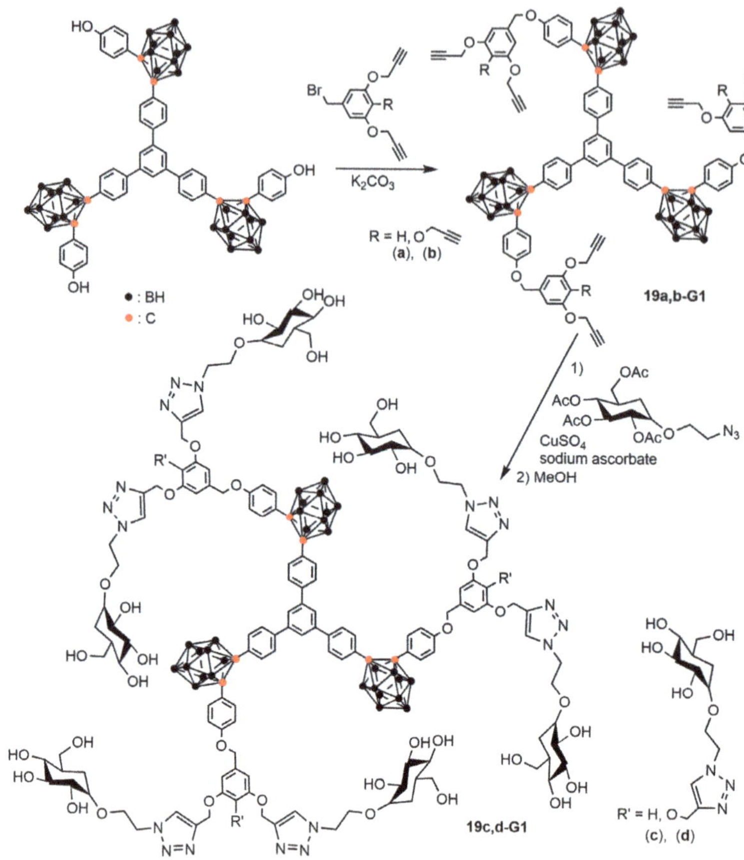

Scheme 19. Dendrimer functionalized with carborane and either 6 (**19c-G1**) or 9 (**19d-G1**) glucose derivatives.

4. Dendrons and Dendritic Structures Functionalized with Boron Clusters

Even if the largest number of dendritic structures functionalized with boron clusters are dendrimers, the very first examples concerned dendrons having a single carborane at the level of the core.

4.1. Boron Clusters at the Core of Dendrons

Small polyether dendrons (generations 0 and 1) bearing benzyl groups on the surface and an alkyne function at the core were reacted with decaborane, to afford dendron **20a-G1** for the first generation, isolated in 47% yield (Scheme 20). The benzyl groups were removed by hydrogenation in the presence of $Pd(OH)_2$ on charcoal under acidic conditions in ethanol to afford the deprotected and water-soluble dendron **20b-G1** (solubility 5.44 mol/L), in 63% yield [45]. The presence of a C–H function on the carborane cluster permitted the performance of different types of functionalizations. In a first attempt, a protected uracyl moiety was grafted to **20a-G1** via a palladium-catalyzed reaction with $Pd(dba)_2$/dppe (dba = dibenzylideneacetone, dppe = 1,2-bis(diphenylphosphino)ethane), to afford dendron **20c-G1** in 47% yield (Scheme 20). Hydrogenation of dendron **20c-G1** with palladium hydroxide on charcoal in ethanol afforded the fully deprotected and hydrogenated dendron **20d-G1** in 75% yield [46].

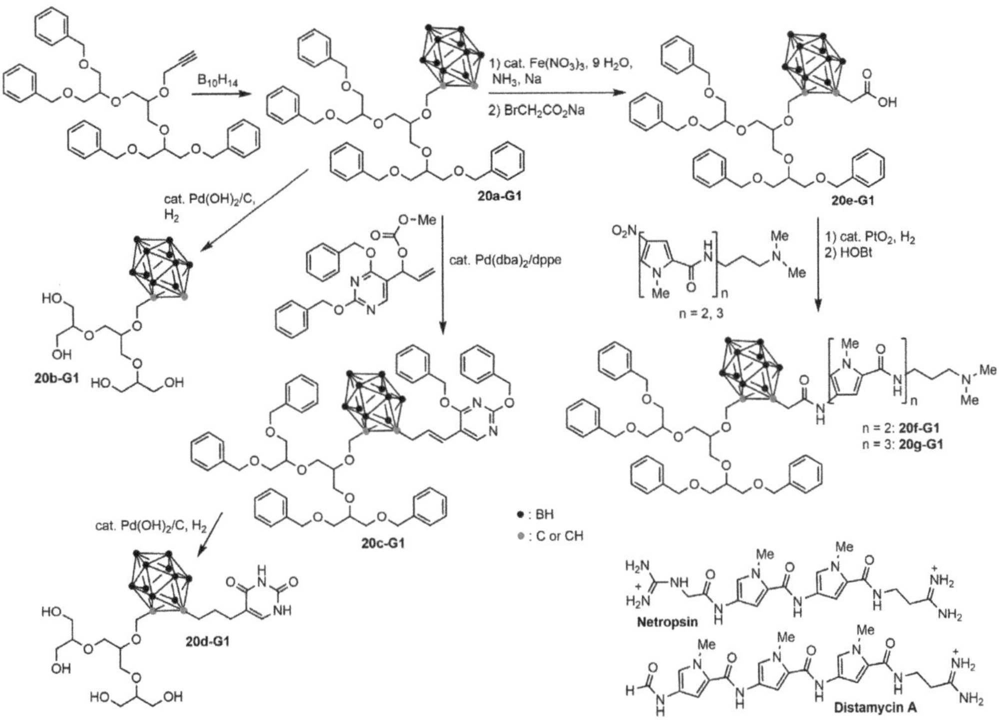

Scheme 20. Examples of polyether dendrons with one carborane attached to the core and a variety of additional functionalities.

In a second attempt, netropsin and distamycin A analogues were grafted to the carboxylic acid dendron **20e-G1**, obtained by coupling the CH of the carborane of dendron **20a-G1** with $BrCH_2CO_2Na$. Netropsin and distamycin A (structure in Scheme 20) are natural products, possessing two or three methylpyrrole moieties, respectively. Both compounds are able to bind to the minor groove of double helical DNA. Their analogues were grafted first by reduction of the nitro group to the corresponding amine, followed by condensation with dendron **20e-G1**, using HOBt (hydroxybenzotriazole) and DCC (N,N′-dicyclohexylcarbodiimide) to give the desired products **20f-G1** and **20g-G1** both isolated in 65% yield (Scheme 20) [47].

Another series of dendrons having a carborane at the core was synthesized by CuAAC reaction between carborane-cored dendrons bearing three or six alkyne groups (dendron **21a-G1**, with six alkyne groups, Scheme 21) and an azide linked to two types of carbohydrates, which are derivatives of protected D-glucose or protected D-galactose. These dendrons were isolated in moderate yields (52–54%). Deprotection of the alcohols with NaOMe in MeOH afforded dendrons functionalized with three (not shown) or six D-glucose (dendron **21b-G1**) or six D-galactose moieties (dendron **21c-G1**), in good yields (86–93%) (Scheme 21). Only dendrons functionalized with six carbohydrates (**21b-G1** and **21c-G1**) were fully soluble in water, contrarily with those functionalized with three carbohydrates [48].

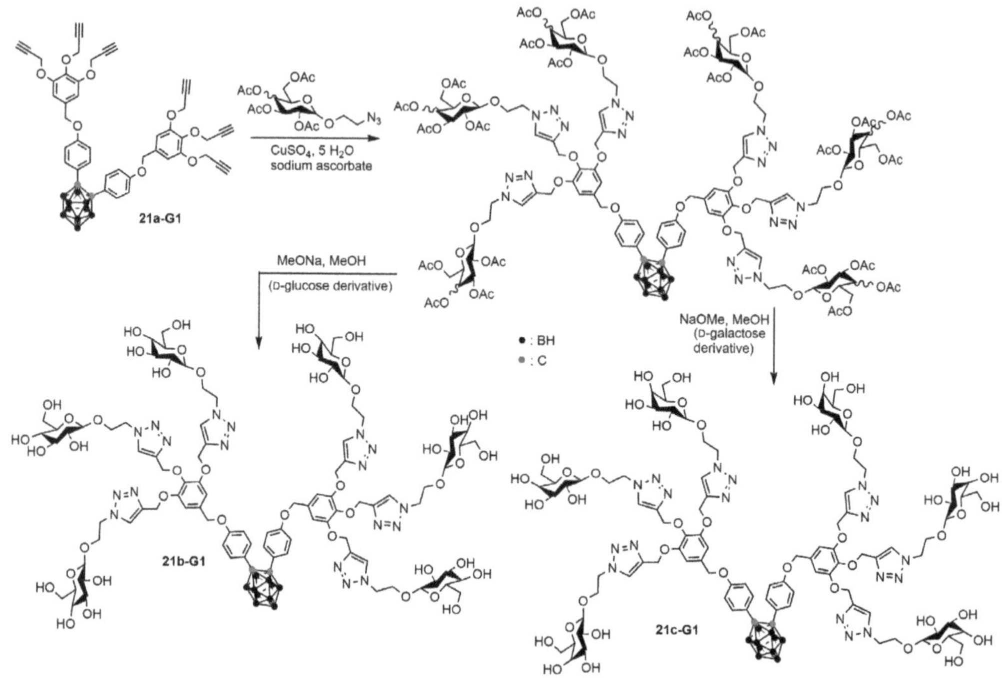

Scheme 21. Carborane dendrons functionalized with D-glucose (**21b-G1**) or D-galactose (**21c-G1**) derivatives.

Special types of dendritic structures are the "dendronized polymers", which are constituted by dendrons grafted to or synthesized on a linear polymer [49]. Two different approaches were used to obtain dendronized carboranyl polymers, using in both cases *para*-carboranes. In the first approach, the *para*-carborane monomer functionalized with a styrene group was polymerized by employing a nitroxide-mediated polymerization (NMP) strategy, using an alkoxyamine initiator, a catalytic amount of free nitroxyde radical and acetic acid in chlorobenzene to afford the polymer **22-G0**. In order to synthesize the dendrons stepwise, the polymer was first treated with n-BuLi and then with an excess of benzylidene-protected anhydride of bisMPA shown in Scheme 22. About 70% of the carboranes were functionalized in this way. Finally, removal of the benzylidene protecting groups was carried out using a Pd-catalyzed hydrogenolysis with $PdOH_2/C/H_2$, followed by an acid-catalyzed deprotection using H_2SO_4, to afford the first generation **22-G1**. In the second method to obtain polymer **22-G1**, the starting compound was a carboranyl monomer already functionalized on one carbon atom with a benzylidene-protecting group, and on the other carbon atom with a styrene group. Polymerization using the NMP strategy obtaining the same type of polymer and subsequent deprotection were carried out as indicated above. This approach yields the dendronized polymer **22-G1** that contains 100% functionalized carboranes, as opposed to the previous method yield of 70%. Polymer **22-G1** obtained by both methods was reacted successively in an iterative esterification with the benzylidene-protected anhydride of bisMPA, DMAP (4-dimethylaminopyridine) and pyridine. The second step was the deprotection of the anhydride, as illustrated in Scheme 22. In both cases, the synthesis was carried out up to the fourth generation of the dendrons, i.e., up to the dendronized polymer **22-G4** [50].

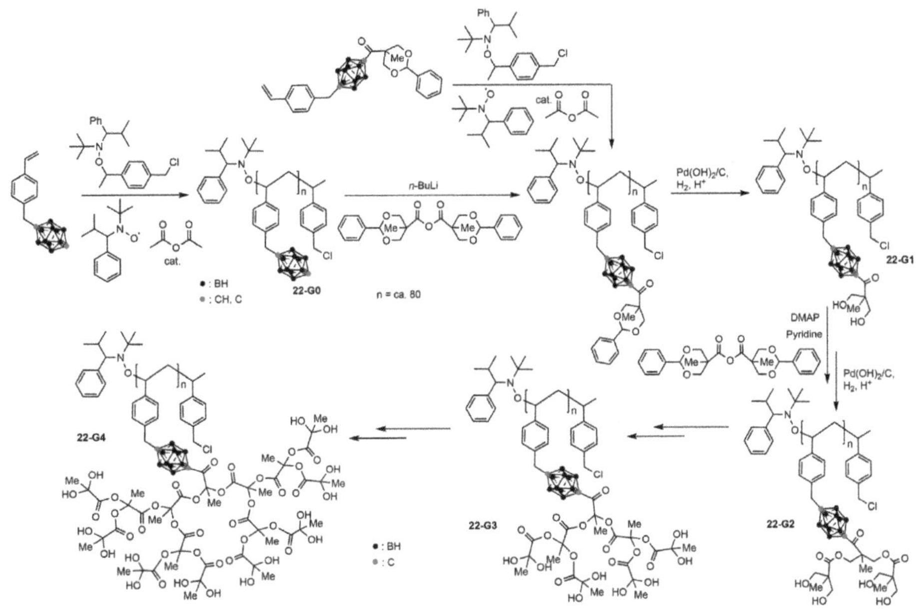

Scheme 22. Synthesis of carborane polymers, followed by the growth of dendritic branches.

4.2. Boron Clusters on the Surface of Dendrons

A second generation poly-L-lysine dendron, obtained by solid state synthesis, was reacted in acylation reactions with (S)-5-(2-methyl)-1,2-dicarba-*closo*-dodecaborane(12)-1-yl)-2-amino pentanoic acid. The resulting dendron **23-G2** was isolated in 81% yield after cleavage and deprotection from the resin. It possesses a relatively long poly (ethyleneglycol) derivative composed of ca. 68 CH_2CH_2O groups at the core to increase the solubility of this dendron in water (Figure 2) [51].

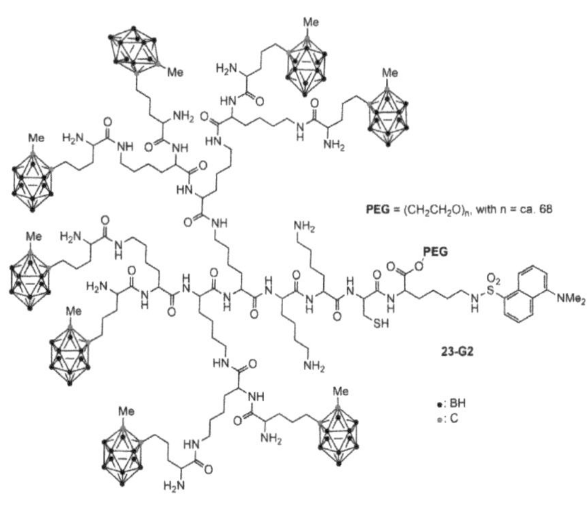

Figure 2. Structure of a poly-L-lysine carborane dendron.

Another type of peptide dendron functionalized with boron clusters on the surface was first obtained by growing different layers of peptides in the solid phase starting from

R11, a cell-penetrating peptide composed of 11 arginine residues, linked to a resin. Prior to the reaction of the surface layer with a Boc-protected cysteine (Boc: *tert*-butyloxycarbonyl), three layers of lysine were constructed. Full deprotection of cysteine enabled also the cleavage of the dendron from the resin. Finally, eight mercaptoundecahydro-dodecaborate units were grafted on the surface, as illustrated in Scheme 23, to afford dendron **24-G2** isolated in 37% yield [52].

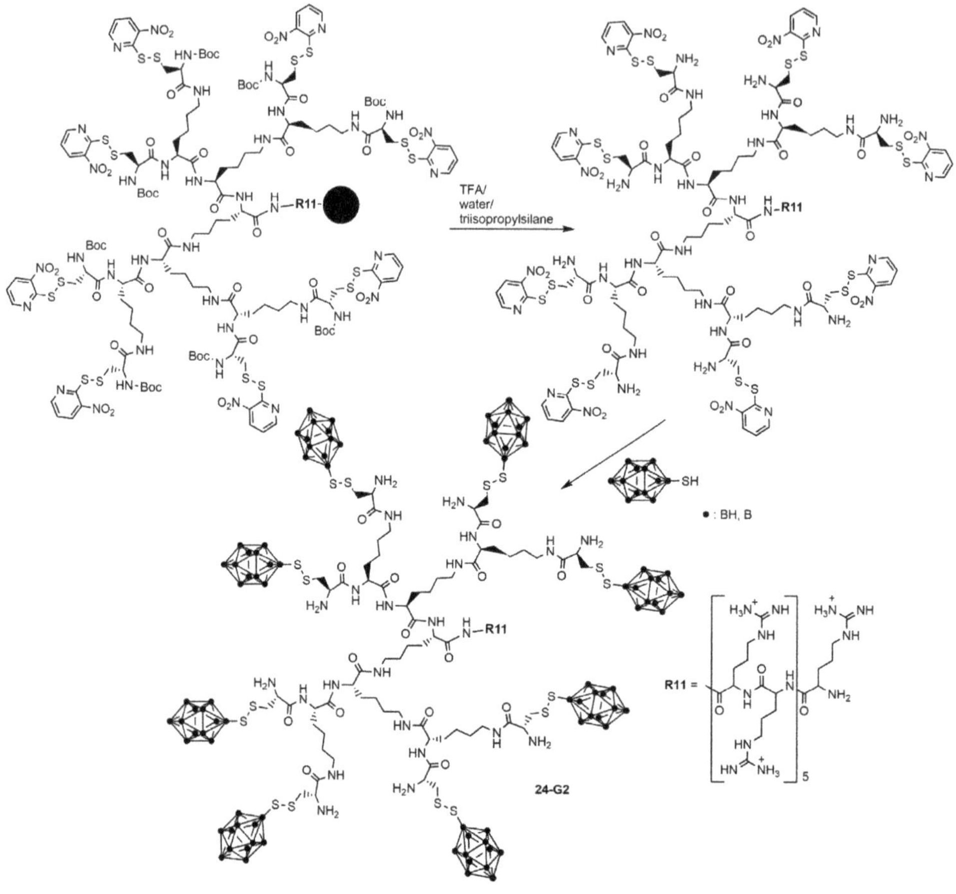

Scheme 23. Another lysine-based peptide dendron functionalized with boron clusters on the surface.

Several types of small polyester dendrons bearing carboranes on their surface were synthesized by a fully divergent process or a mixture of divergent and convergent steps. A first example concerns a generation 2 polyester dendron reacted with a carborane functionalized with a carboxylic acid, in the presence of EDC and DMAP to afford dendron **25a-G2**, isolated in 75% yield (Scheme 24A). Deprotection of the benzyl group at the core was carried out with palladium on carbon, under H_2, to afford dendron **25b-G2**. Attempts to react the carboxylic acid at the core with an alcohol failed, thus another way was used. The starting reagent was a surface-protected small dendron having a carboxylic acid as core, which was first reacted with benzyl-10-hydroxydecanoate, in the presence of EDC and DMAP. The next step was the deprotection of the surface with Dowex H^+ in MeOH, followed by the grafting of a carborane functionalized with a carboxylic acid, as in Scheme 24A, to afford the dendron **25c-G2** (Scheme 24B) [53].

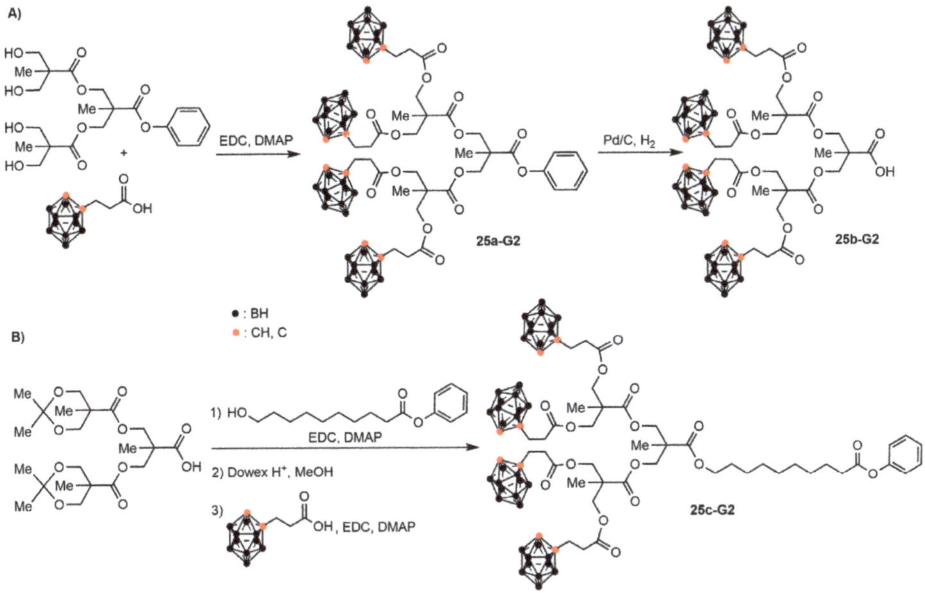

Scheme 24. Several types of polyester carborane dendrons having either a carboxylic acid (**A**) or a benzyl-10-hydroxydecanoate (**B**).

Another type of polyester carborane dendron was obtained by a convergent process, which consisted first in adding the $B_{10}H_{14}$ cluster to a trialkinyl compound, for which the core was modified to graft a carboxylic acid. In the next step, the carboxylic acid was coupled to a diol, for which the core was modified in the last step to have again a carboxylic acid (see Scheme 25 for the last steps of the process). Dendron **26-G2** was obtained in this way in 90% yield. It is potentially suitable for further reactions, but the synthetic process was stopped at this step [54].

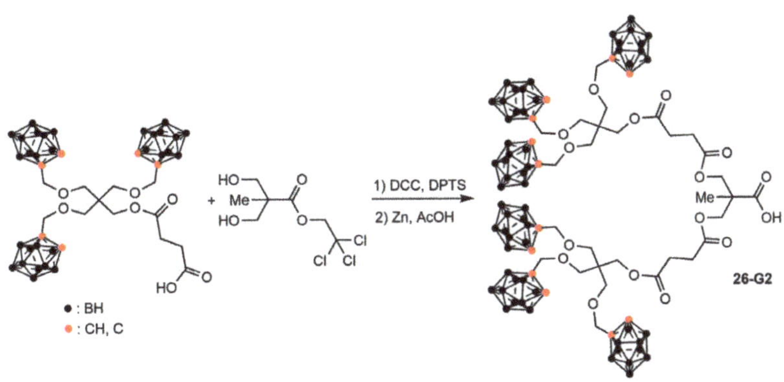

Scheme 25. Polyester carborane dendron obtained by a convergent process.

4.3. Carboranes on a Part of the Surface of Janus Dendrimers

Janus dendrimers are constituted of two halves of different compositions at least on the surface [55]. They are frequently obtained by association of two dendrons through their core. Only very few examples of small Janus dendrimers functionalized with carboranes on a part of their surface have been reported. In a first example, a dendron bearing three galatosyl derivatives on the surface and an alkyne at the core was reacted with a dendron bearing three carboranes on the surface and an azide at the core. The association of both dendrons was carried out employing CuAAC, with CuI, $CuSO_4$, sodium ascorbate, and NEt_3 to afford compound **27**, isolated in 98% yield (Scheme 26) [56].

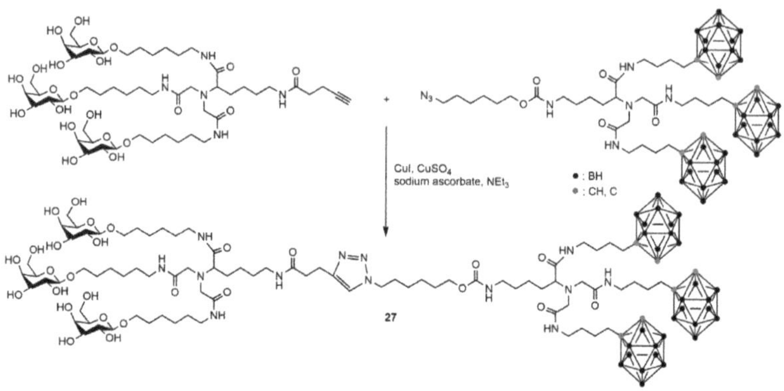

Scheme 26. A small Janus dendrimer bearing carboranes on one side synthesized by CuAAC.

The second example of a Janus dendrimer bearing carboranes on one side was obtained by a multi-step process, for which the last steps are shown in Scheme 27. The preliminary synthesis of a compound bearing an integrin ligand, two amines protected with Boc, and one amine protected with Cbz (carbobenzyloxy) was the starting point for the grafting of six carboranes. In the very last step, a monomethine cyanine dye for visible-light fluorescent imaging was grafted. Selective and sequential deprotection of the amines, using TFA, HBTU (2-(1H-benzotriazol-1-yl)-1,1,3,3-tetramethyluronium hexafluoro phosphate) as coupling agent, DIEA (N,N-diisopropylethylamine), and Pd black, H_2 in acidic media, permitted the synthesis of the sophisticated Janus dendrimer **28** isolated in 25% yield [57].

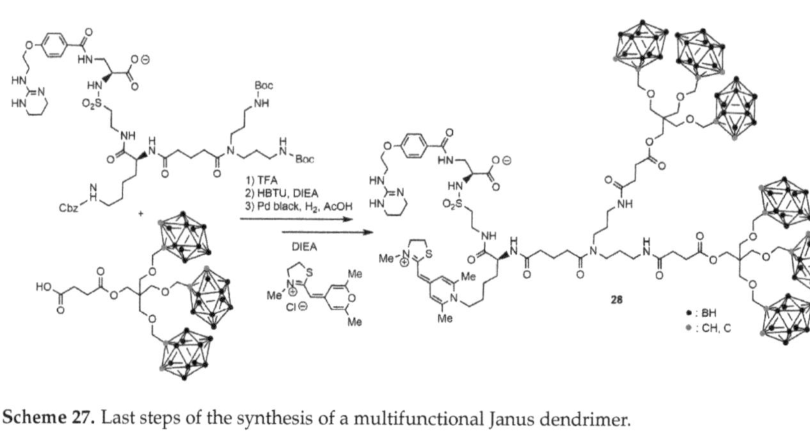

Scheme 27. Last steps of the synthesis of a multifunctional Janus dendrimer.

5. Biological Properties of Dendritic Compounds Having Boron Clusters Somewhere in Their Structure

Practically all types of dendritic compounds incorporating boron clusters somewhere in their structure, as shown in this review, were synthesized to be used for BNCT. However, BNCT experiments were carried out only in a limited number of cases, due to the necessity to have a nuclear reactor laboratory in close proximity until only recently [58]. On the other hand, the anti-cancer properties of some of the dendritic structures shown in the previous paragraphs were tested in vitro or in vivo, without BNCT experiments.

5.1. Anti-Cancer Properties of Dendritic Structures Functionalized with Boron Clusters

Preliminary experiments concerned the possibility of localizing boron in the DNA of target (cancer) cells. For this purpose, analogs of netropsin and distamycin A that bind in the minor groove of double helical DNA were introduced into dendrons **20f-G1** and **20g-G1** (Scheme 20). It was shown that not only the presence of the methylpyrrole moieties, but also that of dendritic branches enhanced the efficiency of binding to the minor groove of DNA [47]. Other anti-cancer experiments were carried out mostly with dendrimers, and in particular with PAMAM dendrimers.

5.1.1. Anti-Cancer Properties and In Vivo Localization of Boronated PAMAM Dendrimers

The in vivo distribution of the PAMAM dendrimer **1b-G4** (Scheme 3) functionalized with a monoclonal antibody (MoAb) IB 16-6, which is directed against the murine B16 melanoma, was studied in normal and tumor-bearing mice carrying sub-cutaneous implants of the B16 melanoma. Unfortunately, a very limited quantity of **1b-G4** was found in the tumor [22]. Another type of MoAb, the chimeric cetuximab (IMC-C225) directed against the epidermal growth factor receptors EGFR and EGFRvIII, was grafted to the fifth generation of the boronated PAMAM dendrimer, as depicted in Figure 3, and using the method shown in Scheme 3. The in vivo localization of this dendrimer **1c-G5** after injection into the tumor of rats bearing intracerebral implants of F98 wild-type ($F98_{WT}$) receptor (−) or EGFR gene-transfected $F98_{EGFR}$ glioma cells demonstrated a much larger localization in $F98_{EGFR}$ versus in $F98_{WT}$ gliomas [59].

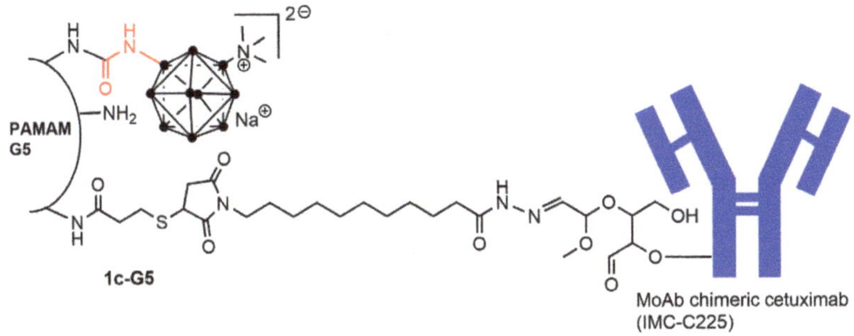

Figure 3. Schematic structure of boronated PAMAM **G5** functionalized with cetuximab.

Another example of boronated PAMAM dendrimer was functionalized with the epidermal growth factor (EGF), since the EGFR gene is found on the cell surface of the majority of high-grade gliomas. It was shown by electron spectroscopic imaging that the dendrimer penetrated in human malignant glioma U-343MG cell line by endocytosis, and accumulated in lysosomes [23]. The third generation boronated PAMAM dendrimer was also reacted with PEGs of varying chain lengths, functionalized on the end with folic acid for targeting the folate receptor on cancer cells. First experiments on KB cells demonstrated a receptor-dependent uptake. However, in vivo experiments in C57BL/6 mice bearing the folate receptor (+) murine 24JK-FBP sarcomas resulted in a slightly selective tumor uptake

(6.0% of the injected dose, ID/g tumor), but unwanted high hepatic (38.8% ID/g) and renal (62.8% ID/g) uptake were also observed [24]. A vascular endothelial growth factor (VEGF) was grafted to a boronated fifth generation PAMAM dendrimer, with the aim of targeting upregulated VEGF receptors (VEGFR), which are overexpressed on tumor neovasculature. This dendrimer was also tagged with a near-IR Cy5 dye for bioimaging. Several dendrimers were grafted per VEGF, as illustrated in Figure 4. Imaging of 4T1 mouse breast carcinoma revealed selective accumulation of VEGF-boronated dendrimer/Cy5, particularly at the tumor periphery where angiogenesis is most active [25].

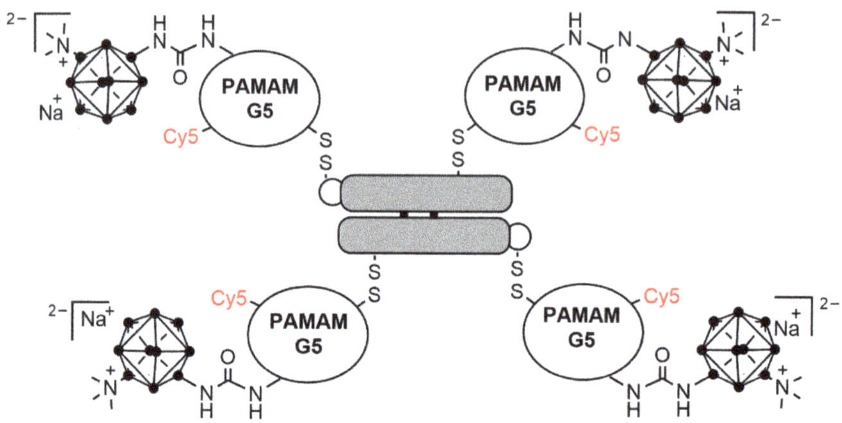

Figure 4. Schematic depiction of VEGF (gray rectangles) and its functionalization with several boronated fluorescent PAMAM dendrimers.

5.1.2. Anti-Cancer Properties and In Vivo Localization of Other Boronated Dendrimers

The biodistribution of the *nido*-carboranylporphyrins issued from **5a-G1** (free) and **5b-G1** (complexing Zn, see Scheme 7) were studied in BALB/c mice bearing EMT-6 mammary tumors. Both compounds were found to be effective tumor localizers, and the zinc(II) *nido*-complex was found to deliver 1.2–1.7 times higher amounts of boron to tumors than the free *nido*-compound [30]. The other *nido*-carboranylporphyrins issued from **6a-G1** and **6b-G1** were readily taken up by human glioblastoma T98G cells in culture, and were localized preferentially in the cell lysosomes. The metal-free *nido*-compound was found to accumulate to a higher extent in these cells compared with its zinc(II) *nido*-complex analog [31].

The dendrimer built from a phenylene core and functionalized with nine carboranes (**9b-G1**, Scheme 10) was tested toward human liver cancer cells (SK-Hep1). This dendrimer accumulated in the SK-Hep1 cancer cells in a concentration dependent manner, the highest accumulation being observed at a 50 μM concentration in **9b-G1** [34]. The biological properties of the triazine-cored dendrimers shown in Scheme 14, having six (**14a-G1**) or nine (**14b-G1**) carboranes on the surface have been evaluated using MCF-7 breast cancer cells. It was shown that the toxicity increased as the number of peripheral carboranes increased. The half maximal inhibitory concentration (IC_{50}) value was found to be 80.67 ng/mL for the largest dendrimer **14b-G1** [38]. Very recently, dendrimers having three carboranes inside the structure and six (**19c-G1**) or nine (**19d-G1**) glucose moieties as surface functions (Scheme 19) were evaluated against MCF-7 breast cancer cell lines. The glycodendrimer **19d-G1** having the highest number of glucose moieties has shown the highest cell death potential via apoptosis, with an IC_{50} value of 41.35 ng/mL (0.01 μM) that is 600 times higher than the cytotoxicity of the chemotherapeutic drug cisplatin (IC_{50} 6 μM) [44].

Besides dendrimers, dendrons bearing a single carborane at the core and functionalized with three or six D-glucose (**21b-G1**) or D-galactose (**21c-G1**) (Scheme 21) were tested against two cancer cell lines (MCF-7 human breast carcinoma cells and A431 skin cancer cells) and one normal cell line (HaCaT skin epidermal cell line). All dendrons showed higher cytotoxicities toward cancer cell lines than toward the normal cell line. Compounds bearing only three glucose or galactose moieties were found to be more cytotoxic than the dendrons **21b-G1** and **21c-G1** [48]. The trifunctional theranostic agent **28**, comprising six carboranes, a monomethine cyanine dye for fluorescent imaging, and an integrin ligand for efficient tumor targeting (Scheme 27), was first tested toward WM115 (human melanoma) and MCF-7 cell lines. Confocal microscopy images indicated that the Janus dendrimer **28** was localized mainly on the cell membrane and in the lysosomes of both cell lines. The same compound was then used in vivo in T-cell deficient nude mice, which were subcutaneously engrafted with WM115 cells. Images show that compound **28** was already localized in the tumor 30 min after injection. A biodistribution study displayed a consistently higher degree of accumulation of compound **28** in the tumor as compared to the other vital organs, namely, lungs, heart, liver, kidneys, and spleen [57].

5.2. BNCT Properties of Dendritic Structures Functionalized with Boron Clusters

The large majority of dendritic structures used in BNCT experiments were based on PAMAM dendrimers, functionalized with boron clusters on the surface, generally together with tumor-targeting moieties. The early publications in the field were previously reviewed [18], whereas a more recent review concerned the current advancements in the field of BNCT, including one paragraph about dendrimers [60].

5.2.1. BNCT Properties of Boronated PAMAM Dendrimers

A boronated PAMAM dendrimer, functionalized with an EGF was first tested toward F98 wild-type ($F98_{WT}$) receptor (−) or EGFR gene-transfected $F98_{EGFR}$ cells implanted into the brains of Fischer rats. Biodistribution studies after 24 h demonstrated that 33.2% of injected dose/g of boronated PAMAM−EGF was retained by $F98_{EGFR}$ gliomas compared with 9.4% of injected dose in $F98_{WT}$ gliomas. Boron concentrations in normal brain, blood, liver, kidneys, and spleen were at nondetectable levels (<0.5 ng/g). Rats were irradiated for BNCT 24 h after injection of boronated PAMAM−EGF in the tumor. Untreated control rats had a mean survival time (MST) of 27 $\pm$ 1 days, and irradiated controls (without dendrimer) had a MST of 31 $\pm$ 1 days. Rats treated with the boronated dendrimer−EGF and which received BNCT had a MST of 33 $\pm$ 2 days for animals bearing $F98_{WT}$ tumors, and of 45 $\pm$ 5 days for animals bearing $F98_{EGFR}$ tumors [61]. In another paper, two types of injections of the same dendrimer bearing EGF were tested, the normal intratumoral (i.t.) injection, and the convection enhanced delivery (CED). Boron concentrations in $F98_{EGFR}$ gliomas were 22.3 and 11.7 μg/g following CED and i.t. injection, respectively. Based on these results, BNCT experiments were carried out on rats that received the dendrimer injected i.v., or not. The MST was 53 $\pm$ 13 days, compared to 31 $\pm$ 4 days for irradiated control animals [62].

The boronated dendrimer functionalized with cetuximab **1c-G5** (Figure 3) was also injected in rats bearing $F98_{EGFR}$ or $F98_{WT}$ gliomas, resulting in the mean boron concentrations of 92.3 $\pm$ 23.3 μg/g and 36.5 $\pm$ 18.8 μg/g, respectively. The MST of rats that received **1c-G5** and were irradiated for BNCT was 45 $\pm$ 3 days, compared to 25 $\pm$ 3 days for untreated control animals [63]. The same dendrimer was also given intracerebrally by CED or direct i.t. injection into the brains of Fischer rats stereotactically implanted with $F98_{EGFR}$ cells. The corresponding MST after BNCT was 54.5 $\pm$ 4.3 days, whereas the MSTs of irradiated and untreated controls were 30.3 $\pm$ 1.6 and 26.3 $\pm$ 1.6 days, respectively [64]. Another paper comparing the efficiency of CED and i.t. injections demonstrated a doubling of the tumor boron concentration (22.3 μg/g for CED vs. 11.7 μg/g for i.t.) [65].

Another monoclonal antibody, L8A4, directed against the receptor EGFRvIII, seems to be a truly tumor-specific target. L8A4 was also linked to the boronated PAMAM dendrimer **1a-G4** or **1a-G5**. This compound was injected in rats bearing F98 wild-type receptor (−) or EGFRvIII human gene-transfected receptor (+) $F98_{npEGFRvIII}$ glioma cells. After

24 h, the amounts of dendrimer retained by receptor (+) gliomas were 60.1% following CED and 43.7% following i.t. injection compared with 14.6% by receptor (−) tumors. BNCT was carried out 24 h after administration of the dendrimer. Rats that received the dendrimer had a mean survival time of 70.4 ± 11.1 days with 10% long-term survivors (>6 months) compared with 30.3 ± 1.6 and 26.3 ± 1.1 days for irradiated and untreated controls, respectively [66]. Another paper compared the efficiency of boronated PAMAM dendrimers linked to cetuximab (**1c-G5**) or L8A4 in a rat glioma composed of a mixture of cells expressing wild-type ($F98_{EGFR}$) or mutant receptors ($F98_{npEGFRvIII}$). After BNCT, the mean survival time was 36 ± 1 days for boronated PAMAM−L8A4 and 38 ± 2 days for boronated PAMAM−cetuximab alone, whereas it was 55 ± 4 days when using the mixture of both dendrimers [67]. A short review summarized the work carried out with both types of boronated dendrimer−MoAb [68].

5.2.2. BNCT Properties of Diverse Boronated Dendritic Structures

Dendrimers of the **16-Gn** series (Scheme 16, n = 3, with four internal carboranes and thirty-two OH terminal functions, and n = 4, with eight or sixteen internal carboranes and sixty-four OH terminal functions) in THF solution were placed in a thermal neutron beam of a nuclear reactor. The characteristic gamma radiation signature at an energy of 480 keV, corresponding to boron neutron capture events was observed in all cases, indicating the possible use of these compounds for BNCT [36].

The small Janus dendrimer **27** (Scheme 26) was used to treat HepG2 cells (human liver cancer cell line) by irradiation with thermal neutrons. In these conditions, the cell killing efficiency of dendrimer **27** was 10-fold greater than that of the monomeric BSH (sodium borocaptate, $Na_2B_{12}H_{11}SH$) [56].

Dendron **24-G2** (Scheme 23) was first added to malignant glioma cells and found to localize at the cell nucleus. It was also administered to nude mice bearing a brain tumor after injection of U87 DEGFR cells. With neutron irradiation, the group that was treated with **24-G2** showed a significant cancer killing effect, even when compared to the group that was treated with a 100 times higher concentration of monomeric BSH, illustrating both the effect of the targeting group and of the concentration in boron due to the dendron [52].

6. Conclusions

The inclusion of boron clusters anywhere in the structure of dendrimers or dendrons has generated a rich chemistry, as illustrated in a large part of this review. About half of the dendritic structures synthesized were of first generations, but larger compounds were also synthesized, up to the fifth generation in some cases. Clearly, the small generations are easier to synthesize and to purify, but they accommodate a small number of boron clusters. On the contrary, high generations need time and money to be synthesized, their purity is sometimes questionable, but they can accommodate a large number of boron clusters. Up to now, most of the boronated dendritic structures tested in biological experiments are based on large PAMAM dendrimers of generations 4 or 5. Thus, having a large quantity of boron, and the possibility of accommodating targeting entities seems to be the most suitable solution for practical uses of boronated dendrimers.

The biological properties of some of these dendritic structures, essentially dendrimers have been assessed against cancer cells, and in some cases in BNCT experiments, generally carried out with mice or rats. The relatively low number of boronated dendritic structures tested is certainly due to difficulty in having a nuclear reactor laboratory in close proximity, until recently. A good efficiency of the boronated dendritic structures in vivo in BNCT is generally observed, with a noticeable increase in the mean survival time of the animals. The presence of multiple functional groups on the surface of dendrimers enables the grafting of a targeting peptide, together with the boron clusters, for an improved localization in the cancer cells, and thus a better efficiency of BNCT. However, there is generally no cure of the cancer in these experiments, in particular concerning brain tumors in animals. This is probably the reason why no BNCT clinical trials have been carried out up to now with boronated dendrimers. However, as several accelerator-based BNCT facilities have been constructed in recent years with many still being under construction and planning [69], there is certainly a demand of improved and selective BNCT agents in future.

Besides dendrimers, other types of carriers of boron clusters are known, such as polymers [70], nanoparticles [71], or liposomes [72]. Polymers can be of natural origin, such as dextrans or glucose polymers, but the structure of polymers is less well defined than that of dendrimers, and their functional groups are less easily accessible. Nanoparticles are frequently composed of toxic metals or of polymer balls, whereas liposomes are quite large compared to the size of dendrimers, but several types of liposomes for drug delivery have been approved by the U.S. Food and Drug Administration (FDA) and European Medicines Agency (EMA) [73]. It should be noted that different types of dendrimers have been and are used in different clinical trials [74], but not in the case of boronated dendrimers until now. In the view of state-of-the-art for the delivery of boron clusters, dendrimers appear to have a large potential, but that needs to be further developed.

Author Contributions: Conceptualization, A.-M.C.; resources, A.-M.C. and E.H.-H.; writing—original draft preparation, A.-M.C.; writing—review and editing, A.-M.C., E.H.-H. and M.M.; supervision, A.-M.C. and E.H.-H.; project administration, A.-M.C. and E.H.-H.; funding acquisition, A.-M.C. and E.H.-H. All authors have read and agreed to the published version of the manuscript.

Funding: This project was funded by European Union's Horizon 2020 Research and Innovation program under the Marie Sklodowska-Curie grant agreement number 860322 for the ITN-EJD "Coordination Chemistry Inspires Molecular Catalysis" CCIMC.

Data Availability Statement: No data available.

Acknowledgments: Thanks are due to the CNRS (Centre National de la Recherche Scientifique) for financial support, to Rinaldo Poli as coordinator of the CCIMC network, and to Alida Lefter as manager of the same network.

Conflicts of Interest: The authors declare no conflict of interest.

References

1. Sergeeva, A.P.; Popov, I.A.; Piazza, Z.A.; Li, W.L.; Romanescu, C.; Wang, L.S.; Boldyrev, A.I. Understanding Boron through Size-Selected Clusters: Structure, Chemical Bonding, and Fluxionality. *Acc. Chem. Res.* **2014**, *47*, 1349–1358. [CrossRef] [PubMed]
2. Grimes, R.N. *Carboranes*, 3rd ed.; Elsevier Academic Press: London, UK, 2016; pp. 1–1041.
3. Heying, T.L.; Ager, J.W., Jr.; Clark, S.L.; Mangold, D.J.; Goldstein, H.L.; Hillman, M.; Polak, R.J.; Szymanski, J.W. A New Series of Organoboranes. I. Carboranes from the Reaction of Decaborane with Acetylenic Compounds. *Inorg. Chem.* **1963**, *2*, 1089–1092. [CrossRef]
4. Zakharkin, L.I.; Stanko, V.I.; Brattsev, V.A.; Chapovskii, Y.A.; Struchkov, Y.T. The structure of B10C2H12 (Barene) and its derivatives. *Bull. Acad. Sci. USSR Div. Chem. Sci.* **1963**, *12*, 1911. [CrossRef]
5. Grafstein, D.; Dvorak, J. Neocarboranes, a New Family of Stable Organoboranes Isomeric with the Carboranes. *Inorg. Chem.* **1963**, *2*, 1128–1133. [CrossRef]
6. Edvenson, G.M.; Gaines, D.F. Thermal Isomerization of Regiospecifically ^{10}B-Labeled Icosahedral Carboranes. *Inorg. Chem.* **1990**, *29*, 1210–1216. [CrossRef]
7. Bregadze, V.I. Fifty years of carborane chemistry: The history of discovery and the first results. *Russ. Chem. Bull.* **2014**, *63*, 1021–1026. [CrossRef]
8. Zhu, Y.; Siwei, X.; Maguire, J.A.; Hosmane, N.S. Application of Cycloaddition Reactions to the Syntheses of Novel Boron Compounds. *Molecules* **2010**, *15*, 9437–9449. [CrossRef]
9. Scholz, M.; Hey-Hawkins, E. Carbaboranes as Pharmacophores: Properties, Synthesis, and Application Strategies. *Chem. Rev.* **2011**, *111*, 7035–7062. [CrossRef]
10. Barth, R.F.; Soloway, A.H. Boron Neutron-Capture Therapy of primary and metastatic brain-tumors. *Mol. Chem. Neuropathol.* **1994**, *21*, 139–154. [CrossRef]
11. Barth, R.F.; Coderre, J.A.; Vicente, M.G.H.; Blue, T.E. Boron neutron capture therapy of cancer: Current status and future prospects. *Clin. Cancer Res.* **2005**, *11*, 3987–4002. [CrossRef]
12. Caminade, A.M.; Turrin, C.O.; Laurent, R.; Ouali, A.; DelavauxNicot, B. *Dendrimers: Towards Catalytic, Material and Biomedical Uses*; Wiley: Chichester, UK, 2011; pp. 1–538. [CrossRef]
13. Tomalia, D.A.; Baker, H.; Dewald, J.; Hall, M.; Kallos, G.; Martin, S.; Roeck, J.; Ryder, J.; Smith, P. A new class of polymers—Starburst-dendritic macromolecules. *Polym. J.* **1985**, *17*, 117–132. [CrossRef]

14. Tomalia, D.A.; Naylor, A.M.; Goddard, W.A. Starburst dendrimers—Molecular level control of size, shape, surface chemistry, topology, and flexibility from atoms to macroscopic matter. *Angew. Chem. Int. Ed. Engl.* **1990**, *29*, 138–175. [CrossRef]
15. Hosmane, N.S.; Zhu, Y.H.; Maguire, J.A.; Kaim, W.; Takagaki, M. Nano and dendritic structured carboranes and metallacarboranes: From materials to cancer therapy. *J. Organomet. Chem.* **2009**, *694*, 1690–1697. [CrossRef]
16. Gao, S.M.; Hosmane, N.S. Dendrimer- and nanostructure-supported carboranes and metallacarboranes: An account. *Russ. Chem. Bull.* **2014**, *63*, 788–810. [CrossRef]
17. Vinas, C.; Nunez, R.; Bennour, I.; Teixidor, F. Periphery Decorated and Core Initiated Neutral and Polyanionic Borane Large Molecules: Forthcoming and Promising Properties for Medicinal Applications. *Curr. Med. Chem.* **2019**, *26*, 5036–5076. [CrossRef]
18. Wu, G.; Barth, R.F.; Yang, W.; Lee, R.J.; Tjark, W.; Backer, M.V.; Backer, J.M. Boron containing macromolecules and nanovehicles as delivery agents for neutron capture therapy. *Anti-Cancer Agents Med. Chem.* **2006**, *6*, 167–184. [CrossRef]
19. Hosmane, N.S.; Zhu, Y.; Maguire, J.A.; Hosmane, S.N.; Chakrabarti, A. Boron nanostructures—From materials to cancer therapy: An account. *Main Group Chem.* **2010**, *9*, 153–166. [CrossRef]
20. Pitto-Barry, A. Polymers and boron neutron capture therapy (BNCT): A potent combination. *Polym. Chem.* **2021**, *12*, 2035–2044. [CrossRef]
21. Liko, F.; Hindre, F.; Fernandez-Megia, E. Dendrimers as Innovative Radiopharmaceuticals in Cancer Radionanotherapy. *Biomacromolecules* **2016**, *17*, 3103–3114. [CrossRef]
22. Barth, R.F.; Adams, D.M.; Soloway, A.H.; Alam, F.; Darby, M.V. Boronated starburst dendrimer monoclonal-antibody immunoconjugates—Evaluations as a potential delivery system for Neutron-Capture Therapy. *Bioconjug. Chem.* **1994**, *5*, 58–66. [CrossRef]
23. Capala, J.; Barth, R.F.; Bendayan, M.; Lauzon, M.; Adams, D.M.; Soloway, A.H.; Fenstermaker, R.A.; Carlsson, J. Boronated epidermal growth factor as a potential targeting agent for boron neutron capture therapy of brain tumors. *Bioconjug. Chem.* **1996**, *7*, 7–15. [CrossRef] [PubMed]
24. Shukla, S.; Wu, G.; Chatterjee, M.; Yang, W.L.; Sekido, M.; Diop, L.A.; Muller, R.; Sudimack, J.J.; Lee, R.J.; Barth, R.F.; et al. Synthesis and biological evaluation of folate receptor-targeted boronated PAMAM dendrimers as potential agents for neutron capture therapy. *Bioconjug. Chem.* **2003**, *14*, 158–167. [CrossRef] [PubMed]
25. Backer, M.V.; Gaynutdinov, T.I.; Patel, V.; Bandyopadhyaya, A.K.; Thirumamagal, B.T.S.; Tjarks, W.; Barth, R.F.; Claffey, K.; Backer, J.M. Vascular endothelial growth factor selectively targets boronated dendrimers to tumor vasculature. *Mol. Cancer Ther.* **2005**, *4*, 1423–1429. [CrossRef] [PubMed]
26. Gonzalez-Campo, A.; Vinas, C.; Teixidor, F.; Nunez, R.; Sillanpaa, R.; Kivekas, R. Modular construction of neutral and anionic carboranyl-containing carbosilane-based dendrimers. *Macromolecules* **2007**, *40*, 5644–5652. [CrossRef]
27. Djeda, R.; Ruiz, J.; Astruc, D.; Satapathy, R.; Dash, B.P.; Hosmane, N.S. "Click" Synthesis and Properties of Carborane-Appended Large Dendrimers. *Inorg. Chem.* **2010**, *49*, 10702–10709. [CrossRef]
28. Minyaylo, E.O.; Anisimov, A.A.; Zaitsev, A.V.; Milenin, S.A.; Tikhonov, P.A.; Vyshivannaya, O.V.; Ol'shevskaya, V.A.; Nikiforova, G.G.; Buzin, M.I.; Peregudov, A.S.; et al. Boron-substituted carborane-carbosilane dendrimers: Synthesis and properties. *React. Funct. Polym.* **2020**, *157*, 104746. [CrossRef]
29. Minyaylo, E.O.; Zubova, V.Y.; Zaitsev, A.V.; Ol'shevskaya, V.A.; Nikiforova, G.G.; Buzin, M.I.; Anisimov, A.A.; Muzafarov, A.M. Studies on the effect of polyhedral carboranes on the physicochemical properties of polycarboranosiloxanes. *Polym. Chem.* **2023**, *14*, 1514–1525. [CrossRef]
30. Vicente, M.G.H.; Wickramasinghe, A.; Nurco, D.J.; Wang, H.J.H.; Nawrocky, M.M.; Makar, M.S.; Miura, M. Synthesis, toxicity and biodistribution of two 5,15-di 3,5-(nido-carboranylmethyl)phenyl porphyrins in EMT-6 tumor bearing mice. *Bioorg. Med. Chem.* **2003**, *11*, 3101–3108. [CrossRef]
31. Gottumukkala, V.; Luguya, R.; Fronczek, F.R.; Vicente, M.G.H. Synthesis and cellular studies of an octa-anionic 5,10,15,20-tetra 3,5-(nido-carboranylmethyl)phenyl porphyrin (H2OCP) for application in BNCT. *Bioorg. Med. Chem.* **2005**, *13*, 1633–1640. [CrossRef]
32. Cabrera-Gonzalez, J.; Xochitiotzi-Flores, E.; Vinas, C.; Teixidor, F.; Garcia-Ortega, H.; Farfan, N.; Santillan, R.; Parella, T.; Nunez, R. High-Boron-Content Porphyrin-Cored Aryl Ether Dendrimers: Controlled Synthesis, Characterization, and Photophysical Properties. *Inorg. Chem.* **2015**, *54*, 5021–5031. [CrossRef]
33. Dash, B.P.; Satapathy, R.; Gaillard, E.R.; Maguire, J.A.; Hosmane, N.S. Synthesis and Properties of Carborane-Appended C-3-Symmetrical Extended pi Systems. *J. Am. Chem. Soc.* **2010**, *132*, 6578–6587. [CrossRef]
34. Dash, B.P.; Satapathy, R.; Bode, B.P.; Reidl, C.T.; Sawicki, J.W.; Mason, A.J.; Maguire, J.A.; Hosmane, N.S. "Click" Chemistry-Mediated Phenylene-Cored Carborane Dendrimers. *Organometallics* **2012**, *31*, 2931–2935. [CrossRef]
35. Gonzalez-Campo, A.; Ferrer-Ugalde, A.; Vinas, C.; Teixidor, F.; Sillanpaa, R.; Rodriguez-Romero, J.; Santillan, R.; Farfan, N.; Nunez, R. A Versatile Methodology for the Controlled Synthesis of Photoluminescent High-Boron-Content Dendrimers. *Chem.-Eur. J.* **2013**, *19*, 6299–6312. [CrossRef]
36. Parrott, M.C.; Marchington, E.B.; Valliant, J.F.; Adronov, A. Synthesis and properties of carborane-functionalized aliphatic polyester dendrimers. *J. Am. Chem. Soc.* **2005**, *127*, 12081–12089. [CrossRef]
37. Lerouge, F.; Vinas, C.; Teixidor, F.; Nunez, R.; Abreu, A.; Xochitiotzi, E.; Santillan, R.; Farfan, N. High boron content carboranyl-functionalized aryl ether derivatives displaying photoluminescent properties. *Dalton Trans.* **2007**, 1898–1903. [CrossRef]

38. Jena, B.B.; Jena, S.R.; Swain, B.R.; Mahanta, C.S.; Samanta, L.; Dash, B.P.; Satapathy, R. Triazine-cored dendritic molecules containing multiple o-carborane clusters. *Appl. Organomet. Chem.* **2020**, *34*, e5754. [CrossRef]
39. Newkome, G.R.; Moorefield, C.N.; Keith, J.M.; Baker, G.R.; Escamilla, G.H. Chemistry within a unimolecular micelle precursor—Boron superclusters by site-specific and depth-specific transformation of dendrimers. 37. Chemistry of micelles. *Angew. Chem. Int. Ed. Engl.* **1994**, *33*, 666–668. [CrossRef]
40. Newkome, G.R.; Moorefield, C.N. Metallo- and metalloido-micellane™ derivatives—Incorporation of metals and nonmetals within unimolecular superstructures. *Macromol. Symp.* **1994**, *77*, 63–71. [CrossRef]
41. Parrott, M.C.; Valliant, J.F.; Adronov, A. Thermally induced phase transition of carborane-functionalized aliphatic polyester dendrimers in aqueous media. *Langmuir* **2006**, *22*, 5251–5255. [CrossRef]
42. Dash, B.P.; Satapathy, R.; Maguire, J.A.; Hosmane, N.S. Synthesis of a new class of carborane-containing star-shaped molecules via silicon tetrachloride promoted cyclotrimerization reactions. *Org. Lett.* **2008**, *10*, 2247–2250. [CrossRef]
43. Minyaylo, E.O.; Zaitsev, A.V.; Ol'shevskaya, V.A.; Peregudov, A.S.; Anisimov, A.A. The CH-functionalization of B-substituted organosilicon derivatives of polyhedral carboranes as a way to obtain new materials. *Mendeleev Commun.* **2023**, *33*, 47–49. [CrossRef]
44. Swain, B.R.; Jena, S.R.; Beriha, S.K.; Mahanta, C.S.; Jena, B.B.; Prasanth, T.; Samanta, L.; Satapathy, R.; Dash, B.P. Synthesis and anticancer properties of dendritic glycoconjugates containing multiple o-carborane clusters. *New J. Chem.* **2023**, *47*, 10296–10308. [CrossRef]
45. Nemoto, H.; Wilson, J.G.; Nakamura, H.; Yamamoto, Y. Polyols of a cascade type as a water-solubilizing element of carborane derivatives for Boron Neutron-Capture Therapy. *J. Org. Chem.* **1992**, *57*, 435. [CrossRef]
46. Nemoto, H.; Cai, J.P.; Yamamoto, Y. Synthesis of a water-soluble o-carborane bearing a uracil moiety via a palladium-catalyzed reaction under essential neutral conditions. *J. Chem. Soc.-Chem. Commun.* **1994**, 577–578. [CrossRef]
47. Yamamoto, Y.; Cai, J.P.; Nakamura, H.; Sadayori, N.; Asao, N.; Nemoto, H. Synthesis of Netropsin and Distamycin analogs bearing O-carborane and their DNA recognition. *J. Org. Chem.* **1995**, *60*, 3352–3357. [CrossRef]
48. Swain, B.R.; Mahanta, C.S.; Jena, B.B.; Beriha, S.K.; Nayak, B.; Satapathy, R.; Dash, B.P. Preparation of dendritic carboranyl glycoconjugates as potential anticancer therapeutics. *RSC Adv.* **2020**, *10*, 34764–34774. [CrossRef] [PubMed]
49. Stocker, W.; Karakaya, B.; Schurmann, B.L.; Rabe, J.P.; Schluter, A.D. Ordered dendritic nanorods with a poly(p-phenylene) backbone. *J. Am. Chem. Soc.* **1998**, *120*, 7691–7695. [CrossRef]
50. Benhabbour, S.R.; Parrott, M.C.; Gratton, S.E.A.; Adronov, A. Synthesis and properties of carborane-containing dendronized polymers. *Macromolecules* **2007**, *40*, 5678–5688. [CrossRef]
51. Qualmann, B.; Kessels, M.M.; Musiol, H.J.; Sierralta, W.D.; Jungblut, P.W.; Moroder, L. Synthesis of boron-rich lysine dendrimers as protein labels in electron microscopy. *Angew. Chem. Int. Ed. Engl.* **1996**, *35*, 909–911. [CrossRef]
52. Michiue, H.; Sakurai, Y.; Kondo, N.; Kitamatsu, M.; Bin, F.; Nakajima, K.; Hirota, Y.; Kawabata, S.; Nishiki, T.-I.; Ohmori, I.; et al. The acceleration of boron neutron capture therapy using multi-linked mercaptoundecahydrododecaborate (BSH) fused cell-penetrating peptide. *Biomaterials* **2014**, *35*, 3396–3405. [CrossRef]
53. Galie, K.M.; Mollard, A.; Zharov, I. Polyester-based carborane-containing dendrons. *Inorg. Chem.* **2006**, *45*, 7815–7820. [CrossRef]
54. Mollard, A.; Zharov, I. Tricarboranyl pentaerythritol-based building block. *Inorg. Chem.* **2006**, *45*, 10172–10179. [CrossRef]
55. Caminade, A.M.; Laurent, R.; Delavaux-Nicot, B.; Majoral, J.P. "Janus" dendrimers: Syntheses and properties. *New J. Chem.* **2012**, *36*, 217–226. [CrossRef]
56. Lai, C.H.; Lin, Y.C.; Chou, F.I.; Liang, C.F.; Lin, E.W.; Chuang, Y.J.; Lin, C.C. Design of multivalent galactosyl carborane as a targeting specific agent for potential application to boron neutron capture therapy. *Chem. Commun.* **2012**, *48*, 612–614. [CrossRef]
57. Dubey, R.; Kushal, S.; Mollard, A.; Vojtovich, L.; Oh, P.; Levin, M.D.; Schnitzer, J.E.; Zharov, I.; Olenyuk, B.Z. Tumor Targeting, Trifunctional Dendritic Wedge. *Bioconjug. Chem.* **2015**, *26*, 78–89. [CrossRef]
58. Hu, N.; Tanaka, H.; Kakino, R.; Yoshikawa, S.; Miyao, M.; Akita, K.; Isohashi, K.; Aihara, T.; Nihei, K.; Ono, K. Evaluation of a treatment planning system developed for clinical boron neutron capture therapy and validation against an independent Monte Carlo dose calculation system. *Radiat. Oncol.* **2021**, *16*, 243. [CrossRef]
59. Wu, G.; Barth, R.F.; Yang, W.L.; Chatterjee, M.; Tjarks, W.; Ciesielski, M.J.; Fenstermaker, R.A. Site-specific conjugation of boron-containing dendrimers to anti-EGF receptor monoclonal antibody cetuximab (IMC-C225) and its evaluation as a potential delivery agent for neutron capture therapy. *Bioconjug. Chem.* **2004**, *15*, 185–194. [CrossRef]
60. Luderer, M.J.; de la Puente, P.; Azab, A.K. Advancements in Tumor Targeting Strategies for Boron Neutron Capture Therapy. *Pharm. Res.* **2015**, *32*, 2824–2836. [CrossRef]
61. Barth, R.F.; Yang, W.L.; Adams, D.M.; Rotaru, J.H.; Shukla, S.; Sekido, M.; Tjarks, W.; Fenstermaker, R.A.; Ciesielski, M.; Nawrocky, M.M.; et al. Molecular targeting of the epidermal growth factor receptor for neutron capture therapy of gliomas. *Cancer Res.* **2002**, *62*, 3159–3166.
62. Yang, W.L.; Barth, R.F.; Wu, G.; Bandyopadhyaya, A.K.; Thirumamagal, B.T.S.; Tjarks, W.; Binns, P.J.; Riley, K.; Patel, H.; Coderre, J.A.; et al. Boronated epidermal growth factor as a delivery agent for neutron capture therapy of EGF receptor positive gliomas. *Appl. Radiat. Isot.* **2004**, *61*, 981–985. [CrossRef]
63. Barth, R.F.; Wu, G.; Yang, W.L.; Binns, P.J.; Riley, K.J.; Patel, H.; Coderre, J.A.; Tjarks, W.; Bandyopadhyaya, A.K.; Thirumamagal, B.T.S.; et al. Neutron capture therapy of epidermal growth factor (plus) gliomas using boronated cetuximab (IMC-C225) as a delivery agent. *Appl. Radiat. Isot.* **2004**, *61*, 899–903. [CrossRef] [PubMed]

64. Wu, G.; Yang, W.L.; Barth, R.F.; Kawabata, S.; Swindall, M.; Bandyopadhyaya, A.K.; Tjarks, W.; Khorsandi, B.; Blue, T.E.; Ferketich, A.K.; et al. Molecular targeting and treatment of an epidermal growth factor receptor-positive glioma using boronated cetuximab. *Clin. Cancer Res.* **2007**, *13*, 1260–1268. [CrossRef] [PubMed]
65. Yang, W.L.; Barth, R.F.; Wu, G.; Huo, T.Y.; Tjarks, W.; Ciesielski, M.; Fenstermaker, R.A.; Ross, B.D.; Wikstrand, C.J.; Riley, K.J.; et al. Convection enhanced delivery of boronated EGF as a molecular targeting agent for neutron capture therapy of brain tumors. *J. Neuro-Oncol.* **2009**, *95*, 355–365. [CrossRef] [PubMed]
66. Yang, W.L.; Barth, R.F.; Wu, G.; Kawabata, S.; Sferra, T.J.; Bandyopadhyaya, A.K.; Tjarks, W.; Ferketich, A.K.; Moeschberger, M.L.; Binns, P.J.; et al. Molecular targeting and treatment of EGFRvIII-positive gliomas using boronated monoclonal antibody L8A4. *Clin. Cancer Res.* **2006**, *12*, 3792–3802. [CrossRef] [PubMed]
67. Yang, W.L.; Wu, G.; Barth, R.F.; Swindall, M.R.; Bandyopadhyaya, A.K.; Tjarks, W.; Tordoff, K.; Moeschberger, M.; Sferra, T.J.; Binns, P.J.; et al. Molecular targeting and treatment of composite EGFR and EGFRvIII-positive gliomas using boronated monoclonal antibodies. *Clin. Cancer Res.* **2008**, *14*, 883–891. [CrossRef]
68. Yang, W.; Barth, R.F.; Wu, G.; Tjarks, W.; Binns, P.; Riley, K. Boron neutron capture therapy of EGFR or EGFRvIII positive gliomas using either boronated monoclonal antibodies or epidermal growth factor as molecular targeting agents. *Appl. Radiat. Isot.* **2009**, *67*, S328–S331. [CrossRef]
69. Available online: https://isnct.net/bnct-boron-neutron-capture-therapy/accelerator-based-bnct-projects-2021/ (accessed on 10 July 2023).
70. Nunez, R.; Romero, I.; Teixidor, F.; Vinas, C. Icosahedral boron clusters: A perfect tool for the enhancement of polymer features. *Chem. Soc. Rev.* **2016**, *45*, 5147–5173. [CrossRef]
71. Sumitani, S.; Nagasaki, Y. Boron neutron capture therapy assisted by boron-conjugated nanoparticles. *Polym. J.* **2012**, *44*, 522–530. [CrossRef]
72. Carlsson, J.; Kullberg, E.B.; Capala, J.; Sjoberg, S.; Edwards, K.; Gedda, L. Ligand liposomes and boron neutron capture therapy. *J. Neuro-Oncol.* **2003**, *62*, 47–59. [CrossRef]
73. Liu, P.; Chen, G.L.; Zhang, J.C. A Review of Liposomes as a Drug Delivery System: Current Status of Approved Products, Regulatory Environments, and Future Perspectives. *Molecules* **2022**, *27*, 1372. [CrossRef]
74. Caminade, A.-M. Dendrimers, an Emerging Opportunity in Personalized Medicine? *J. Pers. Med.* **2022**, *12*, 1334. [CrossRef] [PubMed]

pharmaceutics

MDPI

Article

Targeted Doxorubicin-Loaded Dendronized Gold Nanoparticles

Lance T. Dockery and Marie-Christine Daniel *

Department of Chemistry and Biochemistry, University of Maryland Baltimore County (UMBC), Baltimore, MD 21250, USA; lado1@umbc.edu
* Correspondence: mdaniel@umbc.edu

Abstract: Dendronized nanoparticles, also called nanoparticle-cored dendrimers, combine the advantages of nanoparticles and dendrimers. These very stable and polyvalent nanoparticles can be used for diverse applications. One such application is drug delivery, because the dendrons can enhance the density of the payload. In this report, we describe the design of multifunctional gold nanoparticles (AuNPs) coated with poly(propylene imine) (PPI) dendrons that contain both prostate cancer active targeting and chemotherapeutic drugs. The PPI dendron is a good candidate for the design of drug delivery vehicles because of its ability to induce a proton sponge effect that will enhance lysosomal escape and intracellular therapeutic delivery. The chemotherapeutic drug used is doxorubicin (DOX), and it was linked to the dendron through a hydrazone acid-sensitive bond. Subsequent acidification of the AuNP system to a pH of 4–5 resulted in the release of 140 DOX drugs per nanoparticles. In addition, the PPI dendron was conjugated via "click" chemistry to an EphA2-targeting antibody fragment that has been shown to target prostate cancer cells. In vitro cell viability assays revealed an IC50 of 0.9 nM for the targeted DOX-bearing AuNPs after 48 h incubation with PC3 cells. These results are very promising upon optimization of the system.

Keywords: dendrons; gold nanoparticles; doxorubicin; targeted delivery; prostate cancer

1. Introduction

Nanocarriers enable the delivery of therapeutic drugs with improved target specificity through a combination of prolonged circulation, active targeting, and payload conjugation chemistry [1,2]. The prolonged circulation of nanoparticles can be tuned with careful attention to size and surface coating; for instance, by using polymers, such as polyethylene glycol (PEG) or other polymers, thereby improving nanoparticle pharmacokinetics and biodistribution [3]. The incorporation of active targeting ligands (e.g., peptides, antibodies, etc.) and the conjugation of cytotoxic therapeutic drugs via stimuli-responsive attachments can further enhance nanocarrier target specificity [4].

The pharmaceutical industry has developed many different nanocarriers that have either already been approved by the Food and Drug Administration (FDA) or are currently undergoing clinical trials for the treatment of cancer and other diseases. Lipid nanoparticles have been approved for the delivery of cytotoxic cancer therapeutics (e.g., Doxil) and have in recent years emerged as an efficient method to deliver nucleic acid therapies, like the vaccines against COVID-19 developed by Pfizer and Moderna [5,6]. Various other polymer-based nanoparticles include polymer–protein conjugates, polymer–small molecule conjugates, dendrimers, and polymer nanoparticles [7,8]. Some recently approved polymer conjugate therapeutics include Jivi (Bayer, hemophilia A) and Palynziq (Biogen, phenylketonuria) [9]. Several dendrimer-based therapeutics are currently undergoing clinical trials for cancer, such as AZD0466 (Starpharma/AstraZeneca, leukemia) and DEP ® cabazitaxel (Starpharma, prostate cancer) [10].

The predominance of polymer conjugates and dendrimers in FDA drug approvals and clinical trials highlights an active area of research and a key focus of the nanomedicine community [11]. Dendrimers are highly branched spherical and symmetrical structures composed of a polymer backbone (e.g., poly(amidoamine), PAMAM and poly(propylene imine), PPI) that grows outward from a core into well-defined generations [12–15]. The well-defined and monodisperse nature of dendrimers allows for the attachment of multivalent molecules, such as therapeutic drugs, active targeting moieties, and imaging agents [16–18]. The synergy of gold nanoparticles (AuNP) with dendrimers or dendrons through either ligand adsorption or covalent–coordinate bonding to gold has led to promising dendritic AuNP hybrids with tunable properties [19], including the potential for efficient drug delivery [20–23]. The ability to densely pack drug-loaded dendritic structures around AuNPs with well-defined sizes can dramatically improve therapeutic efficacy over dendrimers on their own [24–26].

Gold nanoparticles are a promising nanomedicine platform because they can be prepared in monodisperse and well-defined sizes and are relatively inert once coated with biocompatible ligands [27–29]. The strong coordinate–covalent interaction between gold nanoparticles and suitable sulfur-containing ligands enables the formation of very stable nanoparticles (NPs). This allows for different thiolated or disulfide ligands to be mixed and imparts multifunctionality (e.g., therapeutic, targeting, imaging) onto the nanoparticle surface. Additionally, AuNPs inherently possess the ability to enhance ultrasound and radiotherapies and to act as contrast agents with X-ray imaging modalities [30,31].

The combination of dendrons (non-spherical asymmetric branched molecules) with AuNPs has been of particular interest to our group. The coating of AuNPs with dendrons offers several advantages. First, the use of dendrons as ligands increases the stability of the resulting gold nanoparticles as well as the density of the functionalities around them. Dendronized AuNPs are stable in biological media towards lyophilization and with respect to shelf life [21,32,33]. Second, adding dendrons onto NPs leads to the formation of giant dendrimers (nanoparticle-cored dendrimers) in one step [21]. Third, the synthesis of dendronized NPs allows for the use of a mixture of dendrons with diverse termini, giving rise to multifunctional nanoconstructs in a single step. Finally, the multifunctionality of the NPs can be easily tuned by varying the ratios of dendrons used to coat them. Dendrons may be synthesized in well-controlled reactions with high yields from commercially available starting materials to give molecules with varied terminal group functionalities and a disulfide (thioctic acid, TA) focal point for attachment to AuNPs [34–36]. We have previously reported the synthesis of poly(propylene imine) (PPI) dendrons having different charges and their incorporation onto the surface of AuNPs to form negatively charged, zwitterionic, and positively charged dendronized AuNPs [21]. These dendronized AuNPs had robust aqueous and serum stability, could withstand several rounds of lyophilization, and showed very low in vitro cytotoxicity. We have also shown that the PPI dendron could be conjugated to doxorubicin (DOX) as a model chemotherapeutic via an acid-labile hydrazone bond at a ratio of three DOX/dendron, giving PPI-DOX [37].

Doxorubicin is one of the most effective antitumor drugs against solid tumors [38], but its clinical usage has been limited due to its low bioavailability and severe side effects, such as cardiotoxicity [39]. Its main mode of action involves intercalation within DNA base pairs resulting in bent DNA strands, which leads to inhibition of both DNA and RNA synthesis, generating the formation of reactive oxygen species and oxidative stress [40].

Herein, we report the preparation of multifunctional dendronized AuNPs possessing acid-labile conjugated DOX drugs and active targeting moieties (Fab) conjugated through copper-free click chemistry. A PPI-N_3 dendron was synthesized and then mixed with PPI-DOX dendrons during a ligand exchange step on AuNPs using different ratios of DOX/N_3. The multifunctional AuNPs reported here were made possible with a novel ligand exchange method starting from PPI-CO_2H-dendronized AuNPs and using a large excess of new dendrons rather than the traditional ligand exchange starting from citrate-coated AuNPs. The stabilizing PPI-CO_2H dendron mixed with PPI-DOX and PPI-N_3 produced multifunctional AuNPs bearing DOX and azide functionality with a good size and polydispersity index (PDI). The increase in size and change in surface charge, as measured by dynamic light scattering (DLS), could be used to monitor the ligand exchange and subsequent bioconjugation to the targeting ligand (Fab). The multifunctional drug-loaded AuNP-DOX-N_3 showed rapid acid-triggered DOX release at a pH of 4.5. The targeted nature of AuNP-DOX/Fab was observed in vitro using transmission electron microscopy (TEM). Finally, in vitro cytotoxicity assays revealed an IC_{50} against PC3 cells of 0.9 nM for AuNP-DOX/Fab.

Although AuNPs have previously been reported for the delivery of DOX [41–43], this is the first study reporting the use of dendronized AuNPs bearing both acid-labile DOX and a Fab ligand targeting prostate tumors.

2. Materials and Methods

2.1. General Methods

Solvents and reagents were obtained from commercial sources (e.g., Sigma Aldrich, St. Louis, MO, USA; Fischer Scientific, Pittsburg, PA, USA; VWR international, Radnor, PA, USA; TCI Chemicals, Portland, OR, USA; etc.) and used without additional purification unless specified otherwise. Glassware, stir bars, and other containers used for gold nanoparticle synthesis and ligand exchange reactions were cleaned with freshly prepared aqua regia and then washed thoroughly (6×) with 18 mΩ ultrapure water from the Milli-Q water purification system. Gold chloride ($HAuCl_4$) and trisodium citrate ($Na_3C_6H_5O_7$) were obtained from Electron Microscopy Sciences (Hatfield, PA, USA) and used without purification. Dendrons used for gold nanoparticle ligand exchange reactions were prepared as described previously [21,34]. Gold nanoparticle centrifugation was performed using either benchtop (Thermo Fisher Sorvall Legend Micro 21R, Waltham, MA, USA) or an Avanti J-E Centrifuge (Beckman Coulter, Brea, CA, USA) and a JA-20 rotor. Gold nanoparticles were purified using either regenerated cellulose dialysis membranes (MWCO 12K-14K Da) obtained from Fisher Scientific (Pittsburg, PA, USA) or with successive rounds of centrifugation and filtration, as described below.

UV-Vis absorbance data were obtained from a Beckman Coulter DU 730 UV-Vis spectrophotometer. Fluorescence measurements were collected using a Horiba Jobin Yvon FluoroMax-3 instrument using the manufacturer's DataMax software (version 32). Unless otherwise specified, excitation wavelength for doxorubicin was set at 470 nm. Dynamic light scattering (DLS) and zeta potential data were collected from a Zetasizer Nano-ZS system (Malvern Instruments, Southborough, MA, USA) using a 633 He-Ne laser and operating on backscatter mode at an angle of 173°. The software used to analyze the data was Zetasizer version number 7.11 by Malvern Instruments.

Next, 1× PBS (pH 7.4) was prepared using volumetric glassware and ultrapure water (resistivity of 18 MΩ·cm). The 1× PBS was filtered through Cytiva Whatman ™ Puradisc 0.2 µm syringe filters prior to use with nanoparticles or diluted to 0.1× PBS (pH 7.4) using ultrapure water. Solutions of NaCl and saturated sodium bicarbonate (Fisher Scientific) were prepared using the corresponding salts and then filtered through Cytiva Whatman ™ Puradisc 0.2 µm syringe filters before use with nanoparticles.

PC-3 prostate cancer cells were provided by Dr. Charles Bieberich (Department of Biology, University of Maryland, Baltimore County). They were grown in Falcon-brand cell culture flasks using RPMI media supplemented with FBS and penstrep (Gibco, Thermo Fisher Scientific, Waltham, MA, USA) at 37 °C in a humidified atmosphere of 5% CO_2. Cytotoxicity studies involving AuNP-CO_2H, AuNP-DOX, AuNP-Fab, and AuNP-DOX/Fab were conducted with PC-3 cells using MTT reagent (Thermo Fisher Scientific) according to the manufacturer's recommended protocol. These studies are described in detail below.

2.2. Synthesis of PPI-N_3 Dendron

PPI-N_3 (2)—A solution of TA-TEG-G2NH_2 [21] (27 mg, 0.03 mmol) was dissolved in 4 mL anhydrous MeOH and stirred in a round-bottom flask. To this stirring solution was added an azide-modified Michael acceptor [44] (121.7 mg, 0.4469 mmol) and LiBr (35 mg, 0.40 mmol). The reaction was stirred vigorously at rt. for 48 h. After 48 h, the reaction was concentrated under reduced pressure to give a yellow oil, which was purified by LH20 size exclusion chromatography in MeOH. The pure product was obtained as a yellow oil (62 mg, 65%). The purity of the product was confirmed by ^{1}H NMR (400 MHz, D20) δ 7.15 (br, 2H), 6.87 (br, 2H), 4.08 (br, 2H), 3.81 (br, 2H), 3.62–3.32 (m, 77H), 3.25–2.10 (m, 63H), and 2.07–0.51 (m, 76H), and FT-IR spectroscopy ν = 3380 cm^{-1}, 2921.3 cm^{-1}, 2851.9 cm^{-1}, 2095 cm^{-1} (N_3), 1732.7 cm^{-1}, 1462 cm^{-1}, 1246.4 cm^{-1}, and 1119 cm^{-1}.

2.3. Synthesis of Dendronized Gold Nanoparticles

AuNP-Citrate (3)—A gold chloride stock solution was prepared by dissolving $HAuCl_4$ (101.7 mg) in 100 mL Millipore ultrapure water in a volumetric flask to give a concentration of 2.99 mM. Separately, 100 mL of a 5% w/v tri-sodium citrate stock solution was prepared using 5 g sodium citrate and Millipore ultrapure water in a volumetric flask. The 2.99 mM 100 mL $HAuCl_4$ stock solution was transferred to a large two-neck round-bottom flask and diluted to a concentration of 0.3 mM using Millipore ultrapure water (~1 L). This solution was stirred and heated to 90 °C. Once the solution reached 90 °C, 14.06 mL of the sodium citrate stock solution (molar ratio 1:6 $HAuCl_4$:Na_3citrate) was added to the reaction in one addition, and the reaction was brought to reflux for 1 h. After 1 h, the reaction was cooled to rt overnight before it was analyzed by UV-Vis and DLS to characterize the formed AuNPs. The particle size (DLS by number) was observed to be 13.6 nm (PDI = 0.067).

AuNP-CO_2H (4)—A solution of AuNP-citrate (269 mL, 6 nM) was stirred in a freshly cleaned glass round-bottom flask. Separately, 37.7 mg PPI-CO_2H [21] (**1**) dendron (25.6 μmol) was dissolved in 1 mL Millipore ultrapure water at a pH of 8 (basified with $NaHCO_3$) and then filtered through a syringe filter (GE Life Sciences, 0.22 μm) to give the dendron solution to be added to the AuNP-citrate solution. An excess of PPI-CO_2H dendron was added such that 20× the total theoretical ligand coating of the AuNP surface area was in the solution. The AuNP-citrate solution was first basified to a pH of 8 (monitored with pH strips) using 1 mL of filtered saturated sodium bicarbonate solution. Then, the previously prepared PPI-CO_2H dendron solution was added to the stirring basic AuNP-citrate solution at rt. The reaction color immediately turned to a darker red. After addition of the dendron solution, an additional 5 mL filtered saturated sodium bicarbonate solution was added to the stirring AuNPs to keep the pH at 8. The reaction was then stirred overnight at rt for a total of 15 h. After 15 h, a 1 mL aliquot was centrifuged twice (15,000× g, 45 min, 4 °C), resuspending in between with Millipore ultrapure water with a pH of 8, and examined via DLS, UV-Vis, and zeta potential, which indicated completion of the reaction. This solution of AuNP-CO_2H was stored without purification until further use. The DLS size by number was 16.8 nm, and the zeta potential was −42.0 mV.

AuNP- Fab (6)—A solution of AuNP-CO_2H was first centrifuged 1× (9k× g, 45 min, 4 °C), the supernatant was removed, and the AuNPs were resuspended in water with a pH of 8 with 0.02% TWEEN20 and 25% DMSO. The solution of AuNP-CO_2H (18 mL, 6.0 nM) was stirred in a 20 mL scintillation vial that had been freshly cleaned with aqua regia. To this stirring solution was added PPI-CO_2H (8 × molar excess) and PPI-N_3 (2 × molar excess) from stock solutions in water with a pH of 8 and DMSO, respectively. The total excess of dendron was added such that 10× the total theoretical ligand coating of the AuNP surface area was in the solution. The AuNPs were stirred for 17 h at room temperature and then centrifuged 1× (11k× g, 1 h, 10 °C) and 2× (9k× g, 45 min, 4 °C), removing the supernatant each time and resuspending the particles in 1× PBS (pH 8) with 0.02% TWEEN20. The washed AuNP-N_3 solution (**5**) was then stirred and Fab-DBCO was added from a stock solution in 1× PBS (est. 20 Fab/AuNP), and the reaction was stirred at room temperature for 1 h. After 1 h, the AuNP-Fab solution was centrifuged 2× (9k× g, 45 min, 4 °C). The AuNPs were characterized by DLS, zeta potential, and UV-Vis spectroscopy. The solution was stored in 1× PBS (pH 8) with 0.02% TWEEN20 in the refrigerator as a stock solution until it was used for TEM experiments. TWEEN20 was removed by 3 rounds of centrifugation and resuspension in 1× PBS prior to in vitro cytotoxicity experiments.

AuNP-DOX—A solution of AuNP-CO_2H (30 mL, 6 nM) was first centrifuged 1× (9k× *g*, 45 min, 4 °C). Then, the supernatant was removed, and the AuNPs were resuspended in pH 8 water with 0.02% TWEEN20 and 25% DMSO. The solution of AuNP-CO_2H (10 mL, 6 nM) was stirred in a 20 mL scintillation vial that had been freshly cleaned with aqua regia. To this stirring solution was added a combined solution (at a pH of 8) of 1.56 mL (1 mg/mL stock) PPI-CO_2H (5 × molar excess) and 1.28 mL (2.51 mg/mL stock) PPI-DOX (5 × molar excess) from stock solutions in pH 8 water and DMSO, respectively. The total excess of dendron was added such that 10x the total theoretical ligand coating of the AuNP surface area was in the solution. The AuNPs were stirred for 22 h at room temperature and then centrifuged 1× (11k× *g*, 1 h, 10 °C) and 2× (9k× *g*, 45 min, 4 °C), removing the supernatant each time and resuspending the particles in 1× PBS (pH 8) with 0.02% TWEEN20. The resulting AuNP-DOX solution was then used for stimuli-responsive acid release experiments.

AuNP-DOX/Fab (8)—A solution of AuNP-CO_2H (10 mL, 6 nM) was first centrifuged 1× (9k× *g*, 45 min, 4 °C). The supernatant was removed, and the AuNP pellet was resuspended in pH 8 water with 0.02% TWEEN20 and 25% DMSO. The resulting solution of AuNP-CO_2H (10 mL, 6 nM) was stirred in a 20 mL scintillation vial that had been freshly cleaned with aqua regia. To this stirring solution was added 2 mg PPI+N_3 (10 × molar excess, from 11.7 mg/mL stock solution in DMSO) and 0.5 mg PPI-DOX (2.5 × molar excess, from 2.51 mg/mL stock solution in DMSO). The total excess of dendron was added such that 12.5× the total theoretical ligand coating of the AuNP surface area was in the solution. The AuNPs were stirred for 22 h at room temperature and then centrifuged 1× (11k× *g*, 1 h, 10 °C) and 2× (9k× *g*, 45 min, 4 °C), removing the supernatant each time and resuspending the particles in 1× PBS (pH 8) with 0.02% TWEEN20. The washed AuNP-DOX/N_3 solution (**7**) was then stirred, Fab-DBCO was added from a stock solution in 1× PBS (est. 20 Fab/AuNP), and the reaction was stirred at room temperature for 1 h. After 1 h, the AuNP-DOX/Fab solution was centrifuged 2× (9k× *g*, 45 min, 4 °C), and the pellet was resuspended in 1× PBS (pH 8) with 0.02% TWEEN20 and characterized by DLS, zeta potential, and UV-Vis spectroscopy. The solution was stored in 1× PBS (pH 8) with 0.02% TWEEN20 in the refrigerator until further experiments. TWEEN20 was removed by 3 rounds of centrifugation and resuspension in 1× PBS prior to in vitro cytotoxicity experiments.

2.4. Stimuli-Responsive DOX Release from AuNPs

A solution of AuNP-DOX (1 mL, 83 pM) was centrifuged and resuspended in 1 mL of 0.1× PBS. The solution was acidified to a pH of 4.5 through the addition of 1M HCl, as monitored by pH test strips. A separate control solution of AuNP-DOX/N_3 (1 mL, 83 pM) in 1× PBS at a pH of 7.4 was also prepared. The solution of acidified solution with a pH of 4.5 was allowed to sit at room temperature in the dark until measuring the fluorescence of the solution (1 h to 19 days). The AuNPs solution was thoroughly mixed using a vortexer prior to each measurement. The AuNP solutions at a pH of 4.5 and a pH of 7.4 were monitored using fluorescence at 15 min, 30 min, 1.5 h, 3 h, 5 h, and 19 days. Rapid release of DOX from AuNP-DOX/N_3 was observed within 5 h at a pH of 4.5. No increase in fluorescence of the AuNP-DOX/N_3 at a pH of 7.4 was observed.

In another experiment, a solution of 1 mL AuNP-DOX was also centrifuged, resuspended in 1 mL of 0.1× PBS, and acidified to a pH of 4.5. However, it was then transferred to a slide-a-lyzer cassette (10,000 MWCO) and dialyzed against 0.1 M PBS at a pH of 4.5. Fluorescence spectra of the dialysate were recorded at 1 h, 2 h, 3 h, 4 h, 5 h, 6 h, 7 h, 24 h, and 48 h. The DOX release trend observed was similar to the release directly measured from the AuNP-DOX solution (see the previous paragraph).

2.5. In Vitro AuNP Experiments

PC3 prostate cancer cells were seeded in a 96-well plate in RPMI media at a density of 10,000 cells/well. After 24 h at 37 °C in a humidified atmosphere of 5% CO_2, AuNPs were added to the wells at the specified concentrations. All experiments were repeated in triplicates. The cells were incubated for 24, 48, and 72 h at 37 °C in a humidified atmosphere of 5% CO_2. At 24, 48, or 72 h time points, 15 µL MTT solution (5 mg/mL in 1× PBS) was added to the cells and incubated for 4 h. After 4 h, the medium was removed, and the formazan crystals were dissolved in 200 µL 1× PBS with sodium dodecyl sulfate (SDS, 5% *v*/*v*). The 96-well plate was read after 3 h on an automated plate reader.

3. Results and Discussion

3.1. Design and Synthesis of AuNP-Fab Bioconjugates

The dendronized AuNP-Fab system contained two dendron components that were prepared separately: a carboxyl-terminated stabilizing dendron (PPI-CO_2H **1**, Figure 1) and an azide-functionalized PPI dendron (PPI-N_3 **2**, Figure 1) capable of bioconjugation to suitable targeting ligands. The third-generation PPI-CO_2H dendron **1** was prepared as described previously starting from TA-TEG-G2NH_2 and methyl acrylate, followed by aqueous hydrolysis of the ester groups and dialysis [21]. The synthesis of the PPI-N_3 dendron **2** was carried out in a similar manner. Starting from TA-TEG-G2NH_2, a custom-made azide-PEG_3 Michael acceptor was reacted to give the corresponding PPI-N_3 dendron **2** with a 65% yield. The PPI-DOX conjugate **3** (Figure 1), bearing three DOX molecules per PPI dendron, was synthesized as described in a previous publication [37].

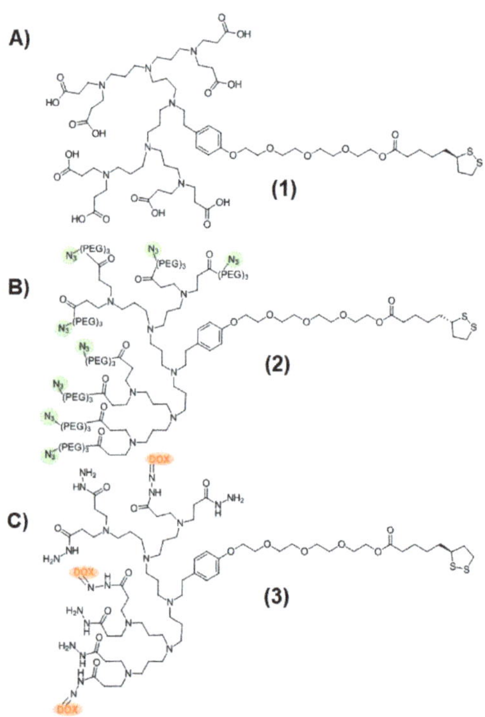

Figure 1. Structures of (**A**) PPI-CO_2H (**1**), (**B**) PPI-N_3 (**2**), and (**C**) PPI-DOX (**3**) poly(propylene imine) dendrons.

As a first attempt to prepare dendronized AuNP-Fab bioconjugates, PPI dendrons **1** and **2** were directly added to a basic solution of AuNP-citrate, as we reported previously, for the preparation of AuNP-CO_2H [21]. However, this reaction did not proceed well, and rapid aggregation of the AuNPs was observed. We hypothesized that the nonpolar nature of azide PPI dendron **2** relative to dendron **1** (evidenced by low aqueous solubility) contributed to the instability of the resulting dendronized AuNPs in the aqueous solution.

To overcome this lack of stability, we developed a novel ligand exchange reaction starting with the more stable AuNP-CO_2H (**4**, Figure 2) itself prepared from AuNP-citrate. A ten-fold molar excess (compared to the theoretical number of ligands per NP) of various ratios of azide and carboxylate PPI dendrons **1** and **2** was added to the reaction, as shown in Figure 2. The addition of 0.02% TWEEN20 overall favored the formation of stable AuNP-N_3 (**5**) by limiting the occurrence of aggregation. The overnight ligand exchange reaction proceeded well when using up to 20% PPI-N_3 dendron, with the size remaining relatively stable at 18 nm (DLS size by volume) and a PDI < 0.15 as measured by DLS. Ratios of between 5% and 20% PPI-N_3 dendrons gave comparable results. However, greater ratios of PPI-N_3 dendron (50–100%) led to some aggregation. The use of 50% PPI-N_3 resulted in partial aggregation, reflected by a significant increase in size (from 21 to 36 nm) and in PDI (from 0.122 to 0.433). And the AuNPs subjected to ligand exchange with 100% PPI-N_3 completely aggregated. The resulting stable AuNP-N_3 (**5**) were purified by centrifugation and washing to remove excess unreacted dendrons and were then conjugated to the targeting ligand. The size of AuNP-N_3 using 20% PPI-N3 dendron increased only slightly compared to AuNP-CO_2H (from 18.8 nm to 19.2 nm), which is in agreement with the small size difference between PPI-CO_2H and PPI-N_3 (PPI-N_3 contains an extra tetraethylene glycol spacer). Also, the zeta potential of AuNP-N_3 is less negative than AuNP-CO_2H (−15.2 mV versus −41.8 mV), reflecting the replacement of some negatively charged PPI-CO_2H dendrons with positively charged PPI-N_3 dendrons (protonated in water).

A)

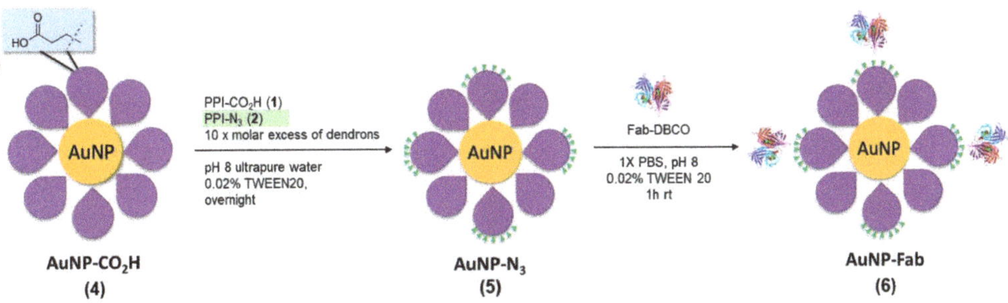

B)

Entry	AuNP-CO_2H start (size by vol., nm)	Start PDI	PPI-N_3 (2)	PPI-CO_2H (1)	AuNP-N_3 (5) (size by vol., nm)	AuNP-N_3 PDI	AuNP-Fab (6) (size by vol., nm)	Final PDI
i	21.31	0.117	100 mol %	0 mol %	aggregated	N/A	N/A	N/A
ii	21.31	0.117	50 mol %	50 mol %	35.60	0.433	N/A	N/A
iii	18.81	0.105	20 mol %	80 mol %	19.22	0.122	28.40	0.349
iv	18.81	0.105	5 mol %	95 mol %	18.57	0.145	26.77	0.335

Figure 2. (**A**) Synthesis of AuNP-N_3 and AuNP-Fab, and (**B**) optimization of ligand exchange ratios for AuNP-N_3 and AuNP-Fab stability.

Bioconjugation of AuNP-N_3 (**5**) to an EphA2-targeting antibody fragment (Fab) derivatized with a clickable DBCO group occurred in 1× PBS with 0.02% TWEEN20 at room temperature over the course of 1 h. AuNP-N_3 solutions with 5% and 20% azide content (Figure 2, entries iii and iv) were reacted with excess Fab-DBCO (20 Fab/AuNP), and the progress of the reaction was monitored by an increase in size by DLS. Both 5% and 20% azide content AuNP-N_3 properly coupled with Fab-DBCO (size ~ 4–5 nm) based on an increase in AuNP size of 8–10 nm for the resulting nanobioconjugate **6** (Figure 2). AuNP-Fab resulting from 5% azide content (Figure 2B, entry iv) displayed the lowest PDI and was less likely to show some aggregation during purification (two to three rounds of successive centrifugation and washing), so this protocol was identified as the optimal bioconjugation to give AuNP-Fab 6.

3.2. Design and Synthesis of Multifunctional AuNP-DOX/Fab

With the protocol to prepare AuNP-Fab (**6**) established, a similar approach was taken to synthesize DOX-loaded AuNP-DOX/Fab. Given the limited polar nature of the PPI-DOX dendron, different conditions were required to achieve efficient ligand exchange and subsequent bioconjugation (Figure 3). As with **6**, the synthesis of AuNP- DOX/N_3 (**7**) required starting with AuNP-CO_2H (**4**), and the ligand exchange with PPI-DOX (**3**) and PPI-N_3 (**2**) dendrons was carried out overnight in a 25% DMSO aqueous solution using 10× molar excess dendrons (compared to the total theoretical number of ligands per NP) to give AuNP-DOX/N_3 (**7**). For this reaction, the best conditions used 80% PPI-N_3 and 20% PPI-DOX (Figure 3, Entry viii) and produced stable nanoparticles with low PDI (0.117), even after two to three rounds of successive centrifugation and washing. After the last round of purification, the AuNP-DOX/N_3 was resuspended in 1× PBS with 0.02% TWEEN20 for targeting ligand conjugation.

A)

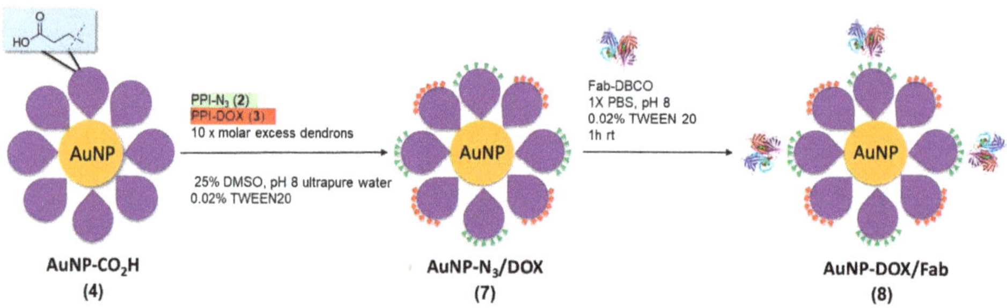

B)

Entry	AuNP-CO_2H start (size by vol., nm)	Start PDI	PPI-N_3 (2)	PPI-DOX (3)	AuNP-N_3/DOX (size by vol., nm)	AuNP-N_3/DOX PDI	AuNP-DOX/Fab (size by vol., nm)	End PDI
v	21.19	0.091	40 mol %	60 mol %	29.00	0.356	103.6	0.500
vi	21.19	0.091	50 mol %	50 mol %	27.18	0.313	40.90	0.439
vii	21.19	0.091	60 mol %	30 mol %	23.44	0.206	36.51	0.375
viii	21.19	0.091	80 mol %	20 mol %	22.95	0.117	28.11	0.230

Figure 3. (**A**) Synthesis of doxorubicin- and azide-functionalized AuNP-N_3/DOX, and (**B**) optimization of ligand exchange ratios for AuNP-N_3/DOX and for AuNP-DOX/Fab stability.

The targeting ligand conjugation of AuNP-N_3/DOX (**7**) to Fab-DBCO was carried out as described with AuNP-N_3 (**5**) using an excess of Fab (20 Fab/AuNP, Figure 3, Entries v–viii). All formulations of AuNP- DOX/N_3 properly coupled with Fab-DBCO, as evidenced by an increase of 5–10 nm in the AuNP-DOX/Fab product, as measured by DLS. However, only entry viii, using 80% PPI-N_3 and 20% PPI-DOX, gave particles with a relatively low PDI (0.230) that were stable during purification by two to three rounds of successive centrifugation and washing. With AuNP-Fab and AuNP-DOX/Fab prepared, a full characterization of the DOX-loaded AuNPs was carried out, and an evaluation of the drug release as well as of the in vitro targeting properties was undertaken.

The reproducibility of the nanoconjugate preparations was assessed by DLS: over six independent experiments, with same ligand ratios, were carried out and showed consistent size increases and PDI values.

3.3. Characterization of Multifunctional AuNP-DOX/Fab

Following the ligand exchange with the PPI-N_3/PPI-DOX dendrons and bioconjugation to the targeting Fab, the final AuNP-DOX/Fab particles were characterized by DLS (size by intensity), zeta potential, UV-vis spectroscopy and transmission electron microscopy (TEM) (Figure 4). The size of the initial citrate-capped AuNPs was observed to be 20 nm (Figure 4A). Ligand exchange with PPI-CO_2H resulted in a small increase in size to 23 nm and a strongly negative zeta potential (−41.8 mV). The 3 nm size increase corresponds to the replacement of citrate with the PPI-CO_2H dendrons. The zeta potential stays negative (AuNP-citrate is also negatively charged with typical zeta potential between −40 and −50 mV) because PPI-CO_2H dendrons predominantly exist as PPI-CO_2^- in water. Further ligand exchange with PPI-N_3/PPI-DOX dendrons resulted in another small increase in the size of the AuNPs to 27 nm. This additional 4 nm size increase can have two explanations: first, the addition of DOX to the dendron increases its size; second, the lower polarity of DOX could lead to the expansion of the previously tight packing of the PPI-CO_2H dendrons at the AuNP surface (Figure 4A). The zeta potential of AuNP-N_3/DOX was also shifted to a less negative value (−11.7 mV), reflecting the decrease in anionic CO_2^- groups in favor of the more positively charged PPI-N_3 and PPI-DOX dendrons on the AuNP. These positive charges come from the protonation of the azide groups and of the primary amine of DOX in water, respectively. The subsequent bioconjugation to give AuNP-DOX/Fab further increased the AuNP size to 30 nm, and the zeta potential shifted to a slightly more negative value (−17.5 mV), indicating successful conjugation of the targeting Fab, as this ligand has been previously observed to impart a negative charge on nanoparticles (Figure 4A) [45,46].

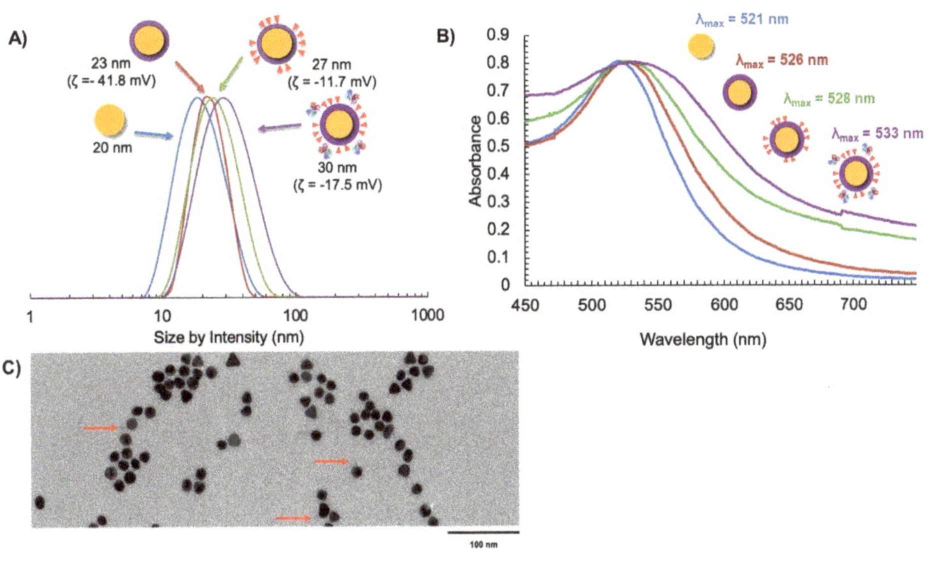

Figure 4. Characterization of AuNP synthesis using (**A**) DLS and zeta potential, (**B**) UV-Vis spectroscopy, and (**C**) TEM with uranyl acetate negative staining (the red arrows indicate the presence of Fab fragments on the surface of AuNPs).

The AuNP-DOX/Fab synthesis was also supported by UV-Vis spectroscopy, as measured by the surface plasmon resonance (SPR) wavelength of absorption as the AuNP coating changed [47]. It was observed that λ_{SPR} = 521 nm for AuNP-citrate (Figure 4B). This value increased to λ_{SPR} = 528 nm for AuNP-DOX/N_3 and further increased to λ_{SPR} = 533 nm for AuNP-DOX/Fab (Figure 4B). The broadening of the SPR peak after the addition of DOX is most likely due to the absorption of PPI-DOX (Figure S2) that occurs at a similar wavelength to AuNP but with a much broader peak (from 440 to 600 nm, with a λ_{max} at around 505 nm) [37,48]. The addition of Fab fragments accentuates this broadening, because these 50 kDa proteins are significantly changing the environment of the AuNP core. The AuNP-DOX/Fab coating was also observed using TEM and negative staining with uranyl acetate. While it is difficult to see targeting ligand attachment for all AuNPs due to the possibility that ligands may be above or below the field of view, some Fab fragments could be observed (Figure 4C).

Next, we characterized the stimuli-responsive nature of these particles in response to acidification. The use of the acid-labile acyl hydrazone bond as a linkage of DOX to the dendron leads to acid-sensitive AuNP-DOX that is expected to release DOX at an acidic pH. To evaluate this release, AuNPs containing DOX dendrons were dissolved in 1× PBS at a pH of 7.4 and then acidified to a pH of 4.5. We chose to carry out the drug release study at a pH of 4.5 in order to mimic the lysosomal environment; indeed, lysosomal compartments are known to have a pH of 4.5 to 5 [49]. The release profile of DOX from this acidic AuNP-DOX system was observed by measuring the direct fluorescence of the AuNP solution as well as through dialysis and observation of aliquots of the dialysate over time (Figure 5). At a pH of 7.4, the AuNP-DOX solutions showed no DOX fluorescence signal (Figure 5A). The lack of fluorescence is due to the quenching of DOX on the AuNP surface due to the closely arranged or π-stacked DOX molecules [50]. In addition, the proximity of DOX to the AuNP core is another possible reason for its fluorescence quenching through energy transfer from DOX to the gold core [51,52]. Acidification to a pH of 4.5 caused the DOX–hydrazone bond to be cleaved, and an initial rapid release of DOX was observed at 15 min (Figure 5A). In the dialysis experiment, the release profile of DOX from AuNP-N_3/DOX obtained by analyzing the dialysate (Figure 5B) matched the release profile using the AuNP-solution-based fluorescence data (Figure 5A). The majority of the DOX cleaved from the AuNPs and found in the dialysate was observed up to 5 h after acidification, and the release curve significantly leveled out after that point. This rapid release profile indicates that the AuNP system may be ideal as a drug delivery platform because rapid release of DOX from AuNPs is necessary during endosome acidification so that it can escape and reach the cytosol and then the nucleus. Indeed, DOX must enter the nucleus and intercalate with DNA to cause cellular cytotoxicity. This release displays similar trends to a recent study using polymeric NPs that encapsulate a pH-sensitive DOX prodrug [53].

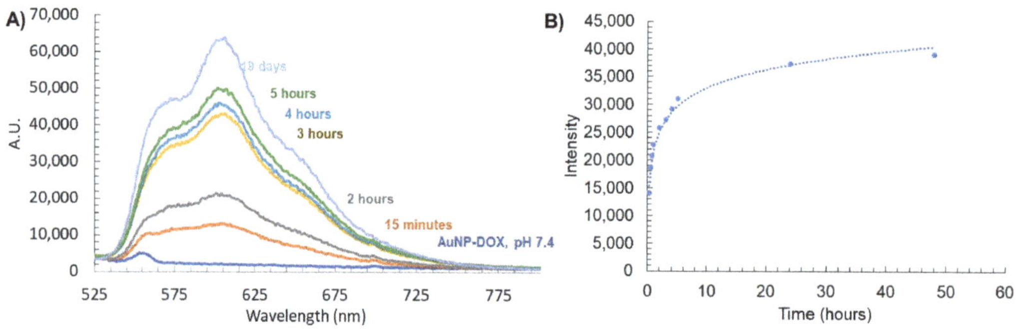

Figure 5. (**A**) Stimuli-responsive release of DOX from AuNP-DOX at a pH of 4.5 measured by fluorescence, and (**B**) fluorescence of free DOX released from AuNPs found in dialysate with a pH of 4.5.

This DOX release study also allowed us to estimate the number of DOX released per AuNP. The fluorescence intensity of the dialysate at 24 h was compared to the corresponding calibration curve, and knowing the concentration of the AuNPs, it was concluded that about 140 DOX were released per AuNP within 24 h.

3.4. *In Vitro Properties of Multifunctional AuNP-DOX/Fab*

As is usually performed for in vitro studies of targeted drug nanocarriers [54,55], we have compared the cellular uptake as well as the cytotoxicity of our targeted and non-targeted AuNPs. To assess the cellular uptake of targeted AuNPs, TEM was used to monitor PC3 prostate cancer cells treated for 24 and 48 h with 0.6 nM AuNP-CO_2H or 0.6 nM AuNP-Fab, respectively. After 24 h or 48 h, respectively, the medium with AuNPs was removed, the PC3 cells were washed with 1× PBS, and the fixative was added. The resulting TEM images showed an increased uptake of AuNP-Fab (Figure 6A ii,iv) compared to AuNP-CO_2H (Figure 6A i,iii) in terms of both the number of AuNPs and the density of the accumulated AuNPs inside the PC3 prostate cancer cells (Figure 6A). This difference is most striking after 24 h, for which the number and density of AuNP-Fab is significantly higher than for AuNP-CO_2H, indicating that the targeting ligand promoted efficient uptake of AuNPs within the first 24 h.

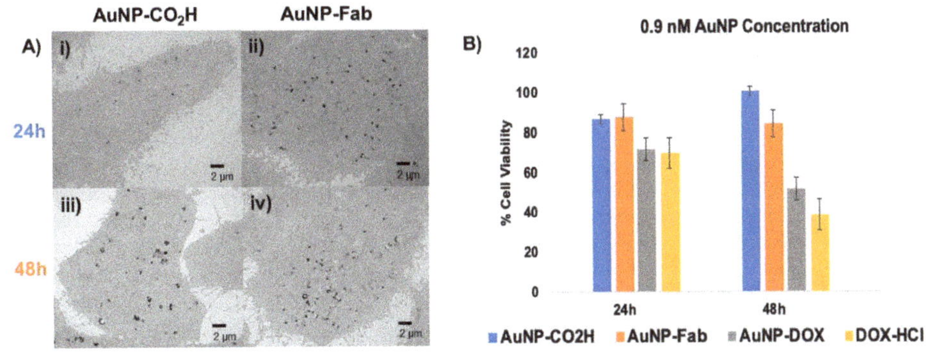

Figure 6. (**A**) In vitro evaluation of Fab-targeted (**ii**,**iv**) AuNPs and untargeted AuNP-CO_2H (**i**,**iii**) using TEM and (**B**) MTT cytotoxicity assay of PC3 cancer cells incubated for 24–48 h with 0.9 nM untargeted AuNP-CO_2H (4), targeted AuNP-Fab (6) and targeted, DOX-loaded AuNP-DOX/Fab (9), with 0.9 µM DOX-HCl as a positive cytotoxicity control.

To further evaluate this AuNP system as a drug delivery platform, an in vitro MTT cytotoxicity assay was performed using AuNP-CO_2H, AuNP-Fab, AuNP-DOX/Fab, and DOX-HCl (as a positive control). PC3 prostate cancer cells were treated with dendronized AuNPs at concentrations of 0.6 or 0.9 nM, and DOX-HCl as a positive control was added at a concentration of 0.9 µM, roughly equivalent to the total DOX loaded on the AuNP-DOX/Fab, as calculated by the AuNP SPR (Supplementary Materials) [47]. At 24 and 48 h after treatment with AuNPs or DOX-HCl, cell viability was measured with an MTT assay (Figure 6B). At 24 and 48 h at both concentrations, the -CO_2H and Fab-conjugated control AuNPs (**4**/**6**) were overall nontoxic to the PC3 prostate cancer cells. However, AuNP-DOX/Fab (**9**) showed a concentration-dependent cytotoxic behavior: while treatment of PC3 cells with 0.6 nM AuNP-DOX/Fab led to lower cytotoxicity (about 70% cell viability after 48 h, Figure S3), the use of 0.9 nM AuNP-DOX/Fab (**9**) gave significantly increased PC3 cell cytotoxicity (about 52% cell viability after 48 h) as compared to AuNPs **4** (about 85% cell viability after 48 h) and **6** (about 94% cell viability after 48 h), and cell death was comparable to the positive DOX control (about 38% cell viability after 48 h) (Figure 6B). This means that the IC_{50} of AuNP-DOX/Fab is around 0.9 nM AuNPs or 0.13 µM DOX (because we found 140 DOX/AuNP). These data also suggest that the control dendronized AuNPs **4** are generally nontoxic to PC3 prostate cancer cells under physiological conditions, while the targeted and drug-loaded AuNP-DOX/Fab shows in vitro potential as a prostate cancer therapeutic. These results are more promising than some obtained by other DOX-loaded NPs, which showed similar potency after 48 h exposure for over 10 times higher concentration than in this study (7 µM DOX in ref. [47] versus 0.13 µM DOX in this work) [52]. In addition, although the antiproliferative activity of AuNP-DOX/Fab is slightly lower than the free DOX one, a main advantage of this nanoparticle formulation is the stimuli-responsive linkage of DOX to the nanoparticle, which keeps DOX as a pro-drug, and thus safe, until it enters the cancer cells. This is a significant advantage over free DOX because this will avoid side effects, especially the cardiotoxicity associated with free DOX.

4. Conclusions

In conclusion, we have successfully prepared a targeted stimuli-responsive DOX-loaded dendronized AuNP platform that has potential as a cancer therapeutic. Using ten times lower concentrations of DOX, it has shown similar potency to other NP formulations at treating castration-resistant prostate cancer, with an IC_{50} around 0.9 nM AuNP (or 0.13 μM DOX). This platform was prepared from a novel ligand exchange reaction between negatively charged dendronized AuNP-CO_2H and azide-functionalized and/or doxorubicin-conjugated PPI dendrons. These dendrons could be added to a solution of AuNP-CO_2H at varied ratios to give multifunctional AuNP-DOX/N_3. The AuNPs prepared here were conjugated through azide/DBCO click chemistry to an antibody fragment to allow for nanoparticle active targeting. Doxorubicin was conjugated to the PPI platform using pH-sensitive acyl hydrazone bonds. The resulting AuNPs were observed to have targeted uptake in PC3 prostate cancer cells, as observed by TEM, and selective cytotoxicity of AuNP-Fab/DOX when compared to AuNP-Fab and AuNP-CO_2H. Overall, these results show that using dendrons on AuNPs can compensate for low ratios of drug-loaded ligands on the NPs (20% DOX ligands on the AuNPs still led to 140 DOX/AuNP) and lead to lower IC_{50} than existing NPs. This opens the door to AuNPs with higher multifunctionality and higher cytotoxicity by combining other drug-loaded dendrons (such as docetaxel or cabazitaxel) with DOX on a single NP using various ratios. This AuNP system may also be expanded to dendrons with MRI contrast agents to afford a powerful theranostic platform.

Supplementary Materials: The following supporting information can be downloaded at: https://www.mdpi.com/article/10.3390/pharmaceutics15082103/s1, Calculation for AuNP ligand exchange reaction; Figure S1: ^1H NMR (D_2O) of TA-TEG-G3N_3 (2); Figure S2: UV-Vis spectrum of PPI-DOX dendron; Figure S3: MTT assay using 0.6 nM AuNPs.

Author Contributions: Data curation, L.T.D.; formal analysis, L.T.D.; funding acquisition, M.-C.D.; investigation, L.T.D. and M.-C.D.; methodology, L.T.D.; project administration, M.-C.D.; resources, M.-C.D.; supervision, M.-C.D.; validation, M.-C.D.; writing—original draft, L.T.D.; Writing—review and editing, L.T.D. and M.-C.D. All authors have read and agreed to the published version of the manuscript.

Funding: This research was funded by the NSF (CBET-1705538). L.T.D. was also supported by the NIH (TT32GM066706-19). The APC was funded by the University of Maryland, Baltimore County (PRFEXC02).

Institutional Review Board Statement: Not applicable.

Informed Consent Statement: Not applicable.

Data Availability Statement: The data presented in this study are available upon request from the corresponding author.

Acknowledgments: The authors thank John Strong (Electron Microscopy Core Imaging Facility (EMCIF), University of Maryland, Baltimore) for the TEM imaging of the PC3 cells. This work utilized an EM sample preparation instrument that was purchased with funding from a National Institutes of Health SIG grant (1S10RR26870-1) awarded to the University of Maryland Baltimore. The authors are also grateful to Charles Bieberich's group for providing the PC3 cells as well as for training L.T.D. for the in vitro assays.

Conflicts of Interest: The authors declare no conflict of interest.

References

1. Villanueva-Flores, F.; Castro-Lugo, A.; Ramírez, O.T.; Palomares, L.A. Understanding cellular interactions with nanomaterials: Towards a rational design of medical nanodevices. *Nanotechnology* **2020**, *31*, 132002. [CrossRef] [PubMed]
2. Peer, D.; Karp, J.M.; Hong, S.; FaroKhzad, O.C.; Margalit, R.; Langer, R. Nanocarriers as an emerging platform for cancer therapy. *Nat. Nanotechnol.* **2007**, *2*, 751–760. [CrossRef]
3. Suk, J.S.; Xu, Q.; Kim, N.; Hanes, J.; Ensign, L.M. PEGylation as a strategy for improving nanoparticle-based drug and gene delivery. *Adv. Drug Deliv. Rev.* **2016**, *99*, 28–51. [CrossRef] [PubMed]
4. Yoo, J.; Park, C.; Yi, G.; Lee, D.; Koo, H. Active Targeting Strategies Using Biological Ligands for Nanoparticle Drug Delivery Systems. *Cancers* **2019**, *11*, 640. [CrossRef]
5. Shan, X.; Gong, X.; Li, J.; Wen, J.; Li, Y.; Zhang, Z. Current approaches of nanomedicines in the market and various stage of clinical translation. *Acta Pharm. Sin. B* **2022**, *12*, 3028–3048. [CrossRef] [PubMed]
6. Rouge, J. RNA and nanocarriers: Next generation drug and delivery platform take center stage. *Trends Biotechnol.* **2023**, *41*, 281–282. [CrossRef]

7. Seidi, F.; Jenjob, R.; Crespy, D. Designing Smart Polymer Conjugates for Controlled Release of Payloads. *Chem. Rev.* **2018**, *118*, 3965–4036. [CrossRef]
8. Begines, B.; Ortiz, T.; Perez-Aranda, M.; Martinez, G.; Merinero, M.; Arguelles-Arias, F.; Alcudia, A. Polymeric Nanoparticles for Drug Delivery: Recent Developments and Future Prospects. *Nanomaterials* **2020**, *10*, 1403. [CrossRef]
9. Ekladious, I.; Colson, Y.L.; Grinstaff, M.W. Polymer-drug conjugate therapeutics: Advances, insights and prospects. *Nat. Rev. Drug Discov.* **2019**, *18*, 273–294. [CrossRef]
10. Wang, J.; Li, B.; Qiu, L.; Qiao, X.; Yang, H. Dendrimer-based drug delivery systems: History, challenges, and latest developments. *J. Biol. Eng.* **2022**, *16*, 18. [CrossRef]
11. Thakor, P.; Bhavana, V.; Sharma, R.; Srivastava, S.; Singh, S.B.; Mehra, N.K. Polymer–drug conjugates: Recent advances and future perspectives. *Drug Discov. Today* **2020**, *25*, 1718–1726. [CrossRef]
12. Tomalia, D.A. Birth of a new macromolecular architecture: Dendrimers as quantized building blocks for nanoscale synthetic polymer chemistry. *Prog. Polym. Sci.* **2005**, *30*, 294–324. [CrossRef]
13. Esfand, R.; Tomalia, D.A. Poly(amidoamine) (PAMAM) dendrimers: From biomimicry to drug delivery and biomedical applications. *Drug Discov. Today* **2001**, *6*, 427–436. [CrossRef]
14. Numai, S.; Yoto, R.; Kimura, M.; Simanek, E.E.; Kitano, Y. Click Chemistry of Melamine Dendrimers: Comparison of "Click-and-Grow" and "Grow-Then-Click" Strategies Using a Divergent Route to Diversity. *Molecules* **2023**, *28*, 131. [CrossRef] [PubMed]
15. Lim, J.; Simanek, E.E. Triazine dendrimers as drug delivery systems: From synthesis to therapy. *Adv. Drug Deliv. Rev.* **2012**, *64*, 826–835. [CrossRef]
16. Menjoge, A.R.; Kannan, R.M.; Tomalia, D.A. Dendrimer-based drug and imaging conjugates: Design considerations for nanomedical applications. *Drug Discov. Today* **2010**, *15*, 171–185. [CrossRef] [PubMed]
17. Lim, J.; Guan, B.; Nham, K.; Hao, G.; Sun, X.; Simanek, E.E. Tumor uptake of triazine dendrimers decorated with four, sixteen, and sixty-four PSMA-targeted ligands: Passive versus active tumor targeting. *Biomolecules* **2019**, *9*, 421. [CrossRef]
18. Falanga, A.; Del Genio, V.; Kaufman, E.A.; Zannella, C.; Franci, G.; Weck, M.; Galdiero, S. Engineering of Janus-like dendrimers with peptides derived from glycoproteins of herpes simplex virus type 1: Toward a versatile and novel antiviral platform. *Int. J. Mol. Sci.* **2021**, *22*, 6488. [CrossRef]
19. Elbert, K.C.; Jishkariani, D.; Wu, Y.; Lee, J.D.; Donnio, B.; Murray, C.B. Design, Self-Assembly, and Switchable Wettability in Hydrophobic, Hydrophilic, and Janus Dendritic Ligand–Gold Nanoparticle Hybrid Materials. *Chem. Mater.* **2017**, *29*, 8737–8746. [CrossRef]
20. Nabavifard, S.; Jalili, S.; Rahmati, F.; Vasseghian, Y.; Ali, G.A.M.; Agarwal, S.; Gupta, V.K. Application of Dendrimer/Gold Nanoparticles in Cancer Therapy: A Review. *J. Inorg. Organomet. Polym. Mater.* **2020**, *30*, 4231–4244. [CrossRef]
21. Saha Ray, A.; Ghann, W.E.; Tsoi, P.S.; Szychowski, B.; Dockery, L.T.; Pak, Y.J.; Li, W.; Kane, M.A.; Swaan, P.; Daniel, M.-C. Set of Highly Stable Amine- and Carboxylate-Terminated Dendronized Au Nanoparticles with Dense Coating and Nontoxic Mixed-Dendronized Form. *Langmuir* **2019**, *35*, 3391–3403. [CrossRef]
22. Dockery, L.; Daniel, M.-C. Dendronized Systems for the Delivery of Chemotherapeutics. *Adv. Cancer Res.* **2018**, *139*, 85–120. [CrossRef] [PubMed]
23. Enciso, A.E.; Doni, G.; Nifosì, R.; Palazzesi, F.; Gonzalez, R.; Ellsworth, A.A.; Coffer, J.L.; Walker, A.V.; Pavan, G.M.; Mohamed, A.A.; et al. Facile synthesis of stable, water soluble, dendron-coated gold nanoparticles. *Nanoscale* **2017**, *9*, 3128–3132. [CrossRef] [PubMed]
24. Zhang, S.; Chen, C.; Xue, C.; Chang, D.; Xu, H.; Salena, B.J.; Li, Y.; Wu, Z.-S. Ribbon of DNA Lattice on Gold Nanoparticles for Selective Drug Delivery to Cancer Cells. *Angew. Chem. Int. Ed.* **2020**, *59*, 14584–14592. [CrossRef]
25. Kalimuthu, K.; Lubin, B.C.; Bazylevich, A.; Gellerman, G.; Shpilberg, O.; Luboshits, G.; Firer, M.A. Gold nanoparticles stabilize peptide-drug-conjugates for sustained targeted drug delivery to cancer cells. *J. Nanobiotechnol.* **2018**, *16*, 34. [CrossRef]
26. Khutale, G.V.; Casey, A. Synthesis and characterization of a multifunctional gold-doxorubicin nanoparticle system for pH triggered intracellular anticancer drug release. *Eur. J. Pharm. Biopharm.* **2017**, *119*, 372–380. [CrossRef]
27. De Souza, C.D.; Nogueira, B.R.; Rostelato, M.E.C.M. Review of the methodologies used in the synthesis gold nanoparticles by chemical reduction. *J. Alloys Compd.* **2019**, *798*, 714–740. [CrossRef]
28. Kimling, J.; Maier, M.; Okenve, B.; Kotaidis, V.; Ballot, H.; Plech, A. Turkevich method for gold nanoparticle synthesis revisited. *J. Phys. Chem. B* **2006**, *110*, 15700–15707. [CrossRef] [PubMed]
29. Enustun, B.V.; Turkevich, J. Coagulation of Colloidal Gold. *J. Am. Chem. Soc.* **1963**, *85*, 3317–3328. [CrossRef]
30. Fu, L.; Ke, H.-T. Nanomaterials incorporated ultrasound contrast agents for cancer theranostics. *Cancer Biol. Med.* **2016**, *13*, 313–324. [CrossRef]
31. Gao, Q.; Zhang, J.; Gao, J.; Zhang, Z.; Zhu, H.; Wang, D. Gold Nanoparticles in Cancer Theranostics. *Front. Bioeng. Biotechnol.* **2021**, *9*, 647905. [CrossRef] [PubMed]
32. Love, C.S.; Ashworth, I.; Brennan, C.; Chechik, V.; Smith, D.K. Dendron-protected Au nanoparticles—Effect of dendritic structure on chemical stability. *J. Colloid Interface Sci.* **2006**, *302*, 178–186. [CrossRef] [PubMed]
33. Cho, T.J.; Zangmeister, R.A.; MacCuspie, R.I.; Patri, A.K.; Hackley, V.A. Newkome-Type Dendron-Stabilized Gold Nanoparticles: Synthesis, Reactivity, and Stability. *Chem. Mater.* **2011**, *23*, 2665–2676. [CrossRef] [PubMed]
34. Pan, H.; Grow, M.E.; Wilson, O.; Daniel, M.-C. A new poly(propylene imine) dendron as potential convenient building-block in the construction of multifunctional systems. *Tetrahedron* **2013**, *69*, 2799–2806. [CrossRef]

35. Ghann, W.E.; Aras, O.; Fleiter, T.; Daniel, M.-C. Syntheses and Characterization of Lisinopril-Coated Gold Nanoparticles as Highly Stable Targeted CT Contrast Agents in Cardiovascular Diseases. *Langmuir* **2012**, *28*, 10398–10408. [CrossRef]
36. Daniel, M.-C.; Grow, M.E.; Pan, H.; Bednarek, M.; Ghann, W.E.; Zabetakis, K.; Cornish, J. Gold nanoparticle-cored poly(propyleneimine) dendrimers as a new platform for multifunctional drug delivery systems. *N. J. Chem.* **2011**, *35*, 2366–2374. [CrossRef]
37. Dockery, L.; Zalesak-Kravec, S.; Kane, M.A.; Daniel, M.-C. Modular and efficient synthesis of a poly (propylene imine) (PPI) dendron applied to acid-sensitive doxorubicin conjugation. *Tetrahedron* **2022**, *125*, 133044. [CrossRef]
38. Ibrahim, A.M.; Nady, S.; Shafaa, M.W.; Khalil, M.M. Radiation and chemotherapy variable response induced by tumor cell hypoxia: Impact of radiation dose, anticancer drug, and type of cancer. *Radiat. Environ. Biophys.* **2022**, *61*, 263–277. [CrossRef]
39. Gomari, H.; Moghadam, M.F.; Soleimani, M.; Ghavami, M.; Khodashenas, S. Targeted delivery of doxorubicin to HER2 positive tumor models. *Int. J. Nanomed.* **2019**, *14*, 5679–5690. [CrossRef]
40. Korga, A.; Ostrowska, M.; Iwan, M.; Herbet, M.; Dudka, J. Inhibition of glycolysis disrupts cellular antioxidant defense and sensitizes HepG2 cells to doxorubicin treatment. *FEBS Open Bio* **2019**, *9*, 959–972. [CrossRef]
41. Aryal, S.; Grailer, J.J.; Pilla, S.; Steeber, D.A.; Gong, S. Doxorubicin conjugated gold nanoparticles as water-soluble and pH-responsive anticancer drug nanocarriers. *J. Mater. Chem.* **2009**, *19*, 7879–7884. [CrossRef]
42. Zhang, C.; Zhang, F.; Han, M.; Wang, X.; Du, J.; Zhang, H.; Li, W. Co-delivery of 5-fluorodeoxyuridine and doxorubicin via gold nanoparticle equipped with affibody-DNA hybrid strands for targeted synergistic chemotherapy of HER2 overexpressing breast cancer. *Sci. Rep.* **2020**, *10*, 22015. [CrossRef]
43. Faid, A.H.; Shouman, S.A.; Badr, Y.A.; Sharaky, M. Enhanced cytotoxic effect of doxorubicin conjugated gold nanoparticles on breast cancer model. *BMC Chem.* **2022**, *16*, 90. [CrossRef] [PubMed]
44. Welser, K.; Perera, M.D.A.; Aylott, J.W.; Chan, W.C. A facile method to clickable sensing polymeric nanoparticles. *Chem. Commun.* **2009**, 6601–6603. [CrossRef]
45. Florinas, S.; Liu, M.; Fleming, R.; Van Vlerken-Ysla, L.; Ayriss, J.; Gilbreth, R.; Dimasi, N.; Gao, C.; Wu, H.; Xu, Z.-Q.; et al. A Nanoparticle Platform to Evaluate Bioconjugation and Receptor-Mediated Cell Uptake Using Cross-Linked Polyion Complex Micelles Bearing Antibody Fragments. *Biomacromolecules* **2016**, *17*, 1818–1833. [CrossRef]
46. Chen, S.; Florinas, S.; Teitgen, A.; Xu, Z.-Q.; Gao, C.; Wu, H.; Kataoka, K.; Cabral, H.; Christie, R.J. Controlled Fab installation onto polymeric micelle nanoparticles for tuned bioactivity. *Sci. Technol. Adv. Mater.* **2017**, *18*, 666–680. [CrossRef]
47. Haiss, W.; Thanh, N.T.K.; Aveyard, J.; Fernig, D.G. Determination of size and concentration of gold nanoparticles from UV−Vis spectra. *Anal. Chem.* **2007**, *79*, 4215–4221. [CrossRef]
48. Chen, C.G.; Nardi, A.N.; Giustini, M.; D'Abramo, M. Absorption behavior of doxorubicin hydrochloride in visible region in different environments: A combined experimental and computational study. *Phys. Chem. Chem. Phys.* **2022**, *24*, 12027–12035. [CrossRef] [PubMed]
49. Chen, R.; Jäättelä, M.; Liu, B. Lysosome as a Central Hub for Rewiring PH Homeostasis in Tumors. *Cancers* **2020**, *12*, 2437. [CrossRef]
50. Sherlock, S.P.; Tabakman, S.M.; Xie, L.; Dai, H. Photothermally Enhanced Drug Delivery by Ultrasmall Multifunctional FeCo/Graphitic Shell Nanocrystals. *ACS Nano* **2011**, *5*, 1505–1512. [CrossRef]
51. Wang, F.; Wang, Y.-C.; Dou, S.; Xiong, M.-H.; Sun, T.-M.; Wang, J. Doxorubicin-Tethered Responsive Gold Nanoparticles Facilitate Intracellular Drug Delivery for Overcoming Multidrug Resistance in Cancer Cells. *ACS Nano* **2011**, *5*, 3679–3692. [CrossRef] [PubMed]
52. Nizamov, T.R.; Garanina, A.S.; Grebennikov, I.S.; Zhironkina, O.A.; Strelkova, O.S.; Alieva, I.B.; Kireev, I.I.; Abakumov, M.A.; Savchenko, A.G.; Majouga, A.G. Effect of Iron Oxide Nanoparticle Shape on Doxorubicin Drug Delivery Toward LNCaP and PC-3 Cell Lines. *Bionanoscience* **2018**, *8*, 394–406. [CrossRef]
53. Czupiel, P.; Delplace, V.; Shoichet, M. Nanoparticle delivery of a pH-sensitive prodrug of doxorubicin and a mitochondrial targeting VES-H8R8 synergistically kill multi-drug resistant breast cancer cells. *Sci. Rep.* **2020**, *10*, 8726. [CrossRef]
54. Muhamad, N.; Plengsuriyakarn, T.; Na-Bangchang, K. Application of active targeting nanoparticle delivery system for chemotherapeutic drugs and traditional/herbal medicines in cancer therapy: A systematic review. *Int. J. Nanomed.* **2018**, *13*, 3921–3935. [CrossRef] [PubMed]
55. Trabulo, S.; Aires, A.; Aicher, A.; Heeschen, C.; Cortajarena, A.L. Multifunctionalized iron oxide nanoparticles for selective targeting of pancreatic cancer cells. *Biochim. Biophys. Acta Gen. Subj.* **2017**, *1861*, 1597–1605. [CrossRef]

pharmaceutics

MDPI

Review

Ferrocene-Based Drugs, Delivery Nanomaterials and Fenton Mechanism: State of the Art, Recent Developments and Prospects †

Catia Ornelas [1,*] and Didier Astruc [2,*]

1 ChemistryX, R&D Department, R&D and Consulting Company, 9000-160 Funchal, Portugal
2 University of Bordeaux, ISM, UMR CNRS, No. 5255, 351 Cours de la Libération, CEDEX, 33405 Talence, France
* Correspondence: catiaornelas@catiaornelaslab.com (C.O.); didier.astruc@u-bordeaux.fr (D.A.)
† This article is dedicated to our distinguished colleague Professor Donald A. Tomalia on the occasion of his 85th birthday.

Abstract: Ferrocene has been the most used organometallic moiety introduced in organic and bioinorganic drugs to cure cancers and various other diseases. Following several pioneering studies, two real breakthroughs occurred in 1996 and 1997. In 1996, Jaouen et al. reported ferrocifens, ferrocene analogs of tamoxifen, the chemotherapeutic for hormone-dependent breast cancer. Several ferrocifens are now in preclinical evaluation. Independently, in 1997, ferroquine, an analog of the antimalarial drug chloroquine upon the introduction of a ferrocenyl substituent in the carbon chain, was reported by the Biot-Brocard group and found to be active against both chloroquine-sensitive and chloroquine-resistant strains of *Plasmodium falciparum*. Ferroquine, in combination with artefenomel, completed phase IIb clinical evaluation in 2019. More than 1000 studies have been published on ferrocenyl-containing pharmacophores against infectious diseases, including parasitic, bacterial, fungal, and viral infections, but the relationship between structure and biological activity has been scarcely demonstrated, unlike for ferrocifens and ferroquines. In a majority of ferrocene-containing drugs, however, the production of reactive oxygen species (ROS), in particular the OH. radical, produced by Fenton catalysis, plays a key role and is scrutinized in this mini-review, together with the supramolecular approach utilizing drug delivery nanosystems, such as micelles, metal–organic frameworks (MOFs), polymers, and dendrimers.

Keywords: ferrocene; metallodrug; anticancer drug; cancer; parasitic; bacterial; fungal and viral diseases; drug delivery; Fenton reaction; hydroxyl radical

1. Introduction

The International Agency for Research on Cancer estimated that the number of cancer cases worldwide reached almost 20 million in 2020, with 10 million deaths [1]. Since conventional treatments, including surgery, radiotherapy, and chemotherapy, cannot cure all categories of cancer, a timely approach to treating solid tumors is the use of tumor-targeting drugs [2]. Likewise, there is an urgent need for environment purification and localized antibacterial treatment because bacterial infections represent the third cause of death worldwide (just after cardiovascular diseases), with an estimated 13.7 million of infectious origin in 2019 [3]. More generally, infectious diseases, in which microorganisms mature or propagate in or on hosts, can be divided into four categories: parasitic (with malaria as the biggest group), bacterial, fungal, and viral. The history of infectious diseases is covered with entire populations being periodically decimated, mostly with pathogenic bacteria or viruses as main infectious agents, as dramatically illustrated by the Black Death epidemic in the 14th century that decimated between a third and half of the European population and by the recent coronavirus COVID-19 that killed around 15 million people in two years, according to the World Health Organization (WHO). The invention of penicillin by A. Fleming in 1928, followed by a variety of antibiotics, subsequently brought considerable relief in the last century. Presently, their excessive use, in particular the prophylactic antibiotic therapy, brings about a dangerous situation because of the adaptability of bacteria, which quickly develop resistance, including sharing of resistant genes between bacteria. Without effective drugs for the prevention and treatment of infections, the human ability to combat common infectious diseases is threatened.

Nanomedicine should largely improve therapeutic strategies using sophisticated targeting of multifunctional drugs. Among a variety of tools, ferrocene chemistry benefits from both numerous possibilities of easy functionalization and stability of the Fe(II) and Fe(III) forms [4] with their easy interconversion in biological media at a mild redox potential [5]. Therefore, this great flexibility of design and physical properties of ferrocene-based drugs should be adaptable to the delicate criteria toward precise and efficient localized chemotherapy. In this mini-review, we will first briefly summarize seminal, early, and recent medical studies utilizing ferrocene-based pharmacophores. Then, we will focus attention on curing strategies utilizing the ferrocene redox system engaging radical mechanisms that involve Fenton chemistry in the production of reactive oxygen species (ROS), in particular OH. radicals. Such ROS provoke disruption of cellular processes via nonspecific attack of proteins, lipids, and DNA. In order to transport drugs, ferrocene-containing nanodrug cargos that can deliver systems onto sick cells, such as micelles, metal–organic frameworks (MOFs), and metallomacromolecules, including polymers and dendrimers, will be discussed. More than a thousand articles and numerous reviews have been published on the anticancer and other biomedical activities of ferrocene-based compounds [6–33].

2. Pioneering and Early Studies

Following a patent from a Soviet Union chemist on ferrocerone in 1971 (no longer in use), in 1976, Brynes et al. discovered the weak antitumor activity against lymphocytic leukemia P-388 of ferrocenyl derivatives containing a substituent that bears amide groups [34]. In 1984, some ferricenium salts were found by Köpf-Maier, Köpf, and Neuse to cure female mice with activity against Ehrlich ascites tumor (EAT) [35] (Figure 1).

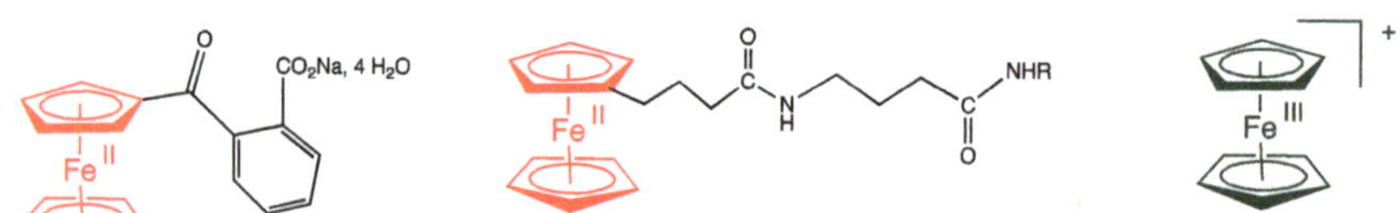

R = H or $(CH_2)_2CONH_2$

X^- = $[CCl_3CO_2]\cdot 2$ CCl_3CO_2H, $[FeCl_4]$ and [Fc] [picrate]

Ferrocerone, USSR, patent, 1971 no longer used

Ferrocenyl bis- and tris- (amide), low activity, Brynes, 1978

Ferricenium salts cure female CF1 mice with Ehrlich ascite tumours. Köpf-Maier, Köpf and Neuse, 1984

Figure 1. Early finding of the antitumoral properties of ferrocene derivatives and ferricenium salts.

It was only more than a decade later that the formation of DNA-damaging OH· radicals from cytotoxic ferricenium and ferrocene derivatives was observed under physiological conditions [36,37]. Since then, the anticancer and antimicrobial activities of ferrocene-containing compounds using OH· radicals generated by ferrocene-based drugs have been the subject of intense scrutiny.

Two properties have appeared essential toward biological activity: (i) the drug delivery design and property of the medicinal cargo [38–41], and (ii) the chemical and electrochemical reversibility provided by the ferrocene/ferricenium redox system (Scheme 1), such as an optimal electron reservoir [42–44].

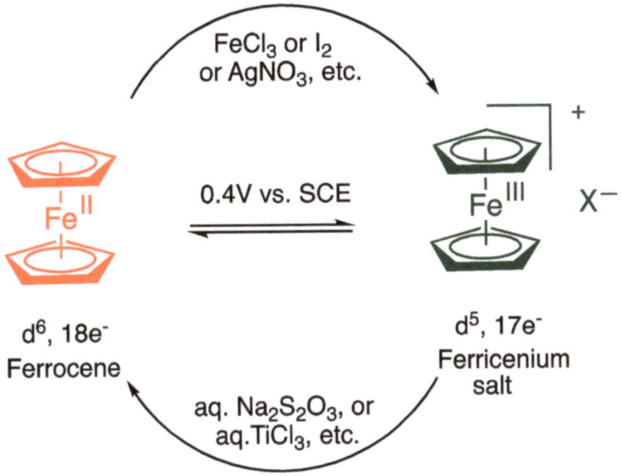

Scheme 1. Ferrocene/ferricenium redox system: redox exchange using common redox reagents.

At an early stage in the field, Neuse, with Köpf-Maier and Köpf, observed activity against Ehrlich ascites tumor (EAT) of some simple water-soluble ferricenium salts (but not all) [44], and with Kanzawa, by in vitro human tumor clonogenic assay, he observed the metabolic oxidation of ferrocene derivatives to ferricenium equivalents in the cell [44]. These seminal works showed that even if the lipophilic sandwich ligands ensured the penetration through biological membranes, the water solubility was very important to the distribution of the drug into the organism. Interestingly, both Fe(III) and Fe(II) derivatives (although not ferrocene by itself) could exhibit antitumor properties.

A very wide variety of ferrocene compounds were reported during the last decade of the last century and the first decade of this century, showing antitumoral properties. These families of active ferrocene derivatives were reviewed in Ornelas' 2011 perspective article [8]. Following Langer's powerful concept of drug delivery [45,46], later emphasized in a review on cancer therapy in 2007 [47], Neuse applied this principle to polyaspartamide–ferrocene conjugates in 1998 [48]. A decade later, the first studies appeared with lipid nanocapsules [8,49] and cyclodextrin complexes (vide infra) [8,50].

On the side of antibacterial, antiparasitic, and antifungal ferrocene-based drugs, several studies appeared near the end of the last century. Epton and Marr et al. reported, in the 1970s, ferrocene analogs of penicillin and cephalosporins, in which the conventional phenyl or heteroaromatic group was replaced by a ferrocene moiety, with antibacterial activity sometimes comparable to that of benzyl-penicillin but lower than that of penicillin [51]. In 1993, Scutaru's group reported activities toward Gram-positive bacteria of ferrocene-containing thioglycolic acid S, the antibacterial activities being similar to those of amoxicillin, cephalothin, and carbenicillin [52].

In 1997, the Biot-Brocard group reported the ferrocene-chloroquine analog, ferroquine, obtained by substituting the carbon chain of the antimalarial agent chloroquine with a ferrocenyl unit, together with its antimalarial activity on mice infected with *Plasmodium berghei N.* and *Plasmodium yoelii NS*. This new drug was 22 times more potent against schizontocides than chloroquine in vitro against a drug-resistant strain of *P. falciparum* [53]. In 2000, the same group also reported the antifungal activity of a ferrocene-fluconazole analog [54]. During that same year, antibacterial properties against *Escherichia coli, Pseudomonas aeruginosa, Staphylococcus aureus*, and *Klebsiella pneumonae* were reported by Chohan and Praveen for symmetric 1,1′-ferrocen-derived Schiff-base ligands and their Co(II), Cu(II), Ni(II), and Zn(II) chelates, the latter performing better than the ligands [55]. During the first decade of the century, a study by the Metzler-Nolte group retained attention on antibacterial activities of metallocene-peptide bioconjugates, in particular [Fc-C(O)WRWRW-NH_2] (Fc = ferrocenyl) that was effective against Gram-positive *Staphylococcus aureus* [25,29,32,34,35,56]. The interest in this study is that numerous plants, insects, and animals possess a wide variety of antibacterial peptides with very different sizes in their immune system. Such research on antibacterial metallodrugs is important because the development of antibiotic resistance to synthetic antibiotics is current, and bacteria are developing resistance very fast, including sharing of resistant genes between bacteria. Numerous ferrocene-appended pharmacophores were reported during the second decade of this century and were summarized in reviews by Patra and Gasser and by Kumar's group in 2016 and 2018, respectively [10,39,56].

3. Antitumoral Ferrocenyl Conjugates

By far, the largest biomedical research activity utilizing the ferrocenyl moiety connected to bioactive molecules has concerned potential anticancer drugs. Artemisinins, peptides (lung cancer), nucleosides and nucleobases (against carcinoma 755), illudine (from mushrooms, extremely toxic), flavonoids, retinoid, curcumin (utilized in the Indian diet), and taxoid derivatives have been derived with ferrocene [12,30]. Ferrocene hybrid anticancer drug research included DNA-targeting compounds (DNA intercalator and inhibitors of topoisomerase II), breast cancer-targeting ferrocifen (prominent examples, analogs of the anti-breast cancer drug tamoxifen, largely developed by Jaouen, Vessières, and Top in Paris) [26,27], raloxifen complexes, prostate cancer-targeting androgens and anti-androgen ferrocenyl complexes, and ferrocenes attached to complexes of first raw (Fe, Co, Ni, Cu) or noble metals (Pt, Pd, Rh, Ir) [8]. Typical examples of ferrocene hybrid anticancer pharmacophores are compounds **1–6** shown in Figure 2.

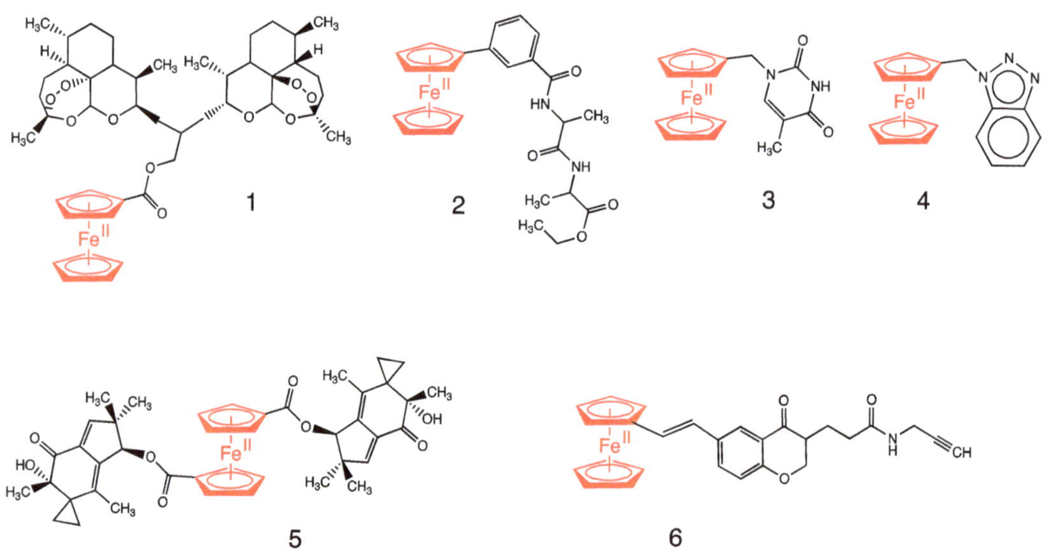

Figure 2. Chemical structures of typical examples of ferrocene-based pharmacophores with anticancer activity.

The di-1,2,4-trioxane-ferrocene hybrid **1** is a very active artemisinin-ferrocene conjugate (IC_{50} = 0.01 μM) against the CCRF-CEM lymphoblastic leukemia cells [57,58]. The N-[meta-(ferrocenyl)benzoyl] dipeptide ethyl ester **2** shows very good antitumor action in vitro against H1299 human lung carcinoma cells with IC_{50} value of 26 μM [59]. Ferrocenyl bioconjugates of adenine, thymine, cytosine, and iodo-cytosine reported by Simenel, such as 1-N-ferrocenylmethyl thymine **3**, showed antitumoral effect against Ca755 cell line (murine adenocarcinoma) with 70% inhibition of tumor growth compared with the control [60,61]. Ferrocenylalkylbenzotriazole **4** showed up to 100% of tumor growth inhibition upon testing against solid tumors and achieved 45% regression. Bis(illudinyl M) 1,10–ferrocenedioate **5** incorporating illudin with ferrocene is not harmful to normal cells but more cell line-specific and highly cancer-selective compared with the parent illudin M [62]. Flavonoid compounds exhibited anticancer mechanisms, such as angiogenesis inhibition, inducing cell cycle. The ferrocene-flavonoid analog **6** (IC_{50}: 23.0–35.0 μM) was sensitive to CCRF-CEM, MCF-7, and HepG2 cancer cell lines [63].

The bioactivity of ferrocene-1,2,3-triazole conjugates, very recently scrutinized and reviewed by Koszytkowska-Stawińska and Buchowicz, revealed the interest in the 1,2,3-triazole link with ferrocene bioconjugates created by facile "click" chemistry from a synthetic point of view and also because the electronic delocalization of the ferrocenyltriazole provides redox potential modulation, thus increasing lipophilicity and π-π staking and hydrogen-bonding facilities that look favorable to bioactivity. These authors emphasized that several ferrocenyltriazole conjugates possessed anticancer properties of the same order of magnitude as those of ferrocifens [12]. Mokhir 's group found that conjugate **7** accumulated in the mitochondria of A2780 ovarian cancer cells more efficiently than the parent clinically approved drug carboplatin **8**. A synergistic effect between the "click"-linked carboplatin group of **7** and the other ferrocene-containing component was postulated since its activity was higher than that of an equimolar mixture of carboplatin **8** and reference compound **9** [64] (Figure 3).

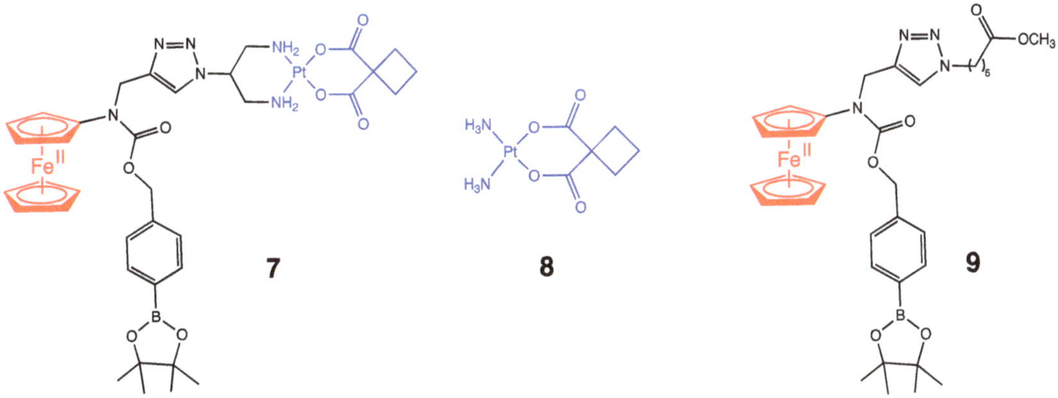

Figure 3. Chemical structures of triazole-containing ferrocenyl-carbopatin conjugate **7**, carboplatin **8**, and triazole-containing ferrocenyl-conjugate reference compound **9**.

Ferrocifens have been designed by Jaouen et al. [26] upon replacing, by a ferrocenyl group, a phenyl group of tamoxifen **10a** (Walpole, Richardson, 1962) and hydroxytamoxifen (TAM-OH, **10b**), which are selective estrogen receptor modulators (SERMs), decreasing the growth of breast cancer cells.

Tamoxifen is used for the treatment of both early and advanced estrogen receptor-positive (ER+) breast cancer [65] and presently is the most sold drug, even as a generic drug in some countries, against this cancer type, but its use suffers from contraindications and serious adverse side effects. Jaouen's ferrocifen broad family of anticancer drugs derived from **11**, first reported in 1996 following synthesis via a tedious route [66], was shortly thereafter made readily accessible using the functional-group-tolerant McMurry coupling (Zn, $TiCl_4$, THF) of two different ketones [67], propionyl ferrocene [26], FcC(O)Et, and a diaryl ketone, in particular di-(4-hydroxyphenyl) ketone, eventually followed by appropriate functionalization at the phenolic group [68]. Ferrocifens, such as **11** ($R^1 = R^2 = OH$) and Fc-Tam-OH **11** ($R^1 = OH$, $R^2 = O(CH_2)_3N(CH_3)_2$ are among the earliest organometallic selective estrogen receptor modulators (SERMs) known since they were described for the first time in 1996 [66]. Whereas tamoxifen shows antiestrogenic activity only on hormone-dependent MCF-7 breast cancer cells, ferrocifens, remarkably, are antiproliferative with dual effects on both hormone-dependent (MCF-7) and hormone-independent (MDA-MB-231) breast cancer cells (IC_{50} of Fc-OH-Tam: 0.8 and 0.5 mM, respectively). Relative binding affinity (RBA) on **11a** and **11b** and Fc-diOH showed at an early stage the possibilities of association with both *a* and *b* isoforms of the estrogen receptor. The antiproliferation effect of the ferrocifens shows that their cytotoxicity is much higher on cancer cells than on normal cells. The ferrocifens **11a** and **12a** were the most active against the NCI panel of 60 cell lines that represent nine cancer types (breast, leukemia, central nervous system, colon, kidney, lung, melanoma, ovary, and prostate) for which there are no satisfactory treatments [69]. The most active ferrocifens were **11a, 11b** (the ferrocifen analog of TAM-OH), and the ansaferrocifen **12a** with, for instance, IC_{50} values on MDA-MB-231 cells (after 5 days of incubation) of 0.64, 0.5 and 0.089 mM, respectively [70]. Interestingly, the IC_{50} values obtained for these complexes were much lower than for their open-chain homologs, despite a less favorable conjugation of the ferrocene ring, due to the bent metallocene structure with the phenol-containing organic group [71]. Nevertheless, conjugation of the ferrocenyl moiety with the double bond plays an important role in optimizing cytotoxicity as, when this double bond is not conjugated to the ferrocenyl group, cytotoxicity becomes an order of magnitude lower. The ruthenocene and osmocene analogs of TAM-OH were also prepared and studied for their pharmacological properties, but they were less active than the corresponding ferrocifens, with their biological properties being essentially related to the amine chain, which emphasized the uniqueness of the ferrocifens [72].

New ferrociphenols **13–15**, synthesized with a polar group on the alkyl chain, showed strong antiproliferative effects, especially against ovarian cancer cells that are resistant to cisplatin. Although, lengthening the ethyl chain with additional CH_2 groups, which increases lipophilicity, resulted in decreased biological activity, introducing a hydroxy group on the propyl chain improved the activity of **13** against all the cell lines tested compared with **11a** [73,74]. With the larger aprotic imide ring group (succinimido in **14** or phthalimido in **15**), an even larger improvement in antitumoral activity on the three ovarian cancer cell lines, compared with **13**, was observed with IC_{50} values below 0.08 μM against A2780 cell line and cisplatin-resistant A2780-Cis cells, for **14** (Figure 4) [75].

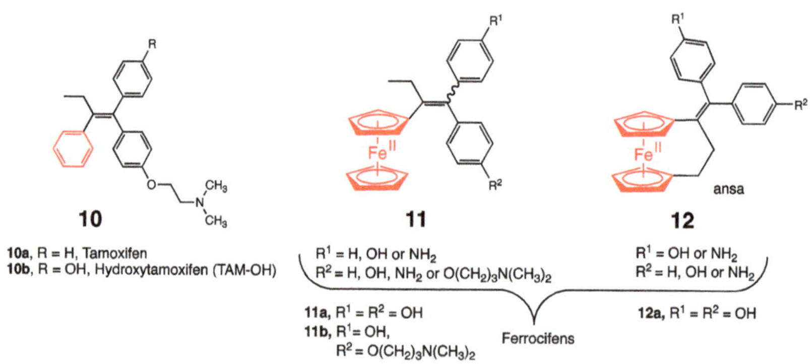

Figure 4. Chemical structures of tamoxifen and ferrocifen derivatives.

The antiproliferative activity of several ferrocifen complexes, including **11a**, **11b**, and **13**, has been evaluated against 15 cell lines obtained from patients, against glioblastoma, the most aggressive type of brain cancer (glioma) (i.e., cancer cells divide very rapidly). These compounds showed a broad diversity of behavior. The study showed that **11a** activated the death receptor signaling pathway in sensitive patient-derived cell lines and acted via the modulation of the expression of FAS (a molecule involved in the regulation of cell death) [76].

Reduction of one of the carbonyl groups of the imide groups of **15** to the corresponding α-hydroxylactam **16** only slightly affected the antiproliferative activity. Conversion of α-hydroxylactam **16** to highly electrophilic *N*-acyliminium ions allowed grafting a wide variety of substituents to the polar imide motif of phthalimido ferrocidiphenol in **17**, which added polarity benefitting diverse cytotoxic activities on two breast cancer cell lines. The compound **17a**, i.e., **17** with XR = $O(CH_2)_3OH$, was the most active compound of the series and was selective against cancer cells (6- or 3-fold less toxic on hTERT-RPE1 with respect to MDA-MB-231 and MCF-7, respectively) (Figure 5) [76].

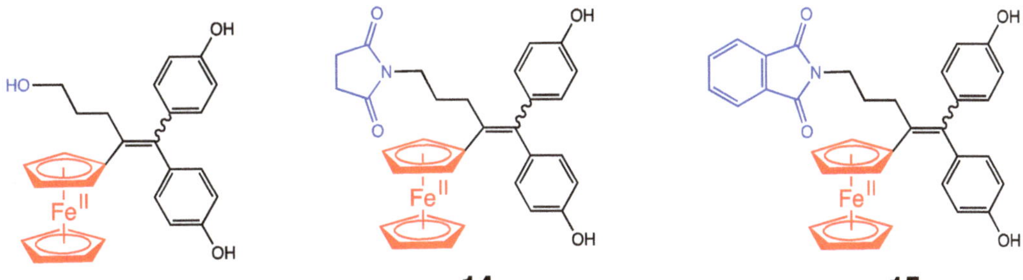

(**a**)

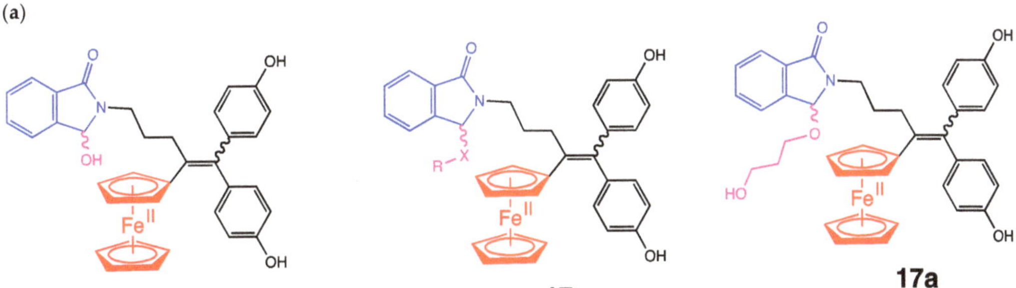

(**b**)

Figure 5. (**a**) Chemical structures of ferrociphenols **13–15**. (**b**) Chemical structure of derivatives of ferrociphenol **15** through reduction of one of the carbonyl groups of the imide groups to the corresponding α-hydroxylactam **16**, followed by conversion of the α-hydroxylactam **16** to highly electrophilic *N*-acyliminium ions with subsequent grafting of a wide variety of substituents.

Most recent publications by Jaouen et al. report antiproliferative activity of ferrocifen derivatives against TNBC (triple-negative breast cancer) cells [77] and the inhibition of cathepsin B by ferrocenyl indenes [78].

Altogether, the design of ferrocifens has involved taking into account, in addition to the starting tamoxifen and tamoxifen-OH pharmacological properties, utilization of the extraordinary flexible ferrocene functionalization and introduction of additional key parameters, such as the refinement of reversible redox site adequate potential for OH. radical generation, the lipophilicity and bulk of the ferrocenyl group (the hydrophobic ferrocenyl group strongly binds the enzyme hydrophobic pockets, which causes inhibition), and solubilizing OH groups at various sites of the molecule, with the ability to provide important H-bonding capacities with the cell components. Over 25 years, Jaouen's group has built up a group of more than 400 diverse ferrocifen derivatives optimizing major anticancer properties, some of which are in preclinical evaluation, and several offer other promising biological functions.

Many other ferrocene pharmacophores have been derived from the structures of natural products or drugs. Other drugs targeting breast cancer with SERMs are the ferrocenyl raloxifens, such as **19** (compare with raloxifen **18**), reported by Marques and showing cytotoxicity against ovarian, cervical, lung, colon, and breast cancer cell lines with IC_{50} values more than one order of magnitude lower than that of cisplatin, with apoptosis cell death mechanism and synergy in **19** between the raloxifen and ferrocenyl moieties [79].

In the category of ferrocenyl androgens and antiandrogens targeting prostate cancer, the metabolite dihydrotestosterone **20**, of testosterone, promotes malignant prostate growth, but the ferrocenyl derivative **21** had low activity. Nevertheless, **21** presented strong antiproliferative activity on hormone-independent PC-3 prostate cancer cells with an IC_{50} value of 8.3 mM [80] (Figure 6).

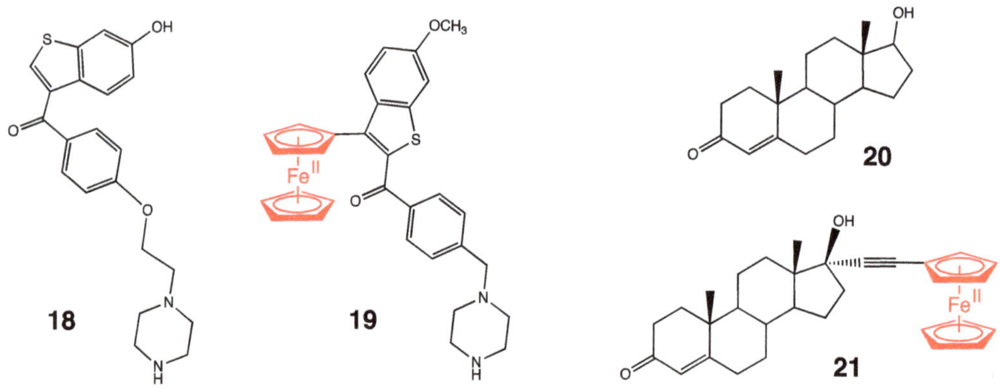

Figure 6. Chemical structures of raloxifen **18** and its ferrocenyl derivative **19**, and of dihydrotestosterone **20** and its ferrocenyl derivative **21**.

Numerous steroid-ferrocene conjugates with variable anticancer properties have been synthesized and evaluated during the last 50 years, including both families of ferrocene-estrogen and ferrocene androgen conjugates, although the first systematic study of ferrocenyl and other organometallic steroidal androgens was reported by the Jaouen group in 2009 [80]. Other ferrocene estrogen [81] and androgen [82] conjugates were recently synthesized and evaluated by the Meléndez group, whereas the Sakač group recently reported new ferrocenyl estrogens [83] and reviewed the field [15].

Kumar's group recently reviewed the advancements in anticancer hybrid drugs, including some ferrocene hybrids [14]. That two parts of a biomolecule exert two distinct functions in synergy toward anticancer properties was inherent to the concept of introduction of a ferrocene group into or branched to a drug in order to improve its antitumoral properties. The most recent examples are ferrocenyl pyrazoles [84] ferrocenyl chalcone amines [85] ferrocenyl chalcono (sugar) triazoles [86], and ferrocene coumarin hybrids [87], which all possess significant cytotoxic activities against various cell lines.

In 2017, Rychlik's group reported several ferrocenyl derivatives of paclitaxel, a diterpene antimitotic agent utilized against ovarian and breast carcinomas and Kaposi's sarcoma. Antiproliferative activity was examined in the human tumor cell lines A549 (alveolar basal epithelial cell adenocarcinoma), COLO 205 (colorectal adenocarcinoma), HCT116 (colorectal adenocarcinoma), Hep G2 (hepatocellular carcinoma), MCF-7 (breast adenocarcinoma), and SW620 (colorectal adenocarcinoma), and efficiency was very dependent on the position of the ferrocenyl group in the molecule. The most promising compound was **22**, with

IC_{50} = 0.005–0.0015 mM against SW620, A549, COLO 205, HCT116, Hep G2, and MCF-7 cells (Figure 7) [88].

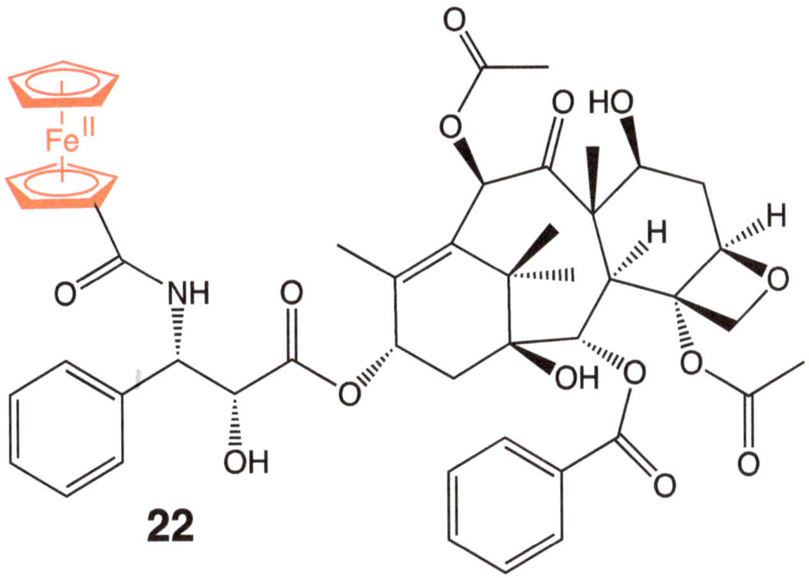

22

Figure 7. Chemical structure of the ferrocenyl derivative of Paclitaxel **22** that showed high anticancer activity.

Recently, several anticancer drugs were reported and evaluated, including aniline derivatives [32] and nucleoside analogs [89]. In the latter example, 1,3-disubstituted ferrocenes were much more cytotoxic than 1,1′-disubstituted isomers. The cytotoxic properties of quinolizidine alkaloids conjugated with ferrocene against cell lines HEK 293, Jurkat, A549, MCF-7, and SH-SY5Y were compared, and their activity against noncancerous HEK 293 cells was shown to be weak [90].

4. Antibacterial Ferrocenyl Conjugates

The dramatic bacterial resistance to antibiotics has motivated an urgent search for metallodrugs with potential antimicrobial activity. Acylation by ferrocene reagents of the commercially available β-lactam antibiotic 6-aminopenicillanic (6-APA), **23**, and 7-aminocephalosporanic acids (7-ACA) **24**, reported in Marr′ seminal work, produced the first ferrocene derivatives antibiotics **25** and **26**, although antibacterial activities were not improved compared with the original organic drugs [51] (Figure 8).

The Metzler-Nolte group has developed very active bioorganometallics, including ferrocenyl-containing antimicrobial peptides (BOAMPs), which were synthesized by attaching the organometallic group to a preformed peptide before liberating the peptide from the solid phase of the peptide synthesizer [9,28,32,56]. For instance, the reaction of $FcCO_2H$ with the peptide **27** attached to the rink amide resin provided the ferrocenyl peptide **28**, after cleavage from the resin and deprotection of the side-chain protecting group, (Figure 9), with an enhanced antibacterial activity compared with that of the original peptide. The hydrophobicity of the ferrocene group was proposed to be responsible for the increased antibacterial activity of peptides, such as **27** in ferrocene-containing peptides, such as **28**, against strains of *Escherichia coli*, *Pseudomonas aeruginosa*, and *Staphylococcus aureus* [91]. Remarkably, the change from L to D of amino acids in the ferrocenyl-BOAMPs also provoked an increase in antibacterial activity, the most active ferrocenyl peptide derivatives sharing a C-terminal-Arg-D-Trp-NH_2 moiety [92].

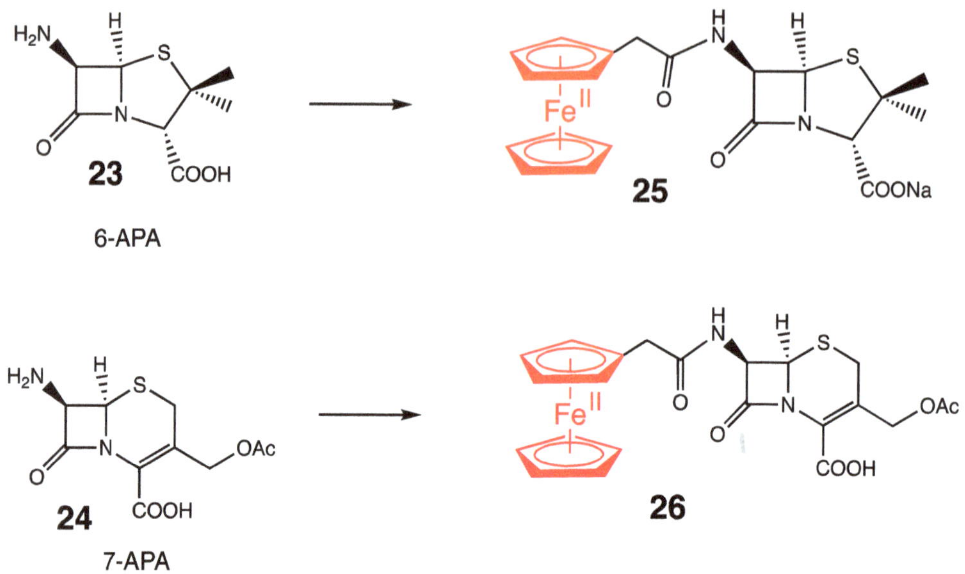

Figure 8. Chemical structures of the antibiotics 6-aminopenicillanic (6-APA) **23**, and 7-aminocephalosporanic acids **24**, and their ferrocenyl derivatives, the first ferrocene-based antibiotics.

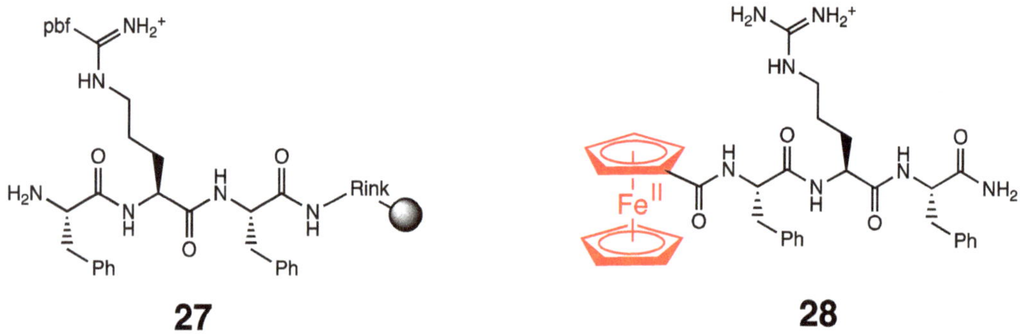

Figure 9. Chemical structure of peptide **27** and a ferrocene-containing derivative **28** that present antimicrobial activity.

The introduction of ferrocene (or other organometallic groups) in the structure of an antibiotic molecule does not always result in an increase in antimicrobial activity. An example of an unfavorable situation was found with the platensimycin mimics **29**, for which the introduction of the ferrocenyl group in **30** resulted in low activity (128 mg/L against *Staphylococcus aureus* Mu50 VISA) [27,93] (Figure 10).

An account of the work by the Metzler-Nolte group on their efficient antibacterial organometallic peptide conjugates was published in 2017 [28], and a comprehensive review by the same group on organometallic-peptide bioconjugates and medicinal applications appeared in 2016 [94]. In addition, Sierra's group published a mini-review on bioorganometallic derivatives of antibacterial drugs in 2017 [27]. In 2022, Hess proposed a selection of concepts to rationally design inorganic and organometallic antibiotics, highlighting their advantages by comparing them to classical drug discovery program [95]. The solid-phase synthesis and antibacterial evaluation of ferrocenyl water-soluble peptides is a subject of continued interest, and the groups of Gomez, Sierra, and Metzler-Nolte recently evaluated water-soluble cyclic metallocenyl, including ferrocenyl hexapeptide bioconjugates derived from the *homo*-sequence H-KKKKKK-NH_2 by substitution of lysine (K) by tryptophan (W) and by orthogonal derivatization of the ε-*N*-amine group of lysine by a metallocene moiety. Insertion of two tryptophan residues and ferrocenyl moieties into linear *homo*-sequence peptides increased antibacterial activity with minimum inhibitory concentration (MIC) down to 5 μM [91].

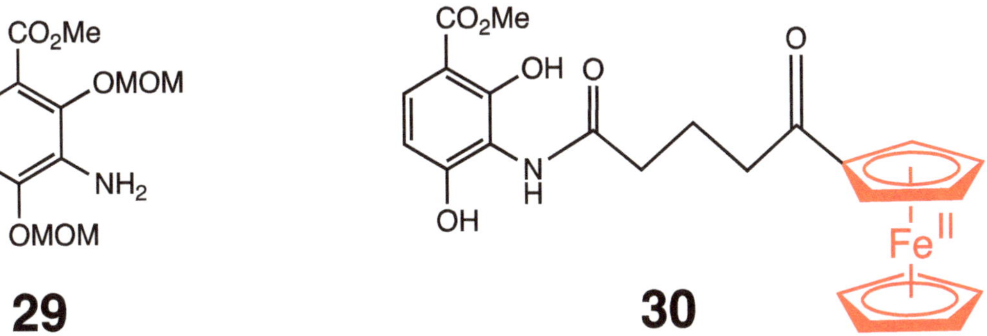

Figure 10. Chemical structures of platensimycin **29** and its ferrocenyl derivative **30**.

Antimicrobial activity of RP-1 peptide (derived from the human chemokine CXCL4) conjugate with ferrocene group has been examined by Cilli and Graminha's group with anti-amastigote activity against *Leishmania amazonensis* (IC_{50} = 0.25 mmol L^{-1}). In comparison with amphotericin B, (IC_{50} = 0.63 mmol L^{-1}), Fc-RP-1 was more active and showed a 2.5-fold higher selectivity index. The RP-1 peptide presented inter alia a MIC of 4.3 mmol L^{-1} against *Streptococcus agalactiae*, while Fc-RP-1 was 4 times more active (MIC = 0.96 mmol L^{-1}), indicating that ferrocene improved the antimicrobial activity against Gram-positive bacteria [92].

The antibiotic ciprofloxacin (**29**, Figure 11), a fluoroquinolone highly active against various microorganisms, is used for the treatment of respiratory and urinary tract infections and as a prophylactic for neutropenia and in veterinary medicine [96–98]. Biot's group examined ferrocenyl-ciprofloxacin derivatives and found an antimalarial efficacy enhancement compared with ciprofloxacin, displaying IC_{50} values between 0.8–3.9 μm in chloroquine-resistant (W2) and chloroquine-sensitive (3D7) parasite strains. These complexes were active against both W2 and 3D7, and **30** (Figure 11) was the most active, with IC_{50} values of 1.0 and 0.8 μm against 3D7 and W2 [97]. A recent study by the group of Stazek and Kowalski elaborated that organometallic ciprofloxacin conjugates showed good antibacterial activity against a set of reference Gram-negative strains (*Escherichia coli* ATCC 25922, *E. coli* NCTC 8196, *Proteus vulgaris* ATCC 49990, and *Klebsiella pneumoniae* ATCC 13883) and Gram-positive strains (*Staphylococcus aureus* ATCC 6538, *Staphylococcus aureus* ATCC 29213, and *Staphylococcus epidermidis* ATCC 12228) and, additionally, against two clinical bone isolates of methicillin-resistant *Staphylococcus aureus* (MRSA) and *Staphylococcus Aureus subsp. Aureus Rosenbach* (ATCC 6538 CIPR). The ferrocenyl ciprofloxacin derivatives were active, in particular **31**, but less so than ciprofloxacin and some cyclopentadienyl manganese tricarbonyl ciprofloxacin derivatives [98].

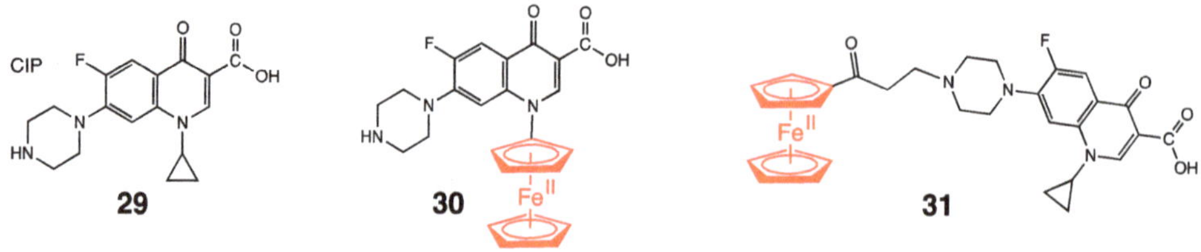

Figure 11. Chemical structures of ciprofloxacin and its ferrocenyl derivatives.

Tirkey et al. reported the synthesis and activity test for bacterial strains *B. subtilis, E. coli, S. aureus, K. pneumoniae,* and *P. aeruginosa* of ferrocenyl hydrazone analogs, such as **33** of the antituberculosis (TB) drug isoniazid **32** (Figure 12). The superior antimicrobial activity of the ferrocenyl conjugate **33** (MIC values: 31.25–125 μg mL^{-1}) compared with the organic drug **32** was assigned to the increased cell permeability and lipophilicity brought about by the ferrocenyl moiety, and possibly additionally to the π-electron delocalization and hindrance of metal binding sites in crucial enzymes [99]. Stringer's group also reported ferrocenyl isoniazid conjugates, such as **34** (Figure 13), and tested them against malarial, trichomonal, and mycobacterial strains, with conjugates showing high antimycobacterial activity toward *Mycobacterium tuberculosis* (H37Rv strain) in the glycerol-based GAST-Fe growth medium (MIC_{90} or MIC_{99} < 1 μm), comparable to that of the free parent drug, **32**; however, **34** was not as active as **32** against *Mycobacterium tuberculosis* [100].

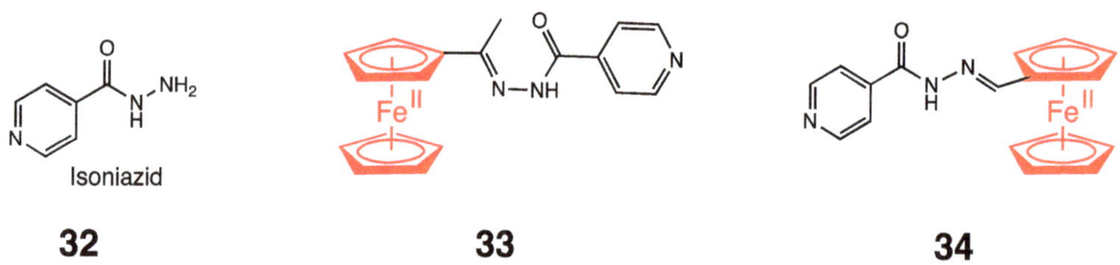

Figure 12. Chemical structure of the antibiotic isoniazid **32** and its ferrocenyl derivatives **33** and **34**.

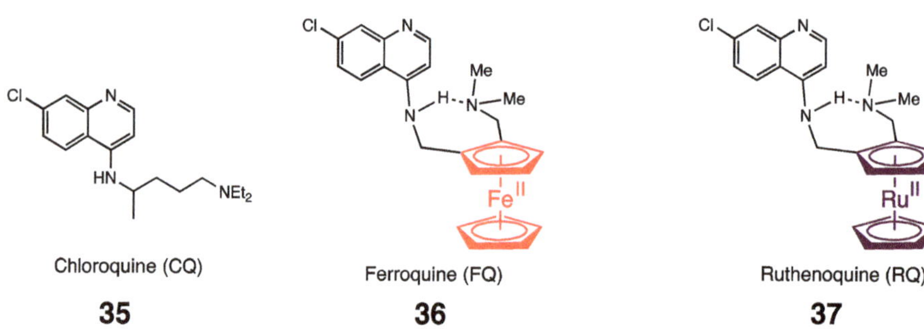

Figure 13. Chemical structures of Chloroquine, Ferroquine, and Ruthenoquine, presenting antimalarial activity.

Trivedi's group recently reported excellent antimicrobial activity of isatin (oxime)-triazole-thiazolidinedione ferrocene conjugates against some selected Gram-positive and Gram-negative strains, with the values comparable to the standard compounds Streptomycin and Flucanazole [101]. Kowalski;s group recently showed that ferrocenyl 7-aminocephalo-sporanic acid (7-ACA) antibiotic conjugate was more active against clinical *Staphylococcus aureus* isolates than the ampicillin reference. Moreover, no undesirable toxic effect in HeLa and L929 cells were observed at the concentrations at which they displayed strong antibacterial effects [102]. Kocak's group recently screened the antimicrobial effect of ferrocene-boronic acid on *Pseudomonas aeruginosa* using proteomics and metabolomics approach and found inter alia that ferrocene-boronic acid affected various antimicrobial targets, such as ATP-dependent DNA helicase RecQ, transcription-repair-coupling factor, and primasome assembly protein PriA [103]. A review of organometallic antibacterial drugs and metal-based materials, including inter alia ferrocene conjugates with antibacterial activity, was recently published by Kowalski et al., and the conclusion was that combination of an organometallic moiety with an organic pharmacophore often resulted in circumventing drug resistance in bacteria, particularly via a bimodal mode of action. The authors also pointed out that the impaired uptake of some organometallic drug derivatives and their potential toxicity against mammalian cells hindered the full exploitation of the antibacterial activity at the clinical stage [104].

5. Antimalarial Ferrocenyl Conjugates

Given the resistance developed by malaria parasites, in particular by *Plasmodium falciparum*, to the main antimalarial drugs artemisinin (see **1**) and chloroquine (CQ) **35**, whose mechanism is inhibition of hemozoin biocrystallization, CQ and all the quinoline-based drugs have become ineffective against these strains. Thus, it was crucial to invent a novel strategy, in particular with metallodrugs, providing new antiparasite mechanisms. This challenge resulted in the 1994 discovery by the Biot-Brocard group of a ferrocenyl CQ derivative **36**, named ferroquine (FQ), in which a ferrocenyl group was incorporated into the alkyl chain binding the amino groups of CQ [105]. FQ was found to be active against both CQ-sensitive and CQ-resistant strains of *Plasmodium falciparum* (the most dangerous malaria species) in vivo and presently remains the most active among more than a hundred related metallodrugs of this series (Figure 13) [30,53,106]. FQ in association with artesunate passed in 2019 to phase IIb clinical trials. Ferroquine is a chiral molecule due to the metallocenyl chirality, but there is no significant difference in the activities of the pure enantiomers of FQ on parasites, and their cytotoxicities are similar. Thus, the racemate is used as an antimalarial drug [107].

In order to provide insight into how FQ acts against the *P. falciparum* parasite, Biot's group has prepared and tested the ruthenocene analog, ruthenoquine (RQ) **37**, of FQ.

Although both FQ and RQ were active against malaria, FQ showed superiority over RQ in vivo in *P. vinckei*-infected mice, taking into account the lack of generation of OH. radicals from RQ, contrary to FQ. This way, FQ induced the breakdown of the parasite digestive vacuole membrane via OH. radicals, contrary to RQ. In addition, the hydrogen bonding in FQ (2.17 Å, broken in acidic media) and RQ between the two amine N atoms was shown to increase the hydrophobicity compared with CQ due to lowering the basicity that generated less protonated, thus more hypophilic species, which, together with the hydrophobicity brought about by the metallocenyl group, accelerated the penetration of the lipophilic digestive vacuole membrane faster than CQ does [108,109]. The authors also prepared and evaluated the methylated derivatives at the metallocenylmethylamine position, FQ-Me **38** and RQ-Me **39**, for which there is no possible hydrogen bonding between the two amine N atoms. Conversely, FQ-Me and RQ-Me, which do not involve this H-bonding between the two amino groups, have a toxicity mechanism related to CQ, contrary to FQ and RuQ (Figure 14).

The fact that FQ-Me and RQ-Me were less active than FQ against CQ-susceptible and CQ-resistant strains shows the crucial role of the H-bonding in the cytotoxicity. The ferrocenyl-lipid structure interaction allows FQ to escape the transport system involved in resistance, concentrating it where the FQ function is ideal for hemozoin formation inhibition. Like SQ, FQ also forms complexes with haematin (log K = 4.95), but it more strongly inhibits haematin crystallization into β-haematin than SQ.

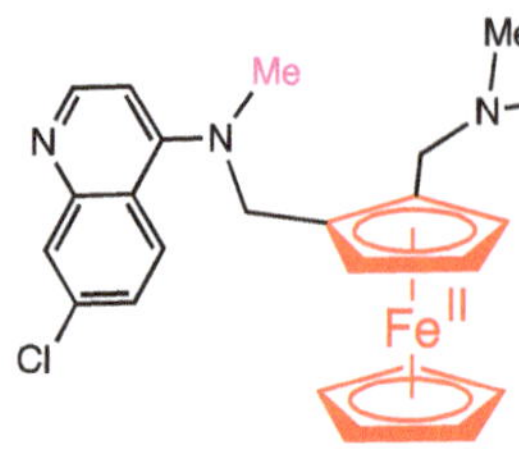

Methyl-Ferroquine (Me-FQ)

38

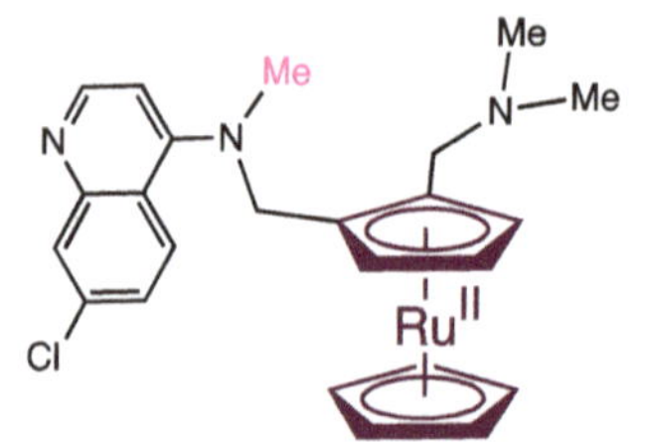

Methyl-Ruthenoquine (Me-RQ)

39

Figure 14. Chemical structures of methyl-ferroquine and methyl-ruthenoquine.

Production of OH. radicals was demonstrated by electron spin resonance (ESR) upon reaction of FQ with H_2O_2 in acidic media, but oxidation of RQ by H_2O_2 did not produce OH. radicals. The difference between ferrocene and ruthenocene in FQ resp. RQ is that ferrocene is reversibly oxidized according to a single-electron transfer, whereas ruthenocene oxidation proceeds with chemical irreversibility according to a two-electron transfer, because following electron transfer, the transient Ru(III) form dismutates to Ru(II) and unstable Ru(IV), and the pairwise reaction does not form OH. radicals. This difference in reactions between FQ and RQ with H_2O_2 matches the fact that FQ is more active than RQ in vivo. Hydroxyl radicals generated upon FQ treatment (contrary to CQ) provoke lesions in cell structures upon oxidation of unsaturated fatty acids in membranes, leading to vacuole membrane destruction and death of the parasite [108,109]. Reviews [109,110] by Biot et al. of their seminal and ongoing work have summarized the properties of the FQ drug families and proposed the overall FQ mechanism. In Figure 15, the mechanism of the intraerythrocytic malaria parasite proposed by Biot et al. is represented.

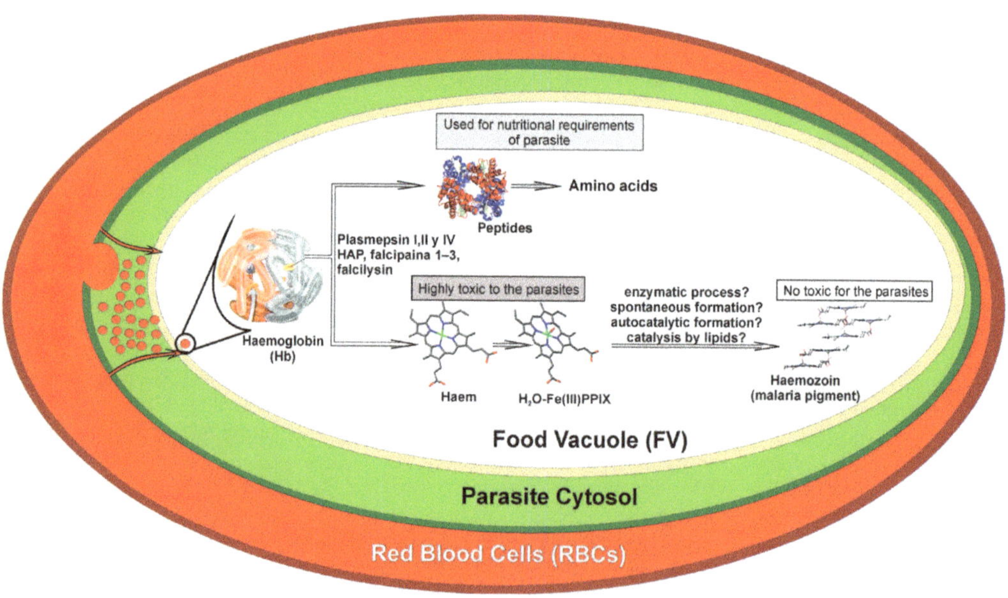

Figure 15. Process of hemoglobin degradation and heme detoxification by intraerythrocytic malaria parasite proposed by Biot et al. Reproduced with permission from Ref. [110]. Copyright 2010 American Chemical Society.

Numerous FQ derivatives, including hydroxychloroquines, chloroquine-bridged ferrocenophane derivatives, trioxaferroquines, ferroquine dual conjugates, 4-*N*-substituted analogs, and other miscellaneous derivatives, have been synthesized and pharmacologically evaluated. Most of them were found to be superior to CQ, but only a few of them, shown in Figure 16, surpassed FQ itself in terms of antimalarial activity [110]. The trimethylsilyl derivatives **47–52** encountered some success because this group increased the FQ lipophilicity, and this series was extended to heterobimetallic derivatives, including FQ ruthenium and rhodium complexes **48–50** and **51–52**, respectively. In vitro, antiplasmodial activity of these compounds was established against the chloroquine-sensitive (NF54) and chloroquine-resistant (Dd2) strains of the malaria parasite *Plasmodium falciparum* [111].

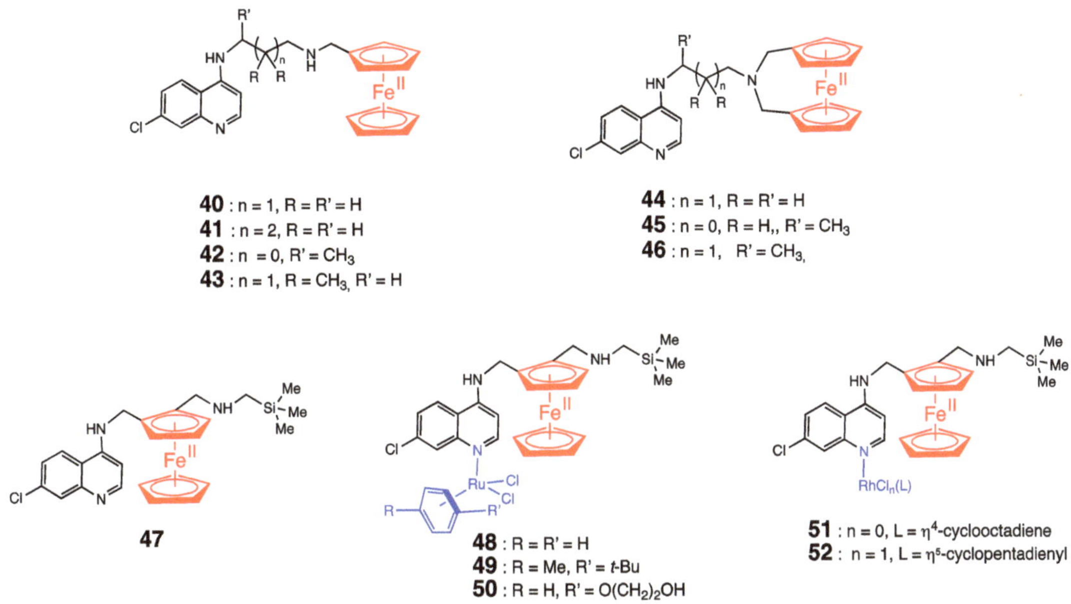

Figure 16. Efficient antimalarial mono-and bimetallic compounds derived from FQ.

Parameters, including the H-bonding, such as in **36**, and the basic and hydrophilic/hydrophobic balance, have been compared and summarized. Briefly, **40–43** were more active than FQ against CQ-resistant K1 strains. The ferrocenophane derivatives **44–46** displayed higher activity than FQ against CQ-resistant K1 strains. The compounds **48**, **49**, **51**, and **52** exhibited better activity than FQ against the NF54 strain of *Plasmodium falciparum*, and the best FQ derivative **50** of this trimethylated series in the bottom of Figure 17 was 10-fold more active than FQ against the same parasitic strain [110,111]. The evaluation of systematic introduction of late transition-metal cation coordinating the amine groups of CQ and FQ has been reviewed very recently [112].

Antimalarial activities of other ferrocenyl derivatives have also been reported in addition to ferroquine. Biot's group, together with the Medebielle's and Bouillon's groups and colleagues from several French laboratories, very recently reported the in vitro and physicochemical evaluation of ferrocenyl-containing hydroxy-lactam-derived tetramates that, interestingly, can exert potent antimalarial activities via a mechanism distinct from that demonstrated for ferroquine [113].

A family of ferrocenyl derivatives containing the antimalarial α-amino-*o*-cresol scaffold (represented in Figure 17 by the two most potent compounds **53** and **54**) showed antiplasmodial and selective antiparasitic activity with a phenolic OH group and rotatable C–NH bond responsible for biological activity and dual mode of action with hemozoin inhibition and DNA interaction. The compounds showed high selectivity toward the malarial 3D7 and Dd2 strains of the *Plasmodium falciparum* parasite, with no indication of cross-resistance and with low cytotoxicity against human umbilical vein endothelium cells (HUVEC). The preferential binding affinity of **53** for the plasmodial DNA over the mammalian DNA, together with hemozoin inhibitory affinity, substantiated the higher selectivity of the compounds for the *P. falciparum* strains. The aminocresol **54** was the most potent compound against the CQS 3D7 strain in the rich series with an IC_{50} value of 0.98 ± 0.10 μM [114].

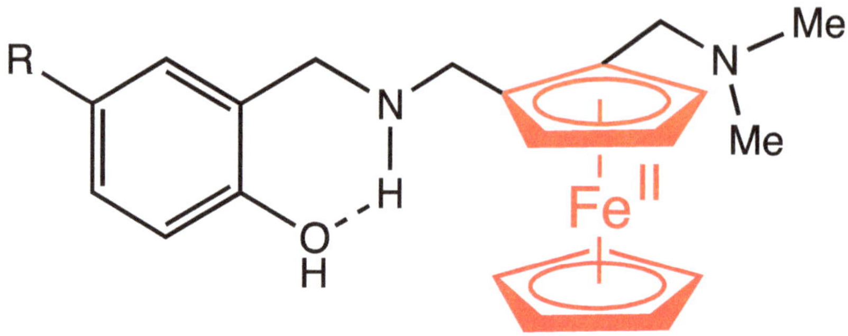

53 : R = 4-Br
54 : R = 4-Me

Figure 17. Potent antimalarial ferrocenyl derivatives containing the α-amino-*o*-cresol scaffold.

Several other antimalarial ferrocene-containing drugs have recently been reported, including betulinic acid/betulin-derived dimers and hybrids [115] and amino-artemisinin-ferrocene derivatives [116–118]. Concerning the latter, artemisinin derivatives are known to promote cancer cell apoptosis, induce cell cycle arrest and autophagy, and inhibit cancer cell invasion and migration. Current artemisinin derivatives (including metal complexes) with potential anticancer activity have been very recently defined [119].

6. Antifungal Ferrocenyl Conjugates

Fungal diseases are also causing global health problems, with treatments becoming ineffective due to the resistant strains of pathogens and high toxicity of drugs currently in use. The scarcity of efficient treatments for fungal diseases should motivate the research of novel drug candidates. In addition to the seminal finding by the Biot-Brocard group of the antifungal activity of a ferrocene derivative of fluconazole **55a** (Figure 18) [54], one of the most common antifungal drugs, active against a large number of mycoses, a recent in vivo study by Gasser's group reported the synthesis and activity of four new fluconazole derivatives. The authors focused on azoles, the mainstay of antifungal drugs, their activity involving their binding via the triazole nitrogen atom marked in blue in **55a** and **55b** to the heme iron atom of the fungal lanosterol 14α-demethylase target enzyme (from computing binding geometry data). The activity of **55b** was shown on clinical isolates, with antimycotic potency up to 400 times higher than fluconazole, and activity toward azole-resistant strains was demonstrated (replacement of the methyl group of **55b** by H or larger groups showed that the methyl group provided the best results). In vivo studies in a mice model of *Candida* infections showed that **55b** not only reduced the fungal growth and dissemination but also improved immunopathology [120].

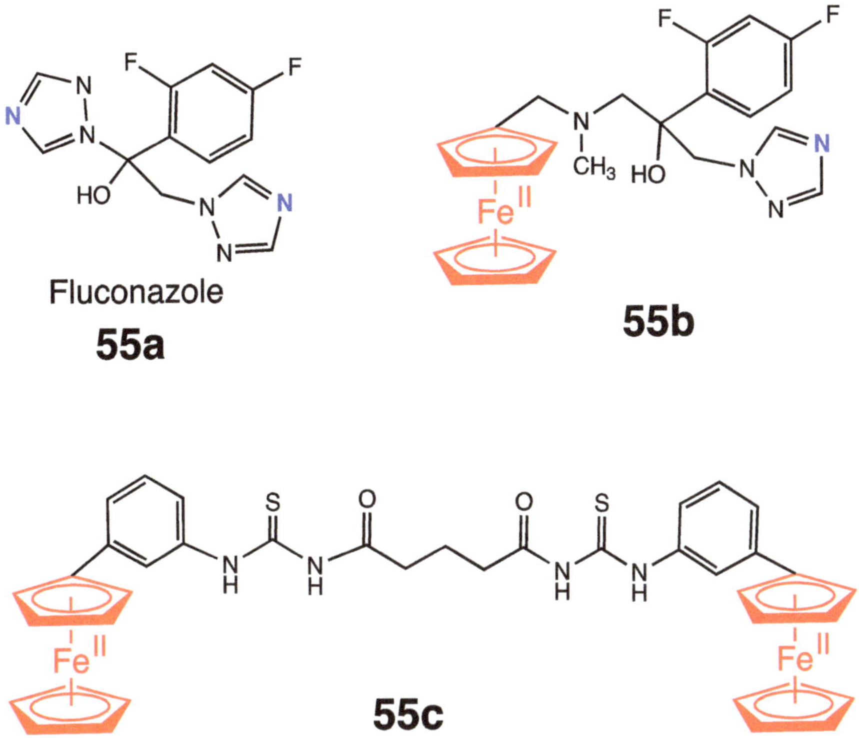

Figure 18. Representative antifungal compounds.

Ferrocenyl drug conjugates showing antifungal activity also show other biological properties, such as antibacterial, antimalarial, and/or anticancer properties. Along this line, additional Schiff-based ligands and their Zn and Cu complexes were found in antibacterial and antifungal agents in vitro, with antifungal properties enhanced by the complexation of the Schiff-based ligand to these metals [62]. Kaliappa's group synthesized ferrocenyl conjugates containing nonsymmetrical tetradentate Schiff-base ligands that were shown to possess antimicrobial activity against four bacterial and two fungal stains [121]. Recently, Cilli et al. developed new strategies for ferrocene-containing antimicrobial RP-1 peptides, synthesized through solid-phase peptide synthesis, with antifungal and antiplasmodial properties with low toxicity in the U87 and HepG2 cell lines [122]. Badshah's group reported new symmetrical ferrocene-based bisthiourea analogs and examined their antibacterial, antifungal, antioxidant, and antidiabetic activities in vitro. In particular, antifungal studies conducted using a disc diffusion method against *Mucor* species (FCBP 0300), *Aspergillus niger* (FCBP 0198), *Aspergillus flavus* (FCBP 0064), and *Fusarium solani* (FCBP 0291) showed activity against all fungal species with maximum activity against *Aspergillus flavus* and *Aspergillus niger*. The most active derivative in the series was **55c** (Figure 19) [123]. Ferrocenyl-containing chalcone derivatives have also been recently shown by various research groups to possess inter alia antifungal properties [82,83,124].

7. The Fenton Reaction with Fe^{2+} and Ferrocene Derivatives

The Fenton reaction, discovered by Fenton at the end of the 19th century [125], involves the reaction of a ferrous (Fe^{2+}) salt (in water, Fe^{2+} is in the form of $[Fe(H_2O)_6]^{2+}$.) [126]

with H_2O_2 (Equation (1)), followed by the slower reaction of the ferric (Fe^{3+}) salt with H_2O_2 (amphoteric role of H_2O_2, Equation (2)). This results in the consumption of Fe^{2+}, via the intermediate $[Fe(III)OOH]^{2+}$, formed according to Equation (3) in a very acidic medium. External energy fields, including light, heat, ultrasound, electric, or magnetic fields, can also promote Fenton reactions. In the photo-Fenton mechanism, the intermediate $[Fe(III)OOH]^{2+}$ is photolyzed to HO_2. and Fe^{2+} (Equation (4)) [127] but, with ferrocene, the Cp ligands are not lost, which inhibits this process. On the other hand, H_2O_2 can be photolyzed to OH. (Equation (5)). The intermediacy of the OH. radicals at pH < 3 was shown much later, in 1934, by Haber and Weiss [128], and observed by EPR in 1979 [129]. In the following equations, the H_2O ligands are omitted.

$$Fe^{2+} + H_2O_2 \rightarrow Fe^{3+} + OH^- + OH^\bullet \quad (1)$$

$$Fe^{3+} + H_2O_2 \rightarrow Fe^{2+} + H^+ + HO_2\bullet \quad (2)$$

$$Fe^{3+} + H_2O_2 \rightarrow [Fe(III)\,OOH]^{2+} + H^+ \quad (3)$$

$$[Fe(III)\,OOH]^{2+} + h\upsilon \rightarrow Fe^{2+} + HO_2\bullet \quad (4)$$

$$H_2O_2 + h\upsilon \rightarrow 2OH^\bullet \quad (5)$$

The pH is crucial to the Fenton reaction, for instance, because of the hydrolysis of Fe^{2+} to $Fe(OH)_n{}^{2-n}$ species (n = 1–4) if the pH is not acidic (including, for n = 2, precipitation of ferrous hydroxide) [130].

Thus, in an acidic medium, Equation (1) becomes Equation (6):

$$Fe^{2+} + H_2O_2 + H^+ \rightarrow Fe^{3+} + H_2O + OH^\bullet \quad (6)$$

For mammalian cells, the intracellular pH value varies from 4.7 in lysosome to 8.0 in mitochondria, and cancer cells are more acidic than healthy cells. The efficiency of the Fenton reaction is optimal in the pH range between 2 and 4. In consequence, the mildly acidic tumor microenvironment is not ideal for the Fenton reaction. Thus, reducing the pH in tumor tissues must be fulfilled by chemodynamic therapy (CDT). Likewise, endogenous H_2O_2 is insufficient to induce an efficient Fenton reaction. An excellent method to decrease the pH and increase the H_2O_2 level in the tumor microenvironment (TME) is to include glucose oxidase (GOx) in the CDT cargo because GOx catalyzes, using the co-factor Flavine Adenine Dinucleotide (FAD), the oxidation of β-D-glucose to H_2O_2 and D-glucoco-1,5-lactone that further hydrolyzes to gluconic acid (vide infra).

The hydroxyl radical OH. produced in the Fenton reaction is an extremely high-energy species [131], its potential E° $(OH\cdot/H_2O)$ being as high as 2.81 V vs. normal hydrogen electrode (NHE). In the presence of excess H_2O_2, the radical OH. is oxidized, yielding the other radical $HO_2\cdot$ (Equation (5)), the protonated form of superoxide radical anion $O_2\cdot^-$ (Equation (7)), with a pK_a value of 4.8 for HO_2.

$$H_2O_2 + OH^\bullet \rightarrow H_2O + HO_2\bullet \quad (7)$$

The superoxide radical anion, $O_2\cdot^-$ [132], and its protonated form HO_2. are also formed, depending on the pH, but the basic and nucleophilic properties of $O_2\cdot^-$ are highly dependent on whether the medium is aqueous or nonaqueous [133]. HO_2 is highly unstable in water and dismutates to H_2O_2 and O_2 (Equation (8)). In a hydrophobic medium, the basic and nucleophilic reactions are favored, and dismutation occurs under the influence of a catalyst, particularly a superoxide dismutase (SOD) enzyme [132].

$$2HO_2\bullet \rightarrow H_2O_2 + O_2\bullet \quad (8)$$

The radical $HO_2\cdot$ also reacts with H_2O_2 to yield $OH\cdot$, but this reaction is too slow to significantly contribute to the production of the radical OH. (Equation (9))

$$H_2O_2 + HO_2\bullet \rightarrow H_2O + OH^{\bullet} + O_2\bullet \tag{9}$$

The radicals $OH\cdot$, $HO_2\cdot$, and $O_2\cdot^-$ belong, together with peroxide (ROOR), singlet oxygen ($^1O_2$), and nitric oxide (NO.), to the so-called reactive oxygen species (ROS) that are byproducts of the normal biological oxygen metabolism, present at low and stationary levels in normal cells, and known for their role in cell signaling and homeostasis; they are also known for causing irreversible damage to intracellular DNA [134]. However, the OH. radical is by far the most reactive among the ROS.

Since both ferricenium and ferrocene derivatives have long been known for their anticancer and antimicrobial activities, it became essential that the redox stability of both redox forms in biological media (Scheme 2) (i.e., the electron-reservoir property of ferrocene) [135] was a key aspect in their pharmacological properties, as noted early in [5,136]. The long-term degradation of ferricenium salts in vivo is still in question. The lipophilic neutral form allows for transferring the derivative through biological membranes, whereas the cationic oxidized form provides solubility in hydrophilic media.

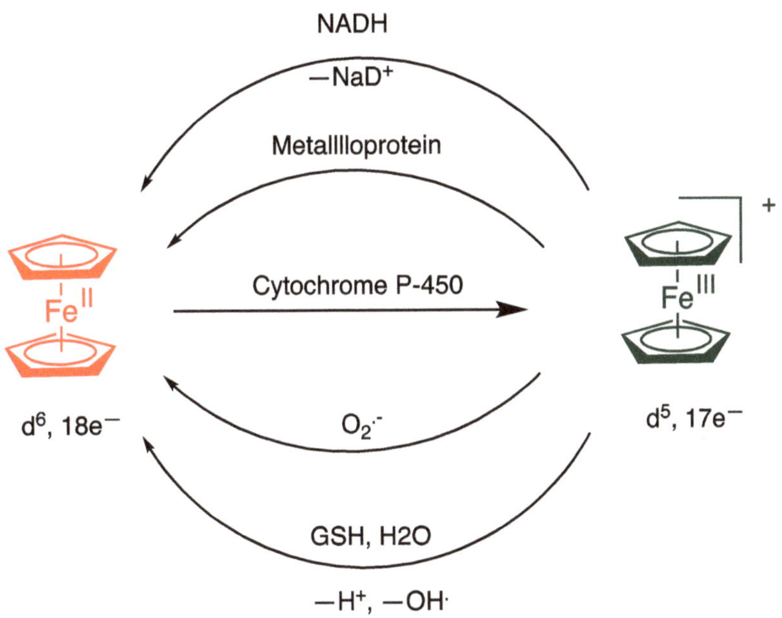

Scheme 2. Ferrocene/Ferricenium redox system: redox exchange by biological reagents. Adapted with permission from Ref. [5]. Copyright 2005 Elsevier.

The ability of the oxidized form of ferrocene, ferricenium, to produce cytotoxic OH. radicals in the Fenton reaction was demonstrated by Hiroshi and Masahiro [36] in 1997 and confirmed by Osella et al. [37] in 2000 by electron paramagnetic resonance (EPR) characterization. Major differences between the oxidation of the two Fe(II) complexes $[Fe(H_2O)_6]^{2+}$ and ferrocene ($FeCp_2$) are the solubilities, the coordination, and the redox potential $E^\circ(Fe^{III/II})$. The salts $[Fe(H_2O)_6]^{2+}(X^-)_2$ are mostly water-soluble, whereas ferrocene is soluble in nonpolar organic solvents and insoluble in water. Another key difference between this classic Fenton reaction of Equations (1)–(3) with Fe^{2+} and the Fenton reaction with ferrocene or ferrocenyl derivatives is that with the latter, Fe(II) in ferrocene is coordinatively saturated ($FeCp_2$ is a robust 18-electron complex), and thus the radicals $OH\cdot$ and

$HO_2\cdot$ cannot bind to the Fe center. This is in contrast with hydrated Fe^{2+}, in which the H_2O ligands are easily deprotonated or displaced by hydroxy anions or radicals.

The redox potential determines the rate of Fe(II) oxidation; $[Fe(H_2O)_6]^{2+}$ is oxidized at 0.77 V vs. NHE in water, whereas ferrocene is oxidized at 0.67 V vs. NHE in DMSO, which means that ferrocene is oxidized slightly more easily than $[Fe(H_2O)_6]^{2+}$, although comparison between reactions in water and organic solvents is difficult (Scheme 3).

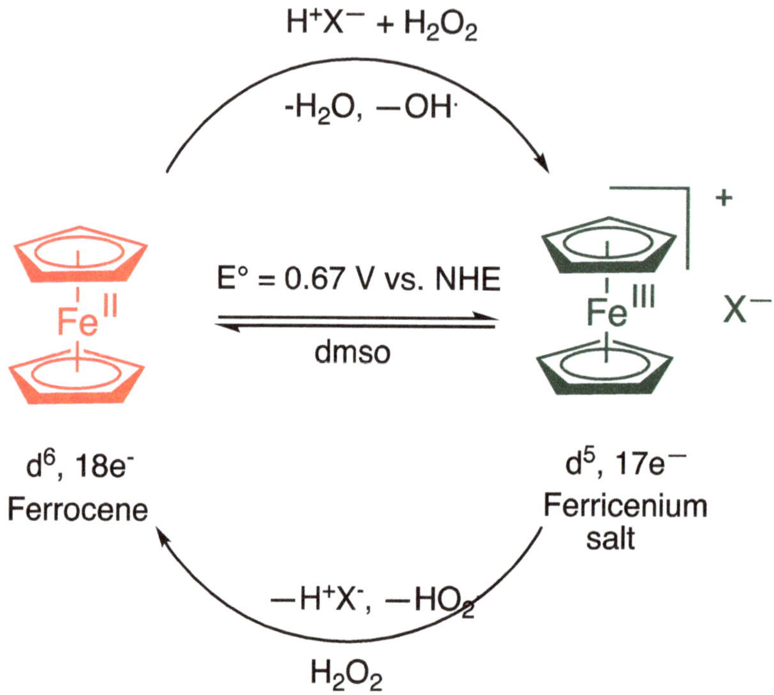

Scheme 3. Fenton reactions involving ferrocene and ferricenium salts.

Another aspect is that ring substituents influence the redox potential of the ferrocenyl group. In particular, when the ferrocenyl moiety bears one or two carbonyl groups on the rings, oxidation becomes more difficult by 0.3 V or 0.6 V, respectively, compared with that of ferrocene [137,138]. Lacina's group reported that the cytotoxicity of ferrocene derivatives and ROS-activated prodrugs based on ferrocenyliminoboronates depended on their redox potential, aminoferrocene with its lowest redox potential exhibiting the highest cytotoxicity [139].

Many ferrocenyl-containing drugs bear a group conjugated (styrenyl, triazole, chalcone, etc.) with the Cp ligand in the Fe(II) and Fe(III) forms, which stabilizes them and lowers the oxidation potential, facilitating the production of hydroxyl radicals. For instance, concerning the ferroxifen of type **11** [7], one can propose that, upon single-electron oxidation, the mono-oxidized species **56** is stabilized by the dual resonant forms (Figure 20), including the fulvalene structure (isolobal to the redox catalysts CpFe(I)arene) [140,141], which explains the proton-coupled electron transfer [142] viewing the strong acidity of the oxenium form (Figure 19).

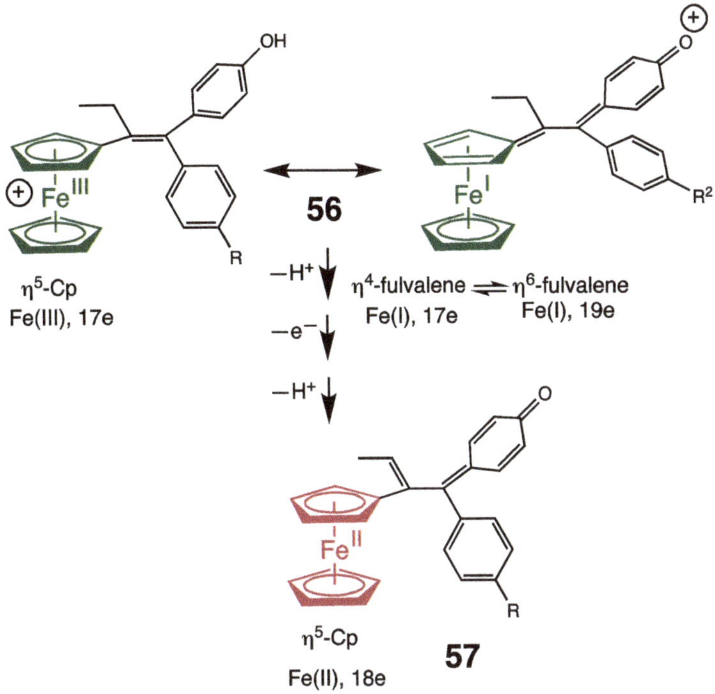

Figure 19. Proposed structure **56** resulting from the single-electron oxidation of ferrocifen **11**. Upon double proton-coupled electron transfer, **11** was oxidized to **57** [7].

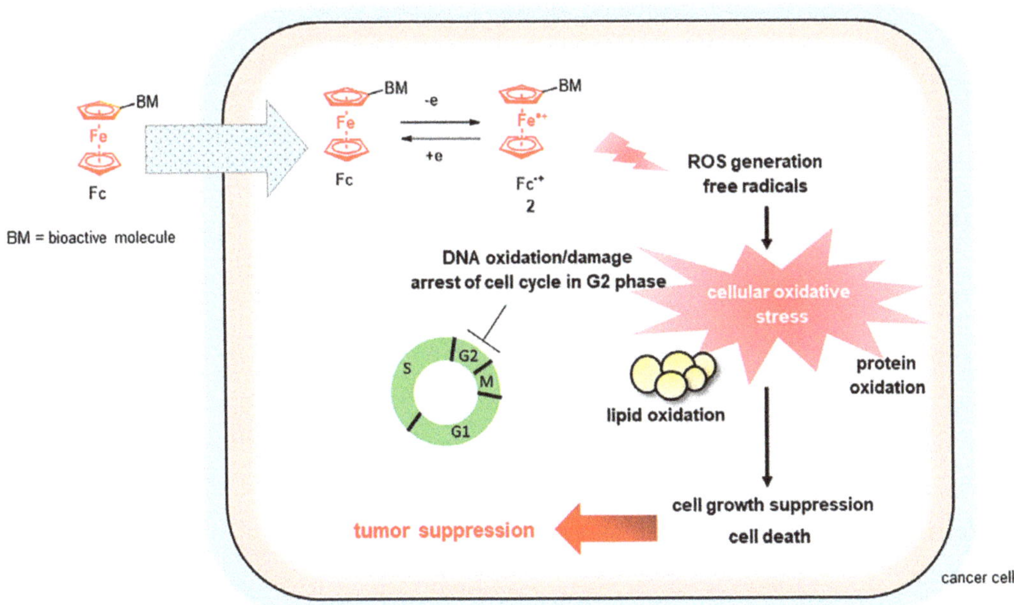

Figure 20. Mechanism of oxidative stress leading to cell death provoked by Fenton reaction with a ferrocenyl conjugate. Reproduced with permission from Ref. [26]. Copyright 2019 Elsevier.

Ultimately, the quinone methide complex **57**, spontaneously obtained at the same potential after two proton-coupled electron transfer sequences, is also more easily oxidized than ferrocene because of the conjugated organic fragment. Complex **57** is thus cytotoxic, responsible for hydroxyl radical generation, and, as a metabolite following treatment with ferrocifen, has been found to likely cause cell death upon interaction with DNA, proteins, and glutathione. Ferrocifen quinone methides are primary metabolites undergoing Michael additions with thiols or selenols of key proteins, which generates a disruption of cell metabolism [143].

This condition is not determining, however; for instance, the ferrocenophane (ansa-ferrocenes) derivatives **12** of the ferrocifen family inhibiting conjugation with the substituent show excellent and sometimes better activity than fully conjugated ferrocifens **11** [7].

The ferrocifens produce ROS at the 1 mM incubation concentration after 10 min incubation, unlike tamoxifen and hydroxytamoxifen. The addition of the antioxidants *N*-acetyl cysteine or vitamin E leads to the loss of antiproliferative effect of ferrocifens, which demonstrates that the toxicity of these ferrocenyl drugs is due to their production of ROS. However, the formation of ROS is not connected to the presence of a phenol group, and the quantity of ROS produced is also independent of the IC_{50} values.

In the mechanism of the oxidation of a series of ferrocene derivatives with hydrogen peroxide, Fomin and Zaitseva observed a shift of λ_{max} of the absorption band of the ferricenium cation toward long wavelengths and its broadening during the reaction, which was assigned to the formation of a {ferricenium cation + OH.} radical pair [144]. Clearly, organoiron radicals play a key role in reactivity [145], especially with such a high-energy species as OH.

ROS at a low level are cellular signaling messengers via modification of protein structure in healthy cells, but high ROS levels disrupt normal cellular processes via nonspecific attack of proteins, lipids, and DNA, thiol groups of proteins and glutathione being privileged targets. The production of ROS by cancer cells is due to increased metabolic rate, mitochondria dysfunction, oncogene expression, increased peroxisome activities, and elevated cell signaling. The Fenton reactions providing excess ROS provoke DNA oxidative damage and cell cycle arrest (Figure 20) [146].

Likewise, with ferroquine, the lipophilic ferrocenyl group produces ROS within the digestive vacuole, provoking membrane damage, due to the specific acidic and oxidative digestive vacuole conditions. The hydroxyl radicals produced upon ferrocenyl group oxidation by H_2O_2 attack unsaturated fatty acids in the phospholipid membrane [110].

Finally, note that the classic and efficient method of ROS generation, tumor irradiation with X-rays, is not without danger for normal tissues on the X-ray path [147,148]. On the chemotherapeutic side, doxorubicin (DOX) is believed to fight tumors through the generation of DNA damage by the DOX-induced direct H_2O_2 generation [149]. In addition to Fe(II), MnO_2-coated mesoporous silica was also reported to yield hydroxyl radicals via glutathione depletion [150]. In general, other chemodynamic therapy (CDT) agents, including Mn^{2+} (vide supra), Ti^{3+}, Cr^{3+}, Ru^{2+}, Cu^{2+}, Co^{2+}, Ce^{3+}, persulfate, and peroxymonosulfate, have been shown to possibly replace Fe^{2+} toward hydroxyl radical production [151]. Along this line, various nanomaterials have also been proposed [152].

8. Drug Delivery Using Ferrocene-Containing Nanomaterials

8.1. Introduction and Early Studies

Recent giant progress in nanomaterials design has allowed for their optimization for drug delivery [38]. Such nanomaterials include organic materials, such as polymers [153], micelles [154], liposomes [155], dendrimers [155–159], cyclodextrin [160], and inorganic materials, such graphene [161], quantum dots [162], gold nanoparticles [163–165], coordination polymers, and metal–organic frameworks (MOFs) [166], and other nanomaterials [41] that can be involved in the generation of ROS [167].

Most of these nanomaterials have been loaded with ferrocenyl groups to increase water-solubility and blood circulation lifetime of small molecules toward Fenton generation of hydroxyl radicals for a therapeutic purpose. This field was pioneered by Neuse with ferrocenyl-containing water-soluble polyaspartamide copolymers probed against HeLa cells and the COLO 320 DM with IC_{50} values in the range of 3.6–36 mM for the best derivatives. In the latter, amine groups provide cationic ammonium for cell entry [5]. The groups of Jaouen [49] and Romao [50] investigated the inclusion of ferrocifens and 1,2-disubstituted ferrocenes, respectively, into b-CD and found an increase in drug solubility without cytotoxicity decrease. Moreover, with heptakis-2,3,6-tri-O-methyl-b-CD (TRIMEB) or 2-hydroxypropyl-b-CD (HPbCD), cytotoxic activity increased by 2.5 times. The shell cross-linked hybrid 1,1′-bis-amidoferrocene-containing self-assembly of poly(N-isopropylacrylamide-co-aminoethyl methacrylate)-b-polymethyl methacrylate (P(NIPAAm-co-AMA)-b-PMMA) polymeric micelle showing reversible dispersion/aggregation in response to temperature cycles exhibited significant cytotoxicity against HeLa cells with a IC_{50} around 0.2 g/L (Figure 21) [168].

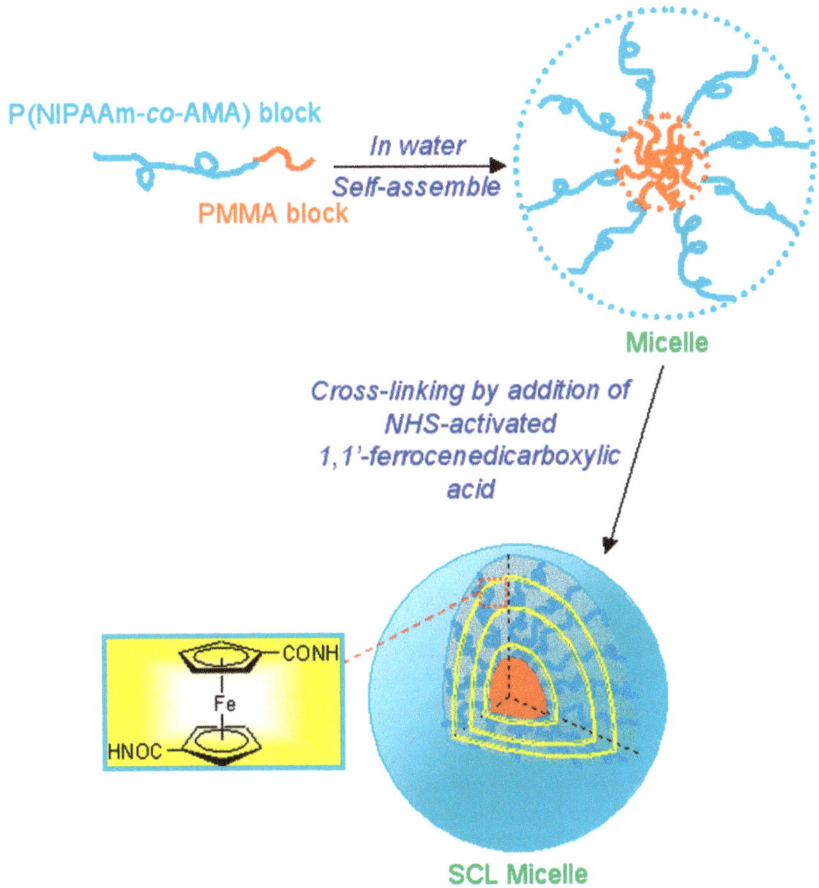

Figure 21. Formation of a shell cross-linked thermoresponsive micelle containing a 1,1′-bis-amidoferrocene. Reproduced with permission from Ref. [168]. Copyright 2010 American Chemical Society.

The Passirani-Benoit group studied local delivery of Jaouen's ferrocifenol **11a** (Figure 4, Fc-diOH) on a 9L glioma model according to two encapsulation strategies: lipid nanocapsules (LNC) and swollen micelles. At the micellar interface, PEG prevented interaction with the cytoplasm membrane, leading to low micelle cell uptake and no biological activity. On the other hand, Fc-diOH (**11a**) cytostatic activity was preserved after encapsulation in LNC, being very effective on 9L-glioma cells (IC_{50}: 0.6 mM). Rat treatment with Fc-diOH-LNC dramatically reduced the tumor mass and glioma volume. Moreover, Fc-diOH-loaded LNCs showed low toxicity levels for healthy cells [49]. Further study by these authors of Fc-diOH in LNC was conducted in combination with external radiotherapy against intracranial 9L glioma. Combining cerebral irradiation (three irradiation of 6 Gy doses, total dose: 18 Gy) with convection-enhanced delivery of Fc-diOH-LNCs led to long-term survivors compared with Fc-diOH-LNCs-treated animals ($p < 0.0001$) and the group treated with blank LNCs + radiotherapy ($p = 0.0079$). Rats survived over 100 days, indicating total eradication of the tumor. This study was the first demonstration of a synergy between these organometallic compounds and external beam radiotherapy [169].

8.2. Polymers, Micelles, and Liposomes

Bio-inspired ferrocene-containing polymers are an emerging field with multiple applications in pharmacotherapy [170,171]. Supramolecular polymers (SP) have been designed to build up nanosized delivery platforms for tumor chemotherapy [172–175]. Supramolecular nanoparticles were assembled via a simple one-step self-assembly process using platinum (IV) complex-modified b-CD-ferrocene conjugates and rapidly dissociated upon exposure to endogenous H_2O_2 in the tumor and release. This way, they released in situ hydroxyl radicals and platinum (IV) prodrug that was reduced to cisplatin, promoting the generation of H_2O_2 in the tumor tissue [172]. There are a few examples reported of SP construct using Fenton reagents as the guests for cancer imaging and treatment [176,177]. Ferrocene-containing amphiphilic block copolymers PEG-b-PMAEFc, synthesized by atom transfer radical polymerization (ATRP) of 2-(methacryloyloxy) ethyl ferrocene-carboxylate (MAEFc) using a PEG-based macro-ATRP agent, self-assembled into various nanostructures in aqueous solution and were treated with H_2O_2 to trigger the release of encapsulated cargo (rhodamine B) from b-CD in the polymeric nanocarriers [178]. A hydrogel with ferrocene groups in a polymer network immersed in water-soluble pillar[6]arene (WP6) aqueous solution was swollen, with approximately 11-fold increase in weight compared with that in pure water, due to the formation of the inclusion complexes between WP6 and ferrocene groups in the hydrogel. It exhibited good responsiveness to temperature, pH, redox, and competitive guests by tuning the dissociation/formation of WP6 ferrocene inclusion complexes [179].

These supramolecular properties of ferrocene-containing polymers have been applied in a few recent cases to the Fenton-like generation of hydroxyl radicals, as follows. Assemblies in the range of 100 nm accumulate around the tumor via the enhanced permeability and retention (EPR) effect and, upon exposure to the TME, ferrocene moieties herein undergo a Fenton-like reaction resulting in size shrinkage to 10 nm, thereby improving the tumor penetration ability of the assembly. These nucleic acid assemblies release hydroxyl radicals into the TME for efficient cancer treatment [180]. In an intracellular acidic environment, a pH/ROS dual-responsive supramolecular polypeptide nanoprodrug, PFW-DOX/GOD, consisting of a pH-responsive ferrocene/pillar[5]arene-containing polypeptide, a ROS-responsive polyprodrug, and encapsulated glucose oxidase (GOx), show pH-triggered disassembly. Simultaneously, the released GOx catalyzes intratumoral glucose into H_2O_2 that is further converted into toxic hydroxyl radicals from the ferrocenyl unit [181]. A biodegradable covalent organic porous polymer (COP), denoted as Fc-Ma, composed of ferrocene and D-mannitol (Ma) with pH-responsive acetal bonds, catalyzes the conversion of cellular H_2O_2 to hydroxyl radicals through a Fenton-like reaction, as an artificial enzyme. It also shows doxorubicin hydrochloride (DOX) drug loading capacity of 64.4 resulting in controlled drug delivery with selective release in acidic media [182]. Green-fluorescent, cancer-cell-targeted, and cationic carbon dots (HP-CDs) were specifically internalized with cancer cells, due to the recognition of surface hyaluronic acid with highly-expressed CD44 receptor. Ferrocenylseleno-dopamine (FcDA) was assembled on the surface of these HP-CDs yielding CDs@FcDA nanoprobe. Upon the cellular-specific uptake, the ferrocene moiety of the nanoprobe was oxidized by intracellular H_2O_2 in a typical Fenton-like reaction producing a toxic hydroxyl radical that provoked cancer cell apoptosis [183].

Amphiphilic PCAE incorporating H_2O_2-generating polymer, consisting of poly [(3-phenylprop-2-ene-1,1-diyl)bis(oxy)bis(ethane-2,1-diyl)diacrylate]-*co*-4,4′(trimethylene dipiperidine)-*co*-poly (ethylene glycol), termed PCAE, in which cinnamaldehyde was covalently incorporated in its backbone through an acid-cleavable linkage and self-assembled into stable micelles encapsulating ferrocene in their hydrophobic core, produced hydroxyl radicals killing *Escherichia coli* and *Pseudomonas aeruginosa* through membrane damage. Intraperitoneally injected ferrocene-loaded PCAE micelles reduced lung damage and increased the survival rate of mice infected with drug-resistant *P. aeruginosa* (Figure 22) [184].

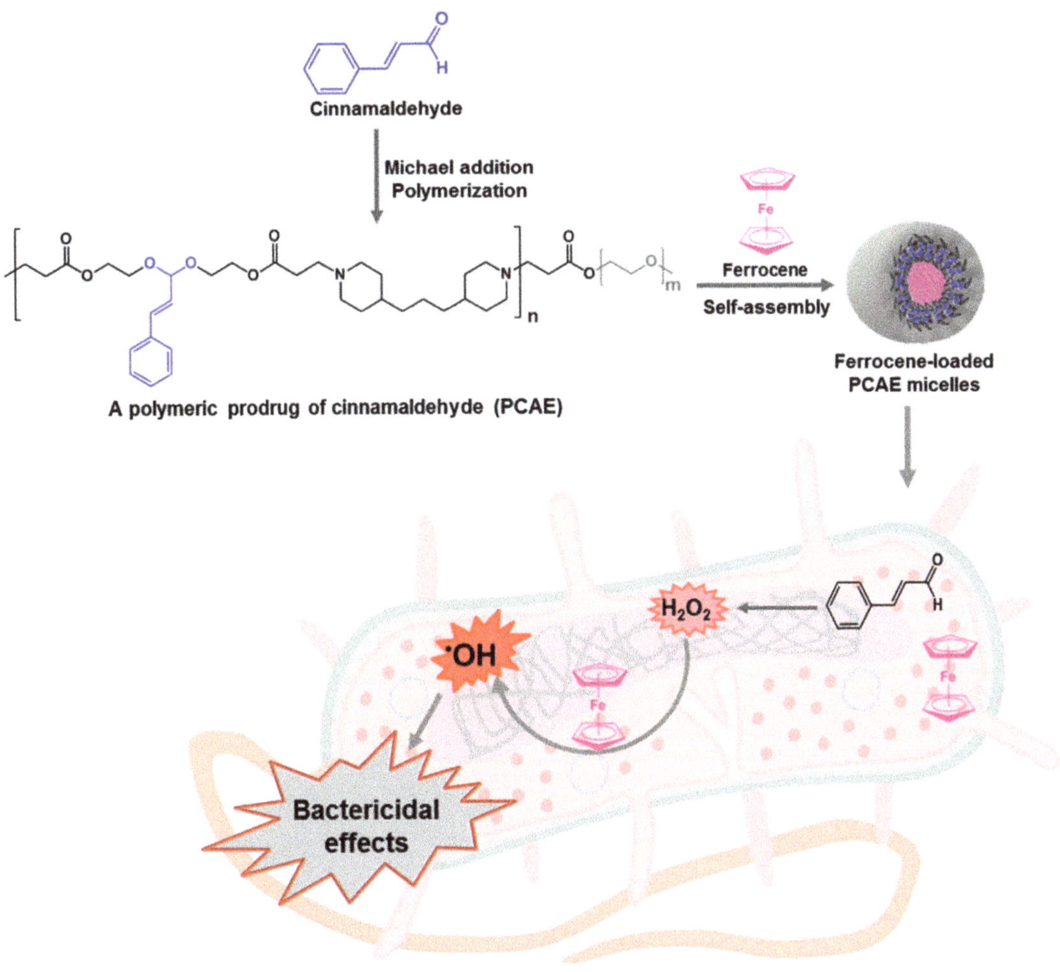

Figure 22. Mechanism of the bactericidal effect of produced hydroxyl radical subsequent to ferrocene@micelle encapsulation, in vivo delivery, and Fenton reaction. Reproduced with permission from Ref. [184]. Copyright 2016 Elsevier.

A micellar system (DOX/FCH), composed of ferrocene and hyaluronic acid (HA), delivered doxorubicin (DOX) in about 50% in 2 h due to disulfide bonds depolymerization in reducing environment simulating tumor intracellular environment, thanks to high affinity between HA and high-expressed CD44 receptors in human cervical carcinoma (HeLa) cells. Hydroxyl radicals produced by the Fenton reaction were detected both extracellularly and intracellularly, showing synergistic effects of chemodynamic therapy of ferrocene and chemotherapy of DOX [185]. Along this line, an amphiphilic copolymer poly(ethylene glycol) (PEG) ferrocenyl monomethyl ether formed stable micelles in water and loading DOX reacted with H_2O_2, which led to hydroxyl radicals via the Fenton reaction, depleting glutathione (GSH) and suppressing the antioxidant capacity of tumor cells. The synergistic effects of DOX and ferrocene optimized the therapeutic impact [186]. Forster resonance energy transfer (FRET) between near-infrared (NIR)-responsive lanthanide-doped upconversion nanoparticles (UCNPs) and ferrocenyl compounds was organized by functionalizing NaYF4:Yb,Tm NPs with ferrocene via the surface coordination followed by encapsulating the NPs inside liposomes for delivery. In vitro and in vivo studies of hydroxyl radical generation by Fc-NPs-liposome showed preferential accumulation in a tumor site followed by enhanced uptake of cancer cells (Figure 23) [187].

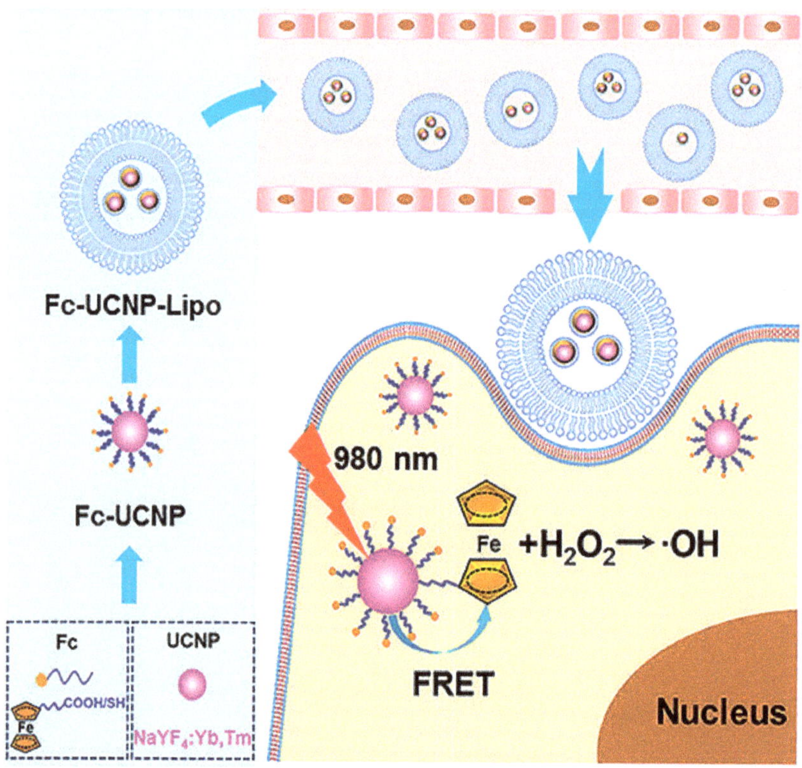

Figure 23. Fenton reaction from FRET between NIR-responsive lanthanide-doped upconversion nanoparticles and ferrocenyl derivative by functionalizing NaYF4:Yb,Tm NPs with ferrocene by encapsulating the NPs inside liposomes for delivery. Reproduced with permission from Ref. [187]. Copyright 2020 American Chemical Society.

8.3. Cyclodextrins and Pillar[6]arenes

Since Breslow' seminal work [188], CDs have been shown to be hosts of choice for the use of ferrocenyl derivatives as guests in biomedicine [180,189–191]. pH-responsive and ferrocene-containing block copolymers, including b-CD, were synthesized to realize pH-stable and multiresponsive glucose oxidase-loaded polymersomes as a permeable membrane providing chemoenzymatic cascade reactions [189]. A polymeric NP that selectively improved H_2O_2 levels in tumor tissue and generated active hydroxyl radicals by the Fenton reaction was proposed. It used a diblock copolymer containing PEG and poly(glutamic acid) modified by b-CD coassembled in aqueous solution with block copolymer, ferrocenecarboxylic acid hexadecyl ester (DFc), and ascorbyl palmitate (PA) yielding a core shell micelle by the complexation of the ferrocenyl group inside the b-CD. Upon intravenous injection, this nanomaterial achieved significant accumulation in tumor tissue where, subsequently, the Fenton reaction between H_2O_2 and Fc groups produced hydroxyl radicals efficiently killing cancer cells and suppressing tumor growth [190]. Dual-responsive supramolecular self-assembled NPs based on polymerized methacrylic acid and polymerized poly(ethylene glycol) dimethyl acrylate-modified 6-CD with Fc-connected (S) (+)-camptothecin was taken up by tumor cells owing to their reversible negative-to-positive charge transition capacity at acidic pH. This supramolecular nanomaterial increased ROS generation, decreased GSH to amplify oxidative stress, improving the therapeutic effect and displaying good drug delivery capabilities to tumor cells or tissues, and inhibited cancer cell proliferation in both the cells and tissues [191].

A nanoplatform polydopamine(PDA)-Pt-CD@RuFc formed by platinum-decorated and CD-modified PDA NPs loaded with a ferrocene-appended ruthenium complex (RuFc) successfully delivered RuFc to the tumor sites, triggered by low pH, photothermal heating, and H_2O_2. The combined photodynamic and photothermal therapy overcame the hypoxic environment of tumors from platinum NP catalysis of $O_2{\cdot}^-$ production from H_2O_2, vasodilation caused by photothermal heating sustaining the oxygen supplement, and photodynamic therapy exerted by RuFc occurring through the Fenton reaction (Figure 24) [192].

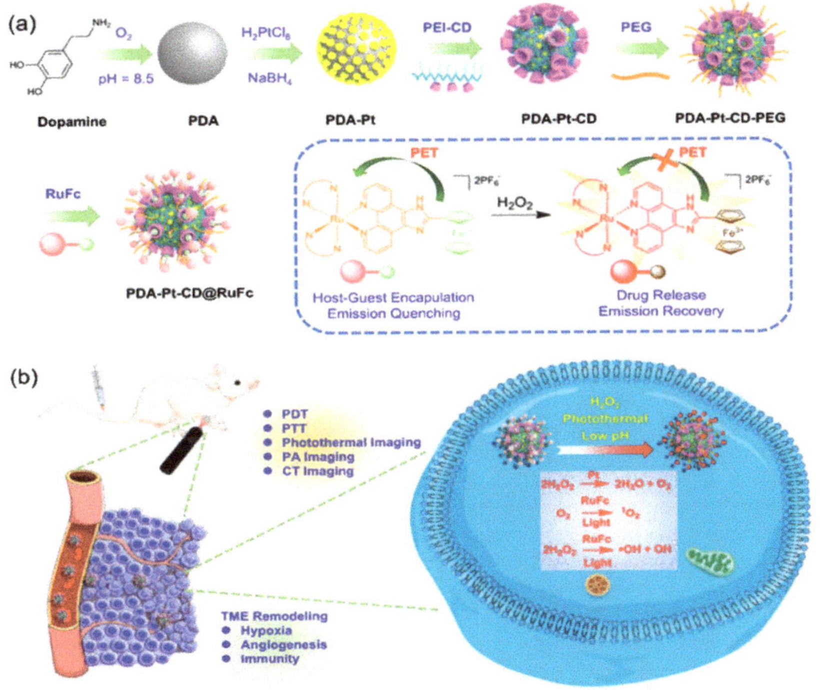

Figure 24. (**a**) Construction of polydopamine (PDA)-Pt-CD@RuFc NPs. Drug release and fluorescence recovery due to oxidation of the ferrocene group in RuFc by H_2O_2 are shown in the frame. (**b**) Proposed action mechanisms of PDA-Pt-CD@RuFc NPs. Reproduced with permission from Ref. [192]. Copyright 2020 Wiley.

As CDs, pillar[6]arene can serve as a supramolecular host for Fc groups inside their hydrophobic cavity. A ternary pillar[6]arene-based supramolecular nanocatalyst (GO*x*@T-NPs) for CDT exhibited a high-efficiency catalytic ability to convert glucose, using GO, into H_2O_2 and gluconic acid, then to hydroxyl radicals via Fc-induced Fenton reaction, and to reduce the pH value inside cancer cells for significant enhancement of the CDT effect. It also showed sensitive glutathione-induced camptothecin (CPT) prodrug release capacity to further improve the efficiency of CDT. Hence, GO*x*@NPs possessed excellent ability to synergistically enhance the CDT [193].

8.4. MOFs

Metal–organic frameworks (MOFs) are promising nanomaterials with abundant micropores and large surface areas [194] that are useful for the delivery of therapeutics; they have been extensively developed in this direction [155] as well as in nanocatalysis [195] and gas storage and separation [196]. Ferrocene-containing MOFs are a recently well-developed area for various applications [197].

A cobalt-ferrocene nanoscale MOF (Co-Fc NMOF), synthesized using $Co(OAc)_2 \cdot 4H_2O$ and $Fc(COOH)_2$ and isostructural to the reported Zn-Fc MOF, of ≈80 nm with the addition of PVP, presented high Fenton activity combined with glucose oxidase (GOx) as a cascade Fenton platform (Co-Fc@GOx) for enhanced tumor treatment, functioning as a biomimetic nanozyme [198]. In the tumor microenvironment, GOx delivered by Co-Fc NMOF was shown to catalyze endogenous glucose to H_2O_2 and gluconic acid, as indicated above with a pillar[6]arene nanomaterial reported in 2021 [193]. The Co-Fc NMOF, scrutinized using various cell lines by cell counting kit-8 (CCK-8) assay, showed the absence of clear in vitro toxicity to normal cells, including HUVEC, HL-7702, and HPNE cell lines, but displayed a dose-dependent cytotoxicity to 4T1 cancer cells due to the induction of intracellular hydroxyl radicals. Both in vitro and in vivo studies showed a remarkable ability of Co-Fc@GOx to inhibit cancer cells and tumor regression [198].

A ferrocene-containing MOF was prepared by reacting $ZrCl_4$ with 1,1′-ferrocene di-carboxylic acid in acetic acid in precise amount (150 °C, 12 h). The resulting thin (16.4 nm thick) MOF (Zr-Fc MOF) nanosheet consisting of $Zr_6(\mu_3\text{-}O)_4(\mu_3\text{-}OH)_4$ clusters as subunits [199] with Fc-di-carboxylate linkers [200,201] has been utilized for synergistic photothermal therapy (PTT) (photo conversion efficiency of 53% at 808 nm) and Fc-induced Fenton reaction-based hydroxyl radical generation as chemodynamic (CDT) therapy to cure cancer. The in situ generation of ROS is checked by ESR using 5,5-dimethyl-1-pyrroline N-oxide (DMPO) as the radical scavenger. UV–Vis absorbance spectroscopy using 5,5′-dithiobis(2-nitrobenzoic acid) (DNTB) as the chromogenic reagent showed that the GSH level decreased by ∼7% after laser irradiation because a hydroxyl radical generated under laser irradiation depleted GSH. In vitro, addition of 100 μg/mL Zr-Fc MOF nanosheet provoked almost 100% cell death. As in vitro, in vivo results with mice showed that PTT dominated the treatment while CDT was enhanced by PTT via the induction of localized hyperthermia. The resultant synergetic PTT and CDT treatment resulted in a very good anticancer therapeutic effect (Figure 25) [201].

Based on a similar 2D Zr-ferrocene (Zr-Fc)-MOF (Zr-Fc-MOF) nanosheet, Cu_2O NPs have recently been grown by reducing Cu^{2+} by hydrazine hydrate in situ on the surface of Zr-Fc-MOF nanosheets to form the 2D Cu_2O/Zr-Fc-MOF composite. The latter showed higher CD activity in the production of hydroxyl radicals via Fenton-like reaction compared with the pristine Zr-Fc-MOF nanosheets. The CD activity of the Cu_2O/Zr-Fc-MOF composite was enhanced by photothermal effect using NIR laser (808 nm) irradiation toward efficient photothermally enhanced CD antibacterial therapy. In vitro, the repression of the Cu_2O/Zr-Fc-MOF composite + H_2O_2 + NIR reached almost 100% on *Staphylococcus aureus* in pH 6.0 PBS buffer. After wound infection in mice with *Staphylococcus aureus*, the combination of PTT and CDT treatment accelerated wound healing that was almost complete on the seventh day without weight change in mice, indicating excellent biocompatibility and safety [13].

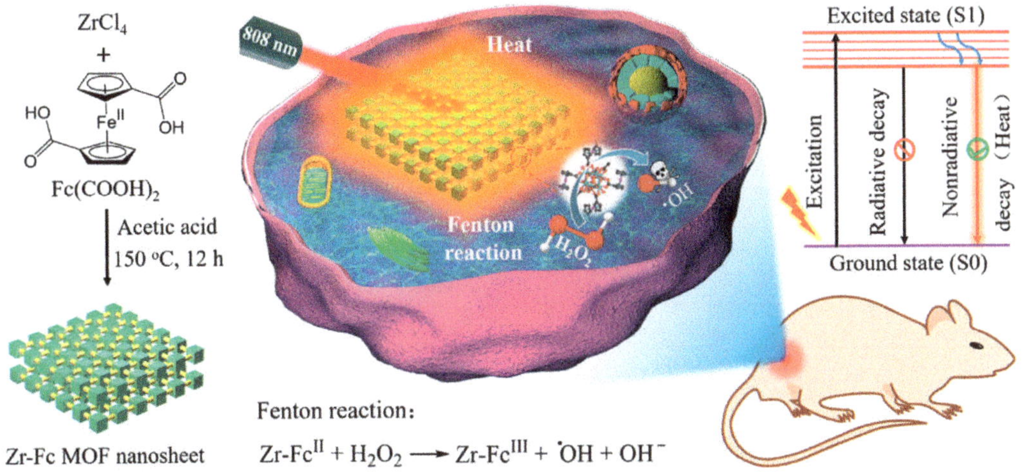

Figure 25. Synthesis of the Zr-Fc MOF nanosheet and illustration of synergetic PTT and Fenton reaction-based CDT. Reprinted with permission from Ref. [201]. Copyright 2020 American Chemical Society.

8.5. Dendrimers

Dendrimers are well-defined nanosized molecules with cauliflower- or tree-shape (dendrons) [149,202–204] that can encapsulate and deliver drugs [110,147–149,204–207], and a few recent publications have reported the production of hydroxyl radicals by the Fenton reaction inside dendrimers [208,209]. Ferrocene-terminated dendrimers that possess numerous ferrocenyl groups and fully reversible redox properties are candidates for the Fenton reaction and drug release [210–213]. Along these studies, it was noticed that large ferrocene dendrimers self-assembled into remarkably discrete regular-sized nanoparticles, just like atoms [213]. Aggregation-induced emission (AIE) from such assemblies was assigned in 2001 by Tang to restriction of intramolecular rotation inhibiting non-radiative decay [214], a concept extended inter alia to collective intra- and inter-chain n–*p* * interactions of heteroatoms [215,216]. It is understandable that large click dendrimers are subjected to such phenomena due to ferrocene termini inhibiting facile intra-branch movements. Indeed, Tomalia has recently associated dendrimer aggregation with a new photoluminescence phenomenon, referred to as non-traditional intrinsic luminescence (NTIL) [217,218]. Various dendritic nanomaterials are known to supramolecularly self-assemble into vesicles with luminescent properties relevant to NTIL [219,220]. The triazolylferrocenyl dendrimer **1** with 81 terminal triazolylferrocenyl groups was shown to self-assemble in aqueous medium into stable low-dispersity spherical-shaped vesosomes, emitting green NTI fluorescence (λ = 525 nm) upon excitation at 469 nm, including in biological medium, and presented cytotoxicity against cancer cells due to the numerous triazolylferrocenyl groups active in the Fenton reaction. Microscopy analysis revealed that formation of the vesosomes was not affected by the presence of enzymes, proteins, amino acids, antibiotics, lipids, hormones, vitamins, and salts present in the cell culture medium (Figure 26) [221].

The cytotoxicity of the vesosomes was evaluated against MCF-7 cells using the cell counting kit-8 (CCK-8) assay. MCF-7 cells were incubated for 24 and 48 h in the presence of the vesosomes. The 150.0 μM concentration tested resulted in 48% cell viability after 24 h (IC_{50}: 168 μM of Fc groups or 2.1 μM of dendrimer), and incubation for 48 h resulted in 38% cell viability (IC_{50}: 124 μM of Fc groups or 1.5 μM of dendrimer) [221].

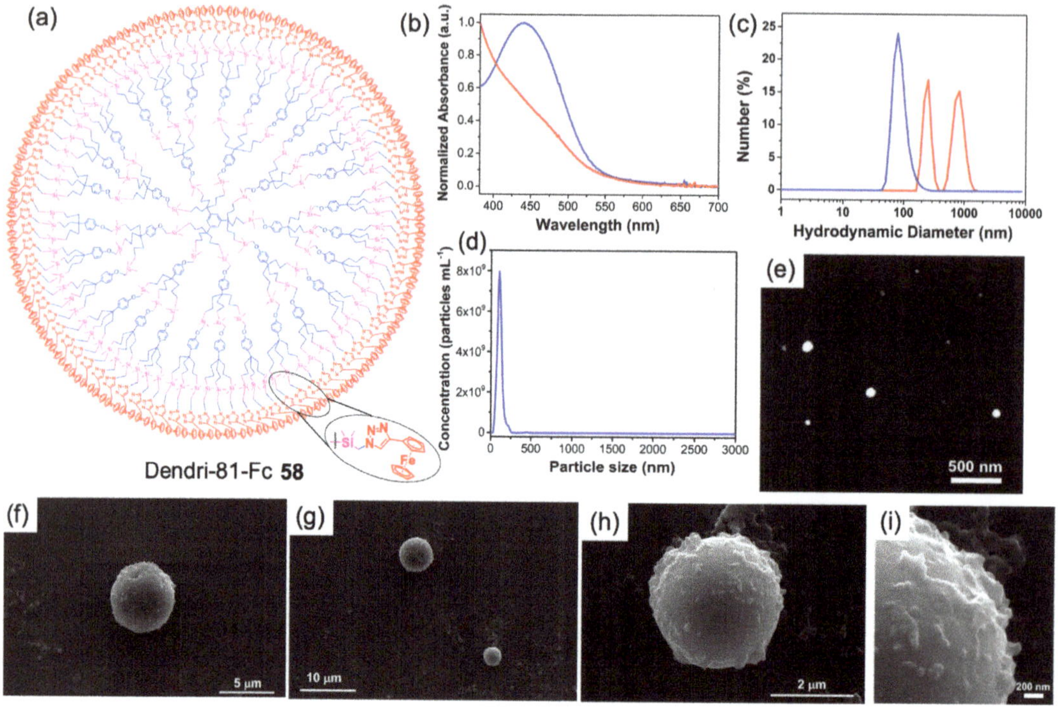

Figure 26. (**a**) Chemical structure of the 81-Fc dendrimer **58**; the inset shows the triazolylferrocenyl termini. (**b**) Absorption spectra of **58** normalized to the ferrocenyl band in $CHCl_3$ (blue) and DMSO (red). (**c**) Hydrodynamic diameter of the self-assemblies formed by **58** in water obtained by DLS: nonfiltered solution (red) and filtered solution (blue). (**d**) Size distribution plot of the nanoassembly formed by **58** in aqueous medium (filtered solution) obtained by NTA. (**e**) Representative NTA video frame of the nanoparticles in solution. (**f–i**) SEM images of the self-assembled microparticles formed by **58**. Reproduced with permission from Ref. [221]. Copyright 2021 American Chemical Society.

The cytotoxicity of a new water-soluble dendrimer with 18 triazolylferrocenyl moieties and 18 free carboxylic acid groups was evaluated against MCF-7 (breast adenocarcinoma), HeLa (cervical cancer), PC3 (prostate adenocarcinoma), Caco-2 (colorectal cancer), and PNT2 (normal prostate cells) cell lines, and the assays showed that the dendrimer exhibited moderate anticancer activity and targeted cancer cells selectively over normal cells [222]. The variety of known and possible precise dendritic structures [157–159,203,204,217,223] is promising for the design of future nanodrugs.

A star-shaped and a dendritic tetranuclear ferrocenylamino complexes were evaluated against two colon cancer cell lines, the wild-type HT-29 and mutant DLD-1, after being treated with 20 µM of complexes and incubated for 24 h, followed by flow cytometry analysis. Moderate micromolar cytotoxic activity in both cell lines was reported, but the cellular uptake demonstrated a good correlation with early induction of apoptosis, and cellular treatment with these complexes increased the number of apoptotic cells [224].

9. Conclusions and Prospects

Due to its robustness in two oxidation states, a redox potential compatible with the Fenton reaction, its lipophilicity, barrel shape, and great possibilities of functionalization, ferrocene has been introduced into numerous drugs for various diseases. The pioneering discovery in 1996–1997 by Jaouen et al. of the anticancer drug ferroxifen adapted from the organic drug tamoxifen and the discovery by the Biot-Brossard group of the antimalarial drug ferroquin adapted from chloroquin resulted from full understanding and exploitation of these key properties. These two success stories in the biorganometallic/bioinorganic community have led to the development of a very large number of bioactive ferrocene-containing pharmacophores, including a number of heterobimetallic compounds, the second metal moiety being Ru, Pd, or Pt, in particular Pt moieties of the cisplatin group [10]. Several anticancer and antiparasitic compounds were often found to be also active against other diseases (antimicrobial and/or antifungal). Synthetic strategies of ferrocene introduction into pharmacophores involved either replacement of a phenyl (ferrocifens), alkyl (ferroquins), or heterocyclic ring of a known drug by a ferrocenyl group or attachment of the latter to a variety of bioactive compounds, natural products, peptides, steroids, betulins, etc. via a functional group. Electronic delocalization by ferrocenyl conjugation with styrenyl, triazole, piperazine, chalcone, etc. is favorable toward oxidation. For instance, ferrocenyl chalcones were also found to be DNA/BSA-interacting agents and inhibitors of DNA topoisomerase I and II activity [225].

The details of the Fenton reaction [226], which is responsible for cytotoxicity, indicate that the $Fe^{III/II}$ redox potential plays a crucial role in the hydroxyl radical generation, and this flexibility does not seem to have been fully controlled and exploited. Other biological studies can include, as recently emphasized by Segur, the evaluation of effects of such ferrocene-containing pharmacophores on the apoptosis and penetration through the blood–brain barrier that is favored by the ferrocene lipophilicity (although nonspecific cellular impermeability should be avoided) [227].

Impaired brain iron homeostatic mechanisms are harmful to the brain due to iron-induced oxidative stress [228]. Along this line, ferrocenecarboxaldoxime was recently found to increase L-ferritin levels in the olfactory bulb, neocortex, pallidum, thalamus, corpus callosum, hippocampal CA3 regions, and substantia nigra [229].

Molecular docking studies have become useful in anticipating optimized structure for protein and DNA interaction with ferrocenyl conjugates, for instance, for anti-coronavirus activity, although no ferrocenyl drug has yet appeared in this case [230].

Another problem is that the endogenous H_2O_2 and the acidity in the tumor microenvironment (TME) are not quite sufficient to provide a very efficient Fenton reaction, which is responsible for slow cytotoxicity. The recent introduction of glucose oxidase into the magic bullets for drug delivery upon glucose ultimate oxidation to H_2O_2 and acid was reported to dramatically accelerate the Fenton reaction (that can even be stimulated by heat and/or light). Along this line, an alternative strategy involves host–guest supramolecular interaction with hydroxyl radical-consuming glutathione to provoke glutathione depletion and thereby elevate the available hydroxyl radical concentration [231].

For this purpose, nanomaterials, such as designed ferrocene-containing polymers, micelles, liposomes, dendritic vesosomes, cyclodextrin (or pillar-arenes), and metal–organic frameworks (MOFs), have been shown to be suitable vectors. This nanomaterial family could expand its utilization to anticancer, antiparasitic, antiviral, antibacterial and antifungal ferrocene conjugates. The use of such nanovectors involves the so-called chemodynamic therapy (CDT) [23]. With such a strategy, hydroxyl radicals are selectively delivered to the TME because, in normal cells, the pH is not low enough and the H_2O_2 concentration is not high enough for damaging hydroxyl-generating Fenton reaction. Nevertheless, such a selectivity will need to be carefully scrutinized in clinical studies for side effects.

The generation of hydroxyl radical leading to tumor destruction can also be generated by radiotherapy (X-ray) and other chemotherapeutic agents, such as doxorubicin, tirapazamine, bleomicin, and the antimalarial drug artimisinin, whose peroxide bridge is a source of hydroxyl radicals. Combined therapies, such as combined DCT and PTT or multiple drug treatment, significantly increase the chances of tumor death. In sum, ferrocene conjugates should hold a privileged place among metallodrugs in various areas of nanomedicine [232]. The diagnostic being essential to drug efficacy on time, a theranostic (i.e., therapy + diagnostic) [233] strategy should be adopted, for example, using gold NPs [163–165] or dendrimers [221]. Finally, given this increasing selectivity and efficacy against a variety of diseases of ferrocene conjugates, it is hoped that the pace of clinical trial will be accelerated toward a dramatic decrease of infected patients.

Funding: This research received no external funding. Financial support from the University of Bordeaux and the Centre National de la Recherche Scientifique (CNRS) is gratefully acknowledged.

Conflicts of Interest: There is no conflict of interest to declare. The company had no role in the design of the study; in the collection, analyses, or interpretation of data; in the writing of the manuscript, and in the decision to publish the results.

References

1. Sung, H.; Ferlay, J.; Siegel, R.L.; Laversanne, M.; Soerjomataram, I.; Jemal, A.; Bray, F. Global cancer statistics 2020: GLOBOCAN estimates of incidence and mortality worldwide for 36 cancers in 185 countries. *CA Cancer J. Clin.* **2021**, *71*, 209–249. [CrossRef] [PubMed] 2
2. Wicki, A.; Witzigmann, D.; Balasubramanian, V.; Huwyler, J. Nanomedicine in cancer therapy: Challenges, opportunities, and clinical applications. *J. Control. Release* **2015**, *200*, 138–157. [CrossRef]
3. Murray, C.J.L.; Ikuta, K.S.; Sharara, F.; Swetschinski, L.; Aguilar, G.R.; Gray, A.; Han, C.; Bisignano, C.; Rao, P.; Wool, E.; et al. Global Burden of Bacterial antimicrobiol resistance in 2019, A Systematic Analysis. *Lancet* **2022**, *399*, 629–655. [CrossRef]
4. Astruc, D. Why is ferrocene so exceptional? *Eur. J. Inorg. Chem.* **2017**, 6–29. [CrossRef]
5. Neuse, E.W. Macromolecular ferrocene compounds as cancer drug models. *J. Inorg. Organomet. Polym. Mater.* **2005**, *15*, 3–32. [CrossRef]
6. Jaouen, G.; Salmain, M. (Eds.) *Bioorganometallic Chemistry: Applications in Drug Discovery, Biocatalysis, and Imaging*; Wiley-VCH: Weinheim, Germany, 2014; ISBN 978-3-527-33527-5.
7. Jaouen, G.; Vessières, A.; Top, S. Ferrocifen type anti cancer drugs. *Chem. Soc. Rev.* **2015**, *44*, 8802–8817. [CrossRef]
8. Ornelas, C. Application of ferrocene and its derivatives in cancer research. *New J. Chem.* **2011**, *35*, 1973–1985. [CrossRef]
9. Gasser, G.; Metzler-Nolte, N. The potential of organometallic complexes in medicinal chemistry. *Curr. Opin. Chem. Biol.* **2012**, *16*, 84–91. [CrossRef]
10. Patra, M.; Gasser, G. The medicinal chemistry of ferrocene and its derivatives. *Nat. Chem. Rev.* **2017**, *1*, 0066. [CrossRef]
11. Braga, S.S.; Silva, A.M.S. A New Age for Iron: Antitumoral Ferrocenes. *Organometallics* **2013**, *32*, 5626–5639. [CrossRef]
12. Koszytkowska-Stawińska, M.; Buchowicz, W. Ferrocene-triazole conjugates: Do we know why they are biologically active? *Dalton Trans.* **2023**, *52*, 1501–1517. [CrossRef] [PubMed]
13. Zhao, X.; He, X.; Hou, A.; Cheng, C.; Wang, X.; Yue, Y.; Wu, Z.; Wu, H.; Liu, B.; Li, H.; et al. Growth of Cu_2O Nanoparticles on Two-Dimensional Zr-Ferrocene- Metal-Organic Framework Nanosheets for Photothermally Enhanced Chemodynamic Antibacterial Therapy. *Inorg. Chem.* **2022**, *61*, 9328–9338. [CrossRef] [PubMed]
14. Singh, A.K.; Kumar, A.; Singh, H.; Sonawane, P.; Paliwal, H.; Thareja, S.; Pathak, P.; Grishina, M.; Jaremko, M.; Emwas, A.-H.; et al. Concept of Hybrid Drugs and Recent Advancements in Anticancer Hybrids. *Pharmaceuticals* **2022**, *15*, 1071. [CrossRef]
15. Raičević, V.; Radulović, N.; Sakač, M. Toward Selective Anticancer Agents: Ferrocene-Steroid Conjugates. *Eur. J. Inorg. Chem.* **2022**, e202100951. [CrossRef]
16. Chaudhary, A.; Poonia, K. The redox mechanism of ferrocene and its phytochemical and biochemical compounds in anticancer therapy: A mini review. *Inorg. Chem. Commun.* **2022**, *134*, 109044. [CrossRef]
17. Idlas, P.; Lepeltier, E.; Jaouen, G.; Passirani, C. Ferrocifen Loaded Lipid Nanocapsules: A Promising Anticancer Medication against Multidrug Resistant Tumors. *Cancers* **2021**, *13*, 2291. [CrossRef] [PubMed]
18. Li, L.; Ma, L.; Sun, J. The Antiproliferative Activity of Ferrocene Derivatives against Drug-Resistant Cancer Cell Lines: A Mini Review. *Curr. Topics Med. Chem.* **2021**, *21*, 1756–1772. [CrossRef]
19. Wang, R.; Chen, H.; Yan, W.; Zheng, M.; Zhang, T.; Zhang, Y. Ferrocene-containing hybrids as potential anticancer agent: Current developments, mechanisms of action and structure-activity relationships. *Eur. J. Med. Chem.* **2020**, *190*, 112109. [CrossRef]
20. Chellan, P.; Sadler, P.J. Enhancing the Activity of Drugs by Conjugation to Organometallic Fragments. *Chem. Eur. J.* **2020**, *26*, 8676–8688. [CrossRef]
21. Xiao, J.; Sun, Z.; Kong, F.; Gao, F. Current scenario of ferrocene-containing hybrids for antimalarial activity. *Eur. J. Med. Chem.* **2020**, *185*, 111791. [CrossRef]
22. Mukaya, E.H.; Mbianda, X.Y. Macromolecular Prodrugs Containing Organoiron-Based Compounds in Cancer Research: A Review. *Mini-Rev. Med. Chem.* **2020**, *20*, 726–738. [CrossRef] [PubMed]
23. Tang, Z.; Liu, Y.; He, M.; Bu, W. Chemodynamic Therapy: Tumour Microenvironment-Mediated Fenton and Fenton-like Reactions. *Angew. Chem. Int. Ed.* **2019**, *58*, 946–956. [CrossRef]
24. Singh, A.; Lumb, I.; Mehra, V.; Kumar, V. Ferrocene-appended pharmacophores: An exciting approach for modulating the biological potential of organic scaffolds. *Dalton Trans.* **2019**, *48*, 2840–2860. [CrossRef] [PubMed]
25. Peter, S.; Aderibigbe, B.A. Ferrocene-Based Compounds with Antimalaria/Anticancer Activity. *Molecules* **2019**, *24*, 3604. [CrossRef] [PubMed]
26. Ludwig, B.S.; Correia, J.D.; Kühn, F.E. Ferrocene derivatives as anti-infective agents. *Coord. Chem. Rev.* **2019**, *396*, 22–48. [CrossRef]

27. Sierra, M.A.; Casarrubios, L.; De La Torre, M.C. Bio-Organometallic Derivatives of Antibacterial Drugs. *Chem. Eur. J.* **2019**, *25*, 7232–7242. [CrossRef]
28. Albada, B.; Metzler-Nolte, N. Highly Potent Antibacterial Organometallic Peptide Conjugates. *Acc. Chem. Res.* **2017**, *50*, 2510–2518. [CrossRef]
29. Chavain, N.; Biot, C. Organometallic Complexes: New Tools for Chemotherapy. *Curr. Med. Chem.* **2010**, *17*, 2729–2745. [CrossRef]
30. Dive, D.; Biot, C. Ferrocene conjugates of chloroquine and other antimalarials: The development of ferroquine, a new antimalarial. *ChemMedChem* **2008**, *3*, 383–391. [CrossRef]
31. Fouda, M.F.R.; Abd-Elzaher, M.M.; Abdelsamaia, R.A.; Labib, A.A. On the medicinal chemistry of ferrocene. *Appl. Organomet. Chem.* **2007**, *21*, 613–625. [CrossRef]
32. Chantson, J.T.; Falzacappa, M.V.V.; Crovella, S.; Metzler-Nolte, N. Solid-phase synthesis, characterization, and antibacterial activities of metallocene-peptide bioconjugates. *ChemMedChem* **2006**, *1*, 1268–1274. [CrossRef] [PubMed]
33. van Staveren, D.R.; Metzler-Nolte, N. Bioorganometallic chemistry of ferrocene. *Chem. Rev.* **2004**, *104*, 5931–5985. [CrossRef] [PubMed]
34. Fiorina, V.J.; Dubois, R.J.; Brynes, S. Ferrocenyl Polyamines as Agents for the Chemoimmunotherapy of Cancer. *J. Med. Chem.* **1976**, *21*, 393. [CrossRef] [PubMed]
35. Neuse, E.W.; Köpf-Maier, P.; Köpf, H. Ferricenium Complexes: A New Type of Water-Soluble Antitumor Agent. *J. Cancer Clin. Oncol.* **1984**, *108*, 336–340. [CrossRef]
36. Hiroshi, T.; Musahiro, M. DNA cleaving activity and cytotoxic activity of ferricenium cations. *Chem. Lett.* **1997**, *26*, 1177–1178. [CrossRef]
37. Osella, D.; Ferrali, M.; Zanello, P.; Laschi, F.; Fontani, M.; Nervi, C.; Cavigiolio, G. On the mechanism of the antitumor activity of ferrocenium derivatives. *Inorganica Chim. Acta* **2000**, *306*, 42–48. [CrossRef]
38. Mitchell, M.J.; Billingsley, M.M.; Haley, R.M.; Wechsler, M.E.; Peppas, N.A.; Langer, R. Engineering precision nanoparticles for drug delivery. *Nat. Rev. Drug Discov.* **2020**, *20*, 101–124. [CrossRef]
39. Patra, J.K.; Das, G.; Fraceto, L.F.; Campos, E.V.R.; del Pilar Rodriguez-Torres, M.; Acosta-Torres, L.S.; Diaz-Torres, L.A.; Grillo, R.; Swamy, M.K.; Sharma, S.; et al. Nano based drug delivery systems: Recent developments and future prospect. *J. Nanobiotechnol.* **2018**, *16*, 71. [CrossRef]
40. Shi, J.; Kantoff, P.W.; Wooster, R.; Farokhzad, O.C. Cancer nanomedicine: Progress, challenges and opportunities. *Nat. Rev. Cancer* **2017**, *17*, 20–37. [CrossRef]
41. Blanco, E.; Shen, H.; Ferrari, M. Principles of nanoparticle design for overcoming biological barriers to drug delivery. *Nat. Biotechnol.* **2015**, *33*, 941–951. [CrossRef]
42. Astruc, D. Electron-Transfer Processes in Dendrimers and their Implication in Biology, Catalysis, Sensing and Nanotechnology. *Nat. Chem.* **2012**, *4*, 255–267. [CrossRef] [PubMed]
43. Aranzaes, J.R.; Daniel, M.-C.; Astruc, D. Metallocenes as references for the determination of redox potentials by cyclic voltammetry: Permethylated iron and cobalt sandwich complexes, inhibition by polyamine dendrimers and the role of hydroxy-containing ferrocenes. *Can. J. Chem.* **2006**, *84*, 288–299. [CrossRef]
44. Neuse, E.W.; Kanzawa, F. Evaluation of the Activity of Some Water-Soluble Ferrocene and Ferricenium Compounds Against Carcinoma of the Lung by the Human Tumor Clonogenic-Assay. *Appl. Organomet. Chem.* **1990**, *4*, 19–26. [CrossRef]
45. Langer, R. Polymeric Delivery Systems for Controlled Drug Release. *Chem. Eng. Commun.* **1980**, *6*, 1–48. [CrossRef]
46. Langer, R.S.; Peppas, N.A. Present and Future Applications of Biomaterials in Controlled Drug DeLivery Systems. *Biomaterials* **1981**, *2*, 201–214. [CrossRef]
47. Peer, D.; Karp, J.M.; Hong, S.; Farokhzad, O.C.; Margalit, R.; Langer, R. Nanocarriers as an emerging platform for cancer therapy. *Nat. Nanotechnol.* **2007**, *2*, 751–760. [CrossRef]
48. Caldwell, G.; Meirim, M.G.; Neuse, E.W.; van Rensburg, C.E.J. Antineoplastic activity of polyaspartamide-ferrocene conjugates. *Appl. Organomet. Chem.* **1998**, *12*, 793–799. [CrossRef]
49. Allard, E.; Passirani, C.; Garcion, E.; Pigeon, P.; Vessières, A.; Jaouen, G.; Benoit, J.-P. Lipid nanocapsules loaded with an organometallic tamoxifen derivative as a novel drug-carrier system for experimental malignant gliomas. *J. Control. Release* **2008**, *130*, 146–153. [CrossRef]
50. Petrovski, Z.; de Matos, M.R.N.; Braga, S.S.; Pereira, C.C.; Matos, M.L.; Gonçalves, I.S.; Pillinger, M.; Alves, P.M.; Romão, C.C. Synthesis, characterization and antitumor activity of 1,2-disubstituted ferrocenes and cyclodextrin inclusion complexes. *J. Organomet. Chem.* **2008**, *693*, 675–684a. [CrossRef]
51. Edwards, E.I.; Epton, R.; Marr, G. The synthesis and Reactions of Homonuclear Ferrocene Acid Anhydrides and their Use in the Preparation of Ferrocenyl-Penicilins and Cephalosporins. *J. Organomet. Chem.* **1979**, *168*, 259–272. [CrossRef]
52. Scutaru, D.; Tataru, L.; Mazilu, I.; Vata, M.; Lixandru, T.; Simionescu, C. Contributions to the synthesis of some ferrocene-containg antibiotics. *Appl. Organomet. Chem.* **1993**, *7*, 225–231. [CrossRef]
53. Biot, C.; Glorian, G.; Maciejewski, L.A.; Brocard, J.S.; Domarle, O.; Blampain, G.; Millet, P.; Georges, A.J.; Abessolo, H.; Dive, D.; et al. Synthesis and antimalarial activity in vitro and in vivo of a new ferrocene–chloroquine analogue. *J. Med. Chem.* **1997**, *40*, 3715–3718. [CrossRef]
54. Biot, C.; François, N.; Maciejewski, L.; Brocard, J.; Poulain, D. Synthesis and Antifungal Activity of a Ferrocene-fluconazole Analogue. *Biorg. Med. Chem. Lett.* **2000**, *10*, 839–841. [CrossRef]

55. Chohan, Z.H.; Praveen, M. Synthesis, characterization and antibacterial properties of symmetric 1,1-ferrocene derived Schiff-base ligands and their Co(II), Cu(II), Ni(II) and Zn(II) chelates. *Appl. Organomet. Chem.* **2000**, *14*, 376–382. [CrossRef]
56. Patra, M.; Gasser, G.; Metzler-Nolte, N. Small organometallic compounds as antibacterial agents. *Dalton Trans.* **2012**, *41*, 6350–6358. [CrossRef]
57. Lam, N.S.; Long, X.; Wong, J.W.; Griffin, R.C.; Doery, J.C. Artemisinin and Its Derivatives: A potential treatment for leukemia. *Anti-Cancer Drugs* **2019**, *30*, 1–18. [CrossRef] [PubMed]
58. XSun, X.; Yan, P.; Zou, C.; Wong, Y.; Shu, Y.; Lee, Y.M.; Zhang, C.; Yang, N.; Wang, J.; Zhang, J. Targeting autophagy enhances the anticancer effect of artemisinin and its derivatives. *Med. Res. Rev.* **2019**, *39*, 2172–2193. [CrossRef]
59. Lal, B.; Badshah, A.; Altaf, A.A.; Khan, N.; Ullah, S. Miscellaneous applications of ferrocene-based peptides/amides. *Appl. Organomet. Chem.* **2011**, *25*, 843–855. [CrossRef]
60. Simenel, A.A.; Morozova, E.A.; Snegur, L.V.; Zykova, S.I.; Kachala, V.V.; Ostrovskaya, L.A.; Bluchterova, N.V.; Fomina, M.M. Simple Route to Ferrocenylalkyl Nucleobases. Antitumor Activity In Vivo. *Appl. Organomet. Chem.* **2009**, *23*, 219–224. [CrossRef]
61. Snegur, L.V.; Nekrasov, Y.S.; Sergeeva, N.S.; Zhilina, Z.V.; Gumenyuk, V.V.; Starikova, Z.A.; Simenel, A.A.; Morozova, N.B.; Sviridova, I.K.; Babin, V.N. Ferrocenylalkylazoles: Bioactivity, synthesis, structure. *Appl. Organomet. Chem.* **2008**, *22*, 139–147. [CrossRef]
62. Knauer, S.; Biersack, B.; Zoldakova, M.; Effenberger, K.; Milius, W.; Schobert, R. Melanoma-Specific Ferrocene Esters of the Fungal Cytotoxin Illudin M. *Anti-Cancer Drugs* **2009**, *20*, 676–681. [CrossRef] [PubMed]
63. Kowalski, K.; Hikisz, P.; Szczupak, Ł.; Therrien, B.; Koceva-Chyła, A. Ferrocenyl and Dicobalt Hexacarbonyl Chromones—New Organometallics Inducing Oxidative Stress and Arresting Human Cancer Cells in G2/M Phase. *Eur. J. Med. Chem.* **2014**, *81*, 289–300. [CrossRef]
64. Reshetnikov, V.; Daum, S.; Janko, C.; Karawacka, W.; Tietze, R.; Alexiou, C.; Paryzhak, S.; Dumych, T.; Bilyy, R.; Tripal, P.; et al. ROS-Responsive N-Alkylaminoferrocenes for Cancer-Cell-Specific Targeting of Mitochondria. *Angew. Chem. Int. Ed.* **2018**, *57*, 11943–11946. [CrossRef]
65. Osborne, C.K. Drug therapy—Tamoxifen in the treatment of breast cancer. *N. Engl. J. Med.* **1998**, *339*, 1609–1618. [CrossRef]
66. Top, S.; Tang, J.; Vessières, A.; Carrez, D.; Provot, C.; Jaouen, G. Ferrocenyl hydroxytamoxifen: A prototype for a new range of oestradiol receptor site-directed cytotoxics. *Chem. Commun.* **1996**, *8*, 955–956. [CrossRef]
67. McMurry, J.E. Carbonyl-Coupling Reactions Using Low-Valent Titanium. *Chem. Rev.* **1989**, *89*, 1513–1524. [CrossRef]
68. Top, S.; Vessières, A.; Leclercq, G.; Quivy, J.; Tang, J.; Vaissermann, J.; Huché, M.; Jaouen, G. Synthesis, biochemical properties and molecular modelling studies of organometallic specific estrogen receptor modulators (SERMs), the ferrocifens and hydroxyferrocifens: Evidence for an antiproliferative effect of hydroxyferrocifens on both hormone-dependent and hormone-independent breast cancer cell lines. *Chem. Eur. J.* **2003**, *9*, 5223–5236. [CrossRef] [PubMed]
69. Görmen, M.; Pigeon, P.; Top, S.; Hillard, E.A.; Huché, M.; Hartinger, C.G.; de Montigny, F.; Plamont, M.-A.; Vessières, A.; Jaouen, G. Synthesis, Cytotoxicity, and Compare Analysis of Ferrocene and [3]Ferrocenophane Tetrasubstituted Olefin Derivatives against Human Cancer Cells. *ChemMedChem* **2010**, *5*, 2039–2050. [CrossRef]
70. de Oliveira, A.C.; Hillard, E.A.; Pigeon, P.; Rocha, D.D.; Rodrigues, F.A.; Montenegro, R.C.; Costa-Lotufo, L.V.; Goulart, M.O.; Jaouen, G. Biological evaluation of twenty-eight ferrocenyl tetrasubstituted olefins: Cancer cell growth inhibition, ROS production and hemolytic activity. *Eur. J. Med. Chem.* **2011**, *46*, 3778–3787. [CrossRef]
71. Plażuk, D.; Vessières, A.; Hillard, E.A.; Buriez, O.; Labbé, E.; Pigeon, P.; Plamont, M.-A.; Amatore, C.; Zakrzewski, J.; Jaouen, G. A [3]Ferrocenophane Polyphenol Showing a Remarkable Antiproliferative Activity on Breast and Prostate Cancer Cell Lines. *J. Med. Chem.* **2009**, *52*, 4964–4967. [CrossRef]
72. Lee, H.Z.S.; Buriez, O.; Chau, F.; Labbé, E.; Ganguly, R.; Amatore, C.; Jaouen, G.; Vessières, A.; Leong, W.K.; Top, S. Synthesis, Characterization, and Biological Properties of Osmium-Based Tamoxifen Derivatives—Comparison with Their Homologues in the Iron and Ruthenium Series. *Eur. J. Inorg. Chem.* **2015**, 4217–4226. [CrossRef]
73. Wang, Y.; Pigeon, P.; Top, S.; McGlinchey, M.J.; Jaouen, G. Organometallic Antitumor Compounds: Ferrocifens as Precursors to Quinone Methides. *Angew. Chem. Int. Ed.* **2015**, *54*, 10230–10233. [CrossRef] [PubMed]
74. Pigeon, P.; Wang, Y.; Top, S.; Najlaoui, F.; Alvarez, M.C.G.; Bignon, J.; McGlinchey, M.J.; Jaouen, G. A New Series of Succinimido-ferrociphenols and Related Heterocyclic Species Induce Strong Antiproliferative Effects, Especially against Ovarian Cancer Cells Resistant to Cisplatin. *J. Med. Chem.* **2017**, *60*, 8358–8368. [CrossRef] [PubMed]
75. Wang, Y.; Dansette, P.M.; Pigeon, P.; Top, S.; McGlinchey, M.J.; Mansuy, D.; Jaouen, G. A new generation of ferrociphenols leads to a great diversity of reactive metabolites, and exhibits remarkable antiproliferative properties. *Chem. Sci.* **2018**, *9*, 70–78. [CrossRef] [PubMed]
76. Pigeon, P.; Gaschard, M.; Othman, M.; Salmain, M.; Jaouen, G. α-Hydroxylactams as Efficient Entries to Diversely Functionalized Ferrociphenols: Synthesis and Antiproliferative Activity Studies. *Molecules* **2022**, *27*, 4549. [CrossRef] [PubMed]
77. Wang, Y.; Pigeon, P.; Li, W.; Yan, J.; Dansette, P.M.; Othman, M.; McGlinchey, M.J.; Jaouen, G. Diversity-oriented synthesis and bioactivity evaluation of N-substituted ferrocifen compounds as novel antiproliferative agents against TNBC cancer cells. *Eur. J. Med. Chem.* **2022**, *234*, 114202. [CrossRef]
78. Garcia, J.S.; Gaschard, M.; Navizet, I.; Sahihi, M.; Top, S.; Wang, Y.; Pigeon, P.; Vessières, A.; Salmain, M.; Jaouen, G. Inhibition of Cathepsin B by Ferrocenyl Indenes Highlights a new Pharmacological Facet of Ferrocifens. *Eur. J. Inorg. Chem.* **2022**, e202101075. [CrossRef]

79. Ferreira, A.P.; da Silva, J.L.F.; Duarte, M.T.; da Piedade, M.F.M.; Robalo, M.P.; Harjivan, S.G.; Marzano, C.; Gandin, V.; Marques, M.M. Synthesis and Characterization of New Organometallic Benzo[b]thiophene Derivatives with Potential Antitumor Properties. *Organometallics* **2009**, *28*, 5412–5423. [CrossRef]
80. Top, S.; Thibaudeau, C.; Vessières, A.; Brulé, E.; Le Bideau, F.; Joerger, J.-M.; Plamont, M.-A.; Samreth, S.; Edgar, A.; Marrot, J.; et al. Synthesis and Structure Activity Relationship of Organometallic Steroidal Androgen Derivatives. *Organometallics* **2009**, *28*, 1414–1424. [CrossRef]
81. Carmona-Negrón, J.A.; Santana, A.; Rheingold, A.L.; Meléndez, E. Synthesis, structure, docking and cytotoxic studies of ferrocene–hormone conjugates for hormone-dependent breast cancer application. *Dalton Trans.* **2019**, *48*, 5952–5964. [CrossRef]
82. Narváez-Pita, X.; Rheingold, A.L.; Meléndez, E. Ferrocene-steroid conjugates: Synthesis, structure and biological activity. *J. Organomet. Chem.* **2017**, *846*, 113–120. [CrossRef]
83. Raičević, V.; Radulović, N.; Jovanović, L.; Rodić, M.; Kuzminac, I.; Jakimov, D.; Wrodnigg, T.; Knedel, T.; Janiak, C.; Sakač, M. Ferrocenylmethylation of estrone and estradiol: Structure, electrochemistry, and antiproliferative activity of new ferrocene–steroid conjugates. *Appl. Organomet. Chem.* **2020**, *34*, e5889. [CrossRef]
84. Huang, X.-F.; Wang, L.-Z.; Tang, L.; Lu, Y.-X.; Wang, F.; Song, G.-Q.; Ruan, B.-F. Synthesis, characterization and antitumor activity of novel ferrocene derivatives containing pyrazolyl-moiety. *J. Organomet. Chem.* **2014**, *749*, 157–162. [CrossRef]
85. Smit, F.J.; Bezuidenhout, J.J.; Bezuidenhout, C.C.; N'da, D.D. Synthesis and in vitro biological activities of ferrocenyl–chalcone amides. *Med. Chem. Res.* **2016**, *25*, 568–584. [CrossRef]
86. Panaka, S.; Trivedi, R.; Jaipal, K.; Giribabu, L.; Sujitha, P.; Kumar, C.G.; Sridhar, B. Ferrocenyl chalcogeno (sugar) triazole conjugates: Synthesis, characterization and anticancer properties. *J. Organomet. Chem.* **2016**, *813*, 125–130. [CrossRef]
87. Wei, J.-N.; Jia, Z.-D.; Zhou, Y.-Q.; Chen, P.-H.; Li, B.; Zhang, N.; Hao, X.-Q.; Xu, Y.; Zhang, B. Synthesis, characterization and antitumor activity of novel ferrocene-coumarin conjugates. *J. Organomet. Chem.* **2019**, *902*, 120968. [CrossRef]
88. Plażuk, D.; Wieczorek, A.; Ciszewski, W.M.; Kowalczyk, K.; Błauż, A.; Pawlędzio, S.; Makal, A.; Eurtivong, C.; Arabshahi, H.J.; Reynisson, J.; et al. Synthesis and in vitro Biological Evaluation of Ferrocenyl Side-Chain-Functionalized Paclitaxel Derivatives. *ChemMedChem* **2017**, *12*, 1882–1892. [CrossRef]
89. Ismail, M.K.; Khan, Z.; Rana, M.; Horswell, S.L.; Male, L.; Nguyen, H.V.; Perotti, A.; Romero-Canelón, I.; Wilkinson, E.A.; Hodges, N.J. Effect of Regiochemistry and Methylation on the Anticancer Activity of a Ferrocene-Containing Organometallic Nucleoside Analogue. *ChemBioChem* **2020**, *21*, 2487–2494. [CrossRef]
90. Tsypysheva, I.P.; Koval'skaya, A.V.; Petrova, P.R.; Lobov, A.N.; Erastov, A.S.; Zileeva, Z.R.; Vakhitov, V.; Vakhitova, Y.V. Synthesis of conjugates of (−)-cytisine derivatives with ferrocene-1-carbaldehyde and their cytotoxicity against HEK293, Jurkat, A549, MCF-7 and SH-SY5Y cells. *Tetrahedron* **2020**, *76*, 130902. [CrossRef]
91. Gómez, J.; Sierra, D.; Ojeda, C.; Thavalingam, S.; Miller, R.; Guzmán, F.; Metzler-Nolte, N. Solid-phase synthesis and evaluation of linear and cyclic ferrocenoyl/ruthenocenoyl water-soluble hexapeptides as potential antibacterial compounds. *J. Biol. Inorg. Chem.* **2021**, *26*, 599–615. [CrossRef]
92. Costa, N.C.S.; Piccoli, J.P.; Santos-Filho, N.A.; Clementino, L.; Fusco-Almeida, A.M.; De Annunzio, S.R.; Fontana, C.R.; Verga, J.B.M.; Eto, S.F.; Pizauro-Junior, J.M.; et al. Antimicrobial activity of RP-1 peptide conjugate with ferrocene group. *PLoS ONE* **2020**, *15*, e0228740. [CrossRef]
93. Patra, M.; Gasser, G.; Wenzel, M.; Merz, K.; Bandow, J.E.; Metzler-Nolte, N. Synthesis and Biological Evaluation of Ferrocene-Containing Bioorganometallics Inspired by the Antibiotic Platensimycin Lead Structure. *Organometallics* **2019**, *29*, 4312–4319. [CrossRef]
94. Albada, B.; Metzler-Nolte, N. Organometallic-peptide bioconjugates: Synthetic strategies and medicinal applications. *Chem. Rev.* **2016**, *116*, 11797–11839. [CrossRef] [PubMed]
95. Hess, J. Rational approaches towards inorganic and organometallic antibacterials. *J. Biol. Chem.* **2021**, *403*, 363–375. [CrossRef]
96. Castro, W.; Navarro, M.; Biot, C. Medicinal potential of ciprofloxacin and its derivatives. *Future Med. Chem.* **2013**, *5*, 81–96. [CrossRef]
97. Dubar, F.; Anquetin, G.; Pradines, B.; Dive, D.; Khalife, J.; Biot, C. Enhancement of the Antimalarial Activity of Ciprofloxacin Using a Double Prodrug/Bioorganometallic Approach. *J. Med. Chem.* **2009**, *52*, 7954–7957. [CrossRef]
98. Szczupak, Ł.; Kowalczyk, A.; Trzybiński, D.; Woźniak, K.; Mendoza, G.; Arruebo, M.; Steverding, D.; Stączek, P.; Kowalski, K. Organometallic ciprofloxacin conjugates with dual action: Synthesis, characterization, and antimicrobial and cytotoxicity studies. *Dalton Trans.* **2020**, *49*, 1403–1415. [CrossRef] [PubMed]
99. Tirkey, V.; Mishra, S.; Dash, H.R.; Das, S.; Nayak, B.P.; Mobin, S.M.; Chatterjee, S. Synthesis, characterization and antibacterial studies of ferrocenyl and cymantrenyl hydrazone compounds. *J. Organomet. Chem.* **2013**, *732*, 122–129. [CrossRef]
100. Stringer, T.; Seldon, R.; Liu, N.; Warner, D.F.; Tam, C.; Cheng, L.W.; Land, K.M.; Smith, P.J.; Chibale, K.; Smith, G.S. Antimicrobial activity of organometallic isonicotinyl and pyrazinyl ferrocenyl-derived complexes. *Dalton Trans.* **2017**, *46*, 9875–9885. [CrossRef] [PubMed]
101. Yagnam, S.; Trivedi, R.; Krishna, S.; Giribabu, L.; Praveena, G.; Prakasham, R.S. Bioactive isatin (oxime)-triazole-thiazolidinedione ferrocene molecular conjugates: Design, synthesis and antimicrobial activities. *J. Organomet. Chem.* **2021**, *937*, 121716. [CrossRef]
102. Lewandowski, E.M.; Szczupak, Ł.; Kowalczyk, A.; Mendoza, G.; Arruebo, M.; Jacobs, L.M.C.; Stączek, P.; Chen, Y.; Kowalski, K. Metallocenyl 7-ACA Conjugates: Antibacterial Activity Studies and Atomic-Resolution X-ray Crystal Structure with CTX-M beta-Lactamase. *ChemBioChem* **2020**, *21*, 2187–2195. [CrossRef] [PubMed]

103. Koçak, E.; Özkul, C.; Önel, G.T.; Nemutlu, E.; Kir, S. Screening the antimicrobial effect of ferrocene-boronic acid on Pseudomonas aeruginosa using proteomics and metabolomics approach. *J. Res. Pharm.* **2020**, *24*, 812–820. [CrossRef]
104. Biegański, P.; Szczupak, Ł.; Arruebo, M.; Kowalski, K. Brief survey on organometalated antibacterial drugs and metal-based materials with antibacterial activity. *Chem. Biol.* **2021**, *2*, 368–386. [CrossRef] [PubMed]
105. Roux, C.; Biot, C. Ferrocene-Based Antimalarials. *Future Med. Chem.* **2012**, *4*, 783–797. [CrossRef]
106. Domarle, O.; Blampain, G.; Agnaniet, H.; Nzadiyabi, T.; Lebibi, J.; Brocard, J.; Maciejewski, L.; Biot, C.; Georges, A.J.; Millet, P. In vitro antimalarial activity of a new organometallic analog, ferrocene-chloroquine. *Antimicrob. Agents Chemother.* **1998**, *42*, 540–544. [CrossRef]
107. Delhaes, L.; Biot, C.; Berry, L.; Delcourt, P.; Maciejewski, L.A.; Camus, D.; Brocard, J.S.; Dive, D. Synthesis of ferroquine enantiomers: First investigation of effects of metallocenic chirality upon antimalarial activity and cytotoxicity. *ChemBioChem* **2002**, *3*, 418–423. [CrossRef]
108. Dubar, F.; Egan, T.J.; Pradines, B.; Kuter, D.; Ncokazi, K.K.; Forge, D.; Paul, J.-F.; Pierrot, C.; Kalamou, H.; Khalife, J.; et al. The Antimalarial Ferroquine: Role of the Metal and Intramolecular Hydrogen Bond in Activity and Resistance. *ACS Chem. Biol.* **2011**, *6*, 275–287. [CrossRef]
109. Dive, D.; Biot, C. Ferroquine as an oxidative shock antimalarial. *Curr. Top. Med. Chem.* **2014**, *14*, 1684–1692. [CrossRef]
110. Navarro, M.; Castro, W.; Biot, C. Bioorganometallic Compounds with Antimalarial Targets: Inhibiting Hemozoin Formation. *Organometallics* **2012**, *31*, 5715–5727. [CrossRef]
111. Li, Y.; de Kock, C.; Smith, P.J.; Chibale, K.; Smith, G.S. Synthesis and evaluation of a carbosilane congener of ferroquine and its corresponding half-sandwich ruthenium and rhodium complexes for antiplasmodial and b-hematin inhibition activity. *Organometallics* **2014**, *33*, 4345–4348. [CrossRef]
112. Abid, M.; Singh, S.; Egan, T.J.; Joshi, M.C. Structural-activity Relationship of Metallo-aminoquines as Next Generation Antimalarials. *Curr. Top. Med. Chem.* **2022**, *22*, 436–472. [CrossRef] [PubMed]
113. Chopin, N.; Bosson, J.; Iikawa, S.; Picot, S.; Bienvenu, A.-L.; Lavoignat, A.; Bonnot, G.; Riou, M.; Beaugé, C.; Guillory, V.; et al. Evaluation of ferrocenyl-containing g-hydroxy- g -lactam-derived tetramates as potential antiplasmodials. *Eur. J. Med. Chem.* **2022**, *243*, 114735. [CrossRef] [PubMed]
114. Mbaba, M.; Dingle, L.M.K.; Swart, T.; Cash, D.; Laming, D.; de la Mare, J.-A.; Taylor, D.; Hoppe, H.C.; Biot, C.; Edkins, A.L.; et al. The in Vitro Antiplasmodial and Antiproliferative Activity of New Ferrocene-Based α-Aminocresols Targeting Hemozoin Inhibition and DNA Interaction. *ChemBioChem* **2020**, *21*, 2643–2658. [CrossRef]
115. Karagöz, A.; Leidenberger, M.; Hahn, F.; Hampel, F.; Friedrich, O.; Marschall, M.; Kappes, B.; Tsogoeva, S.B. Synthesis of new betulinic acid/betulin-derived dimers and hybrids with potent antimalarial and antiviral activities. *Bioorg. Med. Chem.* **2019**, *27*, 110–115. [CrossRef]
116. Reiter, C.; Fröhlich, T.; Zeino, M.; Marschall, M.; Bahsi, H.; Leidenberger, M.; Friedrich, O.; Kappes, B.; Hampel, F.; Efferth, T.; et al. New efficient artemisinin derived agents against human leukemia cells, human cytomegalovirus and Plasmodium falciparum: 2nd generation 1,2,4-trioxane-ferrocene hybrids. *Eur. J. Med. Chem.* **2015**, *97*, 164–172. [CrossRef] [PubMed]
117. de Lange, C.; Coertzen, D.; Smit, F.; Wentzel, J.; Wong, H.N.; Birkholtz, L.-M.; Haynes, R.K.; N'Da, D.D. Synthesis, in vitro antimalarial activities and cytotoxicities of amino-artemisinin-ferrocene derivatives. *Bioorg. Med. Chem. Lett.* **2018**, *28*, 289–292. [CrossRef]
118. de Lange, C.; Coertzen, D.; Smit, F.; Wentzel, J.; Wong, H.N.; Birkholtz, L.-M.; Haynes, R.K.; N'Da, D.D. Synthesis, antimalarial activities and cytotoxicities of amino-artemisinin-1,2-disubstituted ferrocene hybrids. *Bioorg. Med. Chem. Lett.* **2018**, *28*, 3161–3163. [CrossRef]
119. Zhang, S.; Yi, C.; Li, W.; Luo, Y.; Wu, Y.; Ling, H. The current scenario on anticancer activity of artemisinin metal complexes, hybrids, and dimers. *Arch. Pharm.* **2022**, *355*, e2200086. [CrossRef]
120. Rubbiani, R.; Weil, T.; Tocci, N.; Mastrobuoni, L.; Jeger, S.; Moretto, M.; Ng, J.; Lin, Y.; Hess, J.; Ferrari, S.; et al. In vivo active organometallic-containg antimycotic agents. *RSC Chem. Biol.* **2021**, *2*, 1263–1273. [CrossRef]
121. Shunmugaperumal, S.; Dhasarathan, S.; Selvaraj, P.K.; Kaliappan, I. Multi Metal Ion Recognizing Unsymmetrical tetra dentate Schiff bases Associated with Antifungal activity. *Orient. J. Chem.* **2021**, *37*, 833–846. [CrossRef]
122. Cilli, E.M.; Costa, N.C.; Santos-Filho, N.A.; Piccoli, J.P.; Fusco-Almeida, A.M.; Santos, C.T.; de Souza, J.O.; Zanini, C.L.; Aguiar, A.C.C.; Oliva, G.; et al. New Strategies for Novel Drugs: Antimicrobial Peptides Containing Ferrocene with Improved Antifungal and Antiplasmodial Biological Activity. *Protein Pept. Lett.* **2022**, *29*, 1088–1098. [CrossRef] [PubMed]
123. Patujo, J.; Azeem, M.; Khan, M.; Muhammad, H.; Raheel, A.; Fatima, S.; Mirza, B.; Hussain, Z.; Badshah, A. Assessing the biological potential of new symmetrical ferrocene based bisthiourea analogues. *Biorg. Chem.* **2021**, *106*, 104180. [CrossRef] [PubMed]
124. Singh, G.; Arora, A.; Kalra, P.; Maurya, I.K.; Ruizc, C.E.; Estebanc, M.A.; Sinha, S.; Goyal, K.; Sehgal, R. A strategic approach to the synthesis of ferrocene appended chalcone linked triazole allied organosilatranes: Antibacterial, antifungal, antiparasitic and antioxidant studies. *Bioorg. Med. Chem.* **2019**, *27*, 188–195. [CrossRef]
125. Fenton, H.J.H. Oxidation of tartric acid in the presence of iron. *J. Chem. Soc.* **1894**, *65*, 899. [CrossRef]
126. Neyens, E.; Baeyens, J. A review of classic Fenton's peroxidation as an advanced oxidation technique. *J. Hazard. Mater.* **2003**, *98*, 33–50. [CrossRef]

127. Zepp, R.G.; Faust, B.C.; Hoigne, J. Hydroxyl Radical formation in aqueous Reactions (pH 3-8) of Iron (II) with Hydrogen Peroxide-The Photo-Fenton Reaction. *Environ. Sci. Technol.* **1992**, *26*, 313–319. [CrossRef]
128. Haber, F.; Weiss, J. The catalytic decomposition of hydrogen peroxide by iron salts. *Proc. R. Soc. Lond. Ser. A* **1934**, *147*, 332–351. [CrossRef]
129. Lai, C.-S.; Piette, L.H. Further evidence for OH radical production in Fenton's reagent. *Tetrahedron Lett.* **1979**, *9*, 775–778. [CrossRef]
130. Gallard, H.; de Laat, J.; Legube, B. Effect of pH on the oxidation rate of organic compounds by Fe-II/H_2O_2. Mechanisms and simulation. *New. J. Chem.* **1998**, *22*, 263–268. [CrossRef]
131. Gligorovski, S.; Strekowski, R.; Barbati, S.; Vione, D. Environmental Implications of Hydroxyl Radicals. *Chem. Rev.* **2015**, *115*, 13051–13092. [CrossRef]
132. Fridovich, I. Superoxide anion radical (O_2^{-}), superoxide dismutases, and related matters. *J. Biol. Chem.* **1997**, *272*, 18515–18517. [CrossRef]
133. Hamon, J.R.; Astruc, D. Dramatic Salt Effects on the Basic and Nucleophilic Properties of Superoxide Radical Anion Generated from O_2 and Iron(I) "Electron Reservoir Complexes". *J. Am. Chem. Soc.* **1983**, *105*, 5951–5953. [CrossRef]
134. Schieber, M.; Chandel, N.S. ROS Function in Redox Signaling and Oxidative Stress. *Curr. Biol.* **2014**, *24*, R453–R462. [CrossRef] [PubMed]
135. Astruc, D. Transition metal sandwiches as reservoirs of electrons, protons, hydrogen atoms and hydrides: Molecular activation and electronics. *New J. Chem.* **1992**, *16*, 305–328.
136. Cable, E.E.; Isom, H.C. Metabolism of 3,5,5-trimethylhexanoyl-ferrocene by rat liver: Release of iron from 3,5,5-trimethylhexanoyl-ferrocene by a microsomal, phenobarbital-inducible cytochrome P-450. *Drug. Metab. Dispos.* **1999**, *27*, 255–260. [PubMed]
137. Connelly, N.G.; Geiger, W.E. Chemical redox agents for organometallic chemistry. *Chem. Rev.* **1996**, *96*, 877–910. [CrossRef]
138. Astruc, D. *Electron Transfer and Radical Processes in Transition Metal Chemistry*; VCH: New York, NY, USA, 1995; ISBN 1-56081-566-3.
139. Věžník, J.; Konhefr, M.; Fohlerová, Z.; Lacina, K. Redox-dependent cytotoxicity of ferrocene derivatives and ROS-activated prodrugs based on ferrocenyliminoboronates. *J. Inorg. Biochem.* **2021**, *224*, 111561. [CrossRef]
140. Astruc, D.; Hamon, J.-R.; Althoff, G.; Román, E.; Batail, P.; Michaud, P.; Mariot, J.-P.; Varret, F.; Cozak, D. Design, Stabilization and Efficiency of Organometallic "Electron Reservoirs". 19-Electron Sandwichs h^5-$C_5R_5Fe(I)h^6$-C_6R_6, a Key Class Active in Redox Catalysis. *J. Am. Chem. Soc.* **1979**, *101*, 5445–5447. [CrossRef]
141. Rajasekharan, M.V.; Giesinski, S.; Ammeter, J.H.; Ostwald, N.; Michaud, P.; Hamon, J.-R.; Astruc, D. Electron Paramagnetic ESR Studies of the Electronic Structure and Dynamic Jahn-Teller Effect in Fe(I) Sandwich Compounds. *J. Am. Chem. Soc.* **1982**, *104*, 2400–2407. [CrossRef]
142. Huynh, M.H.V.; Meyer, T.J. Proton-Coupled Electron Transfer. *Chem. Rev.* **2007**, *107*, 5004–5064. [CrossRef]
143. Vessières, A.; Wang, Y.; McGlinchey, M.J.; Jaouen, G. Multifaceted chemical behaviour of metallocene (M = Fe, Os) quinone methides. Their contribution to biology. *Coord. Chem. Rev.* **2021**, *430*, 213658. [CrossRef]
144. Fomin, F.M.; Zaitseva, K.S. Mechanism of the oxidation of ferrocene and its derivatives with hydrogen peroxide: A new effect. *Russ. J. Phys. Chem.* **2014**, *88*, 466–470. [CrossRef]
145. Astruc, D. Transition Metal Radicals: Chameleon Structure and Catalytic Function. *Acc. Chem. Res.* **1991**, *24*, 36. [CrossRef]
146. Schumacker, P.T. Reactive Oxygen Species in Cancer: A Dance with the Devil. *Cancer Cell* **2015**, *27*, 156–157. [CrossRef]
147. Hall, E.J.; Wuu, C.-S. Radiation-induced second cancers: The impact of 3D-CRT and IMRT. *Int. J. Rad. Oncol. Biol. Phys.* **2003**, *56*, 83–88. [CrossRef]
148. Favaudon, V.; Caplier, L.; Monceau, V.; Pouzoulet, F.; Sayarath, M.; Fouillade, C.; Poupon, M.-F.; Brito, I.; Hupé, P.; Bourhis, J.; et al. Ultrahigh dose-rate FLASH irradiation increases the differential response between normal and tumor tissue in mice. *Sci. Translat. Med.* **2014**, *6*, 245ra93. [CrossRef]
149. Mizutani, H.; Tada-Oikawa, S.; Hiraku, Y.; Kojima, M.; Kawanishi, S. Mechanism of apoptosis induced by doxorubicin through the generation of hydrogen peroxide. *Life Sci.* **2005**, *76*, 1439–1453. [CrossRef]
150. Lin, L.-S.; Song, J.; Song, L.; Ke, K.; Liu, Y.; Zhou, Z.; Shen, Z.; Li, J.; Yang, Z.; Tang, W.; et al. Simultaneous Fenton-like Ion Delivery and Glutathione Depletion by MnO_2-Based Nanoagent to Enhance Chemodynamic Therapy. *Angew. Chem. Int. Ed.* **2018**, *57*, 4902–4906. [CrossRef]
151. Bokare, A.D.; Choi, W. Review of iron-free Fenton-like systems for activating H_2O_2 in advanced oxidation processes. *J. Hazard. Mater.* **2014**, *275*, 121–135. [CrossRef]
152. Tang, Z.; Zhao, P.; Wang, H.; Liu, Y.; Bu, W. Biomedicine Meets Fenton Chemistry. *Chem. Rev.* **2021**, *121*, 1981–2019. [CrossRef]
153. Kamaly, N.; Yameen, B.; Wu, J.; Farokhzad, O.C. Degradable Controlled-Release Polymers and Polymeric Nanoparticles: Mechanisms of Controlling Drug Release. *Chem. Rev.* **2016**, *116*, 2602–2663. [CrossRef]
154. Cabral, H.; Miyata, K.; Osada, K.; Kataoka, K. Block Copolymer Micelles in Nanomedicine Applications. *Chem. Rev.* **2018**, *118*, 6844–6892. [CrossRef]
155. Allen, T.M.; Cullis, P.R. Liposomal drug delivery systems: From concept to clinical applications. *Adv. Drug. Deliv. Rev.* **2013**, *65*, 36–48. [CrossRef] [PubMed]
156. Kannan, R.M.; Nance, E.; Kannan, S.; Tomalia, D.A. Emerging concepts in dendrimer-based nanomedicine: From design principles to clinical applications. *J. Intern. Med.* **2014**, *276*, 579–617. [CrossRef] [PubMed]
157. Caminade, A.-M.; Turrin, C.-O. Dendrimers for drug delivery. *J. Mater. Chem. B* **2014**, *2*, 4055–4066. [CrossRef]

158. Rolland, O.; Turrin, C.-O.; Caminade, A.-M.; Majoral, J.-P. Dendrimers and nanomedicine: Multivalency in action. *New J. Chem.* **2009**, *33*, 1809–1824. [CrossRef]
159. Astruc, D.; Boisselier, E.; Ornelas, C. Dendrimers Designed for Functions: From Physical, Photophysical, and Supramolecular Properties to Applications in Sensing, Catalysis, Molecular Electronics, Photonics, and Nanomedicine. *Chem. Rev.* **2010**, *110*, 1857–1959. [CrossRef] [PubMed]
160. Tian, B.; Liu, Y.; Liu, J. Smart stimuli-responsive drug delivery systems based on cyclodextrin: A review. *Carbohydr. Polym.* **2021**, *251*, 116871. [CrossRef]
161. Liu, J.; Cui, L.; Losic, D. Graphene and graphene oxide as new nanocarriers for drug delivery applications. *Acta Biomater.* **2013**, *9*, 9243–9257. [CrossRef]
162. Zhou, J.; Yang, Y.; Zhang, C.-Y. Toward Biocompatible Semiconductor Quantum Dots: From Biosynthesis and Bioconjugation to Biomedical Application. *Chem. Rev.* **2015**, *115*, 11669–11717. [CrossRef]
163. Ghosh, P.; Han, G.; De, M.; Kim, C.K.; Rotello, V.M. Gold nanoparticles in delivery applications. *Adv. Drug. Deliv. Rev.* **2008**, *60*, 1307–1315. [CrossRef] [PubMed]
164. Daniel, M.-C.; Astruc, D. Gold Nanoparticles: Assembly, supramolecular chemistry, quantum-size-related properties, and applications toward biology, catalysis, and nanotechnology. *Chem. Rev.* **2004**, *104*, 293–346. [CrossRef] [PubMed]
165. Boisselier, E.; Salmon, L.; Ruiz, J.; Astruc, D. How to very efficiently functionalize gold nanoparticles by "click" chemistry. *Chem. Commun.* **2008**, *44*, 5788–5790. [CrossRef] [PubMed]
166. Horcajada, P.; Gref, R.; Baati, T.; Allan, P.K.; Maurin, G.; Couvreur, P.; Férey, G.; Morris, R.E.; Serre, C. Metal-Organic Frameworks in Biomedicine. *Chem. Rev.* **2012**, *112*, 1232–1268. [CrossRef] [PubMed]
167. Yang, B.; Chen, Y.; Shi, J. Reactive Oxygen Species (ROS)-Based Nanomedicine. *Chem. Rev.* **2019**, *119*, 4881–4985. [CrossRef]
168. Wei, H.; Quan, C.-Y.; Chang, C.; Zhang, X.-Z.; Zhuo, R.-X. Preparation of Novel Ferrocene-Based Shell Cross-Linked Thermoresponsive Hybrid Micelles with Antitumor Efficacy. *J. Phys. Chem. B* **2010**, *114*, 5309–5314. [CrossRef]
169. Allard, E.; Jarnet, D.; Vessières, A.; Vinchon-Petit, S.; Jaouen, G.; Benoit, J.-P.; Passirani, C. Local Delivery of Ferrociphenol Lipid Nanocapsules Followed by External Radiotherapy as a Synergistic Treatment Against Intracranial 9L Glioma Xenograft. *Pharm. Res.* **2010**, *27*, 56–64. [CrossRef]
170. Yang, K.; Yu, G.; Yang, Z.; Yue, L.; Zhang, X.; Sun, C.; Wei, J.; Rao, L.; Chen, X.; Wang, R. Supramolecular Polymerization-Induced Nanoassemblies for Self-Augmented Cascade Chemotherapy and Chemodynamic Therapy of Tumor. *Angew. Chem. Int. Ed.* **2021**, *60*, 17570–17578. [CrossRef]
171. Gu, H.; Mu, S.; Qiu, G.; Liu, X.; Zhang, L.; Yuan, Y.; Astruc, D. Redox-stimuli-responsive drug delivery systems with supramolecular ferrocenyl-containing polymers for controlled release. *Coord. Chem. Rev.* **2018**, *364*, 51–85. [CrossRef]
172. Su, H.; Cui, Y.; Wang, F.; Zhang, W.; Zhang, C.; Wang, R. Theranostic supramolecular polymers formed by the self-assembly of a metal-chelating prodrug. *Biomater. Sci.* **2021**, *9*, 463–470. [CrossRef]
173. Huo, Y.; He, Z.; Wang, C.; Zhang, L.; Xuan, Q.; Wei, S.; Wang, Y.; Pan, D.; Dong, B.; Wei, R.; et al. The recent progress of synergistic supramolecular polymers: Preparation, properties and applications. *Chem. Commun.* **2021**, *57*, 1413–1429. [CrossRef]
174. Luo, Q.; Dong, Z.; Hou, C.; Liu, J. Protein-based supramolecular polymers: Progress and prospect. *Chem. Commun.* **2014**, *50*, 9997–10007. [CrossRef]
175. Wang, H.; Yan, Y.-Q.; Yi, Y.; Wei, Z.-Y.; Chen, H.; Xu, J.-F.; Wang, H.; Zhao, Y.; Zhang, X. Supramolecular Peptide Therapeutics: Host–Guest Interaction-Assisted Systemic Delivery of Anticancer Peptides. *CCS Chem.* **2020**, *2*, 739–748. [CrossRef]
176. Chen, X.-M.; Chen, Y.; Yu, Q.; Gu, B.-H.; Liu, Y. Supramolecular Assemblies with Near-Infrared Emission Mediated in Two Stages by Cucurbituril and Amphiphilic Calixarene for Lysosome-Targeted Cell Imaging. *Angew. Chem. Int. Ed.* **2018**, *57*, 12519–12523. [CrossRef] [PubMed]
177. Yu, G.; Zhao, X.; Zhou, J.; Mao, Z.; Huang, X.; Wang, Z.; Hua, B.; Liu, Y.; Zhang, F.; He, Z.; et al. Supramolecular Polymer-Based Nanomedicine: High Therapeutic Performance and Negligible Long-Term Immunotoxicity. *J. Am. Chem. Soc.* **2018**, *140*, 8005–8019. [CrossRef]
178. Liu, L.; Rui, L.; Gao, Y.; Zhang, W. Self-assembly and disassembly of a redox-responsive ferrocene-containing amphiphilic block copolymer for controlled release. *Polym. Chem.* **2014**, *6*, 1817–1829. [CrossRef]
179. Ni, M.; Zhang, N.; Xia, W.; Wu, X.; Yao, C.; Liu, X.; Hu, X.-Y.; Lin, C.; Wang, L. Dramatically Promoted Swelling of a Hydrogel by Pillar[6]arene-Ferrocene Complexation with Multistimuli Responsiveness. *J. Am. Chem. Soc.* **2016**, *138*, 6643–6649. [CrossRef]
180. Tan, J.; Li, H.; Hu, X.; Abdullah, R.; Xie, S.; Zhang, L.; Zhao, M.; Luo, Q.; Li, Y.; Sun, Z.; et al. Size-Tunable Assemblies Based on Ferrocene-Containing DNA Polymers for Spatially Uniform Penetration. *Chem* **2019**, *5*, 1775–1792. [CrossRef]
181. Ding, Y.; Wang, C.; Ma, Y.; Zhu, L.; Lu, B.; Wang, Y.; Wang, J.; Dong, C.-M.; Yao, Y. Tumor microenvironment responsive polypeptide-based supramolecular nanoprodrugs for combination therapy. *Acta Biomater.* **2022**, *146*, 396–405. [CrossRef]
182. Lou, H.; Fang, H.; Wang, T.; Wang, D.; Han, Q.; Zhou, W.; Song, Y.; Tan, W.; Zhou, B. Biodegradable Porous Polymeric Drug with pH-Stimuli-Responsive Delivery Capacity for Combined Cancer Therapy. *ACS Appl. Polym. Mater.* **2021**, *4*, 714–724. [CrossRef]
183. Lu, X.; Wang, X.; Li, A.; Zhou, T.; Zhang, L.; Qu, J.; Mao, Z.; Gu, X.; Zhang, X.; Jing, S. Ferrocenylseleno-dopamine functionalized carbon dots for redox-gated imaging and drug delivery in cancer cells. *Dyes Pigm.* **2022**, *205*, 110586. [CrossRef]
184. Park, S.-C.; Kim, N.-H.; Yang, W.; Nah, J.-W.; Jang, M.-K.; Lee, D. Polymeric micellar nanoplatforms for Fenton reaction as a new class of antibacterial agents. *J. Control. Release* **2016**, *221*, 37–47. [CrossRef] [PubMed]

185. Yang, F.; Wei, P.; Yang, M.; Chen, W.; Zhao, B.; Li, W.; Wang, J.; Qiu, L.; Chen, J. Redox-sensitive hyaluronic acid-ferrocene micelles delivering doxorubicin for enhanced tumor treatment by synergistic chemo/chemodynamic therapy. *J. Drug Deliv. Sci. Technol.* **2022**, *77*, 103851. [CrossRef]
186. Yang, F.; Song, C.; Ji, R.; Song, X.; Yang, B.; Lv, Y.; Wei, Z. Increasing the Production of Reactive Oxygen Species through a Ferroptosis Pathway Disrupts the Redox Balance of Tumor Cells for Cancer Treatment. *ACS Appl. Polym. Mater.* **2022**, *4*, 5001–5011. [CrossRef]
187. Zhou, J.; Zhu, X.; Cheng, Q.; Wang, Y.; Wang, R.; Cheng, X.; Xu, J.; Liu, K.; Li, L.; Li, X.; et al. Ferrocene Functionalized Upconversion Nanoparticle Nanosystem with Efficient Near-Infrared-Light-Promoted Fenton-Like Reaction for Tumor Growth Suppression. *Inorg. Chem.* **2020**, *59*, 9177–9187. [CrossRef] [PubMed]
188. Thiem, H.J.; Brandl, M.; Breslow, R. Molecular modeling calculations on the acylation of beta-cyclodextrin by ferrocenylacrylate esters. *J. Am. Chem. Soc.* **1988**, *110*, 8612–8616. [CrossRef]
189. Moreno, S.; Hübner, H.; Effenberg, C.; Boye, S.; Ramuglia, A.; Schmitt, D.; Voit, B.; Weidinger, I.M.; Gallei, M.; Appelhans, D. Redox- and pH-Responsive Polymersomes with Ferrocene Moieties Exhibiting Peroxidase-like, Chemoenzymatic Activity and H_2O_2-Responsive Release Behavior. *Biomacromolecules* **2022**, *23*, 4655–4667. [CrossRef]
190. Wang, Y.; Yin, W.; Ke, W.; Chen, W.; He, C.; Ge, Z. Multifunctional Polymeric Micelles with Amplified Fenton Reaction for Tumor Ablation. *Biomacromolecules* **2018**, *19*, 1990–1998. [CrossRef]
191. Xing, C.; Chen, H.; Guan, Y.; Zhang, S.; Tong, T.; Ding, N.; Luo, T.; Kang, Y.; Pang, J. Cyclodextrin-based supramolecular nanoparticles break the redox balance in chemodynamic therapy-enhanced chemotherapy. *J. Colloid Interface Sci.* **2022**, *628*, 864–876. [CrossRef]
192. Liang, J.; Zheng, Y.; Wu, X.; Tan, C.; Ji, L.; Mao, Z. A Tailored Multifunctional Anticancer Nanodelivery System for Ruthenium-Based Photosensitizers: Tumor Microenvironment Adaption and Remodeling. *Adv. Sci.* **2020**, *7*, 1901992. [CrossRef]
193. Liu, X.; Liu, J.; Meng, C.; Zhu, P.; Liu, X.; Qian, J.; Ling, S.; Zhang, Y.; Ling, Y. Pillar[6]arene-Based Supramolecular Nanocatalysts for Synergistically Enhanced Chemodynamic Therapy by the Intracellular Cascade Reaction. *ACS Appl. Mater. Interfaces* **2021**, *13*, 53574–53585. [CrossRef]
194. Furukawa, H.; Cordova, K.E.; O'Keeffe, M.; Yaghi, O.M. The Chemistry and Applications of Metal-Organic Frameworks. *Science* **2013**, *341*, 1230444. [CrossRef] [PubMed]
195. Wang, Q.; Astruc, D. State of the Art and Prospects in Metal–Organic Framework (MOF)-Based and MOF-Derived Nanocatalysis. *Chem. Rev.* **2020**, *120*, 1438–1511. [CrossRef] [PubMed]
196. Li, J.-R.; Kuppler, R.J.; Zhou, H.-C. Selective gas adsorption and separation in metal-organic frameworks. *Chem. Soc. Rev.* **2009**, *38*, 1477–1504. [CrossRef] [PubMed]
197. Huang, Z.; Yu, H.; Wang, L.; Liu, X.; Lin, T.; Haq, F.; Vatsadze, S.Z.; Lemenovskiy, D.A. Lemenovskiy, Ferrocene-contained metal organic frameworks: From synthesis to applications. *Chem. Rev.* **2021**, *430*, 213737. [CrossRef]
198. Fang, C.; Deng, Z.; Cao, G.; Chu, Q.; Wu, Y.; Li, X.; Peng, X.; Han, G. Co–Ferrocene MOF/Glucose Oxidase as Cascade Nanozyme for Effective Tumor Therapy. *Adv. Funct. Mater.* **2020**, *30*, 1910085. [CrossRef]
199. Deng, Z.; Yu, H.; Wang, L.; Liu, J.; Shea, K.J. Ferrocene-based metal–organic framework nanosheets loaded with palladium as a super-high active hydrogenation catalyst. *J. Mater. Chem. A* **2019**, *7*, 15975–15980. [CrossRef]
200. Ma, J.; Wong-Foy, A.G.; Matzger, A.J. The Role of Modulators in Controlling Layer Spacings in a Tritopic Linker Based Zirconium 2D Microporous Coordination Polymer. *Inorg. Chem.* **2015**, *54*, 4591–4593. [CrossRef]
201. Deng, Z.; Fang, C.; Ma, X.; Li, X.; Zeng, Y.-J.; Peng, X. One Stone Two Birds: Zr-Fc Metal–Organic Framework Nanosheet for Synergistic Photothermal and Chemodynamic Cancer Therapy. *ACS Appl. Mater. Interfaces* **2020**, *12*, 20321–20330. [CrossRef]
202. Tomalia, D.A.; Naylor, A.M.; Goddard, W.A. Starburst dendrimers- Molecular-level control of size, shape, surface chemistry, topology and flexibility from atoms to macroscopic matter. *Angew. Chem. Int. Ed.* **1990**, *29*, 138–175. [CrossRef]
203. Newkome, G.R.; Moorefield, C.N.; Vögtle, F. Dendrimers and Dendrons. In *Concepts, Syntheses, Applications*; Wiley-VCH: Wenheim, Germany, 2001; ISBN 3-527-2997-1.
204. Caminade, A.-M.; Turin, C.-O.; Laurent, R.; Ouali, A.; Delavaut-Nicot, B. Dendrimers. In *Towards Catalytic, Material and Biomedical Uses*; Wiley: Chichester, UK, 2011; ISBN 978-0-470-74881-7.
205. Lee, C.C.; Mackay, J.A.; Frechet, J.M.; Szoka, F.C. Designing dendrimers for biological applications. *Nat. Biotechnol.* **2005**, *23*, 1517–1526. [CrossRef]
206. Boas, U.; Heegaard, P.M.H. Dendrimers in drug research. *Chem. Soc. Rev.* **2004**, *33*, 43–63. [CrossRef] [PubMed]
207. Astruc, D. Research avenues on dendrimers towards molecular biology: From biomimetism to medicinal engineering. *C. R. Acad. Sci. Ser. B* **1996**, *322*, 757–766.
208. Guo, Y.; Zhang, X.; Sun, W.; Jia, H.-R.; Zhu, Y.-X.; Zhang, X.; Zhou, N.; Wu, F.-G. Metal-Phenolic Network-Based Nanocomplexes that Evoke Ferroptosis by Apoptosis: Promoted Nuclear Drug Influx and Reversed Drug Resistance of Cancer. *Chem. Mater.* **2019**, *31*, 10071–10084. [CrossRef]
209. Wang, Z.; Guo, Y.; Fan, Y.; Chen, J.; Wang, H.; Shen, M.; Shi, X. Metal-Phenolic-Network-Coated Dendrimer-Drug Conjugates for Tumor MR Imaging and Chemo/Chemodynamic Therapy via Amplification of Endoplasmic Reticulum Stress. *Adv. Mater.* **2022**, *34*, 2107009. [CrossRef]
210. Casado, C.M.; Cuadrado, I.; Morán, M.; Alonso, B.; García, B.; González, B.; Losada, J. Redox-active ferrocenyl dendrimers and polymers in solution and immobilised on electrode surfaces. *Coord. Chem. Rev.* **1999**, *185–186*, 53–79. [CrossRef]

211. Daniel, M.-C.; Ruiz, J.; Blais, J.-C.; Daro, N.; Astruc, D. Synthesis of five generations of redox-stable pentamethylamidoferrocenyl dendrimers and comparison of amidoferrocenyl- and pentamethylamidoferrocenyl dendrimers as electrochemical exoreceptors. *Chem. Eur. J.* **2003**, *9*, 4371–4379. [CrossRef]
212. Ornelas, C.; Aranzaes, J.R.; Cloutet, E.; Alves, S.; Astruc, D. Click assembly of 1,2,3-triazole-linked dendrimers, including ferrocenyl dendrimers, which sense both oxo anions and metal cations. *Angew. Chem. Int. Ed.* **2007**, *46*, 872–877. [CrossRef]
213. Ornelas, C.; Ruiz, J.; Belin, C.; Astruc, D. Giant Dendritic Molecular Electrochrome Batteries with Ferrocenyl and Pentamethylferrocenyl Termini. *J. Am. Chem. Soc.* **2009**, *131*, 590–601. [CrossRef]
214. Luo, J.; Xie, Z.; Xie, Z.; Lam, J.W.Y.; Cheng, L.; Chen, H.; Qiu, C.; Kwok, H.S.; Zhan, X.; Liu, Y.; et al. Aggregation-induced emission of 1-methyl-1,2,3,4,5-pentaphenylsilole. *Chem. Commun.* **2001**, *18*, 1740–1741. [CrossRef]
215. Mei, J.; Leung, N.L.C.; Kwok, R.T.K.; Lam, J.W.Y.; Tang, B.Z. Aggregation-Induced Emission: Together We Shine, United We Soar! *Chem. Rev.* **2015**, *115*, 11718–11940. [CrossRef]
216. Liu, S.; Feng, G.; Tang, B.Z.; Liu, B. Recent advances of AIE light-up probes for photodynamic therapy. *Chem. Sci.* **2021**, *12*, 6488–6506. [CrossRef]
217. Tomalia, D.A.; Klajnert-Maculewicz, B.; Johnson, K.A.-M.; Brinkman, H.F.; Janaszewska, A.; Hedstrand, D.M. Non-Traditional Intrinsic Luminescence: Inexplicable Blue Fluorescence Observed For Dendrimers, Macromolecules And Small Molecular Structures Lacking Traditional/Conventional Luminophores. *Prog. Polym. Sci.* **2019**, *90*, 35–117. [CrossRef]
218. Studzian, M.; Działak, P.; Pułaski, Ł.; Hedstrand, D.M.; Tomalia, D.A.; Klajnert-Maculewicz, B. Synthesis, Internalization and Visualization of N-(4-Carbomethoxy) Pyrrolidone Terminated PAMAM [G5:G3-TREN] Tecto(dendrimers) in Mammalian Cells. *Molecules* **2020**, *25*, 4406. [CrossRef] [PubMed]
219. Al-Jamal, K.T.; Sakthivel, T.; Florence, A.T. Solubilisation And Transformation of Amphipathic Lipidic Dendron Vesicles (Dendrisomes) Into Mixed Micelles. *Colloids Surf. A* **2005**, *268*, 52–59. [CrossRef]
220. Xiao, Q.; Rubien, J.D.; Wang, Z.; Reed, E.H.; Hammer, D.A.; Sahoo, D.; Heiney, P.A.; Yadavalli, S.S.; Goulian, M.; Wilner, S.E.; et al. Self-Sorting and Coassembly of Fluorinated, Hydrogenated, and Hybrid Janus Dendrimers into Dendrimersomes. *J. Am. Chem. Soc.* **2016**, *138*, 12655–12663. [CrossRef]
221. Perli, G.; Wang, Q.; Braga, C.B.; Bertuzzi, D.L.; Fontana, L.A.; Soares, M.C.P.; Ruiz, J.; Megiatto, J.D.; Astruc, D.; Ornelas, C. Self-Assembly of a Triazolylferrocenyl Dendrimer in Water Yields Nontraditional Intrinsic Green Fluorescent Vesosomes for Nanotheranostic Applications. *J. Am. Chem. Soc.* **2021**, *143*, 12948–12954. [CrossRef]
222. Bertuzzi, D.L.; Braga, C.B.; Perli, G.; Ornelas, C. Water-Soluble Well-Defined Bifunctional Ferrocenyl Dendrimer with Anti-Cancer Activity. *Eur. J. Inorg. Chem.* **2022**, e202101084. [CrossRef]
223. Ornelas, C. Brief Timelapse on Dendrimer Chemistry: Advances, Limitations, and Expectations. *Macromol. Chem. Phys.* **2016**, *217*, 149–174. [CrossRef]
224. Baartzes, N.; Szabo, C.; Cenariu, M.; Imre-Lucaci, F.; Dorneanu, S.A.; Fischer-Fodor, E.; Smith, G.S. In vitro antitumour activity of two ferrocenyl metallodendrimers in a colon cancer cell line. *Inorg. Chem. Commun.* **2018**, *98*, 75–79. [CrossRef]
225. Konkoľová, E.; Janočková, J.; Perjési, P.; Vašková, J.; Kožurková, M. Selected ferrocenyl chalcones as DNA/BSA-interacting agents and inhibitors of DNA topoisomerase I and II activity. *J. Organomet. Chem.* **2018**, *861*, 1–9. [CrossRef]
226. Thomas, N.; Dionysiou, D.D.; Pillai, S.C. Heterogeneous Fenton catalysts: A review of recent advances. *J. Hazard. Mater.* **2021**, *404*, 124082. [CrossRef] [PubMed]
227. Snegur, L.V. Modern Trends in Bio-Organometallic Ferrocene Chemistry. *Inorganics* **2022**, *10*, 226. [CrossRef]
228. Peters, D.G.; Purnell, C.J.; Haaf, M.P.; Yang, Q.X.; Connor, J.R.; Meadowcroft, M.D. Dietary lipophilic iron accelerates regional brain iron-load in C57BL6 mice. *Brain Struct. Funct.* **2018**, *223*, 1519–1536. [CrossRef] [PubMed]
229. Sharma, B.; Kumar, V. Has ferrocene really delivered its role in accentuating the bioactivity of organic scaffolds? *J. Med. Chem.* **2021**, *64*, 16865–16921. [CrossRef]
230. Abbas, G.; Irfan, A.; Ahmed, I.; Al-Zeidaneen, F.K.; Muthu, S.; Fuhr, O.; Thomas, R. Synthesis and investigation of anti-COVID-19 ability of ferrocene Schiff base derivatives by quantum chemical and molecular docking. *J. Mol. Struct.* **2022**, *1253*, 132242. [CrossRef]
231. Bai, Y.; Pan, Y.; An, N.; Zhang, H.; Wang, C.; Tian, W.; Huang, T. Host-guest interactions based supramolecular complexes self-assemblies for amplified chemodynamic therapy with H_2O_2 elevation and GSH consuption properties. *Chin. Chem. Lett.* **2023**, *34*, 107552. [CrossRef]
232. Anthony, E.J.; Bolitho, E.M.; Bridgewater, H.E.; Carter, O.W.L.; Donnelly, J.M.; Imberti, C.; Lant, E.C.; Lermyte, F.; Needham, R.J.; Palau, M.; et al. Metallodrugs are unique: Opportunities and challenges of discovery and development. *Chem. Sci.* **2020**, *11*, 12888–12917. [CrossRef]
233. McNerney, M.P.; Doiron, K.E.; Ng, T.L.; Chang, T.Z.; Silver, P.A. Theranostic cells: Emerging clinical applications of synthetic biology. *Nat. Rev. Genet.* **2021**, *22*, 730–746. [CrossRef]

pharmaceutics

MDPI

Article

Screening Libraries to Discover Molecular Design Principles for the Targeted Delivery of mRNA with One-Component Ionizable Amphiphilic Janus Dendrimers Derived from Plant Phenolic Acids †

Juncheng Lu [1,2,‡], Elena N. Atochina-Vasserman [2,‡], Devendra S. Maurya [1,‡], Muhammad Irhash Shalihin [1], Dapeng Zhang [1], Srijay S. Chenna [1], Jasper Adamson [1], Matthew Liu [1], Habib Ur Rehman Shah [1], Honey Shah [1], Qi Xiao [1], Bryn Queeley [2], Nathan A. Ona [2], Erin K. Reagan [2], Houping Ni [2], Dipankar Sahoo [1,2], Mihai Peterca [1], Drew Weissman [2,*] and Virgil Percec [1,*]

1 Roy & Diana Vagelos Laboratories, Department of Chemistry, University of Pennsylvania, Philadelphia, PA 19104-6323, USA; junchlu@sas.upenn.edu (J.L.); maurya@sas.upenn.edu (D.S.M.); shalihin@sas.upenn.edu (M.I.S.); zhdp9114@126.com (D.Z.); srijay.chenna@gmail.com (S.S.C.); jasper.adamson@kbfi.ee (J.A.); liumatt@sas.upenn.edu (M.L.); habib.ur.rehman@iub.edu.pk (H.U.R.S.); honey@sas.upenn.edu (H.S.); qxiao@ethealthcareinc.com (Q.X.); dipankar.sahoo@pennmedicine.upenn.edu (D.S.); mpeterca@gmail.com (M.P.)

2 Department of Medicine, Perelman School of Medicine, University of Pennsylvania, Philadelphia, PA 19104-6323, USA; atochina@pennmedicine.upenn.edu (E.N.A.-V.); queeleyb@pennmedicine.upenn.edu (B.Q.); nathan.ona@pennmedicine.upenn.edu (N.A.O.); ereagan@pennmedicine.upenn.edu (E.K.R.); houping@pennmedicine.upenn.edu (H.N.)

* Correspondence: dreww@pennmedicine.upenn.edu (D.W.); percec@sas.upenn.edu (V.P.)

† Dedicated to the 85th Anniversary of Donald A. Tomalia.

‡ These authors contributed equally to this work.

Abstract: Viral and synthetic vectors to deliver nucleic acids were key to the rapid development of extraordinarily efficient COVID-19 vaccines. The four-component lipid nanoparticles (LNPs), containing phospholipids, PEG-conjugated lipids, cholesterol, and ionizable lipids, co-assembled with mRNA via a microfluidic technology, are the leading nonviral delivery vector used by BioNTech/Pfizer and Moderna to access COVID-19 mRNA vaccines. LNPs exhibit a statistical distribution of their four components when delivering mRNA. Here, we report a methodology that involves screening libraries to discover the molecular design principles required to realize organ-targeted mRNA delivery and mediate activity with a one-component ionizable multifunctional amphiphilic Janus dendrimer (IAJD) derived from plant phenolic acids. IAJDs co-assemble with mRNA into monodisperse dendrimersome nanoparticles (DNPs) with predictable dimensions, via the simple injection of their ethanol solution in a buffer. The precise location of the functional groups in one-component IAJDs demonstrated that the targeted organs, including the liver, spleen, lymph nodes, and lung, are selected based on the hydrophilic region, while activity is associated with the hydrophobic domain of IAJDs. These principles, and a mechanistic hypothesis to explain activity, simplify the synthesis of IAJDs, the assembly of DNPs, handling, and storage of vaccines, and reduce price, despite employing renewable plant starting materials. Using simple molecular design principles will lead to increased accessibility to a large diversity of mRNA-based vaccines and nanotherapeutics.

Keywords: targeted mRNA delivery; one-component vector; ionizable Janus dendrimer; dendrimersome nanoparticles; molecular design principles; vaccines; nanotherapeutics; plant phenolic acids; simplified preparation and handling; reduced vaccine price

1. Introduction

The efficient delivery of nucleic acids via viral [1–3] and synthetic [4–12] vectors has remarkably impacted genetic nanomedicine, as illustrated by the great success of

COVID-19 vaccines [13–18]. Recent reviews [19–23] and three publications from our laboratories [24–26] summarized in great detail the advantages and disadvantages of viral and nonviral delivery systems. Therefore, some of these advantages and disadvantages will only be briefly repeated here. This recapitulation has as its main goal a clarification of the scope, properties, and limitations of viral and synthetic vectors for the delivery of DNA and RNA, and of the main functions of the nucleic acids. DNA must be delivered to the nucleus, while RNA is delivered to the cytoplasm. At the same time, due to enzymatic degradation, neither DNA nor RNA is stable, although RNA needs more careful handling since it is single-stranded and is much less stable than DNA. This dissimilar stability of nucleic acids and location of delivery endows the difference between the methodology principles for the delivery of DNA and RNA.

Viral vectors have high transfection efficacy (95%) and higher specificity for cell targeting, including for unnatural cells. The drawbacks of viral gene delivery include immunogenicity, cytotoxicity, the difficulty of assembly, inflammatory responses to repeated administration, and potential risk for insertional mutagenesis [24–26].

Delivery via nonviral vectors is safer and exhibits lower toxicity and immunogenicity but exhibits much lower transfection efficiency (1–2%), and the synthetic vectors are less stable than the viral vectors. The unlimited synthetic capabilities of synthetic vectors represent, most probably, their main advantage over viral vectors. Taking all these features into account, we can understand why covalent and supramolecular dendrimers, as well as other permanently charged synthetic vectors complexed on their cationic periphery groups with nucleic acids, have pioneered the field of nonviral vectors for the cell transfection of DNA. Due to the relatively higher stability of DNA, no protection–deprotection methodology is required during the delivery of DNA. However, a protection–deprotection methodology is required for the delivery of RNA. More details on these principles and methodologies will be briefly summarized in a later part of this report.

Four-component lipid nanoparticles (LNPs) [27–29] consisting of ionizable lipids [27,28], phospholipids [29], cholesterol, and a PEG-conjugated lipid [26–28], represent the state-of-the-art technology employed by BioNTech/Pfizer [16] and Moderna [17] for the production of their mRNA vaccines (Figure 1A). The protection–deprotection is accomplished in this case through a reversible encapsulation of the mRNA mediated by an ionizable lipid rather than by the permanently charged cationic components employed in the delivery of DNA. The stability of the nanoparticle is aided through co-assembly with cholesterol and PEG-conjugated lipids. The statistical distribution of the four components in the LNPs is responsible for some of their limitations and difficulties of molecular design since the exact location of their four components within LNPs is not known. For example, the segregation of the neutral ionizable lipid as droplets in the core of LNPs [28,30] and the "PEG dilemma" [31–34] are two of the main outcomes induced by the lack of their precise location. An additional deficiency is optimal stability at temperatures of about −70 °C. The detailed structure of the LNP is also not yet known in great detail, but it will be discussed, together with alternative methods of delivery and their evolution, in a later subsection.

Recently, we took advantage of the unlimited synthetic capabilities of nonviral vectors and elaborated a simple one-component sequence-defined ionizable amphiphilic Janus dendrimer (IAJD) [24–26] concept that relies not only on precise composition but also, most importantly, on the exact location and placement of its functional groups (Figure 1B) [24–26]. In addition, one-component IAJDs do not require the microfluidic or T-tube technology employed by four-component LNPs to co-assemble with mRNA. One-component IAJDs are co-assembled with mRNA into vesicles named dendrimersome nanoparticles (DNPs). They exhibit 97% nucleic acid encapsulation efficiency [24] and are assembled via the simple injection of their ethanol solution into an acidic buffer containing mRNA rather than via the microfluidic or T-tube technology required using LNPs. This simple assembly methodology provides rapid access to screening libraries of IAJDs with different compositions and sequences, both in their hydrophilic and hydrophobic parts.

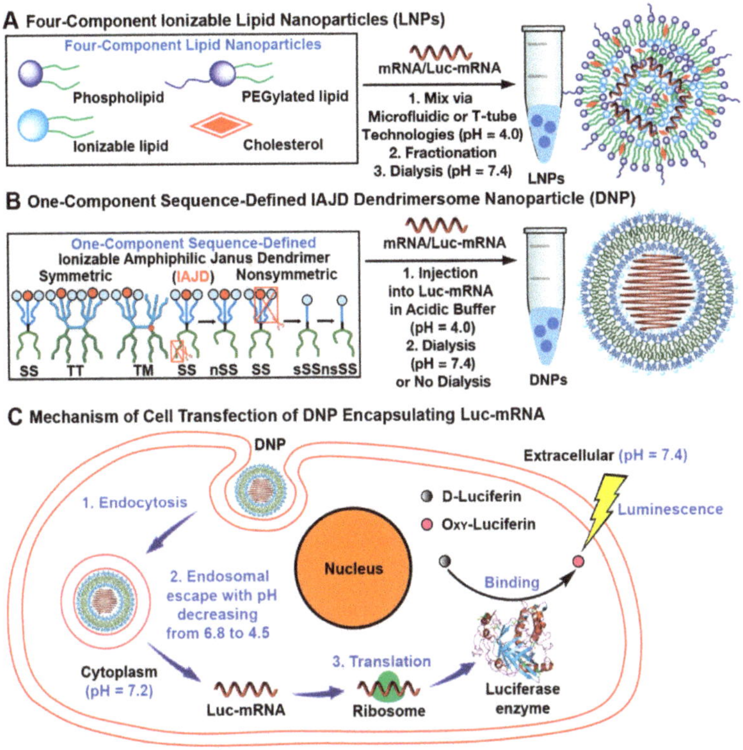

Figure 1. Schematic representation of four-component LNPs, one-component IAJD-based DNPs, and the cell transfection mechanism of LNPs and DNPs encapsulating Luc-mRNA: (**A**) four-component LNPs; (**B**) one-component IAJDs and their DNPs; (**C**) cell transfection mechanism of LNPs and DNPs encapsulating Luc-mRNA.

Here, we will elaborate on a methodology for screening libraries to discover, and later even predict, the molecular design principles required to accomplish organ-targeted mRNA delivery and engineer activity with a one-component ionizable multifunctional amphiphilic Janus dendrimer (IAJD) derived from plant phenolic acids. Quantitative experiments on this topic are outside the scope of this report but will become available soon.

Since this is an invited publication by the Guest Editors of a Special Issue dedicated to the 85th anniversary of Donald A. Tomalia, we decided to organize a more unusual manuscript that represents a combination of an original research paper, as the title indicates, in the first part, combined with a perspective on the discovery, evolution, and the immense role of Don on the discovery, evolution, and the current status of covalent and supramolecular dendrimers, in the second part.

2. Materials and Methods

2.1. Materials

3,5-Dihydroxybenzoic acid (Acros, 97%), 1-bromononane (Lancaster, 99%), 1-bromododecane (Alfa Aesar, 99%),1-bromotetradecane (Acros, 98%), 1-bromohexadecane (TCI, 96%), 1-heptadecanol (TCI, 97%) (*rac*)-3-(bromomethyl)heptane, 1-bromooctadecane (Acros, 96%), 2-ethylhexyl bromide, (Aldrich, 95%), 1-bromooctane (Aldrich, 99%), 1-bromodecane (Acros, 98%), 1-bromoundecane (Aldrich, 99%), 1-bromopentadecane (Aldrich, 98%), benzyl chloride (Alfa Aesar, 99%), 4-toluenesulfonyl chloride (Alfa Aesar, 98%), palladium on activated carbon catalyst (Spectrum, 10 wt% loading), lithium aluminum hydride

($LiAlH_4$, TCI, 95%), 4-bromobutyric acid (Acros, 98%), thionyl chloride (Alfa Aesar, 99+%), potassium phthalimide (Chem Impex, 99.8%), 1-methylpiperazine (Alfa Aesar, 98%), 1-(2-hydroxyethyl)piperazine (Acros, 99%), and triethylamine (TCI, 99%) were used as received. Heptadecyl 4-methylbenzenesulfonate ($C_{17}H_{35}OTs$) was synthesized according to a literature procedure reported by our laboratory [26]. All other reagents and solvents were obtained from commercial sources and were used as received. CH_2Cl_2 (DCM) was dried over CaH_2 and distilled before use. 4-(Dimethylamino)pyridinium 4-toluenesulfonate (DPTS) was prepared according to a literature method [35]. Acetate buffer (10 mM) was prepared by dissolving sodium acetate (2.3 mM) and acetic acid (7.7 mM) in ultra-pure water. The final pH of the buffer was adjusted with 0.1 M HCl or 0.1 M NaOH solution. Nucleoside-modified messenger RNA encoding firefly luciferase (Luc-mRNA) was produced as reported [36]. Human embryonic kidney (HEK) 293T cells (American Type Culture Collection, Manassas, VA, USA) were cultured in Dulbecco's modified Eagle's medium (DMEM) supplemented with 10% inactivated fetal bovine serum (FBS) (Gemini Bio-Products, West Sacramento, CA, USA), 2 mM L–glutamine and 100 U/mL penicillin/streptomycin (Life Technologies, Carlsbad, CA, USA). DPBS (Corning, Corning, NY, USA), OptiMEM (Gibco, Carlsbad, CA, USA), UltraPure DNase/RNase-free distilled water (Invitrogen, Carlsbad, CA, USA), Trypsin-EDTA (0.25%, Gibco, Carlsbad CA, USA), Trypan Blue (Sigma-Aldrich, St. Louis, MO, USA), Cell Culture Lysis 5X Reagent (Promega, Madison, WI, USA), Luciferase Assay System (Promega, Madison, WI, USA), and D-luciferin sodium salt (Regis Technologies, Morton Grove, IL, USA) were used as received.

2.2. Characterization and Methods

The purity and structure of intermediate compounds and final products were determined using a combination of techniques, including thin-layer chromatography (TLC), ^1H and ^{13}C NMR, high-pressure liquid chromatography (HPLC), and matrix-assisted laser desorption ionization–time-of-flight (MALDI-TOF) mass spectrometry.

2.2.1. ^1H and ^{13}C NMR

^1H and ^{13}C NMR spectra were recorded at 400 MHz and 101 MHz, respectively, on a Bruker (Billerica, MA, USA) NEO (400 MHz) NMR spectrometer equipped with an autosampler, or 500 MHz and 126 MHz, respectively, on a Bruker DRX (500 MHz) NMR spectrometer. All NMR values were measured at 23 °C in $CDCl_3$. Chemical shifts (δ) are reported in ppm. The resonance multiplicities in the ^1H NMR spectra are indicated as "s" (singlet), "d" (doublet), "t" (triplet), "m" (multiplet), and "br" (broad resonance). A residual protic solvent of $CDCl_3$ (^1H, δ 7.26 ppm; ^{13}C, δ 77.16 ppm) and tetramethylsilane (TMS, δ 0 ppm) were used as the internal reference in the ^1H and ^{13}C NMR spectra. NMR spectra were analyzed using MNova 14 or TopSpin 4.07 (Bruker). More details are available in previous publications from our laboratory [24–26].

2.2.2. Thin-Layer Chromatography (TLC)

TLC was used to monitor the evolution of the extent of the reaction by using silica gel 60 F_{254} precoated plates (E. Merck, Darmstadt, Germany). The individual compounds with aromatic groups were visualized using UV light (λ = 254 nm). For compounds without aromatic groups, the TLC plate was stained with iodine vapor to help visualization. Purification via flash column chromatography (SiO_2) was performed using silica gel from Silicycle (60 Å, 40–63 μm), with the eluent partially mentioned in the experimental part for each compound. More details are available in previous publications from our laboratory [24–26].

2.2.3. High-Pressure Liquid Chromatography (HPLC)

The determination of the purity of individual compounds via HPLC was performed by using a Shimadzu LC-20AD high-performance liquid chromatograph pump, a PE Nelson Analytical 900 Series integration data station, a Shimadzu SPD-10A VP (UV–vis,

λ = 254 nm), and three AM gel columns (a guard column, two 500 Å, 10 μm columns). THF with 5% of NEt3 was used as the solvent, and characterization was carried out at 23 °C. The detection of the compounds was determined using UV absorbance (λ = 254 nm) or an RI (refractive index) detector. More details are available in previous publications from our laboratory [24–26].

2.2.4. Matrix-Assisted Laser Desorption Ionization–Time-of-Flight (MALDI-TOF) Mass Spectrometry

The molar mass of all molecules was determined via MALDI-TOF mass spectrometry employing a Perseptive Biosystem-Voyager-DE (Framingham, MA, USA) mass spectrometer equipped with a nitrogen laser (337 nm) and operating in linear mode. Angiotensin II and Bombesin were used as standards for calibration. For the preparation of the sample solution, the corresponding compound was first dissolved in THF (5–10 mg/mL). Subsequently, the matrix (2,5-dihydroxybenzoic acid) was dissolved in THF 10 mg/mL, and the two solutions were mixed with a 1/5 (v/v, compound solution/matrix solution) ratio. Then, one drop of solution was placed on the MALDI plate and dried at 23 °C. Afterward, the plate was inserted into the vacuum chamber of the instrument for analysis. The laser intensity and voltages applied for the analysis were adjusted based on the molar mass and nature of each compound. More details are available in previous publications from our laboratory [24–26].

2.2.5. Dynamic Light Scattering (DLS)

DLS for the dimensions (sizes and polydispersities) of DNPs was performed on a Malvern Instruments particle sizer (Zetasizer Nano S, Malvern Instruments, Malvern, UK) equipped with 4 mW He–Ne laser 633 nm and avalanche photodiode positioned at 175° to the beam and temperature-controlled cuvette holder. Instrument parameters were set up automatically along with measurement times. The sample solution (c.a. 0.4 mL) was placed in a semi-micro cuvette (1.6 mL, polystyrene, 10 × 10 × 45 mm, Greiner Bio-One, Monroe, NC, USA), and the experiments were performed at 23 °C. More details are available in previous publications from our laboratory [24–26].

2.2.6. pKa Measurements of Individual IAJDs

IAJDs were dissolved in ethanol (sat. with NaCl) at a concentration of 1.5 mg/mL and in a volume of 3 mL. Then, a 0.1 M HCl solution was added to the ethanol solution, with an increment of 7.5 μL. The resulting pH, after each addition of HCl solution, was measured using a Thermo Scientific Orion Star A121 (Waltham, MA, USA) meter with a Thermo Scientific Orion 8220BNWP pH probe. pK_a was determined using the half equivalence point titration. More details are available in previous publications from our laboratory [24–26].

2.2.7. Production of Nucleoside-Modified Luc-mRNA

mRNA was produced as previously described [36] using T7 RNA polymerase on linearized DNA encoding codon-optimized firefly luciferase and a 101 nt poly(A) tail. 1-methylpseudouridine-5′-triphosphate was used instead of UTP. A trinucleotide cap1 analog was added co-transcriptionally. Purification was performed as previously described [37]. mRNA was analyzed for RNase, dsRNA, endotoxin, and other forms of contamination and stored frozen at −20 °C.

2.2.8. Formulation of DNPs Co-Assembled from IAJDs and Luc-mRNA

Nucleoside-modified mRNA encoding firefly luciferase (Luc-mRNA) was dissolved in UltraPure DNase/RNase-free distilled water with an initial concentration of 4.0 mg/mL. IAJDs were dissolved in ethanol at an initial concentration of 80 mg/mL. Luc-mRNA solution (12.5 μL) was placed into a clean RNA-free Eppendorf (1.5 mL), and 463 μL of acetate buffer (10 mM, pH 4.0) was added. The IAJD stock solution in ethanol was taken (25 µL) and rapidly injected into the above Luc-mRNA solution in acetate buffer, followed by vortex for 5 s. More details are available in previous publications from our laboratory [24–26].

2.2.9. Luminescence Characterization for In Vivo Transfection Experiments

Bioluminescence imaging was performed with an IVIS Spectrum imaging system (PerkinElmer, Waltham, MA, USA). Mice were anesthetized with 3% of isoflurane (Piramal Healthcare Limited) and intraperitoneally (i.p.) administered with D-luciferin (Regis Technologies) at a dose of 150 mg/kg of body weight. Ten minutes after the administration of D-luciferin, mice were placed on the imaging platform while being maintained on isoflurane via a nose cone and imaged using a certain exposure time (60, 30, or 15 s). Bioluminescence values were quantified by measuring photon flux (photons/second, p/s) in the region of interest (ROI) on mice, where the bioluminescence signal emanated was analyzed using the Living Image Software (PerkinElmer). To quantify luminescent flux, an oval ROI was placed over each organ of interest and analyzed. More details are available in previous publications from our laboratory [24–26].

2.2.10. In Vivo mRNA Delivery in Mice with DNPs

All the mice used were in accordance with the guidelines and approval from the Pennsylvania University Institution of Animal Care and Use Committee. Female or male BALB/c mice (6–8 weeks old, from Charles River Laboratories, Wilmington, MA, USA) were anesthetized with isoflurane (Piramal Healthcare Limited) and injected via retro-orbital sinus with 100 µL of a DNP solution containing 10 µg of Luc-mRNA. Then, 4 to 6 h after injection, mice were i.p. injected with D-luciferin (150 mg/kg of body weight, Regis Technologies) and imaged on a PerkinElmer IVIS Spectrum CT system (PerkinElmer, Waltham, MA). The tissue luminescence signal was measured on the IVIS imaging system using a certain exposure time (60, 30, or 15 s) and medium binning (binning = 8) to ensure that the signal obtained was within the operative detection range. For the IVIS imaging of the organs, mice were sacrificed, and the heart, lungs, liver, and spleen were immediately collected; then, bioluminescence imaging was performed as described above. Image analysis was conducted with the Living Image software (PerkinElmer). Bioluminescence values were quantified by measuring photon flux (photons/second) in the region of interest (ROI) using the Living Image software. More details are available in previous publications from our laboratory [24–26].

2.2.11. Molecular Modelling

Molecular models of the IAJD bilayers were drawn using the DS ViewerPro (version 5.0) software. The Material Studio Modeling (version 3.1) software from Accelrys was used to perform energy minimization analyses of the built models on supramolecular structures. BIOVIA Discovery Studio Visualizer (version 2019) was used for display style and coloring. Color codes were used similarly to those in the ChemDraw (Waltham, MA, USA) structure (hydrophilic part in blue; hydrophobic part in light and dark green; oxygen and OH in pink; carbons in the aromatic ring in gray; and H groups on aromatic in white).

2.3. *Synthesis of IAJDs*

2.3.1. Synthesis of the Monoprotected Benzyl Ether of Methyl 3,5-Dihydroxybenzoate, **2**

Methyl 3,5-dihydroxybenzoate, **1**, (10.00 g, 59.5 mmol, 1.0 equiv) (Scheme 1), benzyl chloride (8.30 g, 65.4 mmol, 1.1 equiv), KI (1.23 g, 7.43 mmol, 0.125 equiv), K_2CO_3 (9.06 g, 65.4 mmol, 1.1 equiv), and DMF (50 mL) were added into a 100 mL round-bottom flask. The reaction mixture was stirred at 600 rpm, at 80 °C under N_2 while monitored for conversion using TLC. After 5 h, methyl 3,5-dihydroxybenzoate was completely consumed, and the reaction mixture was poured into ice/water (150 mL). The aqueous layer was extracted with ethyl acetate 4 times. The organic phase was dried over $MgSO_4$, and the solvent was removed in a rotary evaporator. The solid product was purified via column chromatography on silica gel with hexane/ethyl acetate = 5/1 as mobile phase to obtain 6.00 g of white crystals (isolated yield, 39%). Mp = 96 °C. ^{1}H NMR (400 MHz, $CDCl_3$) δ 7.46–7.34 (m, 5 H, Ph*H*), 7.28 (s, 1 H, Ph*H*), 7.17 (s, 1 H, Ph*H*), 6.71 (s, 1 H, Ph*H*), 5.10 (s, 2 H, $PhCH_2O$-), 3.93 (s, 3 H, $PhCOOCH_3$). ^{13}C NMR (101 MHz, $CDCl_3$) δ 167.6, 160.0, 157.2, 136.5, 131.8, 128.7, 128.2, 127.7, 109.8, 108.0, 107.7, 70.3, 52.6. Purity by HPLC: 99+%. MALDI-TOF MS *m/z* of $[M + H]^+$ calculated for $C_{15}H_{15}O_4$: 259.1; found: 259.4. $[M + Na]^+$ calculated for $C_{15}H_{14}NaO_4$: 281.1; found: 281.3. $[M + K]^+$ calculated for $C_{15}H_{14}KO_4$: 297.1; found: 297.2 (Figure S1).

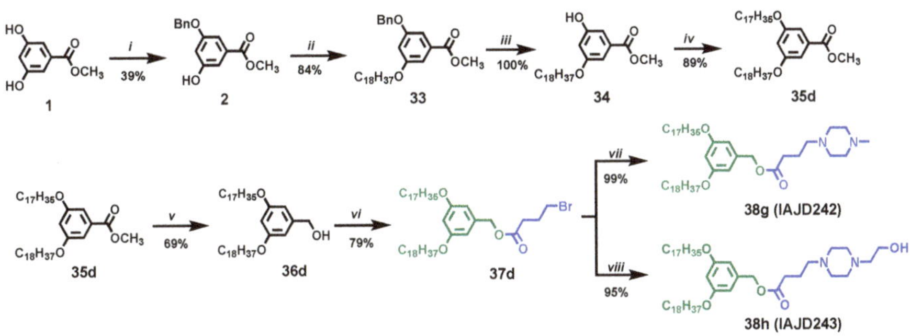

Scheme 1. Synthesis of 3,5-nonsymmetric nsSS IAJDs: (i) BnCl, K_2CO_3, KI, DMF, 80 °C, 5 h; (ii) $C_{18}H_{37}Br$, K_2CO_3, DMF, 120 °C, 2 h; (iii) H_2, Pd/C, DCM, MeOH, 12 h; (iv) $C_{17}H_{35}OTs$, K_2CO_3, DMF, 120 °C, 2 h; (v) $LiAlH_4$, THF, 0–23 °C, 1 h; (vi) DCC, DPTS, DCM 12 h; (vii) methylpiperazine, K_2CO_3, MeCN, 95 °C, 3 h; (viii) 1-(2-hydroxyethyl)piperazine, K_2CO_3, MeCN, 95 °C, 3 h.

2.3.2. Synthesis of Methyl 3-(benzyloxy)-5-(octadecyloxy)benzoate, **33**

Methyl 3-(benzyloxy)-5-hydroxybenzoate, 2, (2.00 g, 7.74 mmol, 1 equiv), 1-bromooctad ecane (2.84 g, 8.52 mmol, 1.1 equiv), K_2CO_3 (2.14 g, 15.48 mmol, 2 equiv), and 30 mL DMF were heated at 120 °C and stirred under a N_2 atmosphere for 2 h. The reaction mixture was cooled to 23 °C poured into 150 mL ice water. The resulting white precipitate was filtered and collected. Then, the precipitate was recrystallized from minimum acetone to afford the title compound as a white solid (3.28 g, 84%). Mp = 65 °C. ^{1}H NMR (400 MHz, $CDCl_3$) δ 7.48–7.29 (m, 5 H, PhH), 7.27 (br, 1 H, PhH), 7.20 (br, 1 H, PhH), 6.73 (t, 1 H, PhH), 5.08 (s, 2 H, $PhCH_2O$-), 3.97 (t, 2 H, $PhOCH_2$-), 3.90 (s, 3 H, $PhCOOCH_3$), 1.78 (m, 2 H, $PhOCH_2CH_2CH_2(CH_2)_{14}CH_3$), 1.44 (m, 2 H, $PhOCH_2CH_2CH_2(CH_2)_{14}CH_3$), 1.28 (m, 28 H, $PhOCH_2CH_2CH_2(CH_2)_{14}CH_3$), 0.89 (t, 3 H, $PhO(CH_2)_{17}CH_3$). ^{13}C NMR (101 MHz, $CDCl_3$) δ 167.0, 160.3, 159.9, 136.7, 132.1, 128.7, 128.2, 127.7, 108.3, 108.0, 107.1, 77.4, 70.4, 68.5, 52.3, 32.1, 29.8, 29.7, 29.7, 29.5, 29.3, 26.4, 26.1, 22.9, 22.8, 14.2. Purity by HPLC: 99+%. MALDI-TOF MS *m/z* of $[M + H]^+$ calculated for $C_{33}H_{51}O_4$: 511.4; found: 512.5. $[M + Na]^+$ calculated for $C_{33}H_{50}NaO_4$: 533.4; found: 534.5. $[M + K]^+$ calculated for $C_{33}H_{50}KO_4$: 549.3; found: 550.4 (Figure S2).

2.3.3. Synthesis of the Methyl 3-hydroxy-5-(octadecyloxy)benzoate, **34**

Methyl 3-(benzyloxy)-5-(octadecyloxy)benzoate, **33**, (3.26 g, 6.42 mmol), DCM (20 mL), and methanol (10 mL) were added in a 50 mL round-bottom flask. Then, Pd/C (0.16 g, 5 wt%) was added to the solution, and the flask was evacuated and filled with hydrogen three times. Afterward, the mixture was stirred at 23 °C under a hydrogen atmosphere for 12 h. The reaction mixture was filtered through Celite, and the filter cake was washed with DCM. The evaporation of the solvent yielded the title compound as a white solid (2.70 g, 100%). Mp = 99 °C. ^{1}H NMR (400 MHz, $CDCl_3$) δ 7.13 (d, 2 H, Ph*H*), 6.64 (t, 1 H, Ph*H*), 3.95 (t, 2 H, $PhOCH_2$-), 3.89 (s, 3 H, $PhCOOCH_3$), 1.75 (m, 2 H, $PhOCH_2CH_2CH_2(CH_2)_{14}CH_3$), 1.44 (m, 2 H, $PhOCH_2CH_2CH_2(CH_2)_{14}CH_3$), 1.26 (m, 28 H, $PhOCH_2CH_2CH_2(CH_2)_{14}CH_3$), 0.88 (t, 3 H, $PhO(CH_2)_{17}CH_3$). ^{13}C NMR (101 MHz, $CDCl_3$) δ 167.0, 160.4, 157.0, 131.9, 109.0, 107.7, 107.1, 68.4, 52.2, 31.9, 29.7, 29.7, 29.6, 29.6, 29.4, 29.4, 29.2, 26.0, 22.7, 14.2. Purity by HPLC: 99+%. MALDI-TOF MS *m*/*z* of $[M + H]^+$ calculated for $C_{26}H_{45}O_4$: 421.3; found: 421.5. $[M + Na]^+$ calculated for $C_{26}H_{44}NaO_4$: 443.3; found: 443.4. $[M + K]^+$ calculated for $C_{26}H_{44}KO_4$: 459.7; found: 459.2 (Figure S3).

2.3.4. Synthesis of Methyl 3-(heptadecyloxy)-5-(octadecyloxy)benzoate (**35d**)

Methyl 3-hydroxy-5-(octadecyloxy)benzoate, **34**, (0.50 g, 1.19 mmol, 1 equiv), $C_{17}H_{35}OTs$ (0.54 g, 1.31 mmol, 1.1 equiv), and K_2CO_3 (0.33 g, 2.38 mmol, 2 equiv) were heated at 120 °C and stirred under a N_2 atmosphere for 2 h. The reaction mixture was cooled to 23 °C and poured into ice/water (150 mL). The resulting white precipitate was filtered and collected. Then, the precipitate was recrystallized from minimum acetone to afford the title compound as a white solid (0.70 g, 89%). Mp = 72 °C. ^{1}H NMR (400 MHz, $CDCl_3$) δ 7.15 (br, 2 H, Ph*H*), 6.63 (t, 1 H, Ph*H*), 3.96 (t, 4 H, $PhOCH_2CH_2CH_2$-), 3.89 (s, 3 H, $PhCOOCH_3$), 1.77 (m, 4 H, $PhOCH_2CH_2CH_2$-), 1.43 (m, 4 H, $PhOCH_2CH_2CH_2$-), 1.26 (m, 54 H, $PhOCH_2CH_2CH_2(CH_2)_{13}CH_3$ and $PhOCH_2CH_2CH_2(CH_2)_{14}CH_3$), 0.88 (t, 6 H, $PhO(CH_2)_{16}CH_3$ and $PhO(CH_2)_{17}CH_3$). ^{13}C NMR (101 MHz, $CDCl_3$) δ 167.1, 160.3, 132.0, 107.8, 106.7, 68.5, 52.3, 34.1, 33.0, 32.1, 29.9, 29.8, 29.8, 29.8, 29.7, 29.7, 29.6, 29.5, 29.3, 28.9, 28.3, 26.2, 22.8, 14.3. Mp = 72 °C. Purity by HPLC: 99+%. MALDI-TOF MS *m*/*z* of $[M + H]^+$ calculated for $C_{43}H_{79}O_4$: 659.6; found: 660.3. $[M + Na]^+$ calculated for $C_{43}H_{78}NaO_4$: 681.6; found: 682.4. $[M + K]^+$ calculated for $C_{43}H_{78}KO_4$: 697.6; found: 699.5 (Figure S4).

2.3.5. Synthesis of (3-(Heptadecyloxy)-5-(octadecyloxy)phenyl)methanol (**36d**)

Methyl 3-(heptadecyloxy)-5-(octadecyloxy)benzoate, **35d**, (0.70 g, 1.06 mmol, 1 equiv) dissolved in 5 mL dry THF, which was added dropwise to a slurry of $LiAlH_4$ (40 mg, 1.06 mmol, 1 equiv) in dry THF (5 mL) at 0 °C under a N_2 atmosphere. Afterward, the resulting mixture was stirred at 23 °C for 1 h. Finally, the reaction was quenched via the successive addition of water (0.2 mL), a 15% NaOH aqueous solution (0.2 mL), and water (1.0 mL). The white precipitate was filtered. The solid filtrate was dissolved in DCM, dried over anhydrous $MgSO_4$, and filtered. The solvent was removed under reduced pressure to afford the title compound as a white solid (0.46 g, 69%). Mp = 62 °C. ^{1}H NMR (400 MHz, $CDCl_3$) δ 6.49 (br, 2 H, Ph*H*), 6.37 (t, 1 H, Ph*H*), 4.61 (s, 2 H, $PhCH_2OH$), 3.93 (t, 4 H, $PhOCH_2CH_2CH_2$-), 1.76 (m, 4 H, $PhOCH_2CH_2CH_2$-), 1.44 (m, 4 H, $PhOCH_2CH_2CH_2$-), 1.29 (m, 54 H, $PhOCH_2CH_2CH_2(CH_2)_{13}CH_3$ and $PhOCH_2CH_2CH_2(CH_2)_{14}CH_3$), 0.88 (t, 6 H, $PhO(CH_2)_{16}CH_3$ and $PhO(CH_2)_{17}CH_3$). ^{13}C NMR (101 MHz, $CDCl_3$) δ 160.7, 160.6, 143.4, 125.7, 105.2, 100.7, 68.2, 65.6, 32.1, 30.5, 29.9, 29.8, 29.8, 29.7, 29.6, 29.5, 29.5, 29.4, 26.2, 25.9, 22.8, 14.3. Mp = 62 °C. Purity by HPLC: 99+%. MALDI-TOF MS *m*/*z* $[M + H]^+$ calculated for $C_{42}H_{77}O_4$: 630.6; found: 631.3. $[M + Na]^+$ calculated for $C_{42}H_{78}NaO_4$: 653.6; found: 653.0. $[M + K]^+$ calculated for $C_{42}H_{78}KO_4$: 670.6; found: 670.6 (Figure S5).

2.3.6. Synthesis of 3-(Heptadecyloxy)-5-(octadecyloxy)benzyl 4-bromobutanoate, **37d**

A solution of (3-(heptadecyloxy)-5-(octadecyloxy)phenyl)methanol, **36d**, (0.46 g, 0.73 mmol, 1 equiv), 4-bromobutyric acid (0.13 g, 0.80 mmol, 1.1 equiv), and DPTS (0.24 g, 0.80 mmol, 1.1 equiv) was dissolved in 8 mL DCM. DCC (0.30 g, 1.46 mmol, 2 equiv) was added to the above mixture. The reaction mixture was stirred at 23 °C for 12 h. Afterward, the resulting precipitate (urea) was filtered out from the reaction mixture. The filtrate was concentrated to around 3 mL and purified via column chromatography (SiO_2) with hexane/DCM = 1/1 as the mobile phase to give the title compound as a white solid (0.45 g, 79%). Mp = 45 °C. ^{1}H NMR (400 MHz, $CDCl_3$) δ 6.46 (br, 2 H, Ph*H*), 6.40 (t, 1 H, Ph*H*), 5.05 (s, 2 H, $PhCH_2OCO$), 3.93 (t, 4 H, $PhOCH_2CH_2CH_2$-), 3.47 (t, 2 H, -$OCOCH_2CH_2CH_2Br$), 2.54 (t, 2 H, -$OCOCH_2CH_2CH_2Br$), 2.20 (m, 2 H, -$OCOCH_2CH_2CH_2Br$), 1.76 (m, 4 H, $PhOCH_2CH_2CH_2$-), 1.45 (m, 4 H, $PhOCH_2CH_2CH_2$-), 1.27 (m, 54 H, $PhOCH_2CH_2CH_2(CH_2)_{13}CH_3$ and $PhOCH_2CH_2CH_2(CH_2)_{14}CH_3$), 0.88 (t, 6 H, $PhO(CH_2)_{16}CH_3$ and $PhO(CH_2)_{17}CH_3$). ^{13}C NMR (101 MHz, $CDCl_3$) δ 172.4, 160.6, 137.9, 106.5, 101.2, 68.2, 66.5, 32.8, 32.6, 32.1, 32.0, 29.8, 29.8, 29.8, 29.7, 29.7, 29.7, 29.5, 29.5, 29.5, 29.4, 27.9, 26.2, 22.8, 14.3. Purity by HPLC: 99+%. MALDI-TOF MS *m*/*z* of $[M + H]^+$

calculated for $C_{46}H_{84}BrO_4$: 779.6; found: 780.5. $[M + Na]^+$ calculated for $C_{46}H_{83}BrNaO_4$: 801.5; found: 802.6. $[M + K]^+$ calculated for $C_{46}H_{83}BrKO_4$: 817.5; found: 818.6 (Figure S6).

2.3.7. Synthesis of 3-(Heptadecyloxy)-5-(octadecyloxy)benzyl 4-(4-methylpiperazin-1-yl)butanoate, **38g**, IAJD242

3-(Heptadecyloxy)-5-(octadecyloxy)benzyl 4-(4-methylpiperazin-1-yl)butanoate, **38g,** IAJD242, was synthesized using a modified literature procedure [38]. A mixture of 3-(heptadecyloxy)-5-(octadecyloxy)benzyl 4-bromobutanoate, **37d,** (0.18 g, 0.23 mmol), 1-methylpiperazine (25 mg, 0.25 mmol), K_2CO_3 (39 mg, 0.28 mmol), and MeCN (10 mL) was stirred at 95 °C for 3 h. The reaction mixture was cooled to 23 °C, and MeCN was removed under reduced pressure. Then, water (20 mL) was added, and the resulting mixture was extracted with DCM (20 mL) three times. The organic phases were collected and dried over anhydrous $MgSO_4$. After filtration, the obtained filtrate was concentrated to around 3 mL and purified via column chromatography (SiO_2) with DCM/MeOH = 30/1 and 15/1 as the eluent. Then, the obtained product was dissolved in DCM (20 mL), which was washed using a $NaHCO_3$ solution (2%, 20 mL). The aqueous phase was extracted via DCM (20 mL) another two times. The organic phases were combined and dried over anhydrous $MgSO_4$. The filtration and evaporation of the solvent yielded the title compound as a colorless oil (0.18 g, 99%). ^{1}H NMR (400 MHz, $CDCl_3$) δ 6.44 (br, 2 H, Ph*H*), 6.37 (t, 1 H, Ph*H*), 5.01 (s, 2 H, PhC*H*$_2$-), 3.90 (t, 4 H, PhOC*H*$_2$-), 2.59–2.25 (m, 15 H, -N(C*H*$_2$C*H*$_2$)$_2$N-, -NC*H*$_2$CH$_2$C*H*$_2$COO- and -NC*H*$_3$), 1.83 (m, 2 H, -OCOCH$_2$C*H*$_2$CH$_2$-), 1.77 (m, 4 H, PhOCH$_2$C*H*$_2$-), 1.42 (m, 4 H, PhOCH$_2$CH$_2$C*H*$_2$-), 1.27 (br, 54 H, PhOCH$_2$CH$_2$CH$_2$(C*H*$_2$)$_{13}$CH$_3$ and PhOCH$_2$CH$_2$CH$_2$(C*H*$_2$)$_{14}$CH$_3$), 0.86 (t, 6 H, -CH$_2$CH$_2$C*H*$_3$). ^{13}C NMR (101 MHz, $CDCl_3$) δ 173.3, 160.5, 138.2, 106.5, 101.0, 68.2, 66.2, 57.6, 55.1, 52.9, 45.9, 32.3, 32.0, 29.8, 29.8, 29.7, 29.7, 29.5, 29.5, 29.4, 26.2, 22.8, 22.2, 14.2. Purity by HPLC: 99+%. MALDI-TOF MS m/z of $[M + H]^+$ calculated for $C_{51}H_{95}N_2O_4$: 799.7; found: 799.8. $[M + Na]^+$ calculated for $C_{51}H_{94}N_2NaO_4$: 821.7; found: 821.7. $[M + K]^+$ calculated for $C_{51}H_{94}KN_2O_4$: 837.6; found: 837.6 (Figure S7).

2.3.8. Synthesis of 3-(Heptadecyloxy)-5-(octadecyloxy)benzyl 4-(4-(2-hydroxyethyl)piperazin-1-yl)butanoate, **38h**, IAJD243

3-(Heptadecyloxy)-5-(octadecyloxy)benzyl 4-(4-(2-hydroxyethyl)piperazin-1-yl)butan oate, **38h,** IAJD243, was synthesized using a modified literature procedure [38]. A mixture of 3-(heptadecyloxy)-5-(octadecyloxy)benzyl 4-bromobutanoate, **37d,** (0.18 g, 0.23 mmol), 1-(2-hydroxyethyl)piperazine (33 mg, 0.25 mmol), K_2CO_3 (39 mg, 0.28 mmol), and MeCN (10 mL) was stirred at 95 °C for 3 h. The reaction mixture was cooled to 23 °C, and MeCN was removed under reduced pressure. Then, water (20 mL) was added, and the resulting mixture was extracted with DCM (20 mL) three times. The organic phases were collected and dried over anhydrous $MgSO_4$. After filtration, the obtained filtrate was concentrated to around 3 mL and purified via column chromatography (SiO_2) with DCM/MeOH = 30/1 and 15/1 as the eluent. Then, the obtained product was dissolved in DCM (20 mL), which was washed using a $NaHCO_3$ solution (2%, 20 mL). The aqueous phase was extracted via DCM (20 mL) another two times. The organic phases were combined and dried over anhydrous $MgSO_4$. The filtration and evaporation of the solvent yielded the title compound as a colorless oil (0.18 g, 95%). ^{1}H NMR (400 MHz, $CDCl_3$) δ 6.45 (br, 2 H, Ph*H*), 6.38 (t, 1 H, Ph*H*), 5.02 (s, 2 H, PhC*H*$_2$-), 3.91 (t, 4 H, PhOC*H*$_2$-), 3.60 (t, 2 H, -CH$_2$C*H*$_2$OH), 2.63–2.31 (m, 14 H, -N(C*H*$_2$C*H*$_2$)$_2$N-, -NC*H*$_2$CH$_2$C*H*$_2$COO- and -C*H*$_2$CH$_2$OH), 1.84 (m, 2 H, -OCOCH$_2$C*H*$_2$CH$_2$-), 1.74 (m, 4 H, PhOCH$_2$C*H*$_2$-), 1.43 (m, 4 H, PhOCH$_2$CH$_2$C*H*$_2$-), 1.25 (br, 54 H, PhOCH$_2$CH$_2$CH$_2$(C*H*$_2$)$_{13}$CH$_3$ and PhOCH$_2$CH$_2$CH$_2$(C*H*$_2$)$_{14}$CH$_3$), 0.87 (t, 6 H, -CH$_2$CH$_2$C*H*$_3$). ^{13}C NMR (101 MHz, $CDCl_3$) δ 173.4, 160.6, 138.2, 106.5, 101.0, 68.2, 66.3, 59.5, 57.8, 57.6, 53.0, 53.0, 32.3, 32.0, 29.8, 29.8, 29.7, 29.7, 29.5, 29.5, 29.4, 26.2, 22.8, 22.2, 14.2. Purity by HPLC: 99+%. MALDI-TOF MS m/z of $[M + H]^+$ calculated for $C_{52}H_{97}N_2O_5$: 829.7; found: 829.8. $[M + Na]^+$ calculated for $C_{52}H_{96}N_2NaO_5$: 851.7; found: 852.0. $[M + K]^+$ calculated for $C_{52}H_{96}KN_2O_5$: 867.7; found: 867.9 (Figure S8).

2.3.9. Synthesis of Methyl 3,5-bis(heptadecyloxy)benzoate), **64d**

Methyl 3,5-dihydroxybenzoate, **1**, (0.40 g, 2.38 mmol, 1 equiv) (Scheme 2), $C_{17}H_{35}OTs$ (2.30 g, 5.23 mmol, 2.2 equiv), K_2CO_3 (0.82 g, 5.95 mmol, 2.5 equiv), and DMF (20 mL) was heated to 120 °C and stirred under a N_2 atmosphere for 2 h. The reaction mixture was cooled to 23 °C and poured into ice water (150 mL). The resulting white precipitate was filtered and collected. The solid precipitate was recrystallized from minimum acetone to afford the title compound as a white solid (1.33 g, 87%). Mp = 70 °C. ^1H NMR (400 MHz, $CDCl_3$) δ 7.16 (br, 2 H, Ph*H*), 6.63 (t, 1 H, Ph*H*), 3.96 (t, 4 H, $PhOCH_2CH_2CH_2$-), 3.89 (s, 3 H, $PhCOOCH_3$), 1.77 (m, 4 H, $PhOCH_2CH_2CH_2$-), 1.45 (m, 4 H, $PhOCH_2CH_2CH_2$-), 1.26 (m, 52 H, $PhOCH_2CH_2CH_2(CH_2)_{13}CH_3$), 0.88 (t, 6 H, $PhO(CH_2)_{16}CH_3$). ^{13}C NMR (101 MHz, $CDCl_3$) δ 167.0, 160.2, 131.8, 107.6, 106.6, 77.2, 68.3, 64.1, 52.2, 31.9, 29.7, 29.7, 29.6, 29.6, 29.4, 29.2, 26.0, 25.8, 22.7, 14.1. Purity by HPLC: 99+%. MALDI-TOF MS m/z of $[M + H]^+$ calculated for $C_{42}H_{77}O_4$: 645.8; found: 646.6. $[M + Na]^+$ calculated for $C_{42}H_{76}NaO_4$: 667.6; found: 668.7. $[M + K]^+$ calculated for $C_{42}H_{76}KO_4$: 683.5; found: 682.6 (Figure S9).

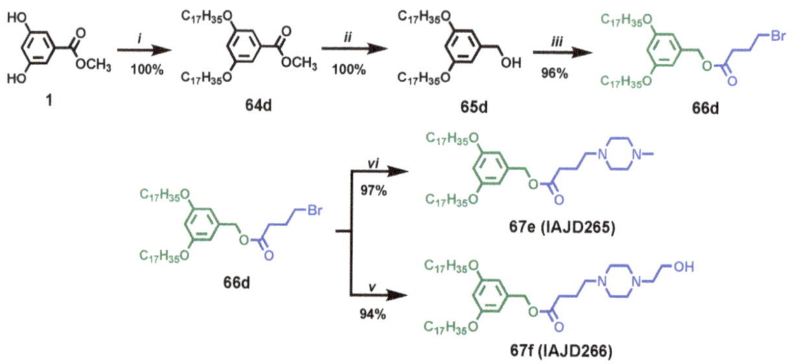

Scheme 2. Synthesis of 3,5-symmetric sSS IAJDs: (i) $C_{17}H_{35}OTs$, K_2CO_3, DMF, 120 °C, 2 h; (ii) $LiAlH_4$, THF, 0–23 °C, 1 h; (iii) DCC, DPTS, DCM 12 h; (iv) methylpiperazine, K_2CO_3, MeCN, 95 °C, 3 h; (v) 1-(2-hydroxyethyl)piperazine, K_2CO_3, MeCN, 95 °C, 3 h.

2.3.10. Synthesis of (3,5-Bis(heptadecyloxy)phenyl)methanol, **65d**

Methyl 3,5-bis(heptadecyloxy)benzoate), **64d**, (0.66 g, 1.02 mmol, 1 equiv) was dissolved in 10 mL dry THF, which was added dropwise to a slurry of $LiAlH_4$ (38 mg, 1.02 mmol, 1 equiv) in dry THF (5 mL) at 0 °C under a N_2 atmosphere. Afterward, the resulting mixture was stirred at 23 °C for 1 h. Finally, the reaction was quenched via the successive addition of water (0.2 mL), a 15% NaOH aqueous solution (0.2 mL), and water (1.0 mL). The white precipitate was filtered. The solid filtrate was dissolved in DCM, dried over anhydrous $MgSO_4$, and filtered. The solvent was removed under reduced pressure to afford the title compound as a white solid (0.62 g, 100%). Mp = 64 °C. ^1H NMR (400 MHz, $CDCl_3$) δ 6.50 (br, 2 H, Ph*H*), 6.37 (t, 1 H, Ph*H*), 4.61 (s, 2 H, $PhCH_2OH$), 3.93 (t, 4 H, $PhOCH_2CH_2CH_2$-), 1.76 (m, 4 H, $PhOCH_2CH_2CH_2$-), 1.45 (m, 4 H, $PhOCH_2CH_2CH_2$-), 1.26 (m, 52 H, $PhOCH_2CH_2CH_2(CH_2)_{13}CH_3$), 0.88 (t, 6 H, $PhO(CH_2)_{16}CH_3$). ^{13}C NMR (101 MHz, $CDCl_3$) δ 160.6, 143.2, 105.1, 100.6, 77.2, 68.1, 65.5, 34.0, 32.9, 31.9, 29.7, 29.7, 29.6, 29.6, 29.6, 29.5, 29.4, 29.4, 29.3, 28.8, 28.2, 26.1, 22.7, 14.1. Purity by HPLC: 99+%. MALDI-TOF MS m/z of $[M + H]^+$ calculated for $C_{41}H_{75}O_4$: 617.6; found: 618.3. $[M + Na]^+$ calculated for $C_{41}H_{76}NaO_4$: 639.6; found: 640.3. $[M + K]^+$ calculated for $C_{41}H_{76}KO_4$: 655.5; found: 656.6 (Figure S10).

2.3.11. Synthesis of 3,5-Bis(heptadecyloxy)benzyl 4-bromobutanoate, **66d**

(3,5-Bis(heptadecyloxy)phenyl)methanol, **65d**, (0.62 g, 1.02 mmol, 1 equiv), 4-bromobut yric acid (0.20 g, 1.22 mmol, 1.2 equiv), DPTS (0.36 g, 1.22 mmol, 1.2 equiv) were dissolved in 10 mL DCM. *N,N′*-Dicyclohexylcarbodiimide, DCC, (0.42 g, 2.04 mmol, 2 equiv) was added into the above mixture. The reaction mixture was stirred at 23 °C for 12 h.

Afterward, the resulting precipitate (urea) was filtered from the reaction mixture. The solid filtrate was concentrated to around 3 mL and purified via column chromatography (SiO_2) with hexane/DCM = 1/1 as the mobile phase to give the title compound as a white solid (0.75 g, 96%). Mp = 55 °C. ^1H NMR (400 MHz, $CDCl_3$)δ 6.47 (br, 2 H, Ph*H*), 6.40 (t, 1 H, Ph*H*), 5.05 (s, 2 H, $PhCH_2OCO$), 3.93 (t, 4 H, $PhOCH_2CH_2CH_2$-), 3.47 (t, 2 H, -$OCOCH_2CH_2CH_2Br$), 2.57 (t, 2 H, -$OCOCH_2CH_2CH_2Br$), 2.20 (m, 2 H, -$OCOCH_2CH_2CH_2Br$), 1.77 (m, 4 H, $PhOCH_2CH_2CH_2$-), 1.45 (m, 4 H, $PhOCH_2CH_2CH_2$-), 1.28 (m, 52 H, $PhOCH_2CH_2CH_2(CH_2)_{13}CH_3$), 0.88 (t, 6 H, $PhO(CH_2)_{16}CH_3$). ^{13}C NMR (101 MHz, $CDCl_3$) δ 172.3, 160.5, 137.8, 106.4, 101.1, 77.2, 68.1, 66.4, 64.8, 32.7, 32.6, 32.5, 32.5, 31.9, 30.3, 29.7, 29.7, 29.6, 29.6, 29.6, 29.5, 29.4, 29.4, 29.3, 27.8, 27.8, 26.1, 25.9, 22.7, 14.1. Purity by HPLC: 99+%. MALDI-TOF MS m/z of $[M + H]^+$ calculated for $C_{45}H_{82}BrO_4$: 765.5; found: 767.0. $[M + Na]^+$ calculated for $C_{45}H_{81}BrNaO_4$: 787.5; found: 790.0. $[M + K]^+$ calculated for $C_{45}H_{81}BrKO_4$: 803.5; found: 805.9 (Figure S11).

2.3.12. Synthesis of 3,5-Bis(pentadecyloxy)benzyl 4-(4-methylpiperazin-1-yl)butanoate, **67e**, IAJD265

3,5-Bis(pentadecyloxy)benzyl 4-(4-methylpiperazin-1-yl)butanoate, **67e**, IAJD265, was synthesized using a modified literature procedure [38]. A solution of 3,5-bis(heptadecyloxy) benzyl 4-bromobutanoate, **66d**, IAJD 264, (300 mg, 0.39 mmol, 1 equiv), 1-methylpiperazine (47 mg, 0.47 mmol, 1.2 equiv), and K_2CO_3 (81 mg, 0.59 mmol, 1.5 equiv) in 20 mL MeCN was heated to 95 °C and stirred for 3 h. The reaction mixture was cooled to 23 °C, and MeCN was removed under reduced pressure. Then, water (20 mL) was added, and the resulting mixture was extracted with DCM (20 mL) three times. The organic phases were collected and dried over anhydrous $MgSO_4$. After filtration, the obtained filtrate was concentrated to around 3 mL and purified via column chromatography (SiO_2) with DCM/MeOH = 30/1 and 15/1 as the eluent. The obtained product was dissolved in DCM (20 mL) and washed using a $NaHCO_3$ solution (2%, 20 mL). The aqueous phase was extracted via DCM (20 mL) another two times. The organic phases were combined and dried over anhydrous $MgSO_4$. The filtration and evaporation of the solvent yielded the title compound as a colorless oil (0.50 g, 97%). ^1H NMR (400 MHz, $CDCl_3$) δ 6.46 (br, 2 H, Ph*H*), 6.39 (t, 1 H, Ph*H*), 5.02 (s, 2 H, $PhCH_2$-), 3.92 (t, 4 H, $PhOCH_2$-), 2.63–2.25 (m, 15 H, -$N(CH_2CH_2)_2N$-, -$NCH_2CH_2CH_2COO$- and -NCH_3), 1.83 (m, 2 H, -$OCOCH_2CH_2CH_2$-), 1.73 (m, 4 H, $PhOCH_2CH_2$-), 1.42 (m, 4 H, $PhOCH_2CH_2CH_2$-), 1.26 (br, 52 H, $PhOCH_2CH_2CH_2(CH_2)_{13}CH_3$), 0.88 (t, 6 H, -$CH_2CH_2CH_3$). ^{13}C NMR (101 MHz, $CDCl_3$) δ 173.3, 160.5, 138.1, 106.4, 100.9, 77.2, 68.1, 66.2, 57.6, 55.2, 53.1, 46.1, 32.3, 31.9, 29.7, 29.7, 29.6, 29.6, 29.4, 29.4, 29.3, 26.1, 22.7, 22.2, 14.1. Purity by HPLC: 99+%. MALDI-TOF MS m/z of $[M + H]^+$ calculated for $C_{50}H_{93}N_2O_4$: 785.7; found: 785.9. $[M + Na]^+$ calculated for $C_{50}H_{92}N_2NaO_4$: 807.7; found: 808.9. $[M + K]^+$ calculated for $C_{50}H_{92}KN_2O_4$: 823.7; found: 835.6 (Figure S12).

2.3.13. Synthesis of 3,5-Bis(pentadecyloxy)benzyl 4-(4-(2-hydroxyethyl)piperazin-1-yl)butanoate, **67f**, IAJD266

3,5-Bis(pentadecyloxy)benzyl 4-(4-(2-hydroxyethyl)piperazin-1-yl)butanoate, **67f**, **IAJD266**, was synthesized using a modified literature procedure [38]. A solution of 3,5-bis(heptadecyloxy)benzyl 4-bromobutanoate, **66d**, IAJD 264, (300 mg, 0.39 mmol, 1 equiv), 1-(2-hydroxyethyl)piperazine (62 mg, 0.47 mmol, 1.2 equiv), and K_2CO_3 (81 mg, 0.59 mmol, 1.5 equiv) in 20mL MeCN was heated to 95 °C and stirred for 3 h. The reaction mixture was cooled to 23 °C, and MeCN was removed under reduced pressure. Then, water (20 mL) was added, and the resulting mixture was extracted with DCM (20 mL) three times. The organic phases were collected and dried over anhydrous $MgSO_4$. After filtration, the obtained filtrate was concentrated to around 3 mL and purified via column chromatography (SiO_2) with DCM/MeOH = 30/1 and 15/1 as the eluent. The obtained product was dissolved in DCM (20 mL) and washed using a $NaHCO_3$ solution (2%, 20 mL). The aqueous phase was extracted via DCM (20 mL) another two times. The organic phases were combined and dried over anhydrous $MgSO_4$. The filtration and evaporation of the solvent yielded the title compound as a colorless oil (0.50 g, 94%). ^1H NMR (400 MHz, $CDCl_3$) δ 6.46 (br, 2 H, Ph*H*),

6.39 (t, 1 H, Ph*H*), 5.01 (s, 2 H, PhCH_2-), 3.89 (t, 4 H, PhOCH_2-), 3.61 (t, 2H, -CH_2CH_2OH), 2.62–2.31 (m, 14 H, -N(CH_2CH_2)$_2$N-, -NCH_2CH$_2$CH_2COO- and -CH_2CH$_2$OH), 1.82 (m, 2 H, -OCOCH$_2$CH_2CH$_2$-), 1.72 (m, 4 H, PhOCH$_2$CH_2-), 1.40 (m, 4 H, PhOCH$_2$CH$_2$CH_2-), 1.28 (br, 52 H, PhOCH$_2$CH$_2$CH$_2$(CH_2)$_{13}$CH$_3$), 0.86 (t, 6 H, -CH$_2$CH$_2$CH_3). ^{13}C NMR (101 MHz, $CDCl_3$) δ 173.3, 160.5, 138.1, 106.4, 100.9, 77.2, 68.1, 66.2, 59.3, 57.6, 57.5, 53.0, 52.8, 32.2, 31.9, 31.8, 29.5, 29.4, 29.4, 29.3, 29.2, 26.1, 22.7, 22.1, 14.1. Purity by HPLC: 99+%. MALDI-TOF MS m/z of $[M + H]^+$ calculated for $C_{51}H_{95}N_2O_5$: 815.7; found: 815.6. $[M + Na]^+$ calculated for $C_{51}H_{94}N_2NaO_5$: 837.7; found: 837.7. $[M + K]^+$ calculated for $C_{51}H_{94}KN_2O_5$: 853.7; found: 853.7 (Figure S13).

3. Results and Discussion

3.1. Concept, Strategy, and Methodology

IAJDs are stable for a long time after being stored in a chemistry laboratory at room temperature in air, while their DNPs are stable and remain active for at least 5 months at the normal refrigerator temperature of 5 °C [24–26]. The original architecture of one-component IAJDs [24–26] was inspired by the structure of amphiphilic Janus dendrimers (JDs) [39–51], Janus glycodendrimers (JGDs) [52–70], and sequence-defined JGDs [71,72] and will be discussed in more detail later.

JDs and JGDs are self-assembled through the simple injection of their ethanol solution into water or buffer to produce monodisperse vesicles known as dendrimersomes and glycodendrimersomes, with predictable dimensions [40]. The physical properties of dendrimersomes are as good as those of three-component stealth liposomes co-assembled from phospholipids, PEG-conjugated lipids, and cholesterol [73–75]. The three-component concept of stealth liposomes [73–76] inspired the elaboration of the four-component LNPs (Figure 1A) currently employed to deliver mRNA. The mechanism for the delivery of mRNA is most probably closely related to the mechanisms of both four-component LNPs and one-component DNPs (Figure 1C), although their structures are quite different (Figure 1A,B).

LNPs contain the mRNA encapsulated together with ionizable lipids in the center of a stealth liposome (Figure 1A), while DNPs may contain the mRNA encapsulated as a spherical helix (Figure 1B) that provides the largest number of contacts between the nucleic acid and dendrimersome.

The ability to molecularly design both the hydrophilic and the hydrophobic parts of one-component IAJDs provides synthetic advantages that will be demonstrated in this publication. Oligooxyethylene fragments were originally employed to design the multifunctional sequence-defined hydrophilic region and generate single–single, (SS, single hydrophilic dendron connected to single hydrophobic dendron), twin–twin (TT, two hydrophilic dendrons connected to two hydrophobic dendrons), and twin–mixed (TM, two different hydrophilic dendrons connected to two hydrophobic dendrons) IAJDs (Figure 1B) [24]. A simplified SS, sSS architecture was also generated, which resulted from the removal of the oligooxyethylene fragments from the hydrophilic dendron while maintaining only its ionizable amine, which, after protonation, becomes hydrophilic and active to mRNA binding (Figure 1B) [24].

In all cases, hydrophobic dendrons were constructed mostly from 3,5-substituted, with only very few preliminary examples of 3,4- and 3,4,5-substituted plant phenolic acids or trisubstituted pentaerythritol containing identical alkyl groups. Sequence-defined JGDs were demonstrated to be extraordinarily important in providing the highest activity of their glycan when binding to sugar-binding proteins known as lectins and galectins [52–57]. Sequence-defined self-assembling dendronized perylenebisimides (PBIs) were also demonstrated to dramatically change their rate of self-organization process via a cogwheel mechanism accompanied by deracemization in a crystal state [76–80]. In addition, phospholipids forming the bilayer of natural cell membranes are generated by a nonsymmetric substitution of their glycerol with alkyl groups containing a different number of *cis*-double bonds to introduce their homochiral stereocenter [81]. This arrangement provides dissimilar chain lengths in the bilayer of vesicles even for an identical number of carbons in their alkyl groups but different numbers of *cis*-double bonds. With the currently available results, the mechanism of the self-assembly of JDs into DNPs was shown to be preferred by the 3,5- rather than 3,4- or 3,4,5-substitution pattern since the 3,5-substitution pattern favors the interdigitation of its alkyl groups in the hydrophobic part of the bilayer of the vesicle and stabilizes the mechanical integrity of the assembly [40].

These literature data prompted us to advance the hypothesis that a sequence-defined arrangement in the hydrophobic part of IAJDs could also be influential, as it was shown to be important in the hydrophilic part, on the activity of targeted delivery of mRNA mediated by IAJDs [24–26]. This was already indicated with preliminary experiments [26] by replacing their identical alkyl group lengths with dissimilar alkyl group lengths in their hydrophobic part to create nonsymmetric SS (nSS) and nonsymmetric simplified SS (nsSS) (Figure 1B) and testing them for their in vitro and in vivo delivery of mRNA.

Originally, this combination of dissimilar alkyl groups in their hydrophobic part was hypothesized to decrease the crystallization tendency of the hydrophobic part of the bilayer containing long alkyl groups and increase the solubility of the IAJD in ethanol. The decreased rate of crystallization and increased solubility of IAJD were indeed accomplished using this methodology, but unexpectedly, it was also accompanied by increased activity of mRNA delivery by the corresponding DNP to specific organs [24–26].

Figure 1A outlines the structure and co-assembly with the mRNA of four-component LNPs [25]. Figure 1B shows the structures of sSS, SS, and TM IAJDs with dissimilar (nsSS, nSS) and similar alkyl groups in their hydrophobic parts and their co-assembly with mRNA into DNPs. Figure 1C illustrates the current mechanism accepted for the in vivo delivery of mRNA with both four-component LNPs and one-component DNPs. This mechanism involves the endocytosis of LNPs or DNPs, followed by the endosomal escape of mRNA and the synthesis of a protein in collaboration with the ribosome.

Since normal mRNA experiments can take extended periods of time, especially in the case of vaccine experiments, we employed firefly luciferase mRNA (Luc-mRNA) that provides important screening results in several hours [24–26]. In this case, the protein translated in the cell is the luciferase enzyme that interacts with D-luciferin to generate oxy-luciferin emitting light that helps to identify rapidly the organ targeted.

3.2. *Accelerated Modular–Orthogonal Synthesis of Two Libraries of nsSS IAJDs*

Figure 2A shows the structures of the 3,5-dihydroxy, 3,4-dihydroxy, and 3,4,5-trihydroxy plant phenolic acids known by common names as α-resorcylic, protocatechuic, and gallic acid, respectively [82], that were used by our laboratory in the synthesis of a larger diversity of complex systems [50] including IAJDs [24–26]. Due to their antioxidant activity, some of these phenolic acid derivatives are used as food additives and are present in vegetable oils, butter, fats, meat, and many other daily components of our food [83].

Here, using the accelerated modular–orthogonal methodology outlined in Figure 2B, we will first report the synthesis of two libraries of nsSS IAJDs containing 78 molecules based on 3,5-dihydroxy phenolic acid containing methyl piperazine and hydroxyethyl piperazine as ionizable amines. The synthesis of a single nSS IAJD-131 (Supporting Scheme S10) is also reported. nsSS IAJDs with various combinations of *n*-alkyl groups containing 18, 17, 16, 14, 12, 10, 9, 8, and 2-ethyl hexyl (EH) were synthesized. Linear and branched alkyl groups were employed since they do not oxidize and therefore dramatically increase the stability of IAJDs by comparison with that of four-component systems containing unsaturated phospholipids.

In the first step of their synthesis, the 3-benzylether of 3,5-dihydroxy methyl benzoate was produced in 40% isolated yield in 5 h via the etherification of **1** with BnCl at 80 °C in DMF with K_2CO_3 base. Subsequently, **2** was alkylated with a 1-bromoalkyl group in DMF, with K_2CO_3 base at 120 °C, to produce a 60% to 98% isolated yield of **3**. The hydrogenolysis of **3** (H_2/Pd, DCM/MeOH, 12 h) generated **4** in 100% isolated yield. The alkylation of **4** with various linear and branched alkyl bromides from 1-bromooctane to 1-bromooctadecane in DMF, with K_2CO_3 base at 120 °C, created the libraries of the nonsymmetric compounds **5** in 75–90% isolated yield.

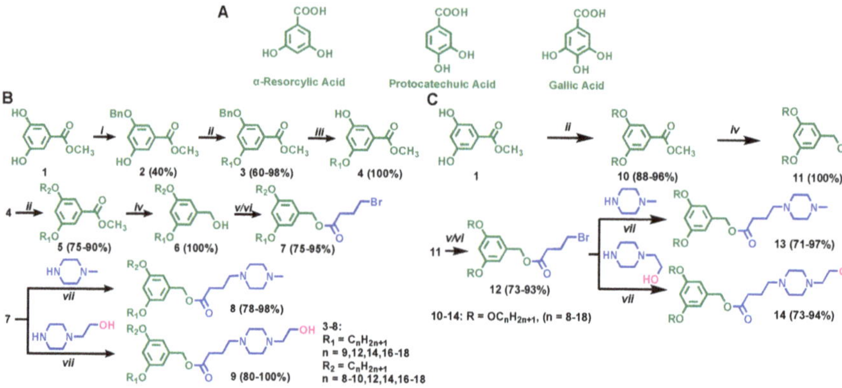

Figure 2. Structures of plant phenolic acids: α-resorcylic acid, protocatechuic acid, and gallic acid and synthesis of nsSS IAJDs containing 3,5-nonsymmetric alkyl groups as well as of sSS IAJDs containing 3,5-symmetric alkyl groups: (**A**) structures of plant phenolic acids employed as starting materials in the synthesis of IAJDs; (**B**) accelerated modular–orthogonal synthesis of nsSS IAJDs based on 3,3-dihydroxybenzoate; (**C**) accelerated modular–orthogonal synthesis of sSS IAJDs based on 3,4-dihydroxybenzoate. Reagents and Conditions: (i) BnCl, K_2CO_3, KI, DMF, 80 °C, 5 h; (ii) RBr, K_2CO_3, DMF, 120 °C, 2 h; (iii) H_2, Pd/C, DCM, MeOH, 12 h; (iv) $LiAlH_4$, THF, 0–23 °C, 1 h; (v) 4-bromobutyric acid, $SOCl_2$, DMF (cat.), DCM, 23 °C, 1 h, then DMAP, NEt_3, DCM, 0–23 °C, 2 h; (vi) DCC, DPTS, 12 h; (vii) methylpiperazine or hydroxyethyl piperazine, K_2CO_3, MeCN, 95 °C, 3 h.

The reduction of compounds **5** with $LiAlH_4$ in THF (0–23 °C, 1 h) generated the benzyl alcohols **6** in 100% isolated yield. Compounds **6** were esterified with 4-bromobutyric acid either via its acid chloride generated with $SOCl_2$ catalyzed via DMF in CH_2Cl_2 at 23 °C followed by reaction in the presence of NEt_3/DMAP (0–23 °C, 2 h) or via the direct esterification of **6** with DCC/DPTS in 12 h to produce compounds **7** in 75% to 95% isolated yield. Compounds **7** were reacted with methyl piperazine or hydroxyethyl piperazine (K_2CO_3, MeCN, 95 °C, 3 h) to give rise to IAJDs **8** (78–98% isolated yields) and **9** (80–100% isolated yields). Their purity using a combination of thin-layer chromatography (TLC), high-pressure liquid chromatography (HPLC), matrix-assisted laser desorption/ionization–time-of-flight (MALDI-TOF) mass spectroscopy, ^{1}H-NMR, and ^{13}C-NMR was higher than 99%.

3.3. Accelerated Modular–Orthogonal Synthesis of a Complete Library of sSS IAJDs

In order to finalize the few experiments reported previously on sSS IAJDs [25,26] and provide a complete library, we employed the methodology from Figure 2C for their synthesis. The dialkylation of **1** was accomplished at 120 °C in DMF with K_2CO_3 as the base in 2 h to produce compounds **10** in 88% to 96% isolated yields. The reduction of **10** with $LiAlH_4$ for 1 h in THF at 0–23 °C generated **11** in 100% yield. Compound **12** (73–93% isolated yields) was prepared as in the case of **7** (Figure 2B,C). Compounds **13** (71–97% isolated yields) and **14** (73–94% isolated yields) were obtained under similar reaction conditions to **8** and **9**. Their structures are shown in Figure 2C.

The structures of all 98 nsSS and sSS IAJDs are shown in Figure 3 (IAJDs 112 to 272) together with IAJD 131. Figure 3 also outlines a simplified cartoon illustration of the structure of each IAJD together with the number of carbons in the pair of their alkyl groups, the number of the IAJD structure, and the pKa values shown in blue under the IAJD numbers in black. The schematic illustration from Figure 3 will simplify the discussion in the rest of this publication. Two libraries of IAJDs containing 85 nsSS, 43 containing methylpiperazine, and 42 hydroxyethyl piperazine ionizable amines were synthesized using the methodology elaborated in Figure 2B. All of them are shown in Figure 3, together with the nSS IAJD 131, whose synthesis is outlined in Supporting Schemes S9 and S11 sSS that were synthesized as outlined in Figure 2B. Therefore, a total of 98 IAJDs together with their complexes with mRNA known as dendrimersome nanoparticles (DNPs) will be discussed in the following subsections. We must clarify again that DNPs are in fact vesicles with a stability closely related to that of viral capsids rather than to the stability of LNPs. As we can see from the structures of Figure 3, all these IAJDs are based on first-generation dendrons that were defined by our laboratory, via analogy with minipeptides and miniproteins as minidendrons and minidendrimers [50]. In this particular case, they contain one or two branching points in their hydrophobic part, while the hydrophilic part contains branching points derived from their ionizable amine.

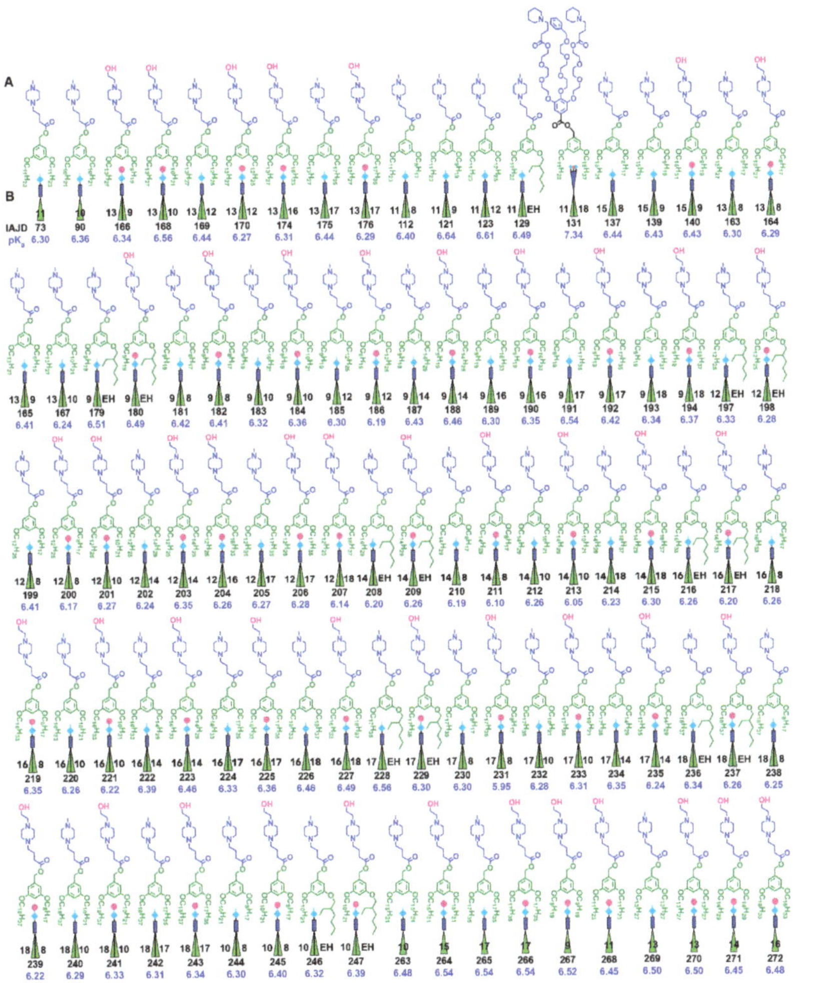

Figure 3. The structures of nsSS IAJDs with 3,5-nonsymmetric alkyl chains and of nSS IAJD 131. IAJD numbers and pK_a values are shown under corresponding schematic representations of nsSS and nSS IAJDs: (**A**) structures of IAJDs; (**B**) schematic representations of IAJDs with the number of carbons in the alkyl groups from their hydrophobic part on the left and right sides of the structure; IAJD numbers in black under the schematic of IAJD, and pKa values in blue under the number of IAJD.

3.4. Co-Assembly of IAJDs with Luc-mRNA into Dendrimersome Nanoparticles (DNPs) via Simple Injection

The injection method elaborated for the self-assembly of dendrimersomes from amphiphilic Janus dendrimers [39] and glycodendrimersomes from Janus glycodendrimers [52] was adopted for the self-assembly of IAJDs [24–26] and their co-assembly with mRNA into DNPs [24–26]. Narrow polydispersity DNPs [24–26] with predictable dimensions, as obtained in the case of dendrimersomes [39] and glycodendrimersomes [52], are accessible via the simple injection of an ethanol solution of IAJD into an acidic solution of Luc-mRNA of molar mass 661,050 daltons. This method facilitates fast access to the DNPs employed for in vivo mice transfection experiments. We must stress that our DNPs are in fact dendrimersome vesicles containing mRNA encapsulated in their interior most probably in a spherical helix conformation (Figure 1B). Their vesicular structure was demonstrated previously [24]. However, the mechanism of mRNA encapsulation and the structure of the DNPs containing mRNA are under investigation. The details of the co-assembly method via injection are described as follows: Nucleoside-modified mRNA encoding firefly luciferase (Luc-mRNA) was dissolved in UltraPure DNase/RNase-free distilled water with an initial concentration of 4.0 mg/mL. IAJDs were dissolved in ethanol with an initial concentration of 80 mg/mL. The Luc-mRNA solution (12.5 μL) was placed into a clean RNA-free Eppendorf tube (1.5 mL). Then, 463 μL of acetate buffer (10 mM, pH 4.0) was added. Afterward, 25 μL of IAJD in the ethanol stock solution was taken and rapidly injected above the Luc-mRNA solution in acetate buffer, followed by vortex for 5 s. The size and the size distribution of the resulting nanoparticles were determined using DLS and are reported in Figure 4 under the schematic illustration of the corresponding IAJDs. More than 98% of Luc-mRNA was encapsulated in the interior of DNPs that are stable and active at 5 °C for more than 135 days. These data will be reported soon.

3.5. In Vivo Delivery of Mice with DNPs Containing Luc-mRNA

Female or male BALB/c mice, 6–8 weeks old, from Charles River Laboratories, were anesthetized with 3% isoflurane from Piramal Healthcare Limited and injected via retro-orbital sinus with 100 μL of DNP solution containing 10 μg of Luc-mRNA. At 4–6 h post-injection, mice were intraperitoneally (i.p.) injected with D-luciferin at a dose of 150 mg/kg of body weight, from Regis Technologies and imaged on a PerkinElmer In Vivo Imaging System (IVIS) Spectrum CT. Ten minutes after the administration of D-luciferin, mice were placed on the imaging platform while being maintained on isoflurane via a nose cone, and whole-body luminescence signal was measured on the IVIS imaging using a certain exposure time (60, 30, or 15 s). The tissue luminescence signal was measured on the IVIS imaging system using a certain exposure time (60, 30, or 15 s) and medium binning (binning = 8) to ensure that the signal obtained was within the operative detection range. For the IVIS imaging of the organs, mice were sacrificed; the heart, lungs, liver, and spleen were immediately collected; and bioluminescence imaging was performed as described above. Image analysis was conducted with the Living Image software from PerkinElmer. Bioluminescence values were quantified by measuring photon flux (photons/second) in the region of interest (ROI) using the Living Image software and were then analyzed. Figure 4 reports the in vivo transfection results for all 78 IAJDs synthesized, together with their organ analysis and total flux luminescence results. The remarkable first conclusion of the complex Figure 4 is that all the IAJDs are active for the delivery of Luc-mRNA, even if these are only fast screening experiments. We must stress that both the co-assembly with mRNA and transfection experiments performed in vivo were not yet optimized.

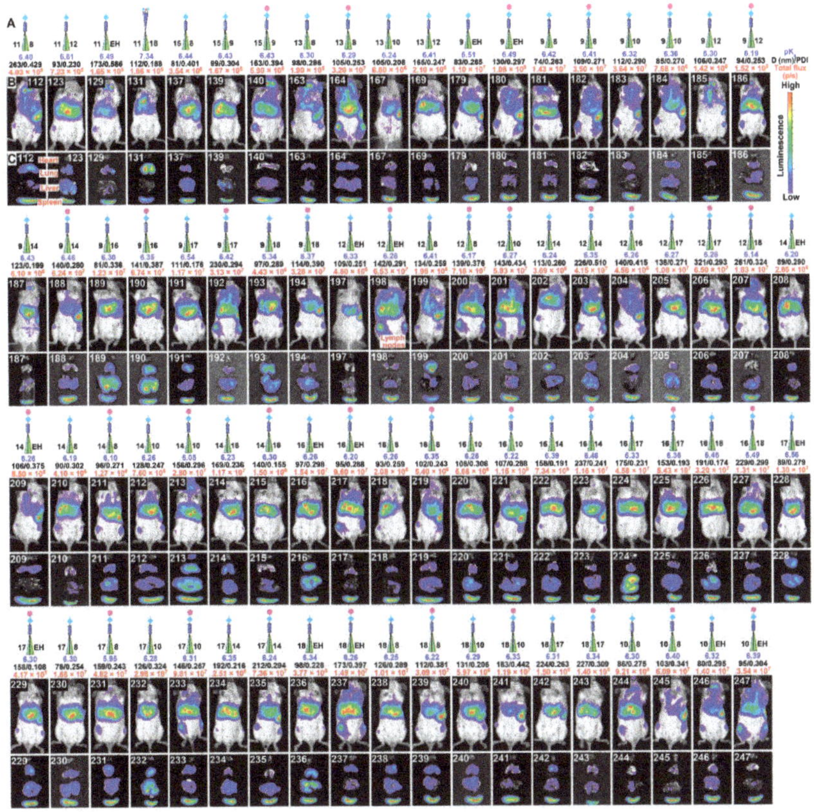

Figure 4. Delivery of Luc-mRNA in vivo by DNPs assembled from IAJDs with 3,5-nonsymmetric alkyl chains: (**A**) schematic representation of the IAJD structures with the number of the carbons in the hydrophobic part on the left and right sides of IAJD, pKa values under the schematic in blue, dimensions and polydispersity under pKa in black, and total flux luminescence activity (p/s) in red; (**B**) the representative image of luciferase expression in the whole body or organs 4–6 h post-intravenous (i.v.) injection of Luc-mRNA co-assembled with various IAJDs; (**C**) the images of organs with luciferase activity shown in the color code from the top right column. Color code: pink is hydroxyethyl, the light blue square is piperazine, and the perpendicular line on the square in blue is methyl, dark blue is the hydrophilic fragment, and green is the hydrophobic fragment of IAJD.

3.6. In Vivo Delivery of Luc-mRNA with nsSS DNPs to Spleen and Liver

A detailed discussion of these results is provided by grouping these results into targeted delivery to specific organs and correlating the molecular structure of the IAJD with the specific target and activity. We decided to group these experiments in specific delivery to the spleen, lymph nodes, liver, and lung. The twenty most active nsSS and sSS IAJDs that deliver predominantly to the spleen are shown in Figure 5A, while the fifteen most active nsSS and SS IAJDs delivering to the liver are presented in Figure 5B. There is a striking difference between the nsSS and sSS IAJDs delivering to the spleen (Figure 5A) vs. the one delivering to the liver (Figure 5B). Seventeen out of the twenty (85%) nsSS IAJDs that deliver to the spleen contain hydroxyethyl piperazine as an ionizable amine in their hydrophilic part, while the other three contain methyl piperazine (Figure 5A). By contrast, twelve out of the fifteen (80%) nsSS JAJDs that deliver to the liver contain the methyl piperazine ionizable amine in their hydrophilic part, two carry hydroxyethyl piperazine, and only one contains dimethyl amino group as ionizable amine (Figure 5B).

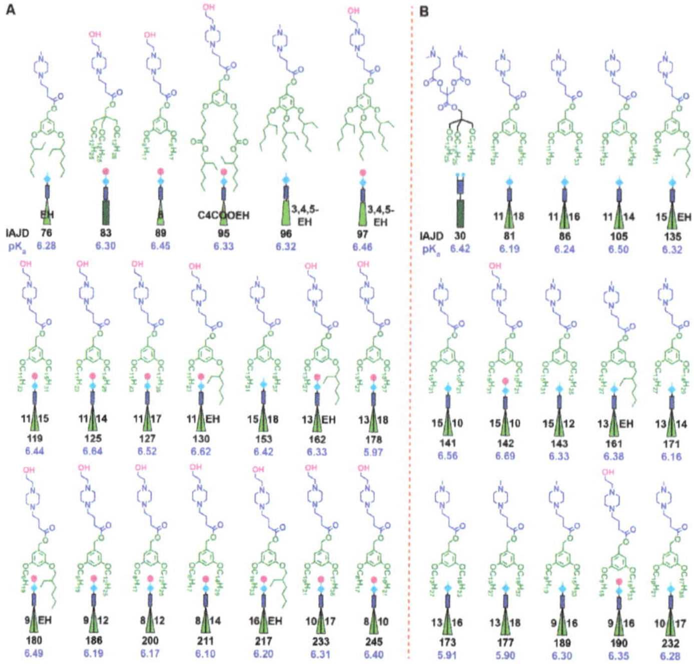

Figure 5. Structures of 15 most active IAJDs for selective delivery of mRNA to the liver and 20 most active IAJDs for selective delivery of mRNA to the spleen: (**A**) IAJDs delivering to the spleen; (**B**) IAJDs delivering to the liver. Legend: schematic representations of IAJDs with the number of carbons in the alkyl groups from their hydrophobic part on the left and right sides of the structure, IAJD numbers in black under the schematic of IAJD, and pKa values in blue under the number of IAJD.

The pKa values of the IAJDs delivering to the spleen are between 6.10 and 6.64, while the pKa values of the compounds targeting the liver are between 5.90 and 6.69. At the extracellular pH of 7.4 (Figure 1C), the exterior of DNPs co-assembled from these IAJDs with Luc-mRNA becomes deprotonated. These results demonstrate that the target of the delivery is provided via the structure of the ionizable amine from the hydrophilic part of the IAJD.

The activity of the IAJDs from Figure 5A in their delivery to the spleen is shown in Figure 6. Most of these IAJDs deliver mRNA to the spleen and lymph nodes. Without any optimization, eleven nsSS IAJDs (55% of them), namely 125, 127, 130, 162, 178, 180, 186, 211, 217, 221, and 233, exhibit the total flux of their luminescence very close to or higher than 10^8 p/s. All the other sSS and nsSS IAJDs display the total flux of their luminescence in the range of high 10^7 p/s values. It is very interesting to observe that the most active of all the IAJDs contain between three and six methylenic units difference between the number of carbons in their nonsymmetric 3,5-disubstituted hydrophobic part. This is a quite remarkable result considering that most of these results were obtained only from screening experiments without any optimization, as shown in the plots from Figure 7.

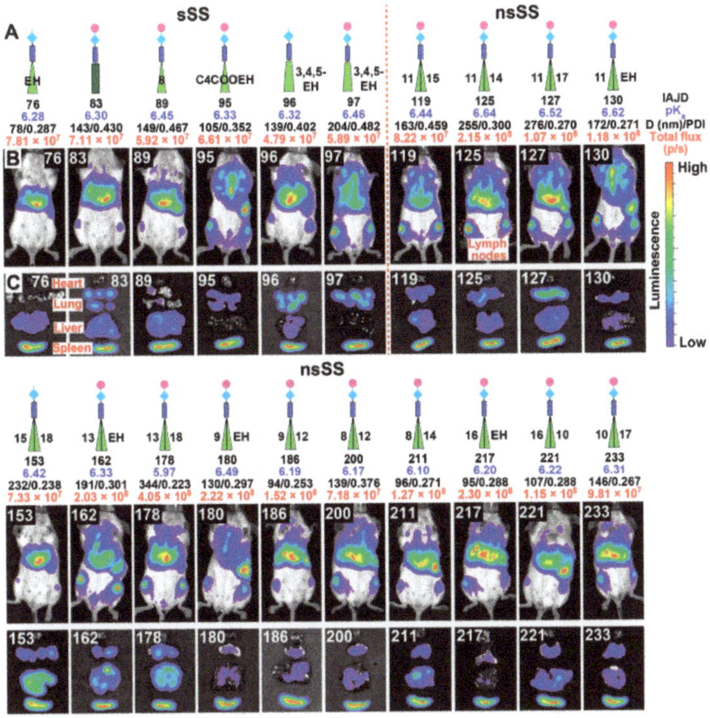

Figure 6. Selective delivery of Luc-mRNA in vivo by 20 most active DNPs to the spleen: (**A**) schematic representation of the IAJD structures with the number of the carbons in the hydrophobic part on the left and right sides of IAJD, pKa values under the schematic in blue, dimensions and polydispersity under pKa in black, and total flux luminescence activity (p/s) in red; (**B**) the representative images of luciferase expression in the whole body or organs after i.v. injection of Luc-mRNA co-assembled with IAJDs; (**C**) the images of organs with luciferase activity shown in color coding from the top right column; color code: pink is hydroxyethyl, the light blue square is piperazine, and the perpendicular line on the square in blue is methyl, dark blue is the hydrophilic fragment, and green is the hydrophobic fragment of IAJD.

Excellent agreement for duplicated or triplicated experiments is shown by the error bars of the statistical analysis illustrated in Figure 7. The experiments, the results of which are shown in Figure 7, revealed the most active synthetic vectors for the delivery of mRNA to the spleen regardless of whether they were generated from four-component LNPs or from one-component DNPs. ***MC3 shows slightly higher activity in delivery to the liver and must not be compared with the spleen since MC3 delivers only to the liver***. Figure 8 illustrates the in vivo delivery of Luc-mRNA with the fifteen most active nsSS IAJDs that deliver to the liver. Delivery to the liver is accomplished successfully with four-component LNPs and is currently part of the technology of BioNTech/Pfizer and Moderna COVID-19 vaccines.

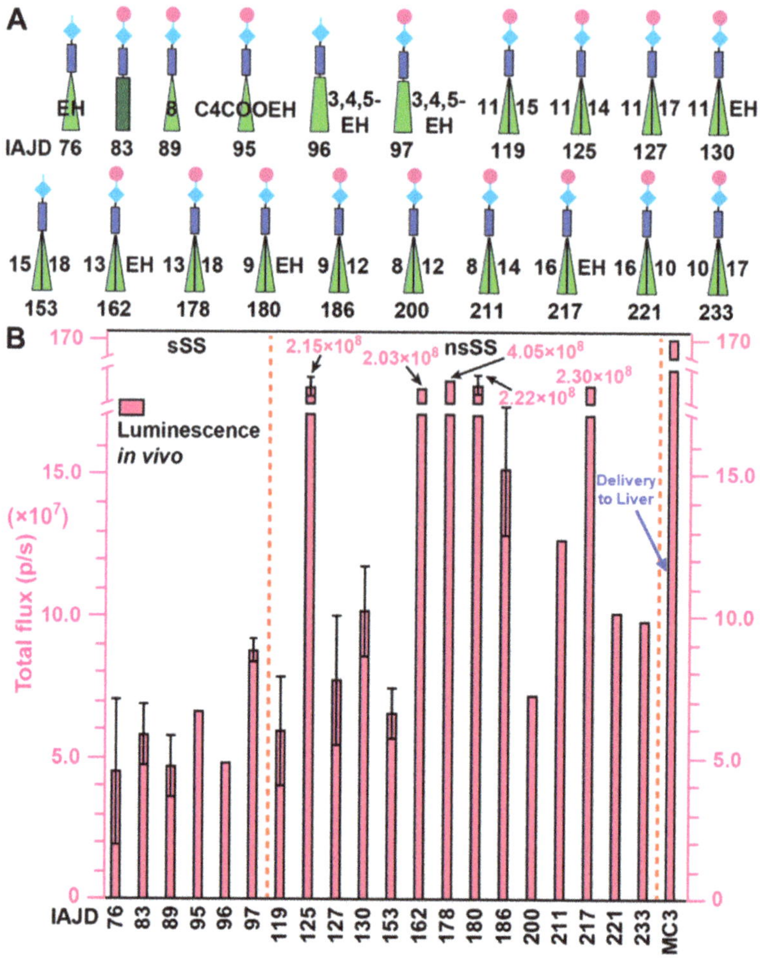

Figure 7. Comparison of the activities of the 20 most active DNPs that deliver mRNA to the spleen: (**A**) schematic representations of IAJDs with the number of carbons in the alkyl groups from their hydrophobic part on the left and right sides of the structure, and IAJD numbers in black under the schematic of IAJD. MC3 delivers mRNA to the liver; (**B**) plots of total flux luminescence (p/s) for the DNPs assembled from the IAJDs from (**A**).

Consequently, to date, we have not invested special effort in delivery experiments to the liver since delivery to the spleen and lymph nodes is more efficient for the design of vaccines. Figure 8 summarizes the most active in vivo mice results accomplished with the nsSS IAJDs from Figure 5B. It is interesting to observe from Figure 8 that the delivery of mRNA to the liver is also accompanied by delivery to lymph nodes. Although only screening experiments were performed in all cases, a total flux of luminescence of 10^8 p/s was observed for the nsSS IAJD 173, which has a combination of 13 and 16 carbons in its nonsymmetric hydrophobic part. This IAJD has a three-carbon difference between the length of the two alkyl groups. This result is in agreement with the results observed for the activity of the delivery to the spleen. Four nsSS IAJDs, i.e., 161, 171, 177, and 190, display almost 10^8 p/s total flux luminescence activity. Without any optimization, screening experiments show that all the other nsSS IAJDs, including the SS IAJD 30, display the total flux of their luminescence in the range of 10^7 p/s.

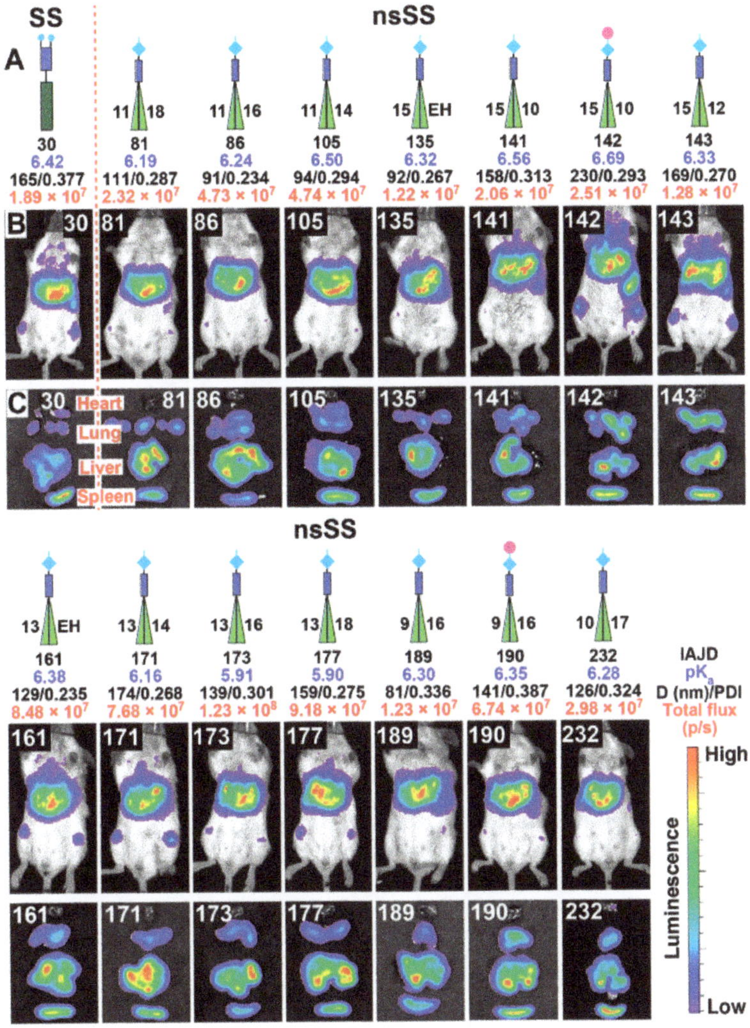

Figure 8. Selective delivery of Luc-mRNA in vivo by 15 most active DNPs to the liver: (**A**) schematic representation of the IAJD structures with the number of the carbons in the hydrophobic part on the left and right sides of IAJD, pKa values under the schematic in blue, dimensions and polydispersity under pKa in black, and total flux luminescence activity (p/s) in red; (**B**) the images of luciferase expression in the whole body 4–6 h after the i.v. injection of Luc-mRNA co-assembled with IAJDs; (**C**) the images of organs with their activity shown using the color code from the bottom right column.

It is interesting to observe that the two pairs of nsSS IAJDs that show activity for delivery to the lung and contain both hydroxyethyl piperazine and methyl piperazine ionizable amines with the identical pairs of alkyl groups (15 and 10 for 141 and 142; 9 and 16 for 189 and 190) follow the same trend of their total flux. The highest activity is for the IAJD containing hydroxyethyl piperazine. The summary of the total flux as a function of IAJD structure is summarized in Figure 9.

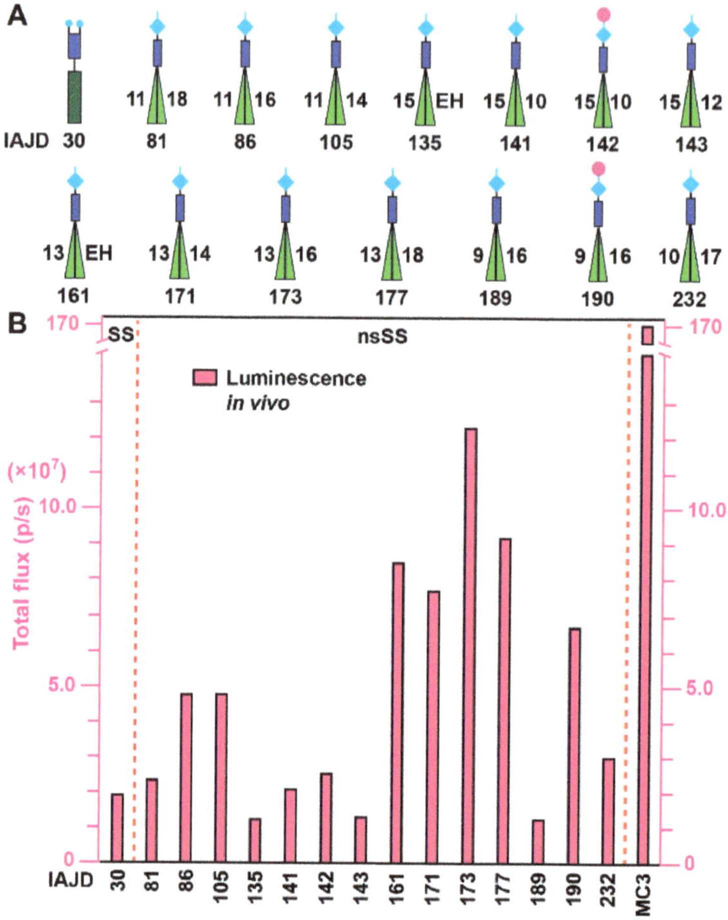

Figure 9. Comparison of the activities of the 15 most active DNPs which deliver mRNA to the liver: (**A**) schematic representations of IAJDs with the number of carbons in the alkyl groups from their hydrophobic part on the left and right sides of the structure, and IAJD numbers in black under the schematic of IAJD; (**B**) plots of total flux luminescence (p/s) for the DNPs assembled from the IAJDs from (**A**).

3.7. In Vivo Delivery of Luc-mRNA with DNPs to Lung

In order to provide a comprehensive discussion on the concept of screening libraries to discover the molecular design principles of IAJDs and correlate their structure with the targeted activity, in this report, we decided to also summarize the twenty IAJDs that display the most active activity in their delivery to the lung [24].

These data represent a combination of results, reported first time here and in our previous publications [24–26]. Figure 10 shows the structures of all these IAJDs. They represent a large diversity of IAJD structures, including SS, TT, TM, sSS, nsSS, and sSS.

Figure 11 shows the mice images for all in vivo experiments performed with the IAJDs from Figure 10. Figure 12 plots the activity data for the IAJDs from Figure 10 with their in vivo mice experiments from Figure 11. Without discussing the details, we see that the hydrophilic part of IAJDs determines the delivery target, while the hydrophobic part of the IAJDs is responsible for the level of activity.

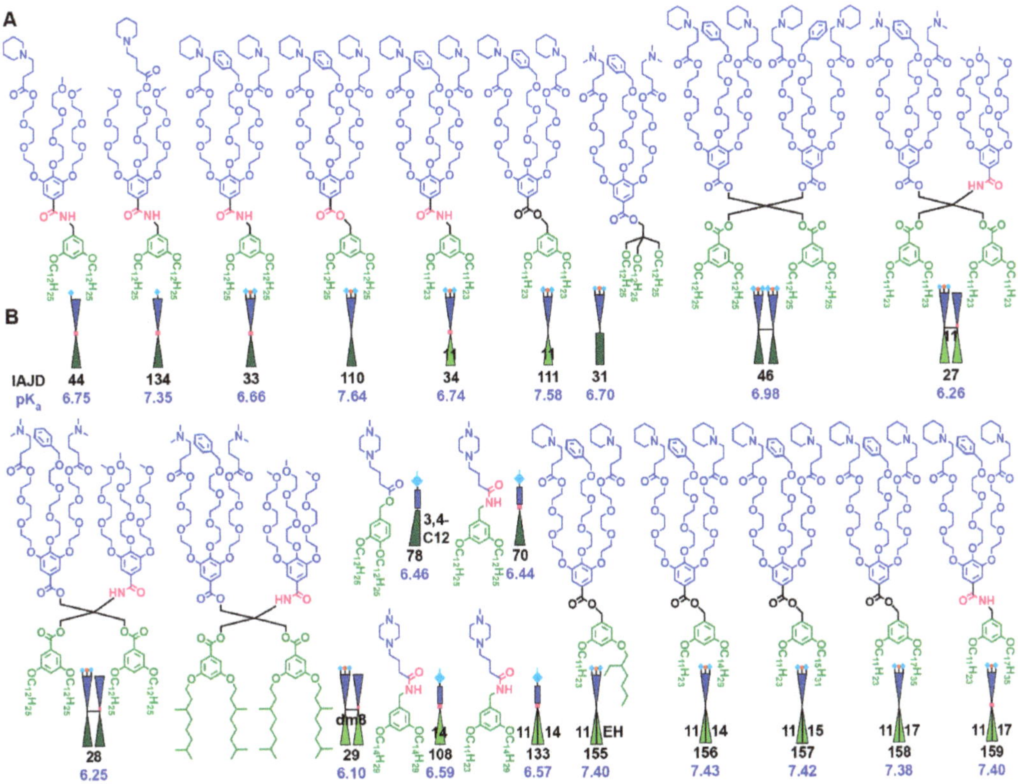

Figure 10. Structures of the 20 most active IAJDs for selective delivery of mRNA to the lung. (**A**) Legend: Schematic representations of IAJDs with the number of carbons in the alkyl groups from their hydrophobic part on the left and right sides of the structure, IAJD numbers in black, under the schematic of IAJD and pKa values in blue under the number of IAJD (**B**).

IAJDs 33, 34, 31, and 155 display activity in the range of 10^8 p/s, while IAJD 33 shows a total flux for the lung of 10^9 p/s, which is similar to that of MC3 to the liver. The comparison with MC3 from Figure 12 is not valid since MC3 delivers mRNA only to the liver. IAJDs 110, 111, 29, and 159 show activity almost equal to 10^8 p/s. We can also compare the SS IAJD 111 containing 11 carbons in its equal alkyl groups of the hydrophobic part and activity of 7.4×10^7 p/s, with nSS IAJD 155 containing a combination of 11 and ethyl hexyl alkyl groups that provide 1.01×10^8 p/s total flux activity.

These unoptimized results demonstrate that the targeted organ is selected according to the structure and sequence of the ionizable amine in the hydrophilic part of the IAJD, while the overall activity is determined mostly based on the structure, composition, and sequence of the hydrophobic part of the IAJD.

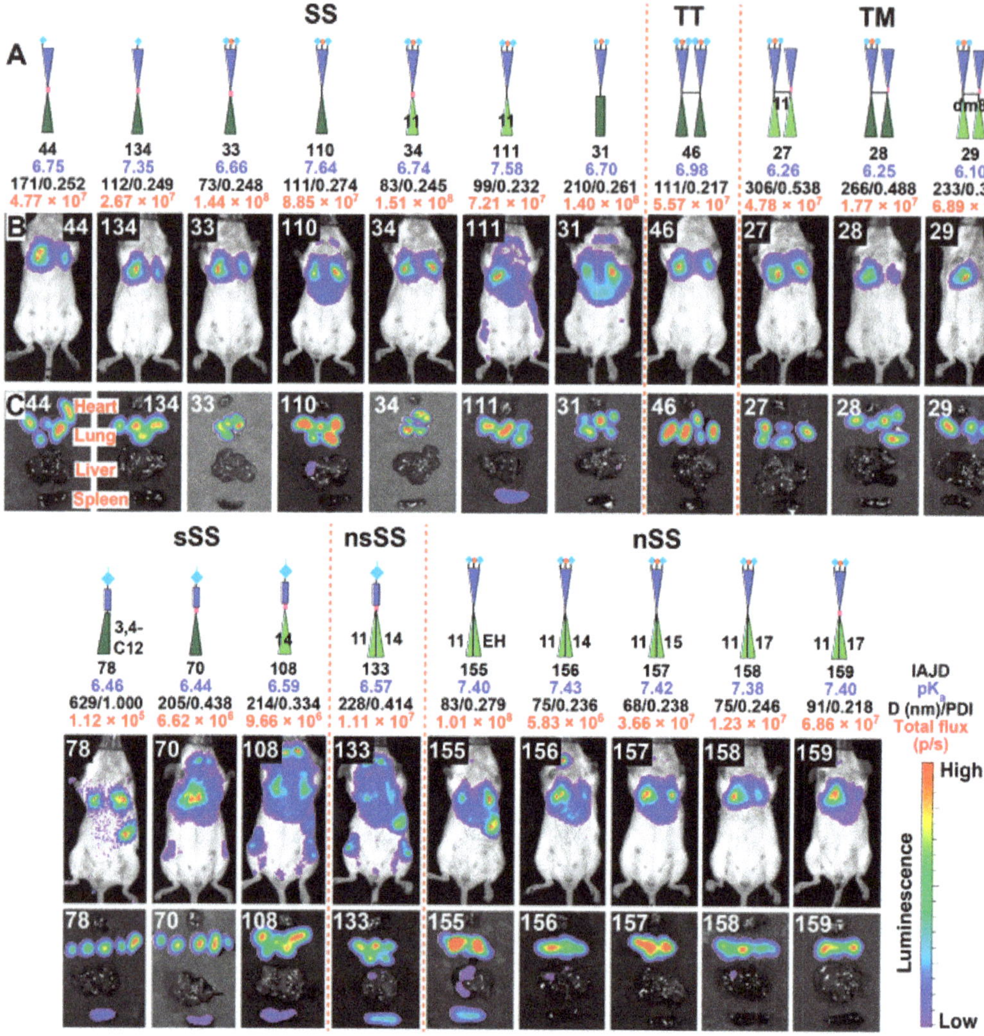

Figure 11. Selective delivery of Luc-mRNA in vivo by 20 most active DNPs to the lung: (**A**) schematic representation of the IAJD structures with the number of the carbons in the hydrophobic part on the left and right sides of IAJD, pKa values under the schematic in blue, dimensions and polydispersity under pKa in black, and total flux luminescence activity (p/s) in red; (**B**) the images of luciferase expression in the whole body 4–6 h after the i.v. injection of Luc-mRNA formulated with IAJDs; (**C**) the images of organs with luciferase activity are shown using color coding from the bottom right column.

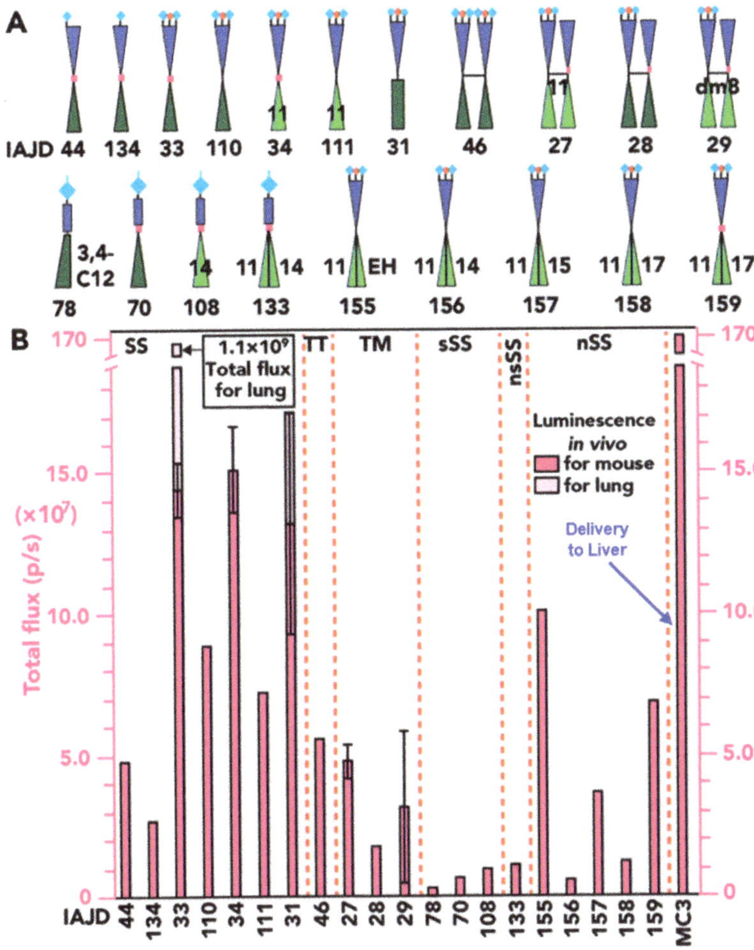

Figure 12. Comparison of the activities of 20 best DNPs that deliver mRNA to the lung: (**A**) schematic representations of IAJDs with the number of carbons in the alkyl groups from their hydrophobic part on the left and right sides of the structure, and IAJD numbers in black under the schematic of IAJD. MC3 delivers mRNA to the liver; (**B**) plots of total flux luminescence (p/s) for the DNPs assembled from the IAJDs from (**A**).

3.8. *In Vivo Delivery of Luc-mRNA with sSS DNPs*

So far, we discussed experiments in which the delivery of mRNA was performed with nsSS-based DNPs. Figure 13A shows the delivery experiments of mRNA with all the 22 sSS IAJD-forming DNPs containing the number of carbons in their alkyl groups that were employed in the construction of the nsSS IAJDs reported in the previous subsections. All the 22 sSS IAJD-based DNPs deliver to the spleen. It is interesting to observe from Figure 13B that the whole-body total flux of the luciferase activity of all the DNPs assembled from sSS IAJDs is in the range of 10^7 p/s, and therefore, it is lower than 10^8 p/s. This demonstrates, as it will be shown more efficiently in three-dimensional figures in the following subsections, that substitution with nonsymmetric alkyl groups in the hydrophobic part of nsSS IAJDs decreases the crystallization and increases the solubility in ethanol of IAJDs with long alkyl groups through comparison with that of sSS IAJDs. At the same time, this concept facilitates a substantial enhancement of the activity of their DNPs.

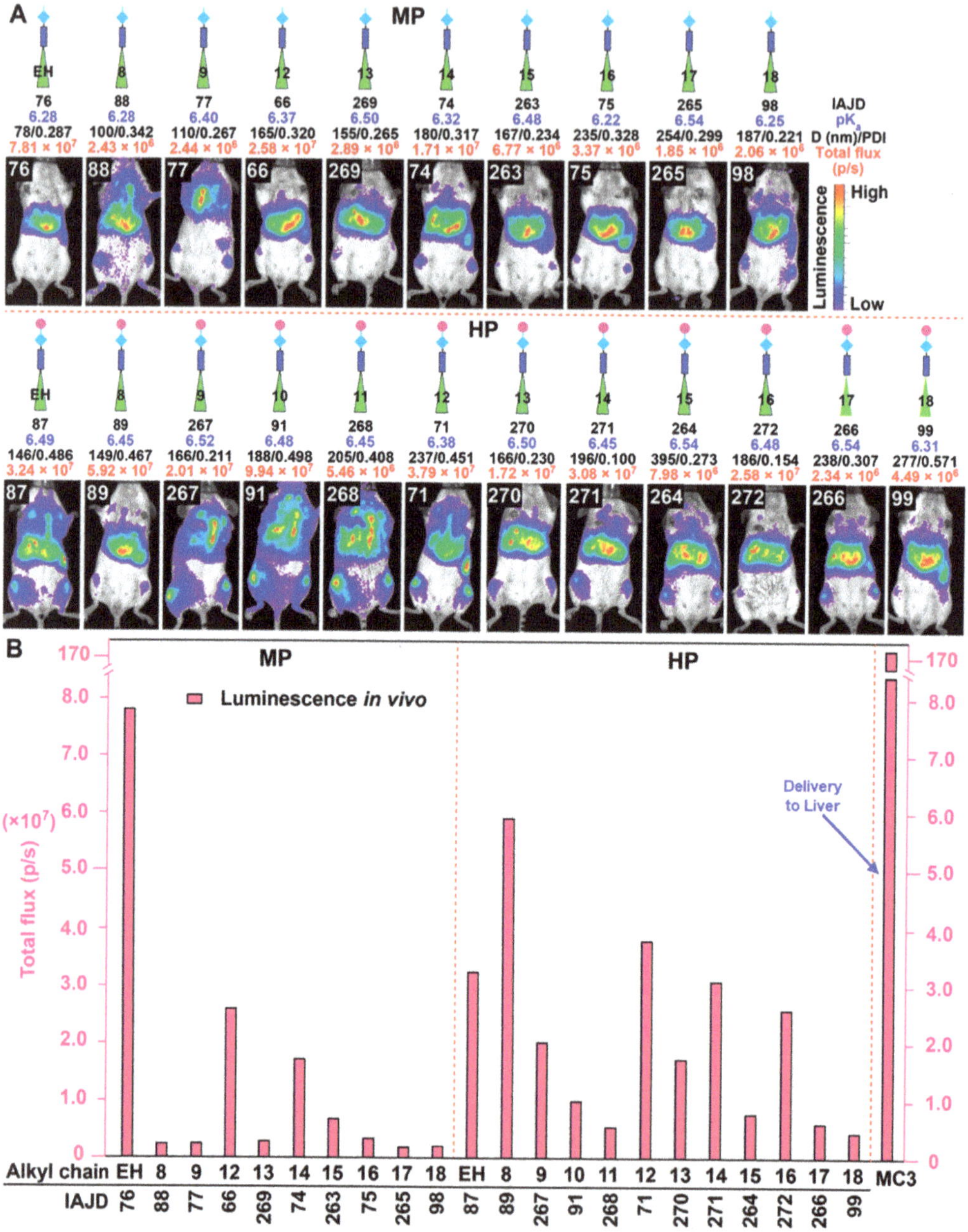

Figure 13. Selective delivery of Luc-mRNA in vivo via all 22 sSS IAJDs-based DNPs: (**A**) the schematic structures of all sSS IAJDs, the number of carbons in their alkyl groups, their numbers, pKa, dimensions and polydispersity of their DNPs and whole-body mice images of delivered Luc-mRNA; (**B**) whole-body luciferase activity (total flux in p/s) as a function of the number of carbons in the alkyl groups of sSS IAJDs derived DNPs.

3.9. A Hypothetic Mechanism Explaining the Activity of mRNA Delivery via the Hydrophobic Part of IAJDs

A model describing the structure of the bilayer of the vesicles named dendrimersomes assembled via the injection of Janus dendrimers in water and in the buffer as well as the prediction of their dimensions was elaborated by one of our laboratories [41]. This method relies on the idea that dendrimersome vesicles are closed bilayer films with identical bilayer structure and bilayer planarity in a solid state that is only slightly curved in the wall of the dendrimersome assembly [84–86].

It has been demonstrated that amphiphilic Janus dendrimers self-assembled from 3,5-disubstituted phenolic acids interdigitate their aliphatic alkyl groups forming dendrimersome vesicles with mechanical properties and prolonged circulation time as good as those of stealth liposomes [73,75,87] and polymersomes [39]. Figure 14A illustrates the interdigitation of the octadecyl alkyl groups of sSS IAJD 99. A perfect bilayer is self-organized during this self-assembly process. This process generates a very compact bilayer of the dendrimersome nanoparticle that in fact is a vesicle with maximum hydrophobic interactions between its alkyl groups. The transition from sSS IAJD 99 to nsSS IAJD 178 and to other nsSS IAJDs was selected originally to improve the solubility of sSS IAJD 99 containing two octadecyl alkyl groups and of other sSS IAJDs containing long alkyl groups. This increased solubility was expected due to the two different alkyl chain lengths in the hydrophobic part of the new nsSS IAJD 178 that will increase the entropy of the bilayer. The expected increased solubility due to decreased tendency towards the crystallization of the IAJDs was indeed accomplished at the transition from sSS IAJDs to nsSS IAJDs, as it was in the case of sSS IAJD 99 to nsSS IAJD 178. This mechanism of increasing solubility by decreasing the tendency towards crystallization provides an excellent opportunity to design IAJDs with long alkyl groups that do not contain *cis*-double bonds as phospholipids contain and, therefore, are oxidatively stable. However, at the time of these preliminary experiments, we could not predict that an increase in DNP activity for the delivery of mRNA from 4.49×10^6 to 4×10^8 will occur by changing the self-assembly of DNPs from sSS IAJD 99 to nsSS IAJD 178. The model for the bilayer of nsSS IAJD 178 responsible for this two orders of magnitude increase in DNP activity is shown in Figure 14B,D,F. This model demonstrates that an increase in nsSS IAJD 178 solubility was accompanied by a decrease in the perfection of the bilayer packing that decreases the hydrophobic interactions between the alkyl groups in the hydrophobic part of the DNP bilayer self-organized from nsSS IAJD 178. This less perfect DNP does not contain empty space in its bilayer, as shown in the model from Figure 14B,D. This "empty space" is in fact filled up with distorted rather than almost all-*trans* alkyl groups. Nevertheless, the "empty space" from Figure 14 helps to indicate the number of methylenes that have to change their all-*trans* conformation, which most probably facilitates a more efficient endosomal escape of the mRNA in the cytoplasm (Figure 1C) due to lower hydrophobic interaction in the bilayer of nsSS IAJDs based DNPs. These preliminary results will be complemented via a comprehensive investigation of this process, which will be published soon. Regardless of the outcome of these more detailed investigations, the model from Figure 14 indicates one of the key contributions of this report: *"an unexpectedly simple design principle for the control of delivery activity by the molecular engineering of the hydrophobic part of DNPs"*.

As already mentioned, a quantitative approach to these molecular design principles requires additional research. For example, the mechanism may be completely different for the case of IAJDs derived from 3,4-dihydroxy and 3,4,5-trihydroxy phenolic acids from the case of the similar structure based on 3,5-dihydroxy homolog since the former do not interdigitate in their bilayer structure. Nevertheless, the synthetic capability of one-component IAJD and DNP delivery systems definitively relies on the ability of molecular design principles based on the precise location of its functional groups rather than on the statistical distribution of its four components from the case of four-component LNPs.

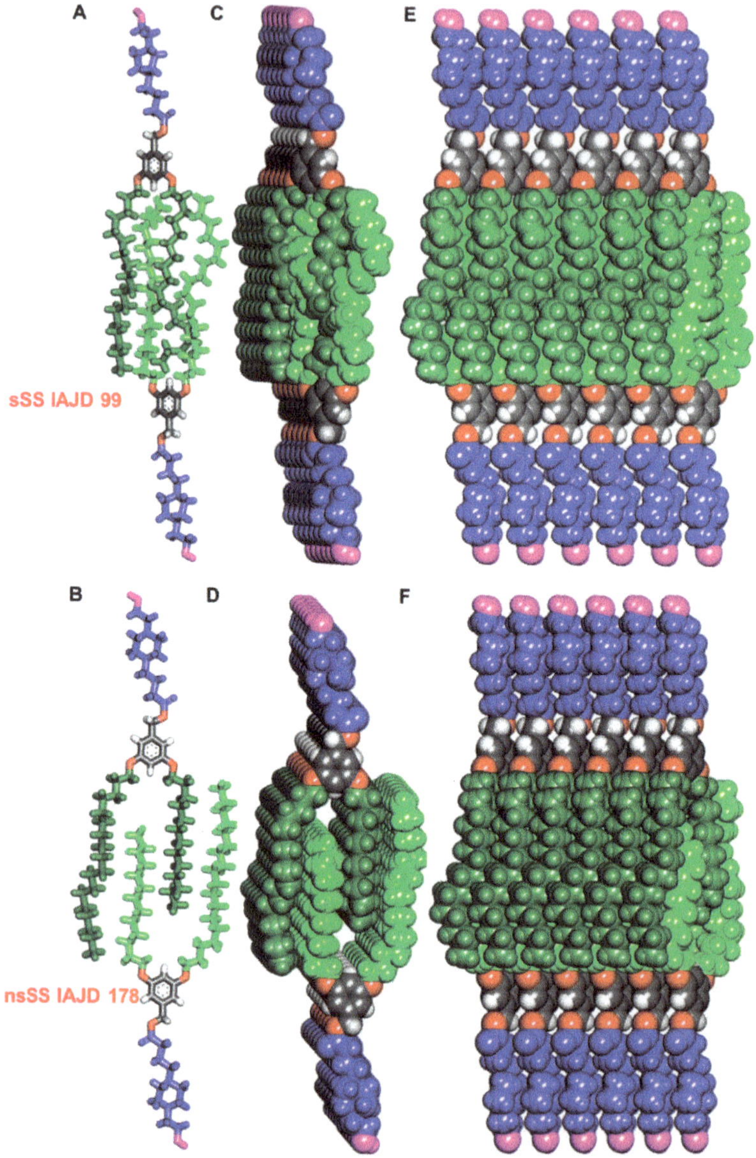

Figure 14. Molecular models of the bilayer structure of sSS IAJD 99 and of nsSS IAJD 178: (**A**,**B**) dimers of sSS IAJD 99 containing 18 carbons in both alkyls and of nsSS IAJD 178 based on 18 and 13 carbons in its alkyls (stick models, side view for both IAJDs); (**C**,**D**) dimers of sSS IAJD 99 and of nsSS IAJD 178 (space-filling models, side view for both IAJDs); (**E**,**F**) bilayers of sSS IAJD 99 and of nsSS IAJD 178 (space-filling models, side views for both IAJDs). Color legends: hydrophilic part in blue; hydrophobic part in light and dark green; oxygen and OH in pink; aromatic ring in gray; H groups on aromatic in white.

3.10. The Current Status of the Molecular Design Principles to Target the Delivery of mRNA Mediated via IAJDs

A three-dimensional (3D) representation of the transfection activity accomplished in vivo with DNPs co-assembled from sSS IAJDs and nsSS IAGDs with mRNA is illustrated in Figure 15 for the case of delivery to the lung (Figure 15A) and to the spleen and lymph nodes (Figure 15B) as a function of the number of carbons in their alkyl groups. The red cylinders from the diagonals of the two 3D plots contain equal numbers of carbons in the alkyl groups located at the 3- and 5- positions of the sSS IAJDs, while the blue and cyan cylinders show the activity results for different numbers of carbons in the same two positions of the nsSS IAJDs derived DNPs.

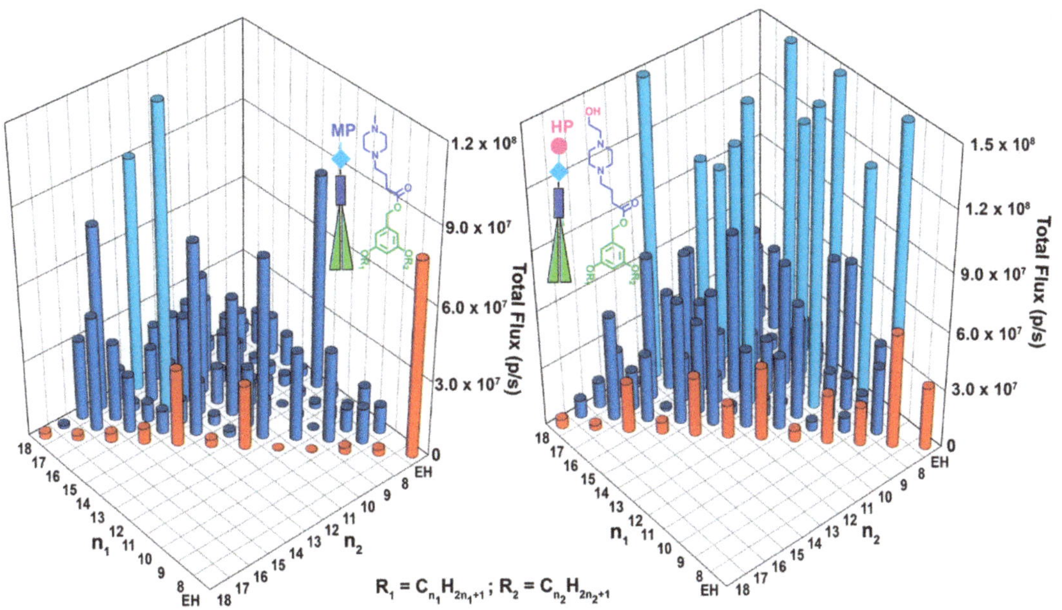

(A) (B)

Figure 15. Comparison of the Luc-mRNA delivery activities (whole-body total flux in p/s) of DNPs exhibiting in the hydrophilic part the methyl piperazine group ((**A**) left side) and hydroxyethylpiperazine group ((**B**) right side). The red cylinders represent the activity of the symmetric sSS IAJDs employed in the assembly of DNPs, and the blue cylinders are the nonsymmetric nsSS IAJDs used to assemble in the hydrophobic part. Cylinders in cyan color represent activity higher than 10^8 (p/s).

A remarkable conclusion results from these 3D plots. The red cylinders that correspond to sDD IAJD-derived DNPs exhibit the lowest activity, while the blue cylinders that correspond to nsSS IAJD-based DNPs display the highest activity. The cyan cylinders exhibit activities that are higher than 10^8 p/s. This structure of IAJD activity of DNP dependence demonstrates the ability to discover molecular design principles for the targeted delivery of mRNA via the rapid screening of DNPs co-assembled through the simple injection of IAJDs with different primary structures with mRNA and to predict their activity. No dialysis and fractionation of the DNP assemblies, as needed in the case of LNPs, is required for these rapid screening experiments.

4. The Early Days of Nucleic Acid Delivery and Their Evolution to the Current Methodologies

According to our knowledge, Figure 16 organizes for the first time the historical development of the viral and synthetic vectors for the delivery of DNA and RNA starting from the early days to the currently employed methodologies. This is not a comprehensive review, and therefore, we apologize to the authors that may have discovered methodologies that we may have missed incorporating in Figure 16. However, the goal of this figure is to illustrate, in a very brief fashion, the conceptual development of this field and the rationale for the direction of its evolution. As shown in the title of Figure 16, delivery vectors for nucleic acids can be classified in the simplest way as viral and nonviral or synthetic. Some of the viruses employed in nucleic acid delivery are the retrovirus which was first used for the delivery of RNA in 2014 [88]. Adenovirus [89], adeno-associated virus [90], and lentivirus [91] were some of the most frequently used viruses for the delivery of DNA that started as early as 1995, 1993, and 1999, respectively. Viral vectors are currently used in commercial vaccines [92–96]. Viral vectors are very efficient, but synthetic vectors rely on their unlimited synthetic capabilities.

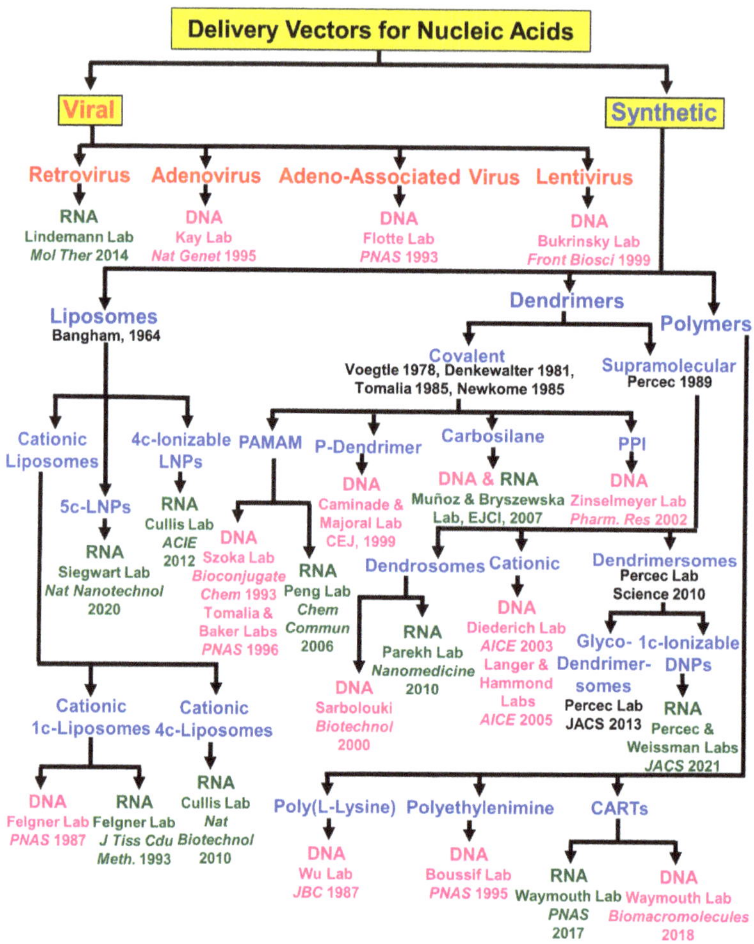

Figure 16. Summary of the viral and nonviral vectors for the delivery of nucleic acids and the evolution of methodology development [2,12,24,29,39,52,88,90,91,95–117].

The discussion on synthetic vectors will rely on demonstrating their synthetic capabilities. The simplest classification of synthetic vectors relies on liposomes, covalent and supramolecular dendrimers, and polymers. The early days of nucleic acid delivery with liposomes employed cationic one-component liposomes. Cationic one-component liposomes were pioneered by the laboratory of Felgner for the delivery of DNA in 1987 [95] and by the same laboratory for the delivery of RNA in 1993 [96]. Cationic liposomes are toxic and bind both DNA and RNA via electrostatic interactions on their exterior surface and in their interior. The nucleic acid from their exterior surface undergoes enzymatic degradation, and therefore, an ideal vector would contain the nucleic acid only in its interior where it is protected against enzymatic degradation. Toxicity and degradation were the limiting features that did not facilitate, according to our knowledge, the commercial development of cationic one-component liposomes in vaccines, although the cationic lipid component is commercially available under the name Lipofectamine transfection reagent and Transfectamine 5000 transfection reagent.

In 2010, Cullis laboratory developed a four-component cationic liposome for the delivery of RNA [97] that is affected by the same features as the one-component cationic liposomes. The solution to the one-component and four-component cationic liposomes was solved in an elegant way also by Cullis laboratory in 2012 [29]. This laboratory elaborated four-component ionizable lipid nanoparticles (LNPs) by expanding the three-component stealth liposomes into four-component lipid nanoparticles. LNPs rely on a combination of phospholipids, cholesterol, ionizable lipids, and PEG-conjugated lipids. The elegance of this concept consists of the presence of an ionizable lipid that, at a certain pH, becomes protonated and, therefore, binds RNA, while at the physiological pH, it becomes deprotonated and, therefore, releases the RNA from the periphery of LNPs but not from its interior and eliminates cationic-derived toxicity. Therefore, LNPs are nontoxic.

However, the ionizable lipid and the PEG-conjugated lipid have their own deficiencies in a four-component LNP, which were briefly mentioned in the introductory part of this paper and in our previous publications [24–26]. Details of these developments and the deficiencies resulting from the statistical distribution of the four components of the LNPs will be discussed in the next subsection. LNPs are currently the most successful RNA delivery vector used in commercial mRNA-based vaccines, although they deliver mostly to the liver. A five-component LNP system was recently developed by Siegwart Laboratory in 2020 [12]. The fifth component of this LNP has either permanently positive or negative charges that can facilitate delivery to organs other than the liver. Cationic covalent dendrimers made their entry into the delivery of nucleic acids in 1993 [98] and 1996 [99], when Szoka and Tomalia, Baker laboratories, reported the delivery of DNA with the cationic covalent PAMAM dendrimers. Both laboratories investigated different generations and observed a strong dependence on the delivery in vitro as a function of generation number. In 2006, Peng Laboratory also employed cationic PAMAM dendrimers to deliver RNA [100]. In 1999, Caminade and Majoral Lab used phosphorus (P)-containing dendrimers to deliver DNA [101]. Cationic carbosilanes were employed to deliver DNA and RNA by Muñoz and Bryszewska laboratories in 2005 [102,118–122], while cationic PPI was used by Sinselmeyer Lab in 2002 [103,123]. Both covalent cationic dendrimers are associated with some of the negative features of cationic liposomes.

A solution to this problem was generated by Sarbolouki's laboratory in 2000 [104]. His laboratory encapsulated the complex of cationic dendrimers with DNA into liposomes named dendrosomes. In 2010, Parekh Lab employed dendrosomes for the delivery of RNA [105]. Dendrosomes eliminate the toxicity and enzymatic degradation of cationic dendrimers but require extensive additional processes for encapsulation in liposomes.

Cationic supramolecular dendrimers obtained via the self-assembly of cationic amphiphilic dendrimers were employed by the laboratory of Diederich starting in 2003 [106] and Langer and Hammond in 2005 [107] for the delivery of DNA. Supramolecular cationic dendrimers are also toxic. Therefore, the Langer and Anderson laboratories elaborated on two- to four-component LNPs in which the ionizable lipid was replaced with amphiphilic ionizable dendrimers based on PAMAM or polyethylene imine (PEI) [124,125].

The most recent progress in this field was in 2021, when Percec and Weissman laboratories [24–26] developed one-component multifunctional sequence-defined ionizable amphiphilic Janus dendrimers (IAJDs) that co-assemble with mRNA into dendrimersome nanoparticles (DNPs). This co-assembly process proceeds by the simple injection of the IAJD into the acidic buffer solution of mRNA. The IAJD concept was developed, as already mentioned in the early part of this paper, based on inspiration from research on amphiphilic Janus dendrimers (JDs) that self-assemble dendrimersomes (DS) [39–51] and sequence-defined amphiphilic Janus glycodendrimers (JGD) that self-assemble glycodendrimersomes (GDSs) [52–70].

As discovered in this report, the structure of the hydrophilic part of IAJD determines the organ targeted, while the structure of the IAJD in its hydrophobic part determines the activity of the in vivo transfection. With these synthetic vector technologies, delivery to the spleen and lymph nodes, liver and lymph nodes, and lung became accessible. One of the most difficult challenges in this field remains the delivery to the nervous system, including the brain, which is under extensive investigation in the laboratory of Cena [126–141].

The final group of synthetic vectors that have been developed are based on synthetic polymers. Cationic poly(L-lysine) and polyethyleneimine were, respectively, both employed for the delivery of DNA in 1987 by Wu's laboratory [108] and in 1995 by Boussif's laboratory [109]. We must recall that polyethyleneimine is a very high-molecular-weight branched polymer obtained via the cationic ring-opening polymerization of ethylene imine. A very elegant strategy was recently developed by Waymouth's laboratory, where Charge–Altering Releasable Transporters (CARTs) were employed for the delivery of RNA in 2017 and for DNA in 2018 [110,111]. A brief illustration of the most important historical developments ranging from liposomes, viral vectors, stealth liposomes, polymersomes, dendrimersomes, four-component LNPs, glycodendrimersomes, and 1c-DNPs is schematically illustrated in Figure 17 [90,112].

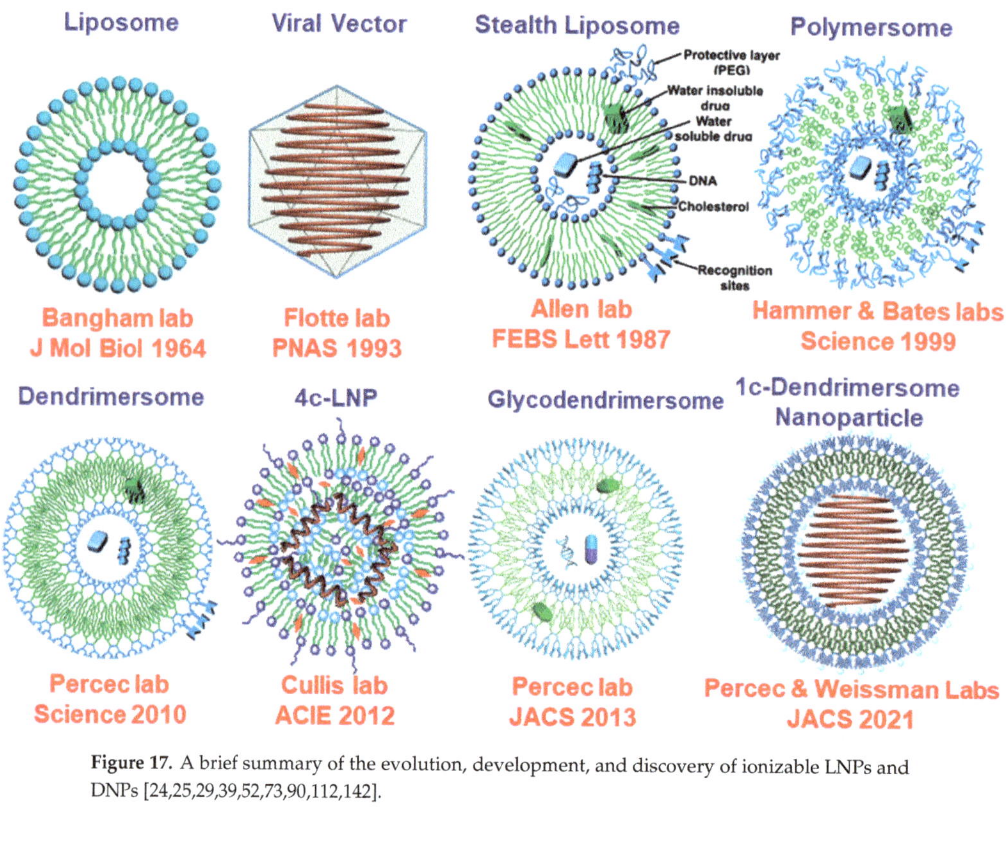

Figure 17. A brief summary of the evolution, development, and discovery of ionizable LNPs and DNPs [24,25,29,39,52,73,90,112,142].

The rationale of Figure 17 is first to illustrate their three-dimensional structures and their structures containing the encapsulated mRNA. Briefly, we can observe that, in the absence of mRNA liposomes, stealth liposomes, polymersomes, dendrimersomes, 4c-LNPs, glycodendrimersomes, and 1c-DNPs are all vesicles. Liposomes are unstable and require cholesterol and PEG-conjugated lipids to increase their stability and circulation time. Polymersomes, 4c-LNPs, glycodendrimersomes, and 4c-DNPs are as stable, or even more stable than, stealth liposomes. Regardless of the method of preparation, liposomes, stealth liposomes, polymersomes, and 4c-LNPs are polydisperse and must be fractionated in order to obtain the desired dimension and polydispersity. Viral vectors are monodispersed, and dendrimersomes, glycodendrimersomes, and 1c-LNPs are obtained with narrow polydispersity and predictable dimensions through simple injection in water or buffer. Therefore, viral vectors and 1c-DNPs are more closely related in both the absence and presence of mRNA. Notably, 4c-LNPs require dialysis after the encapsulation of mRNA. During this process, the neutral ionizable lipids get encapsulated together with the mRNA inside of their external vesicle, generating a complex internal mixture containing ionizable lipids, mRNA, and cholesterol [28,142–147]. Therefore, an ideal synthetic nonviral vector would have to be closely related to the structure of viral vectors in order to provide the very high activity of the viral vectors and the flexibility of the synthetic vectors. Although substantial research is required to accomplish a system like this, we believe that the strategy of 1c-IAJD-DNP is conceptually suitable to accomplish it. Alternative dendrimer fragments such as carbosilane, PPI, and others can also be incorporated into IAJDs [101,102,118–122].

5. Inspiration from and Collaboration with Donald A. Tomalia

The history of the discovery of covalent dendrimers was published repeatedly, and it is well known to all contributors and readers of this Special Issue dedicated to the 85th anniversary of Donald A. Tomalia. However, in spite of being well known, we will repeat it briefly here. Dendrimers were discovered independently in four different laboratories. In 1978, Fritz Voegtle from the University of Bonn [113] reported the bis-cyanoethylation of primary aliphatic amines and of bifunctional secondary amines, followed by the reduction of the cyano groups and the subsequent iteration of these two steps to synthesize two generations of "**cascade**" molecules. In a series of US patents starting in 1981, Denkewalter, Kolc, and Lukasavage of Allied Corporation [114] produced branching monodisperse spherical poly(lysine)s that were found by Aharoni from the same company to be indeed globular and monodisperse [148]. In 1985, Tomalia, Baker, Dewald, Hall, Kallos, Martin, Roeck, Ryder, and Smith from Dow Chemical Company reported the synthesis and characterization of a new class of polymers named **starburst–dendritic macromolecules** [115]. Seven generations of starburst–dendritic macromolecules were synthesized via the iterative Michael addition of methyl acrylate to ethylenediamine or ammonia, followed by extensive amidation with excess ethylene diamine and reiteration of this methodology. Additionally, in 1985, Newkome, Yao, Baker, and Gupta reported a new "**cascade**" molecule that provided a synthetic approach to unimolecular micelles. This molecule was named **arborol** [116]. These laboratories reported excellent synthesis methods, identified side reactions to structural imperfections in the designed compound, and employed careful analysis of the final products.

However, neither "**cascades**" nor "**arborols**" but rather "**dendrimers**" provided the name for the new field of perfectly branched and monodisperse synthetic macromolecules. In fact, **The First International Dendrimer Symposium (IDS-1)**, a conference that became biannual, was organized by Professor Fritz Voegtle, the person who invented "**cascade**" molecules, between 3 and 5 October 1999, in Frankfurt, Germany [149].

Many review articles and books on covalent dendrimers were published by Tomalia, Voegtle, and Newkome laboratories and by many other groups that joined the field soon after [7,8,149–166].

In an attempt to synthesize a biaxial nematic thermotropic liquid crystal, in the late 1980s, Percec's laboratory discovered self-assembling dendrons, self-assembling dendrimers, and self-organizable dendronized polymers [167]. Percec's laboratory, in collaboration with top experts in the field, developed and employed a combination of structural analysis through X-ray diffraction, transmission electron microscopy, electron density maps, and reconstruction of the X-ray diffractograms using the method elaborated by Watson and Crick to solve the structure of DNA, to elucidate the three-dimensional (3D) structure of supramolecular dendrimers [167–174]. This combination of diffraction methodologies added a new dimension to the characterization of dendrimers and created the complementary subfield of supramolecular dendrimers. Helical chirality resembling the mechanism used by rod-like or columnar and polygonal including icosahedral viruses [175–178], Frank–Kasper phases [175,176,178–203], liquid quasicrystals [173,204–209], amphiphilic Janus dendrimers [39–51], Janus glycodendrimers [52–70] and one-component sequence-defined ionizable amphiphilic Janus dendrimers (IAJDs) [24–26] are just a few of the new concepts via which supramolecular dendrimers impacted a diversity of disciplines of soft and living matter.

Tomalia's leading role, characterized by enthusiasm, creativity, and modesty, inspired, encouraged, and attracted new contributors to the field of dendrimers. He supported us when we discovered that supramolecular dendrimers can form conventional thermotropic liquid crystal phases [210–212], rod-like or columnar shape assemblies [117,213–250], and ultimately, spherical and even chiral spherical or spherical helical shapes generating Frank–Kasper [175,176,178–202] and quasicrystal [173,203–209] phases. He also inspired and encouraged us to generate the first nanoperiodic tables of supramolecular dendrimers [198] and to continue the pathway to the discovery of new concepts in supramolecular dendrimers by solving their 3D structure, elucidating the mechanism, and ultimately predicting additional primary structures behaving in a similar way. Don also inspired Percec's laboratory to select the name dendrimersome out of several other options when we discovered the self-assembly of amphiphilic Janus dendrimers into monodisperse vesicles with predictable dimensions [39]. While the readers of this Special Issue are familiar with the contributions of Tomalia to dendrimers, not many of them may know that in 1966, the laboratories of Tomalia, Kagia, Seeliger, and Litt, independently from each other, discovered the cationic ring-opening polymerization of 2-substituted-2-ozazolines and their living polymerization [205,251–257]. Self-organizable dendronized polymers obtained through the living cationic ring-opening polymerization of dendronized 2-oxazolines allowed Percec's laboratory to establish some of the most fundamental dependences of primary structure–tertiary structure [255–257], including the discovery of liquid quasicrystal, A15, and σ Frank–Kasper phases within only five monomer repeat units of the degree of polymerization of the dendronized polymer [205] (Figure 18).

A series of self-accelerated [187,189] and self-interrupted processes [190] during the synthesis of supramolecular dendrimers, some of them inspired by Tomalia's work [149], culminated in the first methodology for the synthesis of monodisperse macromolecules via the self-interrupted living ring-opening polymerization of a dendronized monomer [190]. We would like to state that our laboratory never wrote a joint paper with Tomalia. However, one of the corresponding authors (V.P.) has never been turned down by Don when he was invited as a plenary or invited speaker at the numerous conferences organized by V.P.

The posters shown in Figure 19 present the list of the invited speakers from the third Frontiers in Macromolecular and Supramolecular Science Symposium dedicated to the memory of V.P.'s PhD mentor that took place at the Romanian Academy between 7 and 9 June 2010 in Bucharest and Iasi. Donald Tomalia is an illuminating and enthusiastic lecturer and a contagiously positive example for the young and even for senior generations of scientists (Figure 20).

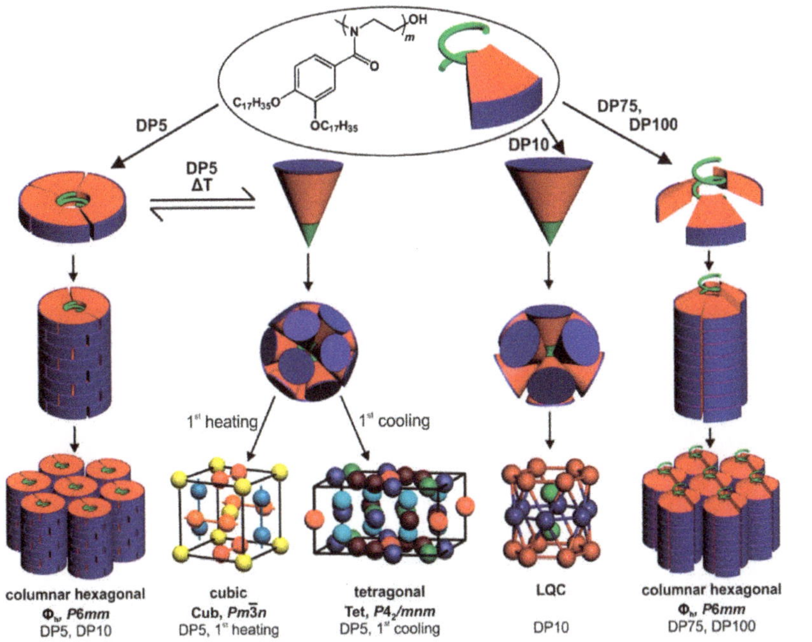

Figure 18. Summary of periodic and quasiperiodic arrays self-organized from assemblies of poly[(3,4)17G1-Oxz] at different degrees of polymerization (DP) and temperature. This Figure is reproduced with permission from reference [205]. Copyright © 2018, American Chemical Society.

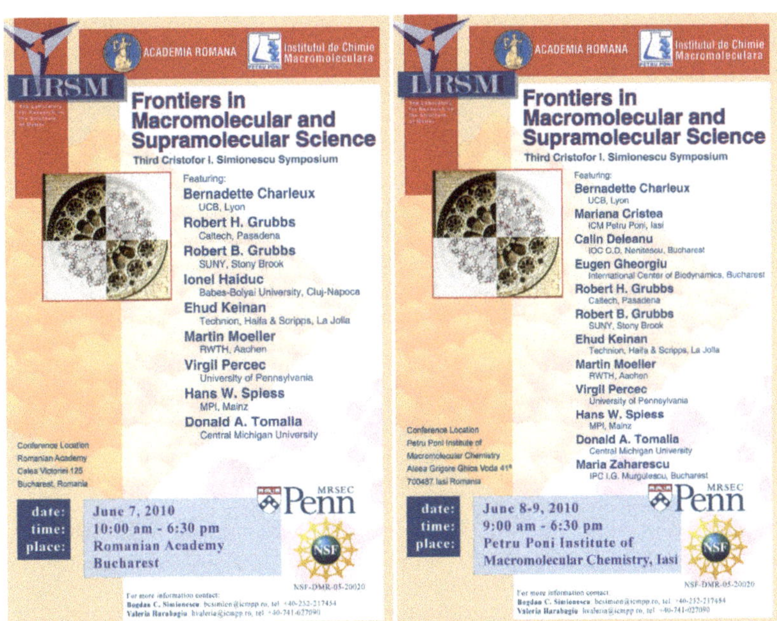

Figure 19. The posters with the names of the invited speakers including Donald A. Tomalia from the 2010 Frontiers in Macromolecular and Supramolecular Science Symposia co-organized by one of us (V.P.) at the Romanian Academy in Bucharest and in Iasi.

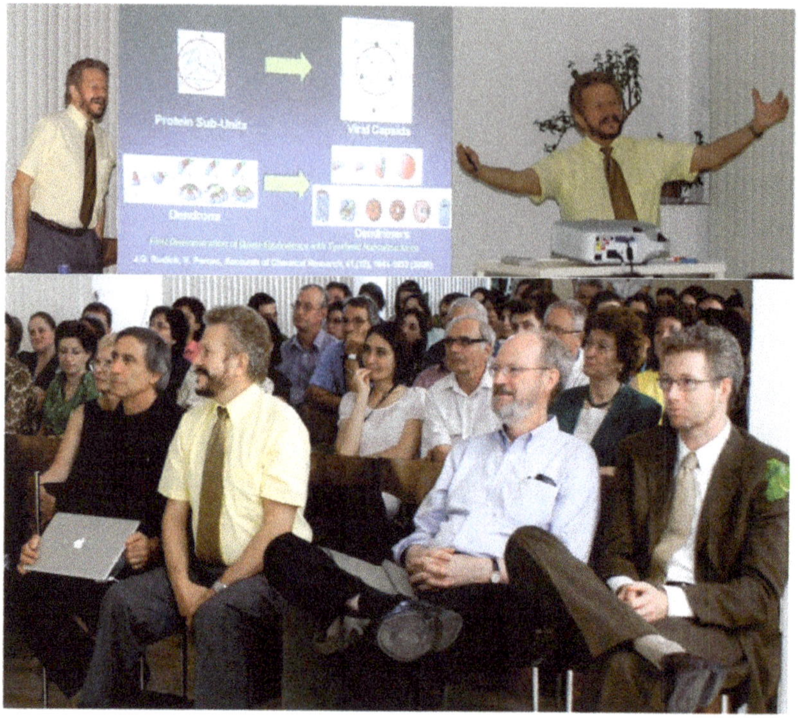

Figure 20. Top part shows the enthusiastic Donald Tomalia giving his lecture at the Romanian Academy in Iasi in 2010. Bottom part, first row from right to left: Robert (Barney) Grubbs, the Nobel Laureate Robert (Bob) Grubbs, Donald Tomalia, and Ehud Keinan, the President of the Israel Chemical Society.

6. Conclusions

Ninety-eight one-component IAJDs based on, mostly plant 3,5-dihydroxy phenolic acid, with different primary structures in both their hydrophilic and hydrophobic parts were synthesized via an accelerated modular–orthogonal methodology. These very simple first-generation amphiphilic Janus dendrimers are constructed from minidendrons, as defined by our laboratory [50,167]. Therefore, they can be named also Janus minidendrimers containing one or two branching points in the hydrophobic part and one or two in the hydrophilic ionizable amine part. In spite of their synthetic simplicity, they are extremely efficient in the construction of IAJDs [24–26]. Their co-assembly with Luc-mRNA was accomplished via injection in an acidic buffer to generate DNPs of well-defined dimensions and narrow polydispersity. This methodology provided rapid access to in vivo transfection experiments in mice, without the need for fractionation or dialysis, and demonstrated that all the IAJDs provided DNPs active in transfection experiments in vivo. This methodology also allowed us to determine that their activity could be grouped in terms of delivery to the spleen and lymph nodes, liver and lymph nodes, and lung.

A primary structure–activity analysis generated by screening libraries allowed the discovery of molecular design principles to target the delivery of mRNA and demonstrate, for this class of IAJDs, that their hydrophilic part determines, through the structure of their ionizable amine and their sequence the targeted organ, with hydroxyethyl piperazine favoring the spleen and methyl piperazine favoring the liver. Piperidine and dimethyl amine favor delivery to the lung. It seems that sterically hindered cyclic ionizable amines display high organ selectivity. The primary structure of the hydrophilic part was shown to determine their activity. A change from sSS IAJDs to nsSS IAJDs demonstrated a mechanism to increase the delivery of mRNA activity by up to two orders of magnitude.

A mechanism explaining the increase in activity via the hydrophobic part was provided. This report generated the first approach to molecular design principles required for mRNA delivery to targeted organs with one-component IAJDs derived from plant phenolic acids and supports the preliminary data reported in previous communications [25,26]. Most experiments reported here were performed with the symmetric 3,5-dihydroxy plant phenolic acid regardless of the substitution pattern in the hydrophobic part. The corresponding 3,4-dihydroxy plant phenolic acids provide two constitutional isomers under the same conditions, thus doubling the discovery capability. The 3,4,5-trihydroxy plant phenolic acid provides four-constitutional isomers, thus quadrupling the power of discovery.

However, in addition to other natural phenolic acids, the 3 phenolic acids reported in Figure 2A were already employed to design and synthesize 30 additional constitutional isomeric symmetric and nonsymmetric AB_2 to AB_9 phenolic acids. All of them can be employed in these IAJD experiments using molecular design principles [83]. Aside from providing access to elucidate some of the most complex systems of fundamental and applied interest for today's society [167,173,174,258–260], we expect that the discovery of the molecular design principle methodology reported here will bestow rapid access to a large diversity of mRNA vaccines and other nanotherapeutics that will require much simpler preparation, handling, and storage at a reduced price, and lower concentration of mRNA while employing renewable plant starting materials.

These results also represent a first step towards the generation of a nanoperiodic table of IAJDs for the delivery of mRNA, similar to those of proteins [261–263], self-assembling dendrons, and dendrimers [198,264,265], that may be able to help expand the fields of genetic medicine and nanomedicine [34,266–269].

We expect that the development of new architectural concepts, including polygonal supramolecular dendrimers and new synthetic methodologies [270–291], as well as the attraction of new creative minds to this field, through a methodology similar to that pioneered by the very enthusiastic Donald A. Tomalia, will help impact this field and take it to a new level of discovery and even prediction that, together with practical applications, will reward education and society. All co-authors of this paper thank the Guest Editors for their kind invitation to contribute, with this special combination of research articles and brief review-perspective to the 85th anniversary of Donald A. Tomalia, one of the most influential inventors of this field.

Supplementary Materials: The following supporting information can be downloaded at: https://www.mdpi.com/article/10.3390/pharmaceutics15061572/s1, Scheme S1: Synthesis of Nonane-Based IAJDs with 3,5-Nonsymmetric Alkyl Chains; Scheme S2: Synthesis of Dodecane-Based IAJDs with 3,5-Nonsymmetric Alkyl Chains; Scheme S3: Synthesis of Tetradecane-Based IAJDs with 3,5-Nonsymmetric Alkyl Chains; Scheme S4: Synthesis of Hexadecane-Based IAJDs with 3,5-Nonsymmetric Alkyl Chains; Scheme S5: Synthesis of Heptadecane-Based IAJDs with 3,5-Nonsymmetric Alkyl Chains; Scheme S6: Synthesis of Octadecane-Based IAJDs with 3,5-Nonsymmetr ic Alkyl Chains; Scheme S7: Synthesis of Undecane and Pentadecane Based IAJDs with 3,5-Nonsymme tric Alkyl Chains; Scheme S8: Synthesis of Tridecane Based IAJDs with 3,5-Nonsymmetric Alkyl Chains; Scheme S9: Synthesis of IAJD131; Scheme S10: Synthesis of Decane-Based IAJDs with 3,5-Nonsymmetric Alkyl Chains; Scheme S11: Synthesis of IAJDs with 3,5-symmetric Alkyl Chains; Figure S1: ^{1}H NMR spectrum (top), MALDI-TOF MS spectrum (bottom left) and HPLC trace (bottom right) of Monoprotected Benzyl Ether of Methyl 3,5-Dihydroxybenzoate **2**; Figure S2: ^{1}H NMR spectrum (top), MALDI-TOF MS spectrum (bottom left) and HPLC trace (bottom right) of Methyl 3-(benzyloxy)-5-(octadecyloxy)benzoate, **33**; Figure S3: ^{1}H NMR spectrum (top), MALDI-TOF MS spectrum (bottom left) and HPLC trace (bottom right) of Methyl 3-hydroxy-5-(octadecyloxy)benzoate, **34**; Figure S4: ^{1}H NMR spectra (top), MALDI-TOF MS spectra (bottom left) and HPLC trace (bottom right) of Methyl 3-(heptadecyloxy)-5-(octadecyloxy)benzoate, **35d**; Figure S5: ^{1}H NMR spectrum (top), MALDI-TOF MS spectrum (bottom left) and HPLC trace (bottom right) of (3-(Heptadecyloxy)-5-(octadecyloxy)phenyl)methanol, **36d**; Figure S6: ^{1}H NMR spectrum (top), MALDI-TOF MS spectrum (bottom left) and HPLC trace (bottom right) of 3-(Heptadecyloxy)-5-(octadecyloxy)benzyl 4-bromobutanoate, **37d**; Figure S7: ^{1}H NMR spectrum (top), MALDI-TOF MS spectrum (bottom left) and HPLC trace (bottom right) of 3-(heptadecyloxy)-5-(octadecyloxy)benzyl 4-(4-methylpiperazin-1-yl)butanoate, **38g**, IAJD242; Figure S8: ^{1}H NMR spectrum (top), MALDI-TOF MS spectrum (bottom left) and HPLC trace (bottom right) of 3-(Heptadecyloxy)-5-(octadecyloxy)benzyl 4-(4-(2-hydroxyethyl)piperazin-1-yl)butanoate, **38h**, IAJD243; Figure S9: ^{1}H NMR spectrum (top), MALDI-TOF MS spectrum (bottom left) and HPLC trace (bottom right) of methyl 3,5-bis(heptadecyloxy)benzo ate), **64d**; Figure S10: ^{1}H NMR spectrum (top), MALDI-TOF MS spectrum (bottom left) and HPLC trace (bottom right) of (3,5-bis(heptadecyloxy)phenyl)methanol, **65d**; Figure S11: ^{1}H NMR spectrum (top), MALDI-TOF MS spectrum (bottom left) and HPLC trace (bottom right) of 3,5-bis(heptadecyloxy) benzyl 4-bromobutanoate, **66d**; Figure S12: ^{1}H NMR spectrum (top), MALDI-TOF MS spectrum (bottom left) and HPLC trace (bottom right) of 3,5-bis(pentadecyloxy)benzyl 4-(4-methylpiperazin-1-yl)butanoate, **67e**, IAJD265; Figure S13: ^{1}H NMR spectrum (top), MALDI-TOF MS spectrum (bottom left) and HPLC trace (bottom right) of 3,5-Bis(pentadecyloxy)benzyl 4-(4-(2-hydroxyethyl)piperazin-1-yl)butanoate, **67f**, IAJD266; Figure S14: DLS data of DNPs assembled from IAJDs 112, 123, 129, 131, 137, 139 and 140; Figure S15: DLS data of DNPs assembled from IAJDs 163, 164, 166–170, 174, 175; Figure S16: DLS data of DNPs assembled from IAJDs 176, 179–185; Figure S17: DLS data of DNPs assembled from IAJDs 186–194; Figure S18: DLS data of DNPs assembled from IAJDs 197–205; Figure S19: DLS data of DNPs assembled from IAJDs 206–214; Figure S20: DLS data of DNPs assembled from IAJDs 224–232; Figure S21: DLS data of DNPs assembled from IAJDs 233–241; Figure S22: DLS data of DNPs assembled from IAJDs 242–247, 263–265; Figure S23: DLS data of DNPs assembled from IAJDs 266–272; Figure S24: Titration curves showing changes in solution pH in response to addition of a strong acid and calculated pKa for IAJDs 73, 90, 112, 121, 123, 129, 131, 137; Figure S25: Titration curves showing changes in solution pH in response to addition of a strong acid and calculated pKa for IAJDs 139, 140, 163–168; Figure S26: Titration curves showing changes in solution pH in response to addition of a strong acid and calculated pKa for IAJDs 169, 170, 174–176, 179–181; Figure S27: Titration curves showing changes in solution pH in response to addition of a strong acid and calculated pKa for IAJDs 182–189; Figure S28: Titration curves showing changes in solution pH in response to addition of a strong acid and calculated pKa for IAJDs 190–194, 197–199; Figure S29: Titration curves showing changes in solution pH in response to addition of a strong acid and calculated pKa for IAJDs 200–207; Figure S30: Titration curves showing changes in solution pH in response to addition of a strong acid and calculated pKa for IAJDs 208–215; Figure S31: Titration curves showing changes in solution pH in response to addition of a strong acid and calculated pKa for IAJDs 261–223; Figure S32: Titration curves showing changes in solution pH in response to addition of a strong acid and calculated pKa for IAJDs 224–231; Figure S33: Titration curves showing changes in solution pH in response to addition of a strong acid and calculated pKa for IAJDs 232–239; Figure S34: Titration curves showing changes in solution pH in response to addition of a strong acid and calculated pKa for IAJDs 240–247; Figure S35: Titration curves showing changes in solution pH in response to addition of a strong acid and calculated pKa for IAJDs 263–270; Figure S36: Titration curves showing changes in solution pH in response to addition of a strong acid and calculated pKa for IAJDs 271, 272; Table S1: pK_a of Individual IAJDs. References [24–26,35,36,38] are cited in the supplementary materials.

Author Contributions: Conceptualization, V.P., E.N.A.-V. and D.W.; methodology, V.P.; investigation, J.L. (40 IAJDs), M.I.S. (15 IAJDs), D.S.M. (10 IAJDs, 96 pKa, 96 DLS, 96 HPLCs), D.Z. (7 IAJDs), J.A. (10 IAJDs), S.S.C. (3 IAJDs), M.L. (8 IAJDs), H.U.R.S. (3 IAJDs with Dev), H.S. (2 IAJDs), Q.X. (1 IAJD), B.Q. (in vivo experiments), E.N.A.-V. (in vivo experiments and data analysis), N.A.O. (in vivo experiments), E.K.R. (Luc-mRNA synthesis and validation), H.N. (Luc-mRNA validation), D.S. (develop molecular models, 1 IAJD) and M.P. (develop molecular models); writing—original draft preparation, V.P.; writing—review and editing, J.L., E.N.A.-V., D.S.M., M.I.S., D.Z., S.S.C., J.A., M.L., H.U.R.S., H.S., Q.X., B.Q., N.A.O., E.K.R., H.N., D.S., M.P., D.W. and V.P.; funding acquisition, V.P. and D.W.; resources, V.P. and D.W.; supervision, V.P., E.N.A.-V. and D.W. All authors have read and agreed to the published version of the manuscript.

Funding: This work was supported by the National Science Foundation, Grants DMR-2104554 and DMR-1720530. The P. Roy Vagelos Chair at the University of Pennsylvania and the Alexander von Humboldt Foundation (all to V.P.); Wellcome Leap R3 Program (to D.W. and V.P.); Fulbright (to J.A.); Vagelos (to M.L.); and Higher Education Commission of Pakistan via the International Research

Support Initiative Program (to H.U.R.S) scholarships are also acknowledged. NMR Instrumentation (NEO400) was supported by The NSF Major Research Instrumentation Program (Award NSF CHE-1827457) and Vagelos Institute for Energy Science and Technology.

Institutional Review Board Statement: All mice were used in accordance with the guidelines and approval from the University of Pennsylvania's Institution of Animal Care and Use Committee (IACUC approval number is: 803941).

Informed Consent Statement: Not applicable.

Data Availability Statement: Data are contained within the article and Supplementary Materials. Additional data will from the lead contact be available upon request.

Conflicts of Interest: The authors declare no conflict of interest.

References

1. Waehler, R.; Russell, S.J.; Curiel, D.T. Engineering Targeted Viral Vectors for Gene Therapy. *Nat. Rev. Genet.* **2007**, *8*, 573–587. [CrossRef] [PubMed]
2. Thomas, C.E.; Ehrhardt, A.; Kay, M.A. Progress and Problems with the Use of Viral Vectors for Gene Therapy. *Nat. Rev. Genet.* **2003**, *4*, 346–358. [CrossRef] [PubMed]
3. Huang, X.; Kong, N.; Zhang, X.; Cao, Y.; Langer, R.; Tao, W. The Landscape of mRNA Nanomedicine. *Nat. Med.* **2022**, *28*, 2273–2287. [CrossRef] [PubMed]
4. Yin, H.; Kanasty, R.L.; Eltoukhy, A.A.; Vegas, A.J.; Dorkin, J.R.; Anderson, D.G. Non-Viral Vectors for Gene-Based Therapy. *Nat. Rev. Genet.* **2014**, *15*, 541–555. [CrossRef] [PubMed]
5. Hajj, K.A.; Whitehead, K.A. Tools for Translation: Non-Viral Materials for Therapeutic mRNA Delivery. *Nat. Rev. Mater.* **2017**, *2*, 17056. [CrossRef]
6. Zhang, Y.; Sun, C.; Wang, C.; Jankovic, K.E.; Dong, Y. Lipids and Lipid Derivatives for RNA Delivery. *Chem. Rev.* **2021**, *121*, 12181–12277. [CrossRef]
7. Mintzer, M.A.; Simanek, E.E. Nonviral Vectors for Gene Delivery. *Chem. Rev.* **2009**, *109*, 259–302. [CrossRef]
8. Mendes, L.P.; Pan, J.; Torchilin, V.P. Dendrimers as Nanocarriers for Nucleic Acid and Drug Delivery in Cancer Therapy. *Molecules* **2017**, *22*, 1401. [CrossRef]
9. Benner, N.L.; McClellan, R.L.; Turlington, C.R.; Haabeth, O.A.W.; Waymouth, R.M.; Wender, P.A. Oligo (Serine Ester) Charge-Altering Releasable Transporters: Organocatalytic Ring-Opening Polymerization and Their Use for In Vitro and In Vivo mRNA Delivery. *J. Am. Chem. Soc.* **2019**, *141*, 8416–8421. [CrossRef]
10. Haabeth, O.A.W.; Lohmeyer, J.J.K.; Sallets, A.; Blake, T.R.; Sagiv-Barfi, I.; Czerwinski, D.K.; McCarthy, B.; Powell, A.E.; Wender, P.A.; Waymouth, R.M.; et al. An mRNA SARS-CoV-2 Vaccine Employing Charge-Altering Releasable Transporters with a TLR-9 Agonist Induces Neutralizing Antibodies and T Cell Memory. *ACS Cent. Sci.* **2021**, *7*, 1191–1204. [CrossRef]
11. Liu, S.; Wang, X.; Yu, X.; Cheng, Q.; Johnson, L.T.; Chatterjee, S.; Zhang, D.; Lee, S.M.; Sun, Y.; Lin, T.-C.; et al. Zwitterionic Phospholipidation of Cationic Polymers Facilitates Systemic mRNA Delivery to Spleen and Lymph Nodes. *J. Am. Chem. Soc.* **2021**, *143*, 21321–21330. [CrossRef] [PubMed]
12. Cheng, Q.; Wei, T.; Fabiak, L.; Johnson, L.T.; Dilliard, S.A.; Siegwart, D.J. Selective Organ Targeting (SORT) Nanoparticles for Tissue-Specific mRNA Delivery and CRISPR-Cas Gene Editing. *Nat. Nanotechnol.* **2020**, *15*, 313–320. [CrossRef] [PubMed]
13. Liu, C.; Zhou, Q.; Li, Y.; Garner, L.V.; Watkins, S.P.; Carter, L.J.; Smoot, J.; Gregg, A.C.; Daniels, A.D.; Jervey, S.; et al. Research and Development on Therapeutic Agents and Vaccines for COVID-19 and Related Human Coronavirus Diseases. *ACS Cent. Sci.* **2020**, *6*, 315–331. [CrossRef] [PubMed]
14. Corbett, K.S.; Edwards, D.K.; Leist, S.R.; Abiona, O.M.; Boyoglu-Barnum, S.; Gillespie, R.A.; Himansu, S.; Schäfer, A.; Ziwawo, C.T.; DiPiazza, A.T.; et al. SARS-CoV-2 mRNA Vaccine Design Enabled by Prototype Pathogen Preparedness. *Nature* **2020**, *586*, 567–571. [CrossRef]
15. Mulligan, M.J.; Lyke, K.E.; Kitchin, N.; Absalon, J.; Gurtman, A.; Lockhart, S.; Neuzil, K.; Raabe, V.; Bailey, R.; Swanson, K.A.; et al. Phase I/II Study of COVID-19 RNA Vaccine BNT162b1 in Adults. *Nature* **2020**, *586*, 589–593. [CrossRef]
16. Ansell, S.M.; Du, X. Preparation of Novel Lipids and Lipid Nanoparticle Formulations for Delivery of Nucleic Acids. WO 2017/075531 A1, 4 May 2017.
17. Sabnis, S.; Kumarasinghe, E.S.; Salerno, T.; Mihai, C.; Ketova, T.; Senn, J.J.; Lynn, A.; Bulychev, A.; McFadyen, I.; Chan, J.; et al. A Novel Amino Lipid Series for mRNA Delivery: Improved Endosomal Escape and Sustained Pharmacology and Safety in Non-human Primates. *Mol. Ther.* **2018**, *26*, 1509–1519. [CrossRef]
18. Ambegia, E.; Ansell, S.; Cullis, P.; Heyes, J.; Palmer, L.; MacLachlan, I. Stabilized Plasmid–Lipid Particles Containing PEG-Diacylglycerols Exhibit Extended Circulation Lifetimes and Tumor Selective Gene Expression. *Biochim. Biophys. Acta Biomembr.* **2005**, *1669*, 155–163. [CrossRef]
19. Chaudhary, N.; Weissman, D.; Whitehead, K.A. mRNA Vaccines for Infectious Diseases: Principles, Delivery and Clinical Translation. *Nat. Rev. Drug Discov.* **2021**, *20*, 817–838. [CrossRef]

20. Kon, E.; Elia, U.; Peer, D. Principles for Designing an Optimal mRNA Lipid Nanoparticle Vaccine. *Curr. Opin. Biotechnol.* **2022**, *73*, 329–336. [CrossRef]
21. Hou, X.; Zaks, T.; Langer, R.; Dong, Y. Lipid Nanoparticles for mRNA Delivery. *Nat. Rev. Mater.* **2021**, *6*, 1078–1094. [CrossRef]
22. Han, X.; Zhang, H.; Butowska, K.; Swingle, K.L.; Alameh, M.-G.; Weissman, D.; Mitchell, M.J. An Ionizable Lipid Toolbox for RNA Delivery. *Nat. Commun.* **2021**, *12*, 7233. [CrossRef]
23. Pardi, N.; Hogan, M.J.; Porter, F.W.; Weissman, D. mRNA Vaccines—A New Era in Vaccinology. *Nat. Rev. Drug. Discov.* **2018**, *17*, 261–279. [CrossRef]
24. Zhang, D.; Atochina-Vasserman, E.N.; Maurya, D.S.; Huang, N.; Xiao, Q.; Ona, N.; Liu, M.; Shahnawaz, H.; Ni, H.; Kim, K.; et al. One-Component Multifunctional Sequence-Defined Ionizable Amphiphilic Janus Dendrimer Delivery Systems for mRNA. *J. Am. Chem. Soc.* **2021**, *143*, 12315–12327. [CrossRef]
25. Zhang, D.; Atochina-Vasserman, E.N.; Maurya, D.S.; Liu, M.; Xiao, Q.; Lu, J.; Lauri, G.; Ona, N.; Reagan, E.K.; Ni, H.; et al. Targeted Delivery of mRNA with One-Component Ionizable Amphiphilic Janus Dendrimers. *J. Am. Chem. Soc.* **2021**, *143*, 17975–17982. [CrossRef] [PubMed]
26. Zhang, D.; Atochina-Vasserman, E.N.; Lu, J.; Maurya, D.S.; Xiao, Q.; Liu, M.; Adamson, J.; Ona, N.; Reagan, E.K.; Ni, H.; et al. The Unexpected Importance of the Primary Structure of the Hydrophobic Part of One-Component Ionizable Amphiphilic Janus Dendrimers in Targeted mRNA Delivery Activity. *J. Am. Chem. Soc.* **2022**, *144*, 4746–4753. [CrossRef] [PubMed]
27. Cullis, P.R.; Hope, M.J. Lipid Nanoparticle Systems for Enabling Gene Therapies. *Mol. Ther.* **2017**, *25*, 1467–1475. [CrossRef] [PubMed]
28. Kulkarni, J.A.; Darjuan, M.M.; Mercer, J.E.; Chen, S.; van der Meel, R.; Thewalt, J.L.; Tam, Y.Y.C.; Cullis, P.R. On the Formation and Morphology of Lipid Nanoparticles Containing Ionizable Cationic Lipids and siRNA. *ACS Nano* **2018**, *12*, 4787–4795. [CrossRef]
29. Jayaraman, M.; Ansell, S.M.; Mui, B.L.; Tam, Y.K.; Chen, J.; Du, X.; Butler, D.; Eltepu, L.; Matsuda, S.; Narayanannair, J.K.; et al. Maximizing the Potency of siRNA Lipid Nanoparticles for Hepatic Gene Silencing In Vivo. *Angew. Chem. Int. Ed.* **2012**, *51*, 8529–8533. [CrossRef]
30. Ramezanpour, M.; Schmidt, M.L.; Bodnariuc, I.; Kulkarni, J.A.; Leung, S.S.W.; Cullis, P.R.; Thewalt, J.L.; Tieleman, D.P. Ionizable Amino Lipid Interactions with POPC: Implications for Lipid Nanoparticle Function. *Nanoscale* **2019**, *11*, 14141–14146. [CrossRef]
31. Hatakeyama, H.; Akita, H.; Harashima, H. A Multifunctional Envelope Type Nano Device (MEND) for Gene Delivery to Tumours Based on the EPR Effect: A Strategy for Overcoming the PEG Dilemma. *Adv. Drug Deliv. Rev.* **2011**, *63*, 152–160. [CrossRef]
32. Sato, Y.; Hatakeyama, H.; Sakurai, Y.; Hyodo, M.; Akita, H.; Harashima, H. A pH-Sensitive Cationic Lipid Facilitates the Delivery of Liposomal siRNA and Gene Silencing Activity In Vitro and In Vivo. *J. Control. Release* **2012**, *163*, 267–276. [CrossRef] [PubMed]
33. Choi, J.S.; MacKay, J.A.; Szoka, F.C. Low-pH-Sensitive PEG-Stabilized Plasmid–Lipid Nanoparticles: Preparation and Characterization. *Bioconjugate Chem.* **2003**, *14*, 420–429. [CrossRef] [PubMed]
34. Pelegri-O'Day, E.M.; Lin, E.-W.; Maynard, H.D. Therapeutic Protein–Polymer Conjugates: Advancing Beyond PEGylation. *J. Am. Chem. Soc.* **2014**, *136*, 14323–14332. [CrossRef] [PubMed]
35. Moore, J.S.; Stupp, S.I. Room Temperature Polyesterification. *Macromolecules* **1990**, *23*, 65–70. [CrossRef]
36. Pardi, N.; Muramatsu, H.; Weissman, D.; Kariko, K. In Vitro Transcription of Long RNA Containing Modified Nucleosides. *Methods Mol. Biol.* **2013**, *969*, 29–42. [CrossRef] [PubMed]
37. Baiersdörfer, M.; Boros, G.; Muramatsu, H.; Mahiny, A.; Vlatkovic, I.; Sahin, U.; Karikó, K. A Facile Method for the Removal of DsRNA Contaminant from In Vitro-Transcribed MRNA. *Mol. Ther. Nucleic Acids* **2019**, *15*, 26–35. [CrossRef]
38. May, J.P.; Undzys, E.; Roy, A.; Li, S.-D. Synthesis of a Gemcitabine Prodrug for Remote Loading into Liposomes and Improved Therapeutic Effect. *Bioconjugate Chem.* **2016**, *27*, 226–237. [CrossRef]
39. Percec, V.; Wilson, D.A.; Leowanawat, P.; Wilson, C.J.; Hughes, A.D.; Kaucher, M.S.; Hammer, D.A.; Levine, D.H.; Kim, A.J.; Bates, F.S.; et al. Self-Assembly of Janus Dendrimers into Uniform Dendrimersomes and Other Complex Architectures. *Science* **2010**, *328*, 1009–1014. [CrossRef]
40. Peterca, M.; Percec, V.; Leowanawat, P.; Bertin, A. Predicting the Size and Properties of Dendrimersomes from the Lamellar Structure of Their Amphiphilic Janus Dendrimers. *J. Am. Chem. Soc.* **2011**, *133*, 20507–20520. [CrossRef]
41. Zhang, S.; Sun, H.-J.; Hughes, A.D.; Moussodia, R.-O.; Bertin, A.; Chen, Y.; Pochan, D.J.; Heiney, P.A.; Klein, M.L.; Percec, V. Self-Assembly of Amphiphilic Janus Dendrimers into Uniform Onion-Like Dendrimersomes with Predictable Size and Number of Bilayers. *Proc. Natl. Acad. Sci. USA* **2014**, *111*, 9058–9063. [CrossRef]
42. Yadavalli, S.S.; Xiao, Q.; Sherman, S.E.; Hasley, W.D.; Klein, M.L.; Goulian, M.; Percec, V. Bioactive Cell-Like Hybrids from Dendrimersomes with a Human Cell Membrane and Its Components. *Proc. Natl. Acad. Sci. USA* **2019**, *116*, 744–752. [CrossRef]
43. Xiao, Q.; Sherman, S.E.; Wilner, S.E.; Zhou, X.; Dazen, C.; Baumgart, T.; Reed, E.H.; Hammer, D.A.; Shinoda, W.; Klein, M.L.; et al. Janus Dendrimersomes Coassembled from Fluorinated, Hydrogenated, and Hybrid Janus Dendrimers as Models for Cell Fusion and Fission. *Proc. Natl. Acad. Sci. USA* **2017**, *114*, E7045–E7053. [CrossRef]
44. Joseph, A.; Wagner, A.M.; Garay-Sarmiento, M.; Aleksanyan, M.; Haraszti, T.; Söder, D.; Georgiev, V.N.; Dimova, R.; Percec, V.; Rodriguez-Emmenegger, C. Zwitterionic Dendrimersomes: A Closer Xenobiotic Mimic of Cell Membranes. In *Advanced Materials*; Wiley Online Library: Hoboken, NJ, USA, 2022; p. 2206288. [CrossRef]
45. Kostina, N.Y.; Rahimi, K.; Xiao, Q.; Haraszti, T.; Dedisch, S.; Spatz, J.P.; Schwaneberg, U.; Klein, M.L.; Percec, V.; Möller, M.; et al. Membrane-Mimetic Dendrimersomes Engulf Living Bacteria via Endocytosis. *Nano Lett.* **2019**, *19*, 5732–5738. [CrossRef]

46. Kostina, N.Y.; Wagner, A.M.; Haraszti, T.; Rahimi, K.; Xiao, Q.; Klein, M.L.; Percec, V.; Rodriguez-Emmenegger, C. Unraveling Topology-Induced Shape Transformations in Dendrimersomes. *Soft Matter* **2021**, *17*, 254–267. [CrossRef]
47. Buzzacchera, I.; Xiao, Q.; Han, H.; Rahimi, K.; Li, S.; Kostina, N.Y.; Toebes, B.J.; Wilner, S.E.; Möller, M.; Rodriguez-Emmenegger, C.; et al. Screening Libraries of Amphiphilic Janus Dendrimers Based on Natural Phenolic Acids to Discover Monodisperse Unilamellar Dendrimersomes. *Biomacromolecules* **2019**, *20*, 712–727. [CrossRef]
48. Li, S.; Xia, B.; Javed, B.; Hasley, W.D.; Melendez-Davila, A.; Liu, M.; Kerzner, M.; Agarwal, S.; Xiao, Q.; Torre, P.; et al. Good. Direct Visualization of Vesicle Disassembly and Reassembly Using Photocleavable Dendrimers Elucidates Cargo Release Mechanisms. *ACS Nano* **2020**, *14*, 7398–7411. [CrossRef]
49. Zhang, D.; Xiao, Q.; Rahimzadeh, M.; Liu, M.; Rodriguez-Emmenegger, C.; Miyazaki, Y.; Shinoda, W.; Percec, V. Self-Assembly of Glycerol-Amphiphilic Janus Dendrimers Amplifies and Indicates Principles for the Selection of Stereochemistry by Biological Membranes. *J. Am. Chem. Soc.* **2023**, *145*, 4311–4323. [CrossRef]
50. Sun, H.-J.; Zhang, S.; Percec, V. From Structure to Function via Complex Supramolecular Dendrimer Systems. *Chem. Soc. Rev.* **2015**, *44*, 3900–3923. [CrossRef]
51. Xiao, Q.; Rubien, J.; Wang, Z.; Reed, E.; Hammer, D.; Sahoo, D.; Heiney, P.; Yadavalli, S.; Goulian, M.; Wilner, S.; et al. Self-Sorting and Co-Assembly of Fluorinated, Hydrogenated, and Hybrid Janus Dendrimers into Dendrimersomes. *J. Am. Chem. Soc.* **2016**, *138*, 12655–12663. [CrossRef]
52. Percec, V.; Leowanawat, P.; Sun, H.-J.; Kulikov, O.; Nusbaum, C.D.; Tran, T.M.; Bertin, A.; Wilson, D.A.; Peterca, M.; Zhang, S.; et al. Modular Synthesis of Amphiphilic Janus Glycodendrimers and Their Self-Assembly into Glycodendrimersomes and Other Complex Architectures with Bioactivity to Biomedically Relevant Lectins. *J. Am. Chem. Soc.* **2013**, *135*, 9055–9077. [CrossRef]
53. Zhang, S.; Xiao, Q.; Sherman, S.E.; Muncan, A.; Ramos Vicente, A.D.M.; Wang, Z.; Hammer, D.A.; Williams, D.; Chen, Y.; Pochan, D.J.; et al. Glycodendrimersomes from Sequence-Defined Janus Glycodendrimers Reveal High Activity and Sensor Capacity for the Agglutination by Natural Variants of Human Lectins. *J. Am. Chem. Soc.* **2015**, *137*, 13334–13344. [CrossRef] [PubMed]
54. Xiao, Q.; Zhang, S.; Wang, Z.; Sherman, S.E.; Moussodia, R.-O.; Peterca, M.; Muncan, A.; Williams, D.R.; Hammer, D.A.; Vértesy, S.; et al. Onion-like Glycodendrimersomes from Sequence-Defined Janus Glycodendrimers and Influence of Architecture on Reactivity to a Lectin. *Proc. Natl. Acad. Sci. USA* **2016**, *113*, 1162–1167. [CrossRef] [PubMed]
55. Rodriguez-Emmenegger, C.; Xiao, Q.; Kostina, N.Y.; Sherman, S.E.; Rahimi, K.; Partridge, B.E.; Li, S.; Sahoo, D.; Perez, A.M.R.; Buzzacchera, I.; et al. Encoding Biological Recognition in a Bicomponent Cell-Membrane Mimic. *Proc. Natl. Acad. Sci. USA* **2019**, *116*, 5376–5382. [CrossRef] [PubMed]
56. Xiao, Q.; Delbianco, M.; Sherman, S.E.; Perez, A.M.R.; Bharate, P.; Pardo-Vargas, A.; Rodriguez-Emmenegger, C.; Kostina, N.Y.; Rahimi, K.; Söder, D.; et al. Nanovesicles Displaying Functional Linear and Branched Oligomannose Self-Assembled from Sequence-Defined Janus Glycodendrimers. *Proc. Natl. Acad. Sci. USA* **2020**, *117*, 11931–11939. [CrossRef]
57. Kostina, N.Y.; Söder, D.; Haraszti, T.; Xiao, Q.; Rahimi, K.; Partridge, B.E.; Klein, M.L.; Percec, V.; Rodriguez-Emmenegger, C. Enhanced Concanavalin A Binding to Preorganized Mannose Nanoarrays in Glycodendrimersomes Revealed Multivalent Interactions. *Angew. Chem. Int. Ed.* **2021**, *60*, 8352–8360. [CrossRef]
58. Kopitz, J.; Xiao, Q.; Ludwig, A.-K.; Romero, A.; Michalak, M.; Sherman, S.E.; Zhou, X.; Dazen, C.; Vértesy, S.; Kaltner, H.; et al. Reaction of a Programmable Glycan Presentation of Glycodendrimersomes and Cells with Engineered Human Lectins to Show the Sugar Functionality of the Cell Surface. *Angew. Chem.* **2017**, *129*, 14869–14873. [CrossRef]
59. Kopitz, J.; Xiao, Q.; Ludwig, A.-K.; Romero, A.; Michalak, M.; Sherman, S.E.; Zhou, X.; Dazen, C.; Vértesy, S.; Kaltner, H.; et al. Reaction of a Programmable Glycan Presentation of Glycodendrimersomes and Cells with Engineered Human Lectins to Show the Sugar Functionality of the Cell Surface. *Angew. Chem. Int. Ed.* **2017**, *56*, 14677–14681. [CrossRef]
60. Ludwig, A.-K.; Michalak, M.; Xiao, Q.; Gilles, U.; Medrano, F.J.; Ma, H.; FitzGerald, F.G.; Hasley, W.D.; Melendez-Davila, A.; Liu, M.; et al. Design–Functionality Relationships for Adhesion/Growth-Regulatory Galectins. *Proc. Natl. Acad. Sci. USA* **2019**, *116*, 2837–2842. [CrossRef]
61. Murphy, P.V.; Romero, A.; Xiao, Q.; Ludwig, A.-K.; Jogula, S.; Shilova, N.V.; Singh, T.; Gabba, A.; Javed, B.; Zhang, D.; et al. Hans-Joachim Gabius Probing Sulfatide-Tissue Lectin Recognition with Functionalized Glycodendrimersomes. *iScience* **2021**, *24*, 101919. [CrossRef]
62. Wilner, S.E.; Xiao, Q.; Graber, Z.T.; Sherman, S.E.; Percec, V.; Baumgart, T. Dendrimersomes Exhibit Lamellar-to-Sponge Phase Transitions. *Langmuir* **2018**, *34*, 5527–5534. [CrossRef]
63. Torre, P.; Xiao, Q.; Buzzacchera, I.; Sherman, S.E.; Rahimi, K.; Kostina, N.Y.; Rodriguez-Emmenegger, C.; Möller, M.; Wilson, C.J.; Klein, M.L.; et al. Encapsulation of Hydrophobic Components in Dendrimersomes and Decoration of Their Surface with Proteins and Nucleic Acids. *Proc. Natl. Acad. Sci. USA* **2019**, *116*, 15378–15385. [CrossRef] [PubMed]
64. Xiao, Q.; Ludwig, A.-K.; Romanò, C.; Buzzacchera, I.; Sherman, S.E.; Vetro, M.; Vértesy, S.; Kaltner, H.; Reed, E.H.; Möller, M.; et al. Exploring Functional Pairing between Surface Glycoconjugates and Human Galectins Using Programmable Glycodendrimersomes. *Proc. Natl. Acad. Sci. USA* **2018**, *115*, E2509–E2518. [CrossRef]
65. Xiao, Q.; Wang, Z.; Williams, D.; Leowanawat, P.; Peterca, M.; Sherman, S.E.; Zhang, S.; Hammer, D.A.; Heiney, P.A.; King, S.R.; et al. Why Do Membranes of Some Unhealthy Cells Adopt a Cubic Architecture? *ACS Cent. Sci.* **2016**, *2*, 943–953. [CrossRef] [PubMed]

66. Zhang, S.; Moussodia, R.-O.; Vértesy, S.; André, S.; Klein, M.L.; Gabius, H.-J.; Percec, V. Unraveling Functional Significance of Natural Variations of a Human Galectin by Glycodendrimersomes with Programmable Glycan Surface. *Proc. Natl. Acad. Sci. USA* **2015**, *112*, 5585–5590. [CrossRef]
67. Zhang, S.; Moussodia, R.-O.; Murzeau, C.; Sun, H.-J.; Klein, M.L.; Vértesy, S.; André, S.; Roy, R.; Gabius, H.-J.; Percec, V. Dissecting Molecular Aspects of Cell Interactions Using Glycodendrimersomes with Programmable Glycan Presentation and Engineered Human Lectins. *Angew. Chem. Int. Ed.* **2015**, *54*, 4036–4040. [CrossRef] [PubMed]
68. Zhang, S.; Moussodia, R.-O.; Sun, H.-J.; Leowanawat, P.; Muncan, A.; Nusbaum, C.D.; Chelling, K.M.; Heiney, P.A.; Klein, M.L.; André, S.; et al. Mimicking Biological Membranes with Programmable Glycan Ligands Self-Assembled from Amphiphilic Janus Glycodendrimers. *Angew. Chem.* **2014**, *126*, 11079–11083. [CrossRef]
69. Zhang, S.; Moussodia, R.-O.; Sun, H.-J.; Leowanawat, P.; Muncan, A.; Nusbaum, C.D.; Chelling, K.M.; Heiney, P.A.; Klein, M.L.; André, S.; et al. Mimicking Biological Membranes with Programmable Glycan Ligands Self-Assembled from Amphiphilic Janus Glycodendrimers. *Angew. Chem. Int. Ed.* **2014**, *53*, 10899–10903. [CrossRef]
70. Zhang, S.; Sun, H.-J.; Hughes, A.D.; Draghici, B.; Lejnieks, J.; Leowanawat, P.; Bertin, A.; De Leon, L.O.; Kulikov, O.V.; Chen, Y.; et al. "Single–Single" Amphiphilic Janus Dendrimers Self-Assemble into Uniform Dendrimersomes with Predictable Size. *ACS Nano* **2014**, *8*, 1554–1565. [CrossRef]
71. Sherman, S.E.; Xiao, Q.; Percec, V. Mimicking Complex Biological Membranes and Their Programmable Glycan Ligands with Dendrimersomes and Glycodendrimersomes. *Chem. Rev.* **2017**, *117*, 6538–6631. [CrossRef]
72. Xiao, Q.; Yadavalli, S.S.; Zhang, S.; Sherman, S.E.; Fiorin, E.; Silva, L.D.; Wilson, D.A.; Hammer, D.A.; André, S.; Gabius, H.-J.; et al. Bioactive Cell-Like Hybrids Coassembled from (Glyco)Dendrimersomes with Bacterial Membranes. *Proc. Natl. Acad. Sci. USA* **2016**, *113*, E1134–E1141. [CrossRef]
73. Allen, T.M.; Chonn, A. Large Unilamellar Liposomes with Low Uptake into the Reticuloendothelial System. *FEBS Lett.* **1987**, *223*, 42–46. [CrossRef]
74. Allen, T.M.; Cullis, P.R. Drug Delivery Systems: Entering the Mainstream. *Science* **2004**, *303*, 1818–1822. [CrossRef] [PubMed]
75. Klibanov, A.L.; Maruyama, K.; Torchilin, V.P.; Huang, L. Amphipathic Polyethyleneglycols Effectively Prolong the Circulation Time of Liposomes. *FEBS Lett.* **1990**, *268*, 235–237. [CrossRef]
76. Papahadjopoulos, D.; Allen, T.M.; Gabizon, A.; Mayhew, E.; Matthay, K.; Huang, S.K.; Lee, K.D.; Woodle, M.C.; Lasic, D.D.; Redemann, C. Sterically Stabilized Liposomes: Improvements in Pharmacokinetics and Antitumor Therapeutic Efficacy. *Proc. Natl. Acad. Sci. USA* **1991**, *88*, 11460–11464. [CrossRef] [PubMed]
77. Olson, F.; Hunt, C.A.; Szoka, F.C.; Vail, W.J.; Papahadjopoulos, D. Preparation of Liposomes of Defined Size Distribution by Extrusion through Polycarbonate Membranes. *Biochim. Biophys. Acta BBA Biomembr.* **1979**, *557*, 9–23. [CrossRef]
78. Roche, C.; Sun, H.-J.; Leowanawat, P.; Araoka, F.; Partridge, B.E.; Peterca, M.; Wilson, D.A.; Prendergast, M.E.; Heiney, P.A.; Graf, R.; et al. A Supramolecular Helix That Disregards Chirality. *Nat. Chem.* **2016**, *8*, 80–89. [CrossRef] [PubMed]
79. Partridge, B.E.; Wang, L.; Sahoo, D.; Olsen, J.T.; Leowanawat, P.; Roche, C.; Ferreira, H.; Reilly, K.J.; Zeng, X.; Ungar, G.; et al. Sequence-Defined Dendrons Dictate Supramolecular Cogwheel Assembly of Dendronized Perylene Bisimides. *J. Am. Chem. Soc.* **2019**, *141*, 15761–15766. [CrossRef]
80. Wang, L.; Partridge, B.E.; Huang, N.; Olsen, J.T.; Sahoo, D.; Zeng, X.; Ungar, G.; Graf, R.; Spiess, H.W.; Percec, V. Extraordinary Acceleration of Cogwheel Helical Self-Organization of Dendronized Perylene Bisimides by the Dendron Sequence Encoding Their Tertiary Structure. *J. Am. Chem. Soc.* **2020**, *142*, 9525–9536. [CrossRef] [PubMed]
81. Darnell, J.; Lodish, H.; Baltimore, D. *Molecular Cell Biology*; Scientific American Books: New York, NY, USA, 1986; pp. 567–615.
82. Garrido, J.; Garrido, E.M.; Borges, F. Studies on the Food Additive Propyl Gallate: Synthesis, Structural Characterization, and Evaluation of the Antioxidant Activity. *J. Chem. Educ.* **2012**, *89*, 130–133. [CrossRef]
83. Percec, V.; Wang, S.; Huang, N.; Partridge, B.E.; Wang, X.; Sahoo, D.; Hoffman, D.J.; Malineni, J.; Peterca, M.; Jezorek, R.L.; et al. An Accelerated Modular-Orthogonal Ni-Catalyzed Methodology to Symmetric and Nonsymmetric Constitutional Isomeric AB_2 to AB_9 Dendrons Exhibiting Unprecedented Self-Organizing Principles. *J. Am. Chem. Soc.* **2021**, *143*, 17724–17743. [CrossRef] [PubMed]
84. Helfrich, W. Elastic Properties of Lipid Bilayers: Theory and Possible Experiments. *Z. Nat. C* **1973**, *28*, 693–703. [CrossRef] [PubMed]
85. Tanford, C. The Hydrophobic Effect and the Organization of Living Matter. *Science* **1978**, *200*, 1012–1018. [CrossRef] [PubMed]
86. Szoka, F.; Papahadjopoulos, D. Comparative Properties and Methods of Preparation of Lipid Vesicles (Liposomes). *Annu. Rev. Biophys. Bioeng.* **1980**, *9*, 467–508. [CrossRef]
87. Gabizon, A.; Papahadjopoulos, D. Liposome Formulations with Prolonged Circulation Time in Blood and Enhanced Uptake by Tumors. *Proc. Natl. Acad. Sci. USA* **1988**, *85*, 6949–6953. [CrossRef] [PubMed]
88. Hamann, M.V.; Stanke, N.; Müllers, E.; Stirnnagel, K.; Hütter, S.; Artegiani, B.; Alonso, S.B.; Calegari, F.; Lindemann, D. Efficient Transient Genetic Manipulation In Vitro and In Vivo by Prototype Foamy Virus-Mediated Nonviral RNA Transfer. *Mol. Ther.* **2014**, *22*, 1460–1471. [CrossRef]
89. Kay, M.A.; Holterman, A.-X.; Meuse, L.; Gown, A.; Ochs, H.D.; Linsley, P.S.; Wilson, C.B. Long–Term Hepatic Adenovirus–Mediated Gene Expression in Mice Following CTLA4Ig Administration. *Nat. Genet.* **1995**, *11*, 191–197. [CrossRef] [PubMed]

90. Flotte, T.R.; Afione, S.A.; Conrad, C.; McGrath, S.A.; Solow, R.; Oka, H.; Zeitlin, P.L.; Guggino, W.B.; Carter, B.J. Stable in Vivo Expression of the Cystic Fibrosis Transmembrane Conductance Regulator with an Adeno-Associated Virus Vector. *Proc. Natl. Acad. Sci. USA* **1993**, *90*, 10613–10617. [CrossRef]
91. Bukrinsky, M.I. HIV-1 Nuclear Import: In Search of a Leader. *Front. Biosci.* **1999**, *4*, 772–781. [CrossRef]
92. Zhao, Z.; Anselmo, A.C.; Mitragotri, S. Viral VECTOR-BASED Gene Therapies in the Clinic. *Bioeng. Transl. Med.* **2022**, *7*, E10258. [CrossRef]
93. Lundstrom, K. Viral Vectors in Gene Therapy: Where Do We Stand in 2023? *Viruses* **2023**, *15*, 698. [CrossRef]
94. Gao, G.-P.; Alvira, M.R.; Wang, L.; Calcedo, R.; Johnston, J.; Wilson, J.M. Novel Adeno-Associated Viruses from Rhesus Monkeys as Vectors for Human Gene Therapy. *Proc. Natl. Acad. Sci. USA* **2002**, *99*, 11854–11859. [CrossRef] [PubMed]
95. Felgner, P.L.; Gadek, T.R.; Holm, M.; Roman, R.; Chan, H.W.; Wenz, M.; Northrop, J.P.; Ringold, G.M.; Danielsen, M. Lipofection: A Highly Efficient, Lipid-Mediated DNA-Transfection Procedure. *Proc. Natl. Acad. Sci. USA* **1987**, *84*, 7413–7417. [CrossRef] [PubMed]
96. Felgner, J.; Martin, M.; Tsai, Y.; Felgner, P.L. Cationic Lipid-Mediated Transfection in Mammalian Cells: "Lipofection". *J. Tissue Cult. Methods* **1993**, *15*, 63–68. [CrossRef]
97. Semple, S.C.; Akinc, A.; Chen, J.; Sandhu, A.P.; Mui, B.L.; Cho, C.K.; Sah, D.W.Y.; Stebbing, D.; Crosley, E.J.; Yaworski, E.; et al. Rational Design of Cationic Lipids for SiRNA Delivery. *Nat. Biotechnol.* **2010**, *28*, 172–176. [CrossRef]
98. Haensler, J.; Szoka, F.C. Polyamidoamine Cascade Polymers Mediate Efficient Transfection of Cells in Culture. *Bioconjugate Chem.* **1993**, *4*, 372–379. [CrossRef]
99. Kukowska-Latallo, J.F.; Bielinska, A.U.; Johnson, J.; Spindler, R.; Tomalia, D.A.; Baker, J.R. Efficient Transfer of Genetic Material into Mammalian Cells Using Starburst Polyamidoamine Dendrimers. *Proc. Natl. Acad. Sci. USA* **1996**, *93*, 4897–4902. [CrossRef]
100. Zhou, J.; Wu, J.; Hafdi, N.; Behr, J.-P.; Erbacher, P.; Peng, L. PAMAM Dendrimers for Efficient SiRNA Delivery and Potent Gene Silencing. *Chem. Commun.* **2006**, *22*, 2362–2364. [CrossRef]
101. Loup, C.; Zanta, M.-A.; Caminade, A.-M.; Majoral, J.-P.; Meunier, B. Preparation of Water-Soluble Cationic Phosphorus-Containing Dendrimers as DNA Transfecting Agents. *Chem. Eur. J.* **1999**, *5*, 3644–3650. [CrossRef]
102. Pedziwiatr, E.; Chonco, L.; Shcharbin, D.; de Jesus, E.; Bermejo, J.F.; Ortega, P.; de la Mata, F.J.; Flores, J.C.; Gomez, R.; Klajnert, B.; et al. Carbosilane Dendrimers as Drug Carriers. *Eur. J. Clin. Investig.* **2007**, *37*, 79. [CrossRef]
103. Zinselmeyer, B.H.; Mackay, S.P.; Schatzlein, A.G.; Uchegbu, I.F. The Lower-Generation Polypropylenimine Dendrimers Are Effective Gene-Transfer Agents. *Pharm. Res.* **2002**, *19*, 960–967. [CrossRef]
104. Sarbolouki, M.N.; Sadeghizadeh, M.; Yaghoobi, M.M.; Karami, A.; Lohrasbi, T. Dendrosomes: A Novel Family of Vehicles for Transfection and Therapy. *J. Chem. Technol. Biotechnol.* **2000**, *75*, 919–922. [CrossRef]
105. Dutta, T.; Burgess, M.; McMillan, N.A.J.; Parekh, H.S. Dendrosome-Based Delivery of SiRNA against E6 and E7 Oncogenes in Cervical Cancer. *Nanomed. Nanotechnol. Biol. Med.* **2010**, *6*, 463–470. [CrossRef]
106. Joester, D.; Losson, M.; Pugin, R.; Heinzelmann, H.; Walter, E.; Merkle, H.P.; Diederich, F. Amphiphilic Dendrimers: Novel Self-Assembling Vectors for Efficient Gene Delivery. *Angew. Chem. Int. Ed.* **2003**, *42*, 1486–1490. [CrossRef] [PubMed]
107. Wood, K.C.; Little, S.R.; Langer, R.; Hammond, P.T. A Family of Hierarchically Self-Assembling Linear-Dendritic Hybrid Polymers for Highly Efficient Targeted Gene Delivery. *Angew. Chem. Int. Ed.* **2005**, *44*, 6704–6708. [CrossRef] [PubMed]
108. Wu, G.Y.; Wu, C.H. Receptor-Mediated In Vitro Gene Transformation by a Soluble DNA Carrier System. *J. Biol. Chem.* **1987**, *262*, 4429–4432. [CrossRef] [PubMed]
109. Boussif, O.; Lezoualc'h, F.; Zanta, M.A.; Mergny, M.D.; Scherman, D.; Demeneix, B.; Behr, J.P. A Versatile Vector for Gene and Oligonucleotide Transfer into Cells in Culture and In Vivo: Polyethylenimine. *Proc. Natl. Acad. Sci. USA* **1995**, *92*, 7297–7301. [CrossRef]
110. McKinlay, C.J.; Vargas, J.R.; Blake, T.R.; Hardy, J.W.; Kanada, M.; Contag, C.H.; Wender, P.A.; Waymouth, R.M. Charge-Altering Releasable Transporters (CARTs) for the Delivery and Release of MRNA in Living Animals. *Proc. Natl. Acad. Sci. USA* **2017**, *114*, E448–E456. [CrossRef]
111. Benner, N.L.; Near, K.E.; Bachmann, M.H.; Contag, C.H.; Waymouth, R.M.; Wender, P.A. Functional DNA Delivery Enabled by Lipid-Modified Charge-Altering Releasable Transporters (CARTs). *Biomacromolecules* **2018**, *19*, 2812–2824. [CrossRef]
112. Bangham, A.D.; Horne, R.W. Negative Staining of Phospholipids and Their Structural Modification by Surface-Active Agents as Observed in the Electron Microscope. *J. Mol. Biol.* **1964**, *8*, 660–668. [CrossRef]
113. Buhleier, E.; Wehner, W.; Voegtle, F. "Cascade"- and "Nonskid-Chain-Like" Syntheses of Molecular Cavity Topologies. *Synthesis* **1978**, *155*, 155–158. [CrossRef]
114. Denkewalter, R.G.; Kole, J.; Lukasavage, W.J. Macromolecular Highly Branched Homogeneous Compound Based on Lysine Units. U.S. Patent 4 289 872, 15 September 1981.
115. Tomalia, D.A.; Baker, H.; Dewald, J.; Hall, M.; Kallos, G.; Martin, S.; Roeck, J.; Ryder, J.; Smith, P. A New Class of Polymers: Starburst-Dendritic Macromolecules. *Polym. J.* **1985**, *17*, 117–132. [CrossRef]
116. Newkome, G.R.; Yao, Z.; Baker, G.R.; Gupta, V.K. Cascade Molecules: A New Approach to Micelles. A [27]-Arborol. *J. Org. Chem.* **1985**, *50*, 2003–2004. [CrossRef]
117. Percec, V.; Heck, J. Side Chain Liquid Crystal Polymers Containing Mesogenic Units Based on Half Disc and Rod-Like Moieties. *Polym. Prepr. Am. Chem. Soc. Div. Polym. Chem.* **1989**, *30*, 450–451.

118. Ortega, P.; Bermejo, J.F.; Chonco, L.; de Jesus, E.; de la Mata, F.J.; Fernández, G.; Flores, J.C.; Gómez, R.; Serramía, M.J.; Muñoz-Fernandez, M.A. Novel Water-Soluble Carbosilane Dendrimers: Synthesis and Biocompatibility. *Eur. J. Inorg. Chem.* **2006**, *2006*, 1388–1396. [CrossRef]
119. Bermejo, J.F.; Ortega, P.; Chonco, L.; Eritja, R.; Samaniego, R.; Müllner, M.; de Jesus, E.; de la Mata, F.J.; Flores, J.C.; Gomez, R.; et al. Water-Soluble Carbosilane Dendrimers: Synthesis Biocompatibility and Complexation with Oligonucleotides; Evaluation for Medical Applications. *Chem. Eur. J.* **2007**, *13*, 483–495. [CrossRef]
120. Chonco, L.; Bermejo-Martín, J.F.; Ortega, P.; Shcharbin, D.; Pedziwiatr, E.; Klajnert, B.; de la Mata, F.J.; Eritja, R.; Gómez, R.; Bryszewska, M.; et al. Water-Soluble Carbosilane Dendrimers Protect Phosphorothioate Oligonucleotides from Binding to Serum Proteins. *Org. Biomol. Chem.* **2007**, *5*, 1886–1893. [CrossRef]
121. Mata, F.D.L.M.D.L.; Ramírez, R.G.; Serrano, J.C.F.; Alcañiz, E.D.J.; López, P.O.; Fernández, M.Á.M.; Martín, J.F.B.; Lobera, M.J.S.; Gómez-Chacón, G.F.; Jiménez, L.C.; et al. Nuevos Dendrímeros Carbosilanos, su Preparación y Sus Usos. WO2007010080A2, 25 January 2007. Available online: https://patents.google.com/patent/WO2007010080A2/en?oq=WO2007010080 (accessed on 18 April 2023).
122. Weber, N.; Ortega, P.; Clemente, M.I.; Shcharbin, D.; Bryszewska, M.; de la Mata, F.J.; Gómez, R.; Muñoz-Fernández, M.A. Characterization of Carbosilane Dendrimers as Effective Carriers of SiRNA to HIV-Infected Lymphocytes. *J. Control. Release* **2008**, *132*, 55–64. [CrossRef]
123. Zinselmeyer, B.H.; Mackay, S.P.; Uchegbu, I.F.; Schatzlein, A.G. Computer Aided Optimisation of Synthetic Gene Delivery Agents Using PPI Dendrimers. *Br. J. Cancer* **2002**, *86*, S105. [CrossRef]
124. Khan, O.F.; Zaia, E.W.; Yin, H.; Bogorad, R.L.; Pelet, J.M.; Webber, M.J.; Zhuang, I.; Dahlman, J.E.; Langer, R.; Anderson, D.G. Ionizable Amphiphilic Dendrimer-Based Nanomaterials with Alkyl-Chain-Substituted Amines for Tunable SiRNA Delivery to the Liver Endothelium In Vivo. *Angew. Chem. Int. Ed.* **2014**, *53*, 14397–14401. [CrossRef]
125. Khan, O.F.; Zaia, E.W.; Jhunjhunwala, S.; Xue, W.; Cai, W.; Yun, D.S.; Barnes, C.M.; Dahlman, J.E.; Dong, Y.; Pelet, J.M.; et al. Dendrimer-Inspired Nanomaterials for the In Vivo Delivery of SiRNA to Lung Vasculature. *Nano Lett.* **2015**, *15*, 3008–3016. [CrossRef]
126. Posadas, I.; Lopez-Hernandez, B.; Clemente, M.I.; Jimenez, J.L.; Ortega, P.; de la Mata, J.; Gomez, R.; Munoz-Fernandez, M.A.; Cena, V. Highly Efficient Transfection of Rat Cortical Neurons Using Carbosilane Dendrimers Unveils a Neuroprotective Role for HIF-1 Alpha in Early Chemical Hypoxia-Mediated Neurotoxicity. *Pharm. Res.* **2009**, *26*, 1181–1191. [CrossRef] [PubMed]
127. Posadas, I.; Guerra, F.; Cena, V. Nonviral Vectors for the Delivery of Small Interfering RNAs to the CNS. *Nanomedicine* **2010**, *5*, 1219–1236. [CrossRef]
128. Rodrigo, A.C.; Rivilla, I.; Perez-Martinez, F.C.; Monteagudo, S.; Ocana, V.; Guerra, J.; Garcia-Martinez, J.C.; Merino, S.; Sanchez-Verdu, P.; Cena, V.; et al. Efficient, Non-Toxic Hybrid PPV-PAMAM Dendrimer as a Gene Carrier for Neuronal Cells. *Biomacromolecules* **2011**, *12*, 1205–1213. [CrossRef] [PubMed]
129. Perez-Martinez, F.; Guerra, J.; Posadas, I.; Cena, V. Barriers to Non-Viral Vector-Mediated Gene Delivery in the Nervous System. *Pharm. Res.* **2011**, *28*, 1843–1858. [CrossRef]
130. Perez-Martinez, F.; Carrion, B.; Cena, V. The Use of Nanoparticles for Gene Therapy in the Nervous System. *J. Alzheimer's Dis.* **2012**, *31*, 697–710. [CrossRef] [PubMed]
131. Perez-Carrion, M.D.; Perez-Martinez, F.C.; Merino, S.; Sanchez-Verdu, P.; Martinez-Hernandez, J.; Lujan, R.; Cena, V. Dendrimer-Mediated SiRNA Delivery Knocks down Beclin 1 and Potentiates NMDA-Mediated Toxicity in Rat Cortical Neurons. *J. Neurochem.* **2012**, *120*, 259–268. [CrossRef]
132. Perez-Martinez, F.; Ocana, A.; Perez-Carrion, M.; Cena, V. Dendrimers As Vectors for Genetic Material Delivery to the Nervous System. *Curr. Med. Chem.* **2012**, *19*, 5101–5108. [CrossRef]
133. Perez-Carrion, M.D.; Cena, V. Knocking Down HMGB1 Using Dendrimer-Delivered SiRNA Unveils Its Key Role in NMDA-Induced Autophagy in Rat Cortical Neurons. *Pharm. Res.* **2013**, *30*, 2584–2595. [CrossRef]
134. Posadas, I.; Monteagudo, S.; Cena, V. Nanoparticles for Brain-Specific Drug and Genetic Material Delivery, Imaging and Diagnosis. *Nanomedicine* **2016**, *11*, 833–849. [CrossRef]
135. Janiszewska, J.; Posadas, I.; Jativa, P.; Bugaj-Zarebska, M.; Urbanczyk-Lipkowska, Z.; Cena, V. Second Generation Amphiphilic Poly-Lysine Dendrons Inhibit Glioblastoma Cell Proliferation without Toxicity for Neurons or Astrocytes. *PLoS ONE* **2016**, *11*, e0165704. [CrossRef]
136. Posadas, I.; Romero-Castillo, L.; El Brahmi, N.; Manzanares, D.; Mignani, S.; Majoral, J.-P.; Cena, V. Neutral High-Generation Phosphorus Dendrimers Inhibit Macrophage-Mediated Inflammatory Response In Vitro and In Vivo. *Proc. Natl. Acad. Sci. USA* **2017**, *114*, E7660–E7669. [CrossRef] [PubMed]
137. Cena, V.; Jativa, P. Nanoparticle Crossing of Blood-Brain Barrier: A Road to New Therapeutic Approaches to Central Nervous System Diseases. *Nanomedicine* **2018**, *13*, 1513–1516. [CrossRef]
138. Stenstrom, P.; Manzanares, D.; Zhang, Y.; Cena, V.; Malkoch, M. Evaluation of Amino-Functional Polyester Dendrimers Based on Bis-MPA as Nonviral Vectors for SiRNA Delivery. *Molecules* **2018**, *23*, 2028. [CrossRef] [PubMed]
139. de la Torre, C.; Cena, V. The Delivery Challenge in Neurodegenerative Disorders: The Nanoparticles Role in Alzheimer's Disease Therapeutics and Diagnostics. *Pharmaceutics* **2018**, *10*, 190. [CrossRef] [PubMed]
140. Mignani, S.; Shi, X.; Cena, V.; Shcharbin, D.; Bryszewska, M.; Majoral, J.-P. In Vivo Therapeutic Applications of Phosphorus Dendrimers: State of the Art. *Drug Discov. Today* **2020**, *26*, 677–689. [CrossRef]

141. Posadas, I.; Romero-Castillo, L.; Ronca, R.-A.; Karpus, A.; Mignani, S.; Majoral, J.-P.; Munoz-Fernandez, M.; Cena, V. Engineered Neutral Phosphorous Dendrimers Protect Mouse Cortical Neurons and Brain Organoids from Excitotoxic Death. *Int. J. Mol. Sci.* **2022**, *23*, 4391. [CrossRef]
142. Discher, B.M.; Won, Y.-Y.; Ege, D.S.; Lee, J.C.-M.; Bates, F.S.; Discher, D.E.; Hammer, D.A. Polymersomes: Tough Vesicles Made from Diblock Copolymers. *Science* **1999**, *284*, 1143–1146. [CrossRef]
143. Leung, A.K.K.; Hafez, I.M.; Baoukina, S.; Belliveau, N.M.; Zhigaltsev, I.V.; Afshinmanesh, E.; Tieleman, D.P.; Hansen, C.L.; Hope, M.J.; Cullis, P.R. Lipid Nanoparticles Containing SiRNA Synthesized by Microfluidic Mixing Exhibit an Electron-Dense Nanostructured Core. *J. Phys. Chem. C* **2012**, *116*, 18440–18450. [CrossRef]
144. Leung, A.K.K.; Tam, Y.Y.C.; Chen, S.; Hafez, I.M.; Cullis, P.R. Microfluidic Mixing: A General Method for Encapsulating Macromolecules in Lipid Nanoparticle Systems. *J. Phys. Chem. B* **2015**, *119*, 8698–8706. [CrossRef]
145. Evers, M.J.W.; Kulkarni, J.A.; van der Meel, R.; Cullis, P.R.; Vader, P.; Schiffelers, R.M. State-of-the-Art Design and Rapid-Mixing Production Techniques of Lipid Nanoparticles for Nucleic Acid Delivery. *Small Methods* **2018**, *2*, 1700375. [CrossRef]
146. Kulkarni, J.A.; Witzigmann, D.; Chen, S.; Cullis, P.R.; van der Meel, R. Lipid Nanoparticle Technology for Clinical Translation of SiRNA Therapeutics. *Acc. Chem. Res.* **2019**, *52*, 2435–2444. [CrossRef]
147. Kulkarni, J.A.; Witzigmann, D.; Leung, J.; Tam, Y.Y.C.; Cullis, P.R. On the Role of Helper Lipids in Lipid Nanoparticle Formulations of SiRNA. *Nanoscale* **2019**, *11*, 21733–21739. [CrossRef]
148. Aharoni, S.M.; Crosby, C.R., III; Walsh, E.K. Size and Solution Properties of Globular tert-Butyloxycarbonyl-poly (α,ω-L-lysine). *Macromolecules* **1982**, *15*, 1093–1098. [CrossRef]
149. Tomalia, D.A.; Naylor, A.M.; Goddard, W.A., III. Starburst Dendrimers: Molecular-Level Control of Size, Shape, Surface Chemistry, Topology, and Flexibility from Atom to Macroscopic Matter. *Angew. Chem. Int. Ed. Engl.* **1990**, *29*, 138–175. [CrossRef]
150. Fischer, M.; Voegtle, F. Dendrimers: From Design to Application-A Progress Report. *Angew. Chem. Int. Ed.* **1999**, *38*, 884–905. [CrossRef]
151. Newkome, G.R.; He, E.; Moorefield, C.N. Suprasupermolecules with Novel Properties: Metallodendrimers. *Chem. Rev.* **1999**, *99*, 1689–1746. [CrossRef] [PubMed]
152. Bosman, A.W.; Jamssen, H.M.; Meijer, E.W. About Dendrimers: Structure, Physical Properties, and Applications. *Chem. Rev.* **1999**, *99*, 1665–1688. [CrossRef]
153. Grayson, S.M.; Frechet, J.M.J. Convergent Dendrons and Dendrimers: From Synthesis to Applications. *Chem. Rev.* **2001**, *101*, 3819–3867. [CrossRef]
154. Majoral, J.-P.; Caminade, A.M. Dendrimers Containing Heteroatoms (Si, P, B, Ge, or Bi). *Chem. Rev.* **1999**, *99*, 845–880. [CrossRef]
155. Watson, M.D.; Fechtenkotter, A.; Muellen, K. Big is Beautiful-"Aromaticity" Revisited from Viewpoint of Macromoilecular and Supramolecular Benzene Chemistry. *Chem. Rev.* **2001**, *101*, 1267–1300. [CrossRef]
156. Astruc, D.; Chardac, F. Dendritic Catalysts and Dendrimers in Catalysis. *Chem. Rev.* **2001**, *101*, 2991–3023. [CrossRef] [PubMed]
157. Astruc, D.; Boisselier, E.; Omelas, C. Dendrimers Designed for Functions: From Physical, Photophysical, and Supramolecular Properties to Applications in Sensis, Catalysis, Molecular Electronics, Photonics, and Nanomedicine. *Chem. Rev.* **2010**, *110*, 1857–1959. [CrossRef] [PubMed]
158. Li, W.-S.; Aida, T. Dendrimer Porphyrins and Phthalocyanines. *Chem. Rev.* **2009**, *109*, 6047–6076. [CrossRef] [PubMed]
159. Carlmark, A.; Hawker, C.; Hult, A.; Malkoch, M. New methodologies in the Constructions of Dendritic Materials. *Chem. Soc. Rev.* **2009**, *38*, 352–362. [CrossRef]
160. Schluter, A.D.; Rabe, J.P. Dendronized Polymers: Synthesis, Characterization, Assembly at Interfaces and Manipulation. *Angew. Chem. Int. Ed.* **2000**, *39*, 864–883. [CrossRef]
161. Voegtle, F.; Richard, G.; Werner, N. *Dendrimer Chemistry*; Wiley-VCH: Weinheim, Germany, 2009.
162. Frechet, J.M.J.; Tomalia, D.A. *Dendrimers and Other Dendritic Polymers*; John Wiley & Sons, Ltd.: Chichester, UK, 2001.
163. Tomalia, D.A.; Christensen, J.B.; Boas, U. *Dendrimers, Dendrons and Dendritic Polymers*; Cambridge University Press: Cambridge, UK, 2012.
164. Klajnert, B.; Peng, L.; Cena, V. (Eds.) *Dendrimers in Biomedical Applications*; RSC Publishing: Cambridge, UK, 2013.
165. Newkome, G.R.; Moorefield, C.N.; Voegtle, F. *Dendritic Molecules*; VCH: Weinheim, Germany, 1996.
166. Newkome, G.R.; Moorefield, C.N.; Voegtle, F. *Dendrimers and Dendrons*; Wiley-VCH: Weinheim, Germany, 2001.
167. Rosen, B.M.; Wilson, C.J.; Wilson, D.A.; Peterca, M.; Imam, M.R.; Percec, V. Dendron-Mediated Self-Assembly, Disassembly, and Self-Organization of Complex Systems. *Chem. Rev.* **2009**, *109*, 6275–6540. [CrossRef]
168. Percec, V.; Xiao, Q. The Legacy of Rosalind E. Franklin: Landmark Contributions to Two Nobel Prizes. *Chem* **2021**, *7*, 529–536. [CrossRef]
169. Percec, V.; Dulcey, A.E.; Balagurusamy, V.S.K.; Miura, Y.; Smidrkal, J.; Peterca, M.; Nummelin, A.; Edlund, U.; Hudson, S.D.; Heiney, P.A.; et al. Self-Assembly of Amphiphilic Dendritic Dipeptides into Helical Pores. *Nature* **2004**, *430*, 764–768. [CrossRef]
170. Percec, V.; Glodde, M.; Bera, T.K.; Miura, Y.; Shiyanowskaya, I.; Singer, K.D.; Balagurusamy, V.S.K.; Heiney, P.A.; Schnell, I.; Rapp, A.; et al. Self-Organization of Supramolecular Helical Dendrimers into Complex Electronic Materials. *Nature* **2002**, *419*, 384–387. [CrossRef]
171. Percec, V. Merging Macromolecular and Supramolecular Chemistry into Bioinspired Synthesis of Complex Systems. *Isr. J. Chem.* **2020**, *60*, 48–66. [CrossRef]

172. Percec, V.; Xiao, Q. Helical Chirality of Supramolecular Columns and Spheres Self-Organizes Complex Liquid Crystals, Crystals and Quasicrystals. *Isr. J. Chem.* **2021**, *61*, 530–556. [CrossRef]
173. Percec, V.; Heck, J.; Johansson, G.; Tomazos, D.; Kawasumi, M.; Ungar, G. Molecular-Recognition-Directed Self-Assembly of Supramolecular Polymers. *J. Macromol. Sci. Part A Pure Appl. Chem.* **1994**, *31*, 1031–1070. [CrossRef]
174. Percec, V.; Xiao, Q. Helical Self-Organizations and Emerging Functions in Architectures, Biological and Synthetic Macromolecules. *Bull. Chem. Soc. Jpn.* **2021**, *94*, 900–928. [CrossRef]
175. Hudson, S.D.; Jung, H.-T.; Percec, V.; Cho, W.-D.; Johansson, G.; Ungar, G.; Balagurusamy, V.S.K. Direct Visualization of Individual Cylindrical and Spherical Supramolecular Dendrimers. *Science* **1997**, *278*, 449–452. [CrossRef]
176. Yeardley, D.J.P.; Ungar, G.; Percec, V.; Holerca, M.N.; Johansson, G. Spherical Supramolecular Minidendrimers Self-Organized in an "Inverse Micellar"-like Thermotropic Body-Centered Cubic Liquid Crystalline Phase. *J. Am. Chem. Soc.* **2000**, *122*, 1684–1689. [CrossRef]
177. Dukeson, D.R.; Ungar, G.; Balagurusamy, V.S.K.; Percec, V.; Johansson, G.A.; Glodde, M. Application of Isomorphous Replacement in the Structure Determination of a Cubic Liquid Crystal Phase and Location of Counterions. *J. Am. Chem. Soc.* **2003**, *125*, 15974–15980. [CrossRef]
178. Balagurusamy, V.S.K.; Ungar, G.; Percec, V.; Johansson, G. Rational Design of the First Spherical Supramolecular Dendrimers Self-Organized in a Novel Thermotropic Cubic Liquid-Crystalline Phase and the Determination of Their Shape by X-ray Analysis. *J. Am. Chem. Soc.* **1997**, *119*, 1539–1555. [CrossRef]
179. Peterca, M.; Imam, M.R.; Hudson, S.D.; Partridge, B.E.; Sahoo, D.; Heiney, P.A.; Klein, M.L.; Percec, V. Complex Arrangement of Orthogonal Nanoscale Columns via a Supramolecular Orientational Memory Effect. *ACS Nano* **2016**, *10*, 10480–10488. [CrossRef]
180. Sahoo, D.; Peterca, M.; Aqad, E.; Partridge, B.E.; Heiney, P.A.; Graf, R.; Spiess, H.W.; Zeng, X.; Percec, V. Tetrahedral Arrangements of Perylene Bisimide Columns via Supramolecular Orientational Memory. *ACS Nano* **2017**, *11*, 983–991. [CrossRef]
181. Sahoo, D.; Peterca, M.; Imam, M.R.; Partridge, B.E.; Xiao, Q.; Percec, V. Conformationally Flexible Dendronized Cyclotetraveratrylenes (CTTV)s Self-Organize a Large Diversity of Chiral Columnar, Frank-Kasper and Quasicrystal Phases. *Giant* **2022**, *10*, 100096. [CrossRef]
182. Sahoo, D.; Peterca, M.; Aqad, E.; Partridge, B.E.; Klein, M.L.; Percec, V. Losing Supramolecular Orientational Memory via Self-Organization of a Misfolded Secondary Structure. *Polym. Chem.* **2018**, *9*, 2370–2381. [CrossRef]
183. Wilson, D.A.; Andreopoulou, A.K.; Peterca, M.; Leowanawat, P.; Sahoo, D.; Partridge, B.E.; Huang, N.; Heiney, P.A.; Percec, V. Supramolecular Spheres Self-Assembled from Conical Dendrons are Chiral. *J. Am. Chem. Soc.* **2019**, *141*, 6162–6166. [CrossRef] [PubMed]
184. Sahoo, D.; Peterca, M.; Aqad, E.; Partridge, B.E.; Heiney, P.A.; Graf, R.; Spiess, H.; Zeng, X.; Percec, V. Hierarchical Self-Organization of Perylene Bisimides into Supramolecular Spheres and Periodic Arrays Thereof. *J. Am. Chem. Soc.* **2016**, *138*, 14798–14807. [CrossRef] [PubMed]
185. Percec, V.; Rudick, J.G.; Peterca, M.; Yurchenko, M.E.; Smidrkal, J.; Heiney, P.A. Supramolecular Structural Diversity among First-Generation Hybrid Dendrimers and Twin Dendrons. *Chem. Eur. J.* **2008**, *14*, 3355–3362. [CrossRef] [PubMed]
186. Percec, V.; Cho, W.-D.; Möller, M.; Prokhorova, S.A.; Ungar, G.; Yeardley, D.J.P. Design and Structural Analysis of the First Spherical Monodendron Self-Organizable in a Cubic Lattice. *J. Am. Chem. Soc.* **2000**, *122*, 4249–4250. [CrossRef]
187. Percec, V.; Ahn, C.-H.; Barboiu, B. Self-Encapsulation, Acceleration and Control in the Radical Polymerization of Monodendritic Monomers via Self-Assembly. *J. Am. Chem. Soc.* **1997**, *119*, 12978–12979. [CrossRef]
188. Percec, V.; Ahn, C.-H.; Ungar, G.; Yeardley, D.J.P.; Möller, M.; Sheiko, S.S. Controlling Polymer Shape through the Self-Assembly of Dendritic Side-Groups. *Nature* **1998**, *391*, 161–164. [CrossRef]
189. Percec, V.; Ahn, C.-H.; Cho, W.-D.; Jamieson, A.M.; Kim, J.; Leman, T.; Schmidt, M.; Gerle, M.; Möller, M.; Prokhorova, S.A.; et al. Visualizable Cylindrical Macromolecules with Controlled Stiffness from Backbones Containing Libraries of Self-Assembling Dendritic Side Groups. *J. Am. Chem. Soc.* **1998**, *120*, 8619–8631. [CrossRef]
190. Holerca, M.N.; Peterca, M.; Partridge, B.E.; Xiao, Q.; Lligadas, G.; Monteiro, M.J.; Percec, V. Monodisperse Macromolecules by Self-Interrupted Living Polymerization. *J. Am. Chem. Soc.* **2020**, *142*, 15265–15270. [CrossRef]
191. Percec, V.; Cho, W.-D.; Mosier, P.E.; Ungar, G.; Yeardley, D.J.P. Structural Analysis of Cylindrical and Spherical Supramolecular Dendrimers Quantifies the Concept of Monodendron Shape Control by Generation Number. *J. Am. Chem. Soc.* **1998**, *120*, 11061–11070. [CrossRef]
192. Percec, V.; Cho, W.-D.; Ungar, G. Increasing the Diameter of Cylindrical and Spherical Supramolecular Dendrimers by Decreasing the Solid Angle of Their Monodendrons via Periphery Functionalization. *J. Am. Chem. Soc.* **2000**, *122*, 10273–10281. [CrossRef]
193. Percec, V.; Cho, W.-D.; Ungar, G.; Yeardley, D.J.P. Synthesis and Structural Analysis of Two Constitutional Isomeric Libraries of AB_2-Based Monodendrons and Supramolecular Dendrimers. *J. Am. Chem. Soc.* **2001**, *123*, 1302–1315. [CrossRef]
194. Percec, V.; Mitchell, C.M.; Cho, W.-D.; Uchida, S.; Glodde, M.; Ungar, G.; Zeng, X.; Liu, Y.; Balagurusamy, V.S.K.; Heiney, P.A. Designing Libraries of First Generation AB_3 and AB_2 Self-Assembling Dendrons via the Primary Structure Generated from Combinations of $(AB)_y$–AB_3 and $(AB)_y$–AB_2 Building Blocks. *J. Am. Chem. Soc.* **2004**, *126*, 6078–6094. [CrossRef] [PubMed]
195. Percec, V.; Holerca, M.N.; Nummelin, S.; Morrison, J.J.; Glodde, M.; Smidrkal, J.; Peterca, M.; Rosen, B.M.; Uchida, S.; Balagurusamy, V.S.K.; et al. Exploring and Expanding the Structural Diversity of Self-Assembling Dendrons through Combinations of AB, Constitutional Isomeric AB_2, and AB_3 Biphenyl-4-Methyl Ether Building Blocks. *Chem. Eur. J.* **2006**, *12*, 6216–6241. [CrossRef]

196. Percec, V.; Peterca, M.; Sienkowska, M.J.; Ilies, M.A.; Aqad, E.; Smidrkal, J.; Heiney, P.A. Synthesis and Retrostructural Analysis of Libraries of AB_3 and Constitutional Isomeric AB_2 Phenylpropyl Ether-Based Supramolecular Dendrimers. *J. Am. Chem. Soc.* **2006**, *128*, 3324–3334. [CrossRef]
197. Percec, V.; Won, B.C.; Peterca, M.; Heiney, P.A. Expanding the Structural Diversity of Self-Assembling Dendrons and Supramolecular Dendrimers via Complex Building Blocks. *J. Am. Chem. Soc.* **2007**, *129*, 11265–11278. [CrossRef]
198. Rosen, B.M.; Wilson, D.A.; Wilson, C.J.; Peterca, M.; Won, B.C.; Huang, C.; Lipski, L.R.; Zeng, X.; Ungar, G.; Heiney, P.A.; et al. Predicting the Structure of Supramolecular Dendrimers via the Analysis of Libraries of AB_3 and Constitutional Isomeric AB_2 Biphenylpropyl Ether Self-Assembling Dendrons. *J. Am. Chem. Soc.* **2009**, *131*, 17500–17521. [CrossRef]
199. Ungar, G.; Liu, Y.; Zeng, X.; Percec, V.; Cho, W.-D. Giant Supramolecular Liquid Crystal Lattice. *Science* **2003**, *299*, 1208–1211. [CrossRef]
200. Sahoo, D.; Imam, M.R.; Peterca, M.; Partridge, B.E.; Wilson, D.A.; Zeng, X.; Ungar, G.; Heiney, P.A.; Percec, V. Hierarchical Self-Organization of Chiral Columns from Chiral Supramolecular Spheres. *J. Am. Chem. Soc.* **2018**, *140*, 13478–13487. [CrossRef]
201. Percec, V.; Huang, N.; Xiao, Q.; Partridge, B.E.; Sahoo, D.; Imam, M.R.; Peterca, M.; Graf, R.; Spiess, H.-W.; Zeng, X.; et al. Self-Organization of Rectangular Bipyramidal Helical Columns by Supramolecular Orientational Memory Epitaxially Nucleated from a Frank-Kasper σ Phase. *Giant* **2022**, *9*, 100084. [CrossRef]
202. Duan, H.; Hudson, S.D.; Ungar, G.; Holerca, M.N.; Percec, V. Definitive Support by Transmission Electron Microscopy, Electron Diffraction and Electron Density Calculations for the Formation of a BCC Lattice from Poly{N-[3,4,5-tris(n-dodecan-1-yloxy)benzoyl]ethyleneimine}. *Chem. Eur. J.* **2001**, *7*, 4134–4141. [CrossRef] [PubMed]
203. Percec, V.; Heck, J.; Johansson, G.; Tomazos, D.; Ungar, G. Towards Tobacco Mosaic Virus-like Self-Assembled Supramolecular Architectures. *Macromol. Symp.* **1994**, *77*, 237–265. [CrossRef]
204. Zeng, X.; Ungar, G.; Liu, Y.; Percec, V.; Dulcey, A.E.; Hobbs, J.K. Supramolecular dendritic liquid quasicrystals. *Nature* **2004**, *428*, 157–160. [CrossRef]
205. Holerca, M.N.; Sahoo, D.; Partridge, B.E.; Peterca, M.; Zeng, X.; Ungar, G.; Percec, V. Dendronized Poly(2-Oxazoline) Displays within Only Five Monomer Repeat Units Liquid Quasicrystal, A15 and σ Frank–Kasper Phases. *J. Am. Chem. Soc.* **2018**, *140*, 16941–16947. [CrossRef] [PubMed]
206. Ungar, G.; Percec, V.; Zeng, X.; Leowanawat, P. Liquid Quasicrystals. *Isr. J. Chem.* **2011**, *51*, 1206–1215. [CrossRef]
207. Imam, M.R.; Peterca, M.; Xiao, Q.; Percec, V. Enhancing Conformational Flexibility of Dendronized Triphenylene via Diethylene Glycol Linkers Lowers Transitions of Helical Columnar, Frank-Kasper, and Quasicrystal Phases. *Giant* **2022**, *10*, 100098. [CrossRef]
208. Yue, K.; Huang, M.; Marson, R.L.; He, J.; Huang, J.; Zhou, Z.; Wang, J.; Liu, C.; Yan, X.; Wu, K.; et al. Geometry Induced Sequence of Nanoscale Frank–Kasper and Quasicrystal Mesophases in Giant Surfactants. *Proc. Natl. Acad. Sci. USA* **2016**, *113*, 14195–14200. [CrossRef]
209. Percec, V.; Sahoo, D. Discotic liquid crystals 45 years later. Dendronized discs and crowns increase liquid crystal complexity to columnar from spheres, cubic Frank-Kasper, liquid quasicrystals and memory-effect induced columnar-bundles. *Giant* **2022**, *12*, 100127. [CrossRef]
210. Percec, V.; Chu, P.; Kawasumi, M. Toward 'Willowlike' Thermotropic Dendrimers. *Macromolecules* **1994**, *27*, 4441–4453. [CrossRef]
211. Percec, V. Molecular Design of Novel Liquid Crystalline Polymers with Complex Architecture: Macrocyclics and Dendrimers. *Pure Appl. Chem.* **1995**, *67*, 2031–2038. [CrossRef]
212. Percec, V.; Kawasumi, M. Synthesis and characterization of a thermotropic nematic liquid crystalline dendrimeric polymer. *Macromolecules* **1992**, *25*, 3843–3850. [CrossRef]
213. Percec, V.; Sahoo, D.; Adamson, J. Stimuli-Responsive Principles of Supramolecular Organizations Emerging from Self-Assembling and Self-Organizable Dendrons, Dendrimers, and Dendronized Polymers. *Polymers* **2023**, *15*, 1832. [CrossRef] [PubMed]
214. Percec, V.; Lee, M.; Heck, J.; Blackwell, H.E.; Ungar, G.; Alvarez-Castillo, A. Re-entrant Isotropic Phase in a Supramolecular Disc-like Oligomer of 4-[3,4,5-Tris(N-Dodecanyloxy)Benzoyloxy]-4′-[(2-Vinyloxy)Ethoxy]Biphenyl. *J. Mater. Chem.* **1992**, *2*, 931–938. [CrossRef]
215. Percec, V.; Heck, J.; Tomazos, D.; Falkenberg, F.; Blackwell, H.; Ungar, G. Self-assembly of Taper-Shaped Monoesters of Oligo(ethylene oxide) with 3,4,5-Tris(p-dodecyloxybenzyloxy)benzoic Acid and of Their Polymethacrylates into Tubular Supramolecular Architectures Displaying a Columnar Mesophase. *J. Chem. Soc. Perkin Trans.* **1993**, *1*, 2799–2811. [CrossRef]
216. Percec, V.; Tomazos, D.; Heck, J.; Blackwell, H.; Ungar, G. Self-assembly of Taper-Shaped Monoesters of Oligo(ethylene oxide) with 3,4,5-Tris(n-dodecan-1-yloxy)benzoic Acid and of Their Polymethacrylates into Tubular Supramolecular Architectures Displaying a Columnar Hexagonal Mesophase. *J. Chem. Soc. Perkin Trans.* **1994**, *2*, 31–44. [CrossRef]
217. Kwon, Y.K.; Chvalun, S.N.; Schneider, A.-I.; Blackwell, J.; Percec, V.; Heck, J.A. Supramolecular Tubular Structures of a Polymethacrylate with Tapered Side Groups in Aligned Hexagonal Phases. *Macromolecules* **1994**, *27*, 6129–6132. [CrossRef]
218. Kwon, Y.K.; Chvalun, S.N.; Blackwell, J.; Percec, V.; Heck, J.A. Effect of Temperature on the Supramolecular Tubular Structure in Oriented Fibers of a Poly(methacrylate) with Tapered Side Groups. *Macromolecules* **1995**, *28*, 1552–1558. [CrossRef]
219. Percec, V.; Schlueter, D.; Kwon, Y.K.; Blackwell, J.; Moeller, M.; Slangen, P.J. Dramatic Stabilization of a Hexagonal Columnar Mesophase Generated from Supramolecular and Macromolecular Columns by the Semifluorination of the Alkyl Groups of Their Tapered Building Blocks. *Macromolecules* **1995**, *28*, 8807–8818. [CrossRef]
220. Kwon, Y.K.; Danko, C.; Chvalun, S.; Blackwell, J.; Heck, J.A.; Percec, V. Comparison of the Supramolecular Structures Formed by a Polymethacrylate with a Highly Tapered Side-Chain and its Monomeric Precursor. *Macromol. Symp.* **1994**, *87*, 103–114. [CrossRef]

221. Chvalun, S.N.; Scherbina, M.A.; Yakunin, A.N.; Blackwell, J.; Percec, V. Structure of gyroid mesophase formed by monodendrons with fluorinated alkyl tails. *Polym. Sci. Ser. A* **2007**, *49*, 158–167. [CrossRef]
222. Blackwell, J.; Chvalun, S.N.; Cho, J.D.; Kwon, Y.K.; Percec, V.; Heck, J.A. *X-ray Analyses of the Supramolecular Structures Formed by Polymers with Highly Tapered Side Groups*; Case Western Reserve University: Cleveland, OH, USA, 1997; Volume 214, p. 32-Poly.
223. Chvalun, S.N.; Blackwell, J.; Cho, J.D.; Kwon, Y.K.; Percec, V.; Heck, J.A. X-ray Analysis of the Internal Rearrangement of the Self-Assembling Columnar Structure Formed by a Highly Tapered Molecule. *Polymers* **1998**, *39*, 4515–4522. [CrossRef]
224. Chvalun, S.N.; Blackwell, J.; Kwon, Y.K.; Percec, V. Small Angle X-ray Analysis of the Effect of Temperature on the Self-Assembling Columnar Structures Formed by a Polymethacrylate with Highly Tapered Side Groups and by One of its Low Molar Mass Precursors. *Macromol. Symp.* **1997**, *118*, 663–675. [CrossRef]
225. Percec, V.; Schlueter, D.; Ronda, J.C.; Johansson, G.; Ungar, G.; Zhou, J.P. Tubular Architectures from Polymers with Tapered Side Groups. Assembly of Side Groups via a Rigid Helical Chain Conformation and Flexible Helical Chain Conformation Induced via Assembly of Side Groups. *Macromolecules* **1996**, *29*, 1464–1472. [CrossRef]
226. Percec, V.; Schlueter, D. Mechanistic Investigations on the Formation of Supramolecular Cylindrical Shaped Oligomers and Polymers by Living Ring Opening Metathesis Polymerization of a 7-Oxanorbornene Monomer Substituted with Two Tapered Monodendrons. *Macromolecules* **1997**, *30*, 5783–5790. [CrossRef]
227. Percec, V.; Johansson, G.; Schlueter, D.; Ronda, J.C.; Ungar, G. Molecular Recognition Directed Self-Assembly of Tubular Supramolecular Architectures from Building Blocks Containing Monodendrons as Exo-Receptors and Crown- or Pseudo-Crown-Ethers as Endo-Receptors. *Macromol. Symp.* **1996**, *101*, 43–60. [CrossRef]
228. Percec, V.; Ahn, C.-H.; Cho, W.-D.; Johansson, G.; Schlueter, D. Design of New Macromolecular Architectures by Using Quasi-Equivalent Monodendrons as Building Blocks. *Macromol. Symp.* **1997**, *118*, 33–43. [CrossRef]
229. Percec, V.; Schlueter, D.; Ungar, G.; Cheng, S.Z.D.; Zhang, A. Hierarchical Control of Internal Superstructure, Diameter, and Stability of Supramolecular and Macromolecular Columns Generated from Tapered Monodendritic Building Blocks. *Macromolecules* **1998**, *31*, 1745–1762. [CrossRef]
230. Percec, V.; Johansson, G.; Ungar, G.; Zhou, J. Fluorophobic Effect Induces the Self-Assembly of Semifluorinated Tapered Monodendrons Containing Crown Ethers into Supramolecular Columnar Dendrimers Which Exhibit a Homeotropic Hexagonal Columnar Liquid Crystalline Phase. *J. Am. Chem. Soc.* **1996**, *118*, 9855–9866. [CrossRef]
231. Johansson, G.; Percec, V.; Ungar, G.; Zhou, J.P. Fluorophobic Effect in the Self-Assembly of Polymers and Model Compounds Containing Tapered Groups into Supramolecular Columns. *Macromolecules* **1996**, *29*, 646–660. [CrossRef]
232. Johansson, G.; Percec, V.; Ungar, G.; Smith, K. Fluorophobic Effect Generates a Systematic Approach to the Synthesis of the Simplest Class of Rodlike Liquid Crystals Containing a Single Benzene Unit. *Chem. Mater.* **1997**, *9*, 164–175. [CrossRef]
233. Percec, V.; Heck, J. Side-Chain Liquid Crystal Polymers Containing Hemiphasmidic Mesogens. *Polym. Prepr. Am. Chem. Soc. Div. Polym. Chem.* **1991**, *32*, 263–264.
234. Percec, V.; Heck, J. Molecular Recognition Directed Supramolecular Polymer Architectures. *Polym. Prepr. Am. Chem. Soc. Div. Polym. Chem.* **1991**, *32*, 698–699.
235. Percec, V.; Heck, J.; Ungar, G. Towards Tobacco Mosaic Virus-Like Supramolecular Synthetic Polymers. *Polym. Prepr. Am. Chem. Soc. Div. Polym. Chem.* **1992**, *33*, 152–153.
236. Percec, V.; Heck, J. Molecular Design of Externally Regulated Self-Assembled Supramolecular Ionic Channels. *Polym. Prepr. Am. Chem. Soc. Div. Polym. Chem.* **1992**, *33*, 217–218.
237. Percec, V.; Heck, J.; Johansson, G.; Ungar, G. Towards Tobacco Mosai Virus-Like Self-Assembled Supramolecular Architectures. *Polym. Prepr. Am. Chem. Soc. Div. Polym. Chem.* **1993**, *34*, 116–117.
238. Percec, V.; Heck, J. Liquid Crystalline Polymers Containing Mesogenic Units Based on Half-Disk and Rod-Like Moieties. 1. Synthesis and Characterization of 4-(11-Undecan-1yloxy)-4′-[3,4,5-Tri(p-n-Dodecan-1-yloxybenzyloxy)benzoate]Biphenyl Side Groups. *J. Polym. Sci. Part A Polym. Chem.* **1991**, *29*, 591–597. [CrossRef]
239. Percec, V.; Heck, J. Liquid Crystalline Polymers Containing Mesogenic Units Based on Half-Disk and Rod-Like Moieties. 2. Synthesis and Characterization of Poly(2-[3,4,5-Tri[p(N-Dodecan-1yloxy)-Benzyloxy)Benzoate]-7-[p-11-Undecan-yloxy)Benzoare]Naphthalene]Methyl Siloxane. *Polym. Bull.* **1990**, *24*, 255–262. [CrossRef]
240. Percec, V.; Heck, J. Liquid Crystalline Polymers Containing Mesogenic Units Based on Half-Disk and Rod-Like Moieties. 3. Synthesis and Characterization of Polymethylsiloxanes and Copolymethysiloxanes Based on 4-[3,4,5-Tri(p-N-Dodecan-1-yloxybenzyloxy)benzoate]-4′-[p-Allyloxybenzoate)biphenyl and 4-(3,4,5-Tri(p-N-dodecan-1-yloxy-benzyloxy)benzoate]-4′-(p-allyloxybenzoate)thiodiphenyl Side Groups. *Polym. Bull.* **1991**, *25*, 55–62. [CrossRef]
241. Percec, V.; Heck, J. Liquid Crystalline Polymers Containing Mesogenic Units Based on Half-Disk and Rod-Like Moieties. 4. Side-Chain Liquid-Crystalline Polymethylsiloxanes Containing Hemiphasmidic Mesogens Based on 4-[3,4,5-Tri(Alkan-1-yloxy)benzoate]Biphenyl Groups. *Polym. Bull.* **1991**, *25*, 431–438. [CrossRef]
242. Percec, V.; Heck, J.; Ungar, G. Liquid Crystalline Polymers Containing Mesogenic Units Based on Half-Disk and Rod-Like Moieties. 5. Side-Chain Liquid-Crystalline Poly(methylsiloxane)s Containing Hemiphasmidic Mesogens Based on 4-[[3,4,5-Tris(Alkan-1-yloxy)benzoyl]oxy]-4′-[[p-(Propan-1-yloxy)benzoyl]oxy]Biphenyl Groups. *Macromolecules* **1991**, *24*, 4957–4962. [CrossRef]
243. Percec, V.; Heck, J. Side-chain liquid-crystal polymers containing mesogenic units based on 1/2 disk and rod-like moieties. In *Abstracts of Papers of the American Chemical Society*; ACS: Washington, DC, USA, 1989; Volume 30, p. 450.

244. Ho, M.-S.; Partridge, B.E.; Sun, H.-J.; Sahoo, D.; Leowanawat, P.; Peterca, M.; Graf, R.; Spiess, H.W.; Zeng, X.; Ungar, G.; et al. Screening Libraries of Semifluorinated Arylene Bisimides to Discover and Predict Thermodynamically Controlled Helical Crystallization. *ACS Comb. Sci.* **2016**, *18*, 723–739. [CrossRef]
245. Peterca, M.; Sahoo, D.; Imam, M.R.; Xiao, Q.; Percec, V. Searching for the simplest self-assembling dendron to study helical self-organization and supramolecular polymerization. *Giant* **2022**, *12*, 100118. [CrossRef]
246. Peterca, M.; Sahoo, D.; Emad, A.; Peterca, M.; Percec, V. Molecular design principles of helical pyramidal chirality self-organized from achiral hexakis(alkyloxy)triphenylene. *Giant* **2023**, *13*, 100138. [CrossRef]
247. Sahoo, D.; Emad, A.; Peterca, M.; Percec, V. A highly ordered 8/1 helical pyramidal column self-organized from the crown conformation of achiral hexa(butyloxy)triphenylene. *Giant* **2023**, *13*, 100135. [CrossRef]
248. Rudick, J.G.; Percec, V. Helical chirality in dendronized in dendronized polyarylacetylenes. *New J. Chem.* **2007**, *31*, 1083–1096. [CrossRef]
249. Rudick, J.G.; Percec, V. Induced Helical Backbone conformations of self-organizable dendronized polymers. *Acc. Chem. Res.* **2008**, *41*, 1641–1652. [CrossRef]
250. Percec, V. Bioinspired supramolecular liquid crystals. *Philos. Trans. R. Soc. A Math. Phys. Eng. Sci.* **2006**, *364*, 2709–2719. [CrossRef] [PubMed]
251. Tomalia, D.A.; Sheetz, D.P. Homopolymerization of 2-Alkyl- and 2-Aryl-2-Oxazolines. *J. Polym. Sci. Part A-1 Polym. Chem.* **1966**, *4*, 2253–2265. [CrossRef]
252. Kagiya, T.; Narisawa, S.; Maeda, T.; Fukui, K. Ring-Opening Polymerization of 2-Substituted 2-Oxazolines. *J. Polym. Sci. Part B Polym. Lett.* **1966**, *4*, 441–445. [CrossRef]
253. Seeliger, W.; Aufderhaar, E.; Diepers, W.; Feinauer, R.; Nehring, R.; Thier, W.; Hellmann, H. Recent Syntheses and Reactions of Cyclic Imidic Esters. *Angew. Chem. Int. Ed. Engl.* **1966**, *5*, 875–888. [CrossRef]
254. Bassiri, T.G.; Levy, A.; Litt, M. Polymerization of Cyclic Imino Ethers. I. Oxazolines. *J. Polym. Sci. Part B Polym. Lett.* **1967**, *5*, 871–879. [CrossRef]
255. Holerca, M.N.; Sahoo, D.; Peterca, M.; Partridge, B.E.; Heiney, P.A.; Percec, V. A Tetragonal Phase Self-Organized from Unimolecular Spheres Assembled from a Substituted Poly(2-Oxazoline). *Macromolecules* **2017**, *50*, 375–385. [CrossRef]
256. Percec, V.; Holerca, M.N.; Magonov, S.N.; Yeardley, D.J.P.; Ungar, G.; Duan, H.; Hudson, S.D. Poly(Oxazolines)s with Tapered Minidendritic Side Groups. The Simplest Cylindrical Models to Investigate the Formation of Two-Dimensional and Three-Dimensional Order by Direct Visualization. *Biomacromolecules* **2001**, *2*, 706–728. [CrossRef] [PubMed]
257. Percec, V.; Holerca, M.N.; Uchida, S.; Yeardley, D.J.P.; Ungar, G. Poly(Oxazoline)s with Tapered Minidendritic Side Groups as Models for the Design of Synthetic Macromolecules with Tertiary Structure. A Demonstration of the Limitations of Living Polymerization in the Design of 3-D Structures Based on Single Polymer Chains. *Biomacromolecules* **2001**, *2*, 729–740. [CrossRef]
258. Lehn, J.-M. Toward Self-Organization and Complex Matter. *Science* **2002**, *295*, 2400–2403. [CrossRef] [PubMed]
259. Lehn, J.-M. Supramolecular Chemistry: Where from? Where to? *Chem. Soc. Rev.* **2017**, *46*, 2378–2379. [CrossRef] [PubMed]
260. Lehn, J.-M. Beyond Chemical Synthesis: Self-Organization? *Isr. J. Chem.* **2018**, *58*, 136–141. [CrossRef]
261. Taylor, W.R. A "Periodic Table" for Protein Structures. *Nature* **2002**, *416*, 657–660. [CrossRef]
262. Moutevelis, E.; Woolfson, D.N. A Periodic Table of Coiled-Coil Protein Structures. *J. Mol. Biol.* **2009**, *385*, 726–732. [CrossRef]
263. Ahnert, S.E.; Marsh, J.A.; Hernández, H.; Robinson, C.V.; Teichmann, S.A. Principles of Assembly Reveal a Periodic Table of Protein Complexes. *Science* **2015**, *350*, aaa2245. [CrossRef]
264. Tomalia, D.A. In Quest of a Systematic Framework for Unifying and Defining Nanoscience. *J. Nanopart. Res.* **2009**, *11*, 1251–1310. [CrossRef] [PubMed]
265. Tomalia, D.A.; Khanna, S.N. A Systematic Framework and Nanoperiodic Concept for Unifying Nanoscience: Hard/Soft Nanoelements, Superatoms, Meta-Atoms, New Emerging Properties, Periodic Property Patterns, and Predictive Mendeleev-like Nanoperiodic Tables. *Chem. Rev.* **2016**, *116*, 2705–2774. [CrossRef] [PubMed]
266. Le Gall, T.; Berchel, M.; Davies, L.; Mottais, A.; Ghanem, R.; Fautrel, A.; Gill, D.; Hyde, S.; Lehn, P.; Lehn, J.-M.; et al. Aerosol-Mediated Non-Viral Lung Gene Therapy: The Potential of Aminoglycoside-Based Cationic Liposomes. *Pharmaceutics* **2022**, *14*, 25. [CrossRef]
267. Esfand, R.; Tomalia, D.A. Poly(Amidoamine) (PAMAM) Dendrimers: From Biomimicry to Drug Delivery and Biomedical Applications. *Drug Discov. Today* **2001**, *6*, 427–436. [CrossRef] [PubMed]
268. Svenson, S.; Tomalia, D.A. Dendrimers in Biomedical Applications—Reflections on the Field. *Adv. Drug Deliv. Rev.* **2005**, *57*, 2106–2129. [CrossRef] [PubMed]
269. Elsabahy, M.; Wooley, K.L. Design of Polymeric Nanoparticles for Biomedical Delivery Applications. *Chem. Soc. Rev.* **2012**, *41*, 2545–2561. [CrossRef]
270. Bergmann, G.H.F.; Finkelmann, H.; Percec, V.; Zhao, M. Liquid-Crystalline Main-Chain Elastomers. *Macromol. Rapid Commun.* **1997**, *18*, 353–360. [CrossRef]
271. Percec, V.; Hahn, B. Liquid Crystalline Polymers Containing Heterocycloalkanediyl Groups as Mesogens. 7. Molecular Weight and Composition Effects on the Phase Transitions of Poly(Methylsiloxane)s and Poly(Methylsiloxane-Co-Dimethylsiloxane)s Containing 2-[4-(2(S)-Methyl-1-Butoxy)Phenyl]-5-(11-Undecanyl)-1,3,2-Dioxaborinane Side Groups. *Macromolecules* **1989**, *22*, 1588–1599. [CrossRef]

272. Johansson, G.; Percec, V.; Ungar, G.; Abramic, D. Molecular Recognition Directed Self-Assembly of Tubular Liquid Crystalline and Crystalline Supramolecular Architectures from Taper Shaped (15-Crown-5)Methyl 3,4,5-Tris(p-Alkyloxybenzyloxy)Benzoates and (15-Crown-5)Methyl 3,4,5-Tris(p-Dodecyloxy)Benzoate. *J. Chem. Soc. Perkin Trans.* **1994**, *1*, 447–459. [CrossRef]
273. Percec, V.; Cho, W.-D.; Ungar, G.; Yeardley, D.J.P. From Molecular Flat Tapers, Discs, and Cones to Supramolecular Cylinders and Spheres Using Fréchet-Type Monodendrons Modified on Their Periphery. *Angew. Chem. Int. Ed.* **2000**, *39*, 1597–1602. [CrossRef]
274. Rosen, B.M.; Percec, V. A Reaction to Stress. *Nature* **2007**, *446*, 381–382. [CrossRef]
275. Ungar, G.; Abramic, D.; Percec, V.; Heck, J.A. Self-Assembly of Twin Tapered Bisamides into Supramolecular Columns Exhibiting Hexagonal Columnar Mesophases. Structural Evidence for a Microsegregated Model of the Supramolecular Column. *Liq. Cryst.* **1996**, *21*, 73–86. [CrossRef]
276. Percec, V.; Grigoras, C.; Kim, H.-J. Toward Self-Assembling Dendritic Macromolecules from Conventional Monomers by a Combination of Living Radical Polymerization and Irreversible Terminator Multifunctional Initiator. *J. Polym. Sci. A Polym. Chem.* **2004**, *42*, 505–513. [CrossRef]
277. Percec, V.; Peterca, M.; Tadjiev, T.; Zeng, X.; Ungar, G.; Leowanawat, P.; Aqad, E.; Imam, M.R.; Rosen, B.M.; Akbey, U.; et al. Self-Assembly of Dendronized Perylene Bisimides into Complex Helical Columns. *J. Am. Chem. Soc.* **2011**, *133*, 12197–12219. [CrossRef] [PubMed]
278. Percec, V.; Asgarzadeh, F. Metal-Catalyzed Living Radical Graft Copolymerization of Olefins Initiated from the Structural Defects of Poly(Vinyl Chloride). *J. Polym. Sci. A Polym. Chem.* **2001**, *39*, 1120–1135. [CrossRef]
279. Percec, V.; Glodde, M.; Peterca, M.; Rapp, A.; Schnell, I.; Spiess, H.W.; Bera, T.K.; Miura, Y.; Balagurusamy, V.S.K.; Aqad, E.; et al. Self-Assembly of Semifluorinated Dendrons Attached to Electron-Donor Groups Mediates Their π-Stacking via a Helical Pyramidal Column. *Chem. Eur. J.* **2006**, *12*, 6298–6314. [CrossRef]
280. Wilson, D.A.; Wilson, C.J.; Rosen, B.M.; Percec, V. Two-Step, One-Pot Ni-Catalyzed Neopentylglycolborylation and Complementary Pd/Ni-Catalyzed Cross-Coupling with Aryl Halides, Mesylates, and Tosylates. *Org. Lett.* **2008**, *10*, 4879–4882. [CrossRef]
281. Rosen, B.M.; Huang, C.; Percec, V. Sequential Ni-Catalyzed Borylation and Cross-Coupling of Aryl Halides via in Situ Prepared Neopentylglycolborane. *Org. Lett.* **2008**, *10*, 2597–2600. [CrossRef]
282. Nguyen, N.H.; Levere, M.E.; Percec, V. SET-LRP of Methyl Acrylate to Complete Conversion with Zero Termination. *J. Polym. Sci. A Polym. Chem.* **2012**, *50*, 860–873. [CrossRef]
283. Moreno, A.; Lligadas, G.; Adamson, J.; Maurya, D.S.; Percec, V. Assembling Complex Macromolecules and Self-Organizations of Biological Relevance with Cu(I)-Catalyzed Azide-Alkyne, Thio-Bromo, and TERMINI Double "Click" Reactions. *Polymers* **2023**, *15*, 1075. [CrossRef]
284. Rosen, B.M.; Percec, V. Single Electron-Transfer and Single-Electron Transfer Degenerative Chain Transfer Living Radical Polymerization. *Chem. Rev.* **2009**, *109*, 5069–5119. [CrossRef] [PubMed]
285. Rosen, B.M.; Quasdorf, K.W.; Wilson, D.A.; Zhang, N.; Resmerita, A.-M.; Garg, N.K.; Percec, V. Nickel-Catalyzed Cross-Couplings Involving Carbon–Oxygen Bonds. *Chem. Rev.* **2011**, *111*, 1346–1416. [CrossRef] [PubMed]
286. Zhang, N.; Samantha, S.R.; Rosen, B.M.; Percec, V. Single-Electron Transfer in Radical and Radical-Mediated Organic, Materials and Polymer Synthesis. *Chem. Rev.* **2014**, *114*, 5848–5958. [CrossRef] [PubMed]
287. Jiang, X.; Rosen, B.M.; Percec, V. Mimicking "Nascent" Cu(0) Mediated SET-LRP of Methyl Acrylate in DMSO Leads to Complete Conversion in Several Minutes: MIMICS of "Nascent" Cu(0) in SET-LRP of MA. *J. Polym. Sci. A Polym. Chem.* **2010**, *48*, 403–409. [CrossRef]
288. Nguyen, N.H.; Kulis, J.; Sun, H.-J.; Jia, Z.; Van Beusekom, B.; Levere, M.E.; Wilson, D.A.; Monteiro, M.J.; Percec, V. A Comparative Study of the SET-LRP of Oligo(Ethylene Oxide) Methyl Ether Acrylate in DMSO and in H_2O. *Polym. Chem.* **2013**, *4*, 144–155. [CrossRef]
289. Percec, V.; Ungar, G.; Peterca, M. Self-Assembly in Action. *Science* **2006**, *313*, 55–56. [CrossRef]
290. Peterca, M.; Percec, V. Recasting Metal Alloy Phases with Block Copolymers. *Science* **2010**, *330*, 333–334. [CrossRef]
291. Peterca, M.; Imam, M.R.; Leowanawat, P.; Rosen, B.M.; Wilson, D.A.; Wilson, C.J.; Zeng, X.; Ungar, G.; Heiney, P.A.; Percec, V. Self-Assembly of Hybrid Dendrons into Doubly Segregated Supramolecular Polyhedral Columns and Vesicles. *J. Am. Chem. Soc.* **2010**, *132*, 11288–11305. [CrossRef]

MDPI AG
Grosspeteranlage 5
4052 Basel
Switzerland
Tel.: +41 61 683 77 34

Pharmaceutics Editorial Office
E-mail: pharmaceutics@mdpi.com
www.mdpi.com/journal/pharmaceutics

www.ingramcontent.com/pod-product-compliance
Lightning Source LLC
Chambersburg PA
CBHW061618220926
51850CB00005B/538
* 9 7 8 3 7 2 5 8 4 8 4 9 2 *